Rehabilitation of the Knee:
A Problem-Solving Approach

Contemporary Perspectives in Rehabilitation

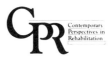

Steven L. Wolf, PhD, FAPTA
Editor-in-Chief

PUBLISHED VOLUMES

The Biomechanics of the Foot and Ankle
Robert Donatelli, MA, PT, OCS

Pharmacology in Rehabilitation
Charles D. Ciccone, PhD, PT

Wound Healing: Alternatives in Management
Luther C. Kloth, MS, PT, Joseph M. McCulloch, PhD, PT, and Jeffrey A. Feedar, PT

Thermal Agents in Rehabilitation, 2nd Edition
Susan L. Michlovitz, MS, PT

Electrotherapy in Rehabilitation
Meryl R. Gersh, MMSc, PT

Dynamics of Human Biologic Tissues
Dean P. Currier, PhD, PT and Roger M. Nelson, PhD, PT

Concepts in Hand Rehabilitation
Barbara G. Stanley, PT, CHT, and Susan M. Tribuzi, OTR, CHT

Cardiopulmonary Rehabilitation: Basic Theory and Application, 2nd Edition
Frances J. Brannon, PhD, Margaret W. Foley, MN, Julie Ann Starr, MS, PT, and Mary Geyer Black, MS, PT

Rehabilitation of the Knee:
A Problem-Solving Approach

Bruce H. Greenfield, MMSc, PT
Instructor
Division of Physical Therapy
Department of Rehabilitation Medicine
Emory University School of Medicine

Private Practice
Physical Therapy Associates of Metro Atlanta
Atlanta, Georgia

F. A. DAVIS COMPANY • Philadelphia

F. A. Davis Company
1915 Arch Street
Philadelphia, PA 19103

Printed in the United States of America

Last digit indicates print number: 10 9 8 7 6 5 4 3 2 1

Senior Allied Health Editor: Jean-François Vilain
Senior Allied Health Developmental Editor: Ralph Zickgraf
Production Editor: Jody Gould

As new scientific information becomes available through basic and clinical research, recommended treatments and drug therapies undergo changes. The author(s) and publisher have done everything possible to make this book accurate, up to date, and in accord with accepted standards at the time of publication. The authors, editors, and publisher are not responsible for errors or omissions or for consequences from application of the book, and make no warranty, expressed or implied, in regard to the contents of the book. Any practice described in this book should be applied by the reader in accordance with professional standards of care used in regard to the unique circumstances that may apply in each situation. The reader is advised always to check product information (package inserts) for changes and new information regarding dose and contraindications before administering any drug. Caution is especially urged when using new or infrequently ordered drugs.

Library of Congress Cataloging-in-Publication Data

Rehabilitation of the knee : a problem-solving approach / [edited by]
  Bruce H. Greenfield.
      p.   cm. — (Contemporary perspectives in rehabilitation)
  Includes bibliographical references and index.
  ISBN 0-8036-4335-7 (hardcover : alk. paper) :
    1. Knee — Wounds and injuries — Physical therapy. 2. Knee — Wounds
and injuries — Patients — Rehabilitation. 3. Knee — Diseases —
Patients — Rehabilitation. I. Greenfield, Bruce H., 1953–
II. Series.
    [DNLM: 1. Knee Injuries — rehabilitation. 2. Knee Injuries —
diagnosis. WE 870 R3453 1993]
  RD561.R434 1993
  617.5'8203 — dc20
  DNLM/DLC
  for Library of Congress   93-324
                                                                   CIP

This book is dedicated to my most significant others: my lovely wife, Amy; my daughters, Heather, Suzanne, and Eleanor; my sister, Meryl Jacobs; my father, Seymour Greenfield; and my late mother, Eleanore Greenfield.

Foreword

Increasingly, health care professionals, including physical therapists and athletic trainers, are asked to shorten the time allocated (and reimbursed) for treatment of many acute conditions, including musculoskeletal disorders. In the contexts of sports- and occupation-related problems, the two areas that probably require the most attention are the knee and low back. Because rehabilitating these types of injuries requires maximal and optimal care in increasingly briefer treatment schedules, the ability of the clinician to render proper and justifiable service hinges now, as never before, on proper and well-conceived treatment plans. Such plans demand clarity of thought and documented support derived from careful review of the literature. And the health care provider who can synthesize these elements into effective management of the rehabilitation patient truly stands on the threshold of that much-talked-about notion, physical diagnosis.

At the risk of embarrassing my friend and former student Bruce Greenfield, editor of *Rehabilitation of the Knee: A Problem-Solving Approach*, I must say that his dedication to orthopedic and sports physical therapy and his vision of a future rehabilitation praxis that embodies the elements of inquiry just noted permeate every aspect of this volume of the *Contemporary Perspectives in Rehabilitation* series. The attention to detail and comprehensibility evident in every chapter will serve as the model for all future "targeted topic" rehabilitation books. Wise readers will keep in mind the probability that their grasp of such issues as rationales for treatment, justification of numbers of treatments prescribed, and supporting reimbursement claims will hinge on the ability of the student to understand and the clinician to express the insights offered in every chapter.

Next to the comprehensive philosophy of treatment that it offers, the greatest strength of *Rehabilitation of the Knee* may well be the makeup of the list of contributors. This is not merely a number of knowledgeable people chosen only for their common interest in the knee but a group of master clinicians, many of whom work together and all of whom know one another. Such a constellation affords the reader a consistent, fluid sequence of topics that minimizes confusion and contradiction. This is a particularly important feature both for those who are studying the knee for the first time and for those who are looking for greater detail.

Bruce Greenfield's treatment of the anatomy of the knee is not only informative but superlative. As a teacher of human anatomy for 23 years, I can avow that this functional approach is one of the best I have ever read. In his second chapter, Bruce applies this approach to illuminate the process of evaluating the injured knee. This presentation, in turn, is a logical antecedent to Mark Albert's excellent treatise on principles of exercise in relation to knee rehabilitation. Section I is rounded out by Pamela Catlin's expert dissection of the elements of the problem-solving sequence. Undoubtedly, all the treatment strategies for pathological knee conditions that follow are based on a clinical decision-making format whose components are embraced in Catlin's chapter.

Sections II and III concentrate on rehabilitation for, respectively, nonprotective or protective knee injuries. Section II, on nonprotective injuries, includes chapters on microtrauma (Johanson, Donatelli, and Greenfield), patellofemoral joint dysfunction (Bennett), and arthritis (Lechner). Each chapter provides a pathophysiological overview and documents the known benefits and limitations of clinical management approaches. Case studies at the end of each chapter highlight the most important ideas and challenge the reasoning skills of the reader.

Chapter 9 (Einhorn, Sawyer, and Tovin) begins the Section III coverage of protective knee injury management with a review of surgical procedures for intra-articular repairs and the rationales for rehabilitation that govern each type of intervention. The authors review the guidelines for rehabilitations and present case studies that highlight essential concerns in knee joint therapy. Kevin Wilk does an outstanding job of describing treatment for medial joint capsule injuries. Michael Wooden follows Wilk's sequencing in describing lateral compartment injuries. Both chapters present functional anatomy and special testing clearly and challenge the reader to think through case presentations.

Treatment following meniscectomy is common in sports-related rehabilitation; in their chapter on the menisci, Seto and Brewster review the relevant biomechanics, the mechanisms of injury, and the evaluation process. Brenda Greene follows a similar format in her presentation on knee joint replacements. As in preceding chapters in this section, Brenda thoroughly elucidates the many considerations pertinent to management of total knee arthroplasties and concludes with superb case study examples.

Bruce Greenfield as editor of the book and I as editor of the *Contemporary Perspectives in Rehabilitation* series have urged and encouraged the contributors to write as though they were lecturing to students while at the same time challenging clinicians currently treating orthopedic or sports-related injuries. We were driven by our desire to make the content as meaningful and useful as possible to the largest possible number of existing and future practitioners. We await your responses to our effort and seek your input in making the next edition even more germane to your needs. In the interim, we trust that the thoughtfulness with which this book was written will add to your evaluative skills and contribute to optimal care for your knee patients.

Steven L. Wolf, PhD, FAPTA
Series Editor, *Contemporary
Perspectives in Rehabilitation*

Preface

When I was asked to edit a book on knee rehabilitation, my first thoughts were as follows: (1) Some very good texts are already available that review the medical management and rehabilitation of the knee. (2) I do *not* want merely to organize and reprint material available elsewhere. (3) Therefore, what is needed for a unique and competitive text? After talking with my colleagues and pondering this dilemma, I identified several important elements of a successful and necessary book:

1. *Comprehensiveness.* One problem in putting together a book on the knee is organizing and limiting the abundant information available. A related concern is deciding which topics to emphasize. For example, should the book include chapters devoted to management of knee injury by both rehabilitation and surgery? Should I limit the text to the more common sports-related knee injuries? Or should I expand the scope to include topics not normally seen in the sports rehabilitation clinic but germane to management of orthopedic knee problems, arthritic knees, and total knee replacement? From a review of the literature I learned that there were both excellent texts reviewing orthopedic surgical care of the knee and chapters devoted to surgery in knee rehabilitation texts written by physical therapists and athletic trainers. Because the medical/surgical management of knee problems has been amply covered, I decided to focus this text on rehabilitation and to exclude chapters devoted to surgical management of the knee. As a result of that decision, every chapter in this book has been written by rehabilitation specialists. Where applicable, the contributors have discussed surgery as a variable that influences rehabilitation decision making. Throughout, they have referred the reader to the relevant medical textbooks for detailed descriptions of surgical procedures. In addition, aware of the many rehabilitation specialists who treat non–sports-related knee injuries, I have included two comprehensive chapters on rehabilitation of the arthritic knee and rehabilitation of the total knee replacement.
2. *Contributors.* To achieve credibility for a book devoted to the review of knee rehabilitation, I assembled a group of recognized clinical experts to contribute chapters on the management of specific knee pathologies or injuries.
3. *Organization.* This was the most important question: How can I organize the book to make it truly unique and educational? The answer became self-evident. What was needed was not only current information on knee rehabilitation but a guide to applying that information to clinical decision making. For that reason, this volume provides the reader with both content and process information. To make the process

information as clear and accessible as possible, I persuaded Dr. Pam Catlin of Emory University to write a chapter that outlines the problem-solving paradigm for clinical decision making. In addition, I asked each contributor to present extensive case studies of patients with diagnosed medical pathologies of the knee, each study incorporating clinical decision making based on the problem-solving paradigm. This book, therefore, is based on the physical therapy model of treatment: making a physical therapy problem list, determining the characteristics and factors that affect the problems, setting goals of treatment, making a treatment plan for reaching those goals, and reevaluating and modifying the treatment. In addition, some contributors have included problematic cases that require unique treatment strategies. As a result of this approach, the book will be relevant and helpful for both practicing clinicians and physical therapy students.

I believe that the completed book has successfully incorporated these elements. Overall, I am extremely pleased with the finished product, grateful to my contributors for their enthusiastic participation, and proud to have made available a book on rehabilitation written entirely by rehabilitation specialists.

Bruce H. Greenfield

Acknowledgments

The opportunity to edit such a book as this is in a certain sense the culmination of training fostered by a number of persons who have, directly or indirectly, influenced the editor. The following individuals have indeed become "a part of all that I have met."

Above all I want to pay tribute to Robert Engle, teacher, mentor, and friend. Bob died before seeing his chapter to this book (Chapter 11) in print; my sorrow is tempered by pride in offering one of the last contributions of an accomplished clinician and educator.

I would like to thank my colleagues and friends at Physical Therapy Associates of Metro Atlanta, especially Marie A. Johanson, Robert Donatelli, Scot Irwin, and Michael J. Wooden. I am also grateful to my most significant educational mentors: Dr. Steve Wolf, Dr. Pam Catlin, and the late Leo Bilancio, all of whom taught me the meaning of academic excellence and integrity. I owe a debt of gratitude also to my in-laws, Florence and Ed Schuman, for their love and support and to my brother-in-law, Andrew Jacobs. In addition, I would like to credit all the physicians who refer patients to Physical Therapy Associates, especially Dr. Joseph Wilkes and Dr. Alan Davis. Their faith in our expertise has allowed my colleagues and me to practice with a high degree of professionalism and autonomy. I and all the contributors owe a great deal to the reviewers of this text, Michael Morrisey, Tab Blackburn, Terry Malone, Cynthia Norkin, Chuck Ciccone, and of course Steve Wolf, whose constructive criticisms were instrumental in shaping this text. Finally, my thanks to F.A. Davis for its support, to Ralph Zickgraf and his punctilio, to Jody Gould, and especially to Senior Editor Jean-François Vilain, who throughout the project kept the necessary and precarious balance between cajolery and nurturance.

Contributors

Mark S. Albert, MEd, PT, ATC, SCS
Director
Physical Therapy Associates
Private Practice Clinic
Instructor
Georgia State University
Physical Therapy Program
Atlanta, Georgia

J. Gregory Bennett, MS, PT
Dominion Physical Therapy, PC
Springfield, Virginia

Clive E. Brewster, MS, PT
Director of Physical Therapy
Kerlan-Jobe Orthopaedic Clinic
Inglewood, California

Gary C. Canner, MD
Director
Sports Medicine
Reading Hospital and Medical Center
Director
Eastern Sports Medicine and
    Orthopedic Institute
West Reading, Pennsylvania

Pamela A. Catlin, EdD, PT
Associate Professor and Director
Division of Physical Therapy
Department of Rehabilitation Medicine
Emory University School of Medicine
Atlanta, Georgia

Robert Donatelli, MA, PT, OCS
Instructor
Division of Physical Therapy
Department of Rehabilitation Medicine
Emory University School of Medicine
Co-Director
Physical Therapy Associates of Metro
    Atlanta
Atlanta, Georgia

Andrew R. Einhorn, PT, ATC
Southern California Center for Sports
    Medicine
Long Beach, California

Robert P. Engle, PT, ATC
Former Adjunct Professor
Department of Physical Therapy
Temple University School of Medicine
Philadelphia, Pennsylvania
Former Director
Knee Rehabilitation Institute
Berwyn, Pennsylvania
Former Director
Center for Sports Physical Therapy
Wyomissing and Berwyn, Pennsylvania

Holly R. Ford, MSEd, PT
President and Founder
Professional Temps
Adjunct Professor
University of Central Florida
Adjunct Professor
Seminole Community College
Orlando, Florida

Brenda Greene, MMSc, PT, OCS
Instructor
Division of Physical Therapy
Department of Rehabilitation Medicine
Emory University School of Medicine
Atlanta, Georgia

Bruce H. Greenfield, MMSc, PT
Instructor
Division of Physical Therapy
Department of Rehabilitation Medicine
Emory University School of Medicine
Private Practice
Physical Therapy Associates of Metro
   Atlanta
Atlanta, Georgia

Marie A. Johanson, MS, PT
Director
Physical Therapy Associates of Metro
   Atlanta
Clinical Instructor
Division of Physical Therapy
Department of Rehabilitation Medicine
Emory University School of Medicine
Laboratory Instructor
Northeast Seminars
Atlanta, Georgia

Deborah E. Lechner, MS, PT
Assistant Professor
Division of Physical Therapy
University of Alabama at Birmingham
Birmingham, Alabama

Terry R. Malone, EdD, PT, ATC
Associate Professor
Director of Physical Therapy
University of Kentucky
Lexington, Kentucky

Thomas D. Meade, MD
Director
Allentown Sports Medicine
Attending Surgeon
Lehigh Valley Hospital
Allentown, Pennsylvania

Michael Sawyer, PT
Director of Physical Therapy
Southern California Center for Sports
   Medicine
Long Beach, California

Malton A. Schexneider, MMSc, PT, OCS
Assistant Professor
Physical Therapy Program
University of Louisville
Co-Director
Orthopaedic Physical Therapy
   Associates
Louisville, Kentucky

Judy L. Seto, MA, PT
Coordinator of Physical Therapy
   Research
Kerlan-Jobe Orthopaedic Clinic
Inglewood, California

Brian Tovin, MMSc, PT, ATC
Private Practice
Physical Therapy Associates of Metro
   Atlanta
Director of Rehabilitation
Georgia Tech Athletic Association
Atlanta, Georgia

Kevin E. Wilk, PT
Director of Research and Clinical
   Education
HealthSouth Rehabilitation Corporation
Associate Clinical Director
HealthSouth Sports Medicine and
   Rehabilitation Center
Director of Rehabilitative Research
American Sports Medicine Institute
Birmingham, Alabama

Michael J. Wooden, MS, PT, OCS
Partner
Donatelli, Irwin and Kraus, P.A.
Clinical Director and Research Associate
Physical Therapy Associates of Metro
   Atlanta
Instructor
Division of Physical Therapy
Department of Rehabilitation Medicine
Emory University School of Medicine
Atlanta, Georgia

Contents

SECTION I

Introduction

CHAPTER 1

Functional Anatomy of the Knee

Bruce H. Greenfield, MMSc, PT

The knee joint consists of the tibiofemoral joint, the patellofemoral joint, and the surrounding soft tissues. The complex arrangement of the knee joint results in a mutually supportive system of osseous, contractile, and noncontractile tissues. Normal function of the knee joint occurs when these tissues interact in a coordinated manner. Dysfunction in one tissue or structure can affect the function of the entire knee joint. An understanding of this structural interrelationship results in the effective and safe use of exercises during rehabilitation.

A review of the functional anatomy of the knee joint is divided into the following sections: osseous; menisci; crucial ligaments; medial compartment; and lateral compartment. The anatomic review is followed by a subsection of examples to describe the mutually supportive nature of the knee joint. The final two sections review basic biomechanics of the tibiofemoral and patellofemoral joints relevant to treatment. The intent of this chapter is to limit the review to clinical biomechanics and to omit arcane biomechanical analysis and constructs less germane to the practicing clinician. This chapter supplements anatomic and biomechanical descriptions of specific knee structures that are presented in subsequent chapters in this text.

OSSEOUS ANATOMY

The articulation between the tibia and femur forms the tibiofemoral joint. The shape of the corresponding joint surfaces is important in the movement of the tibia on the femur. The femur courses medially and distally from its articulation with the acetabulum in the pelvis to the condyles of the knee joint.[1] The distal end of the femur undergoes a medial torsion of 30 degrees, which corresponds to the angle of torsion (version) of the femoral neck. The femoral neck forms an angle that is between 10 and 30 degrees anterior to the transverse axis of the femoral condyles (Fig. 1–1A).[1] The

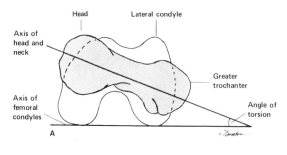

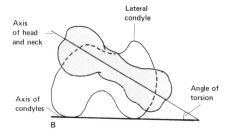

FIGURE 1-1. *A*) A bird's-eye view of the angle of torsion of the right femoral neck. The angle ranges between 10 and 30 degrees anterior to the transcondylar plane of the distal femur. *B*) A pathologic increase in the angle of torsion is called anteversion. *C*) A pathologic decrease in the angle of torsion is called retroversion. (From Norkin, CC and Levangie, PK: Joint Structure and Function: A Comprehensive Analysis, ed 2. FA Davis, Philadelphia, 1991, p 306.)

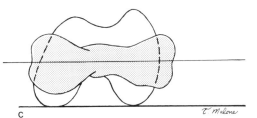

distal end of the tibia is oriented approximately 25 to 30 degrees anterior to the frontal plane. Therefore, the medial torsion of the distal femur orients the femoral condyles close to the frontal plane, the patellae face straight ahead, and the longitudinal axes of the feet are directed 5 to 10 degrees outward.[2] An angle of torsion of the femoral neck that exceeds 30 degrees results in an abnormal condition called *femoral anteversion* (Fig. 1–1B). Conversely, an angle of torsion that is less than 10 degrees results in a *femoral retroversion* (Fig. 1–1C). Clinically, the patient with an anteverted hip lacks external rotation, and a patient with a retroverted hip lacks internal rotation. Individuals who exhibit femoral anteversion or retroversion usually develop torsional and/or frontal plane changes in their lower extremities. These changes can affect the stresses within the tibiofemoral joint, as well as the function and stresses within the patellofemoral joint. The effects of lower extremity malalignment on the knee are described in Chapter 6.

As shown in Figure 1–2, because the femoral neck overhangs the femoral shaft, the axis of the femoral shaft does not coincide with that of the leg but forms with it an obtuse angle of 170 degrees, opening outward. The result is that when standing with the distal surfaces of the condyles level, the femur and tibia normally form a valgus angle of approximately 10 degrees.[2] This angle is called the *physiologic valgus angle of the knee.* A physiologic valgus angle that exceeds the normal 10 degrees results in an abnormal condition called *genu valgum.* Conversely, if the physiologic valgus angle is less than 10 degrees, the resulting abnormality is called *genu varum.*

The angulation formed between the axis of the femoral neck and femoral shaft in the frontal plane is called the *angle of inclination* and can affect the physiologic valgus angle of the knee joint. The angle of inclination in the adult is approximately 125 degrees (Fig. 1–3A). A pathologic increase in the angle is called *coxa valga* (Fig. 1–3B), whereas a pathologic decrease is called *coxa vara* (Fig. 1–3C). Clinically, patients with

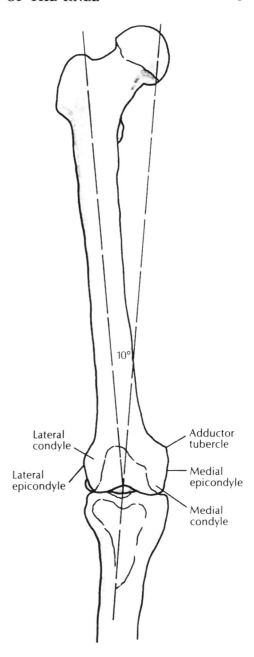

FIGURE 1-2. Anterior view of the right femur illustrating the physiologic valgus angle. (From Kessler MR and Hertling D: Management of Common Musculoskeletal Disorders: Physical Therapy Principles and Methods, ed 2. JB Lippincott, Philadelphia, 1990, p 299, with permission.)

coxa valga usually present with a decrease in the physiologic valgus angle of the knee (genu varum), while patients with coxa vara present with an increase in the physiologic valgus angle (genu valgum). In patients with either genu valgum or genu varum, there is asymmetric loading in the lateral and medial compartments of the tibiofemoral joint, respectively. Over time, this asymmetric loading may result in arthritic changes between the articulating joint surfaces.

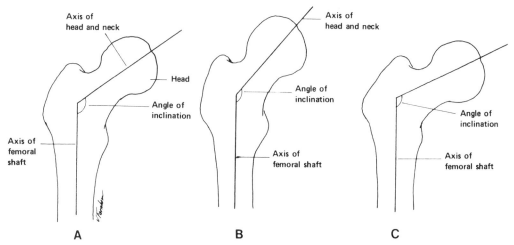

FIGURE 1-3. The axis of the femoral neck forms an angle with the axis of the femoral shaft, called the angle of inclination. *A*) The drawing shows a normal angle of inclination. *B*) A pathologic increase in the angle of inclination is called coxa valga. *C*) A pathologic decrease in the angle is called coxa vara. (From Norkin, CC and Levangie, PK: Joint Structure and Function: A Comprehensive Analysis, ed 2. FA Davis, Philadelphia, 1991, p 305.)

Femoral Condyles

The distal femur flares into two condyles separated posteriorly by an intercondylar notch. Anteriorly, the femoral condyles blend to form the concave trochlear groove, providing an articulating surface with the patella. When viewed from below, the femoral condyles form two prominences (Fig. 1-4). These prominences are convex in both the frontal and sagittal planes and longer in the sagittal (anteroposterior) direction than in the frontal (mediolateral) direction. Furthermore, the long axes of the two condyles are not parallel but diverge in a posterior direction. The medial femoral condyle leaves the midline of the femur at a greater angle than the lateral but is narrower in width (see Fig. 1-4). According to Frankel and Nordin,[3] the medial femoral condyle is approximately 1.7 cm longer than the lateral femoral condyle.

The structure of the femoral condyles was examined by Müller.[4] Viewed from the axial position, the medial femoral condyle is distinguished by the presence of a weight

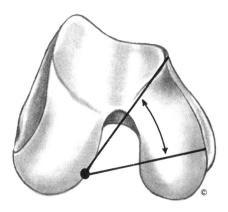

FIGURE 1-4. Distal femoral condyles are convex in both the sagittal and frontal planes and diverge posteriorly. The medial femoral condyle is approximately 1.7 cm longer than the lateral femoral condyle and contains an extra weight bearing area oriented approximately 60 degrees to the horizontal plane. This is called the annular sector of the medial femoral condyle. The condyles project anteriorly to form the trochlear groove, which articulates with the patella. The lateral condyle of the lateral trochlear groove projects approximately 7 mm higher than the medial condyle. This lateral projection affords osseous stability to the patella during range of motion of the knee joint. (Illustration: Abby Drue, Inc.)

bearing surface or an annular sector of 50 to 60 degrees to the horizontal plane (see Fig. 1–4). The annular sector of the medial femoral condyle influences the arthrokinematic movement between the tibia and femur and is reviewed later in this chapter (see Biomechanics of the Tibiofemoral Joint).

Tibial Plateau

The proximal end of the tibia flares into a plateau with a medial and lateral section separated by a prominent tibial spine. The tibial spine forms an articulation with the corresponding femoral intercondylar notch. An investigation of the topography of the proximal tibial surface performed by McLeod and associates[5] found that the surface along the region where most of the tibiofemoral contact occurs slopes approximately 9 degrees in a posterior direction (Fig. 1–5).

Both tibial plateaus are concave in the frontal plane. The medial tibial plateau is concave in the sagittal plane, and the total surface area is larger than that of the lateral tibial plateau to accommodate the wider flare and anteroposterior dimensions of the medial femoral condyle. The medial tibial plateau is oval and does not extend over the shaft of the tibia (Fig. 1–6).

Conversely, the lateral tibial plateau is convex in the sagittal plane and has a posterolateral corner that overhangs the shaft of the tibia (see Fig. 1–6). The posterolateral corner contains a facet which articulates with the fibula.[6] The radii of curvature of the corresponding femoral condyles and tibial plateaus are unequal, resulting in incongruency between the articular surfaces of the tibiofemoral joint. Additionally, the convex configuration of the lateral tibial plateau articulating with the convex lateral femoral condyle creates an unstable osseous lateral compartment of the knee joint. Fortunately, the presence of fibrocartilaginous menisci seated along the medial and lateral tibial plateaus form a trough for the corresponding femoral condyles.

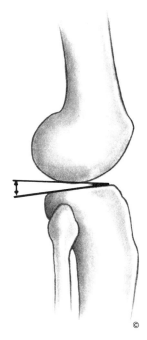

FIGURE 1–5. Posterior slope of tibial plateaus. With the tibial shaft oriented vertically, the tibial plateaus slope 9 degrees posteriorly. (Illustration: Abby Drue, Inc. Adapted from McLeod, WD and Hunter, S: Biomechanical analysis of the knee: Primary functions as elucidated by anatomy. Phys Ther 60:1563, 1980. Reprinted from PHYSICAL THERAPY with the permission of the American Physical Therapy Association.)

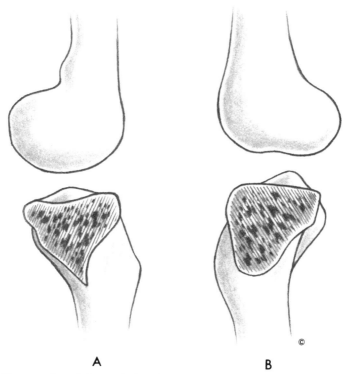

FIGURE 1-6. Topography of the medial and lateral tibial plateaus. *A*) Medial tibial plateau is concave in the sagittal plane. *B*) Lateral tibial plateau is convex in the sagittal plane. (Illustration: Abby Drue, Inc. Adapted from Kapandji,[1] p 87, with permission.)

The tibial spine forms a ridge that separates the medial and lateral tibial plateaus. The tibial spine is covered by hyaline cartilage capable of bearing loads. Equally thick cartilage is found along the opposing inner surfaces of the femoral condyles. The posterior horns of the menisci and the anterior horns are connected with the tibial spine. The result is that the tibial spine forms a central pivot during flexion and rotation of knee joint. According to Goodfellow and colleagues,[7] the tibial spine exerts optimum guidance precisely in the position of midflexion and thus at a point where a high degree of rotational freedom is combined with high axial loads.

Fibrous Capsule

The fibrous capsule surrounding the tibiofemoral joint contains vertical fibers that are attached above the margins of the femoral condyles and the posterior margins of the tibial plateaus and the posterior border of the intercondylar spine. According to Kapandji,[1] the general form of the capsule can be understood when compared to a cylinder which is invaginated posteriorly, as shown in Figure 1-7. This invagination leads to the formation of a partition in a sagittal plane, which divides the joint cavity into a medial and lateral half. On the anterior surface of the cylinder a window is cut to receive the patella. The attachment of the capsule on the tibia is between the two intercondylar

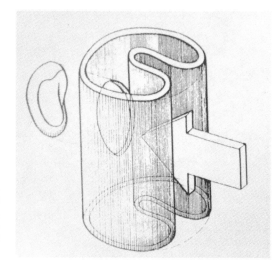

FIGURE 1-7. Capsule of the knee joint. The general form of the capsule compares to a cylinder which is invaginated posteriorly. A window is cut out along the anterior surface to receive the patella. (From Kapandji,[1] p 93, with permission.)

tubercles separating the tibial condyles and inserting in the middle of the anterior intercondylar area (see Fig. 1-7). The insertion of the capsule is therefore in front of the tibial attachment of the anterior cruciate ligament. Thus, according to Kapandji,[1] the tibial attachments of the anterior and posterior cruciate ligaments are extracapsular. However, Arnoczky[8] found that the synovial membrane is reflected from the fibrous capsule. The synovial membrane incompletely divides the knee joint in the sagittal plane and forms an envelope about the cruciate ligaments. Therefore the cruciate ligaments are actually situated within the fibrous capsule but are extrasynovial.

Plicae

The synovial membrane of the knee joint develops from three separate pouches. Seams from fusion are present in the synovial membrane. These seams are termed *plicae* and are somewhat inconstant in nature.[9-12] For example, in a series of 371 clinical arthroscopies, Patel[9] found that only 18 percent contained plicae. This finding is compared with that of Sakakibara,[11] who found plicae in 35 percent of 100 arthroscopic surgical knees, and Iino,[12] who found plicae in 50 percent of 67 cadaveric knees. The differences in the reported incidences of plicae may result from the historical differences in the definition and location of plicae in the knee joint. Generally, three distinct plicae are identified in the knee joint: suprapatellar, medial, and infrapatellar (Fig. 1-8). According to Patel,[9] rarely does a lateral plica exist. The suprapatellar plica is a crescent-shaped septum that lies between the suprapatellar bursa and undersurface of the quadriceps femoris muscle tendon. The suprapatellar plica attaches along the supero-medial and lateral aspect of the knee joint. The medial plica originates along the medial aspect of the knee joint and courses obliquely toward and inserts into the synovium covering the medial infrapatellar fat pad. The suprapatellar and medial plicae can be considered as one continuous structure.[13] The infrapatellar plicae is commonly called the *ligamentum mucosum* and traverses from the intercondylar notch to the infrapatellar fat pad.

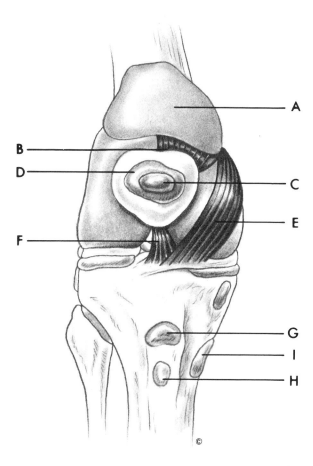

FIGURE 1-8. The bursae and plicae around the knee joint. *A*) Suprapatellar pouch. *B*) Suprapatellar plica. *C*) Superficial prepatellar bursa. *D*) Deep prepatellar bursa. *E*) Medial plica. *F*) Infrapatellar plica. *G*) Deep infrapatellar bursa. *H*) Superficial infrapatellar bursa. *I*) Pes anserinus bursa. (Illustration: Abby Drue, Inc. Adapted from Ficat, P and Hungerford, DS: Disorders of the Patello-Femoral Joint. Williams & Wilkins, 1977, p 118, with permission. © 1977, the Williams & Wilkins Co., Baltimore.)

Irritation of a plica can result either from direct trauma or by chronic impingement of a tight medial plicae between the superior medial femoral condyle and medial facet of the patella. A symptomatic medial plica may be palpated one finger-breadth from the medial border of the patella along the medial femoral condyle. A pathologic plica is usually tender and thickened. Clicking or popping of the thickened medial plica occurs during flexion and extension of the knee joint.[14]

Bursae and Infrapatellar Fat Pad

Numerous bursae are located about the knee joint. Bursae are small sacs that contain synovial fluid and are interposed between tissues or structures that glide along each other during normal functional movement, which results in reduced friction and smooth gliding between tissues. Irritation of a bursa may result in knee pain and dysfunction. The clinician must locate and palpate these structures during evaluation of the knee joint. Figure 1-8 presents the common bursae located around the knee joint. The suprapatellar bursa is located between the femur and the quadriceps femoris muscle tendon and helps reduce friction between these two structures during extension of the knee joint. The prepatellar bursa lies over the patella; it functions to cushion the anterior surface of the patella against direct blows and to reduce friction between the skin and the patella surface. Irritation of this bursa, either from a direct blow or prolonged kneeling, may result in swelling along the anterior patella surface and is commonly referred to as "housemaid's knee."[2] The deep and superficial infrapatellar bursae are interposed between the tibia and infrapatellar tendon, and the infrapatellar tendon and skin, respectively. During extension of the knee joint, these bursae facilitate gliding between these structures. The pes anserinus bursa is located between the proximal anteromedial aspect of the tibia and the undersurface of the pes anserinus muscle tendons (gracilis, semitendinosus, and sartorius muscles).[2] Two bursae not depicted in Figure 1–8 are the subpopliteus and gastrocnemius bursae. These bursae are situated along the posterior aspect of the knee joint. The gastrocnemius bursa lies deep to the tendon of the medial head of the gastrocnemius muscle and thus separates the muscle tendon from the femur. The subpopliteus bursa lies between the tendon of the popliteus muscle and the lateral condyle of the tibia. These bursae often communicate with the knee joint capsule and may become effused. This condition is referred to as a *Baker's cyst.*[2] The infrapatellar fat pad is located in the anterior aspect of the knee joint and sometimes results in pathologic changes. Specifically, the infrapatellar fat pad is located between the patellar tendon and the underlying synovial tissue and bone. Infrapatellar contracture syndrome is described by Paulos and associates[15] as a distinct clinical entity that occurs primarily as an exaggerated pathologic fibrous hyperplasia of the fat pad beyond that associated with normal healing. Occasionally, in the presence of prolonged knee joint immobilization the infrapatellar fat pad will become fibrotic and interfere with the normal gliding of the patella during movement of the knee joint. Any attempt to fully extend the knee is painful due to the entrapment of the fibrotic fat pad between the articulating surfaces of the tibia and femur bones. Surgical removal of the fat pad is sometimes required to restore full range of motion to the knee joint.

MENISCUS

Most authors today agree that a knee joint with two healthy menisci has a far better long-term prognosis than a knee joint after meniscectomy.[16–21] The preservation and restoration of normal meniscal function are therefore important surgical and rehabilitation goals.

Anatomy of the Meniscus

The menisci are biconcave fibrocartilaginous tissues interposed between the articulating surfaces of the tibia and femur (Fig. 1–9). The menisci are formed in the eighth embryonic week along with the cruciate ligaments from interposed mesenchymal tissue.[22] The common origin between the menisci and cruciate ligaments suggests a coordinated meniscoligamentous complex.[23]

The medial meniscus is semilunar in shape and is wider posteriorly than anteriorly. By contrast, the lateral meniscus is circular. The medial meniscus possesses important peripheral attachments to the femur, anteromedially by the capsule reinforced with the medial retinaculum, centrally by the medial capsule, and posteriorly by the posteromedial capsular complex. The capsular attachment includes the meniscotibial (coronary) ligaments and meniscofemoral ligaments (see Fig. 1–9). As shown in Figure 1–9, the medial or tibial collateral ligament runs external to the deep capsular ligaments, entirely

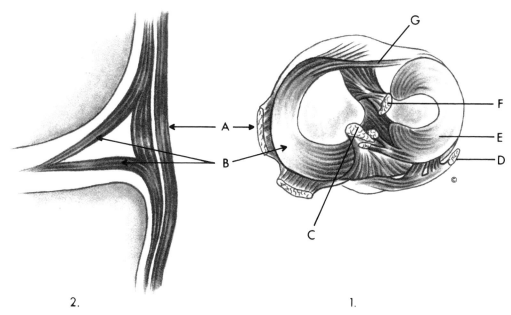

FIGURE 1–9. 1) Bird's-eye view of medial and lateral menisci. The medial meniscus is semilunar in shape while the lateral meniscus is circular. 2) Cross-sectional view of medial meniscus. *A)* Tibial collateral ligament. Note that the tibial collateral ligament is separate from the deep medial capsule. *B)* Medial meniscus with its deep capsular attachments called the meniscofemoral ligaments (attaches from the femur to the meniscus), and meniscotibial ligaments (attaches from the tibia to the meniscus). These ligaments are also called the coronary ligaments. *C)* Posterior cruciate ligament. *D)* Popliteus muscle tendon. *E)* Lateral meniscus. *F)* Anterior cruciate ligament. *G)* Transverse ligament. (Illustration: Abby Drue, Inc.)

separate from the meniscus. In between the deep capsule and the tibial collateral ligament are blood vessels that supply the periphery of the meniscus. Anteriorly, the medial meniscus receives attachment from the meniscopatellar ligament while the posterior horn of the medial meniscus receives a slip from the semimembranosus tendon. By virtue of these attachments, contraction of the quadriceps femoris muscles and hamstring muscles helps pull the medial meniscus forward and backward, respectively.

The attachment of the lateral meniscus along the lateral capsule is not as extensive as that of the medial side. Anteriorly, the lateral meniscus receives a slip of the meniscopatellar ligament and a slip of the transverse ligament. The transverse ligament, which also attaches to the anterior horn of the medial meniscus, forms a connection between the anterior horns of the medial and lateral menisci. Laterally, the meniscus is thinly attached to the capsule and does not connect to the lateral collateral ligament. Posterolaterally, the popliteus tendon passes up and over the rim of the lateral femoral condyle and separates the deep lateral capsule from the posterior horn of the lateral meniscus (Fig. 1–10). This area is known as the *popliteal hiatus* and results in increased mobility of the lateral meniscus compared with the medial meniscus. The popliteus tendon also sends a slip into the posterolateral meniscus, and therefore contraction of popliteus muscle assists in pulling the lateral meniscus posteriorly during flexion of the knee joint. The meniscofemoral ligaments of Humphry and Wrisberg demonstrate the close relationship of the lateral meniscus to the posterior cruciate ligament (see Fig

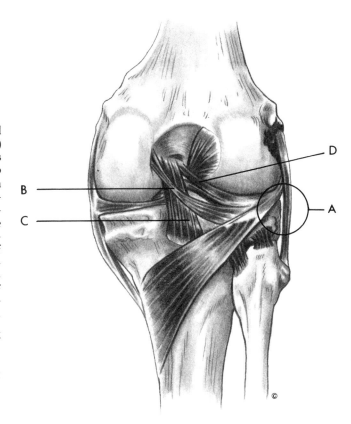

FIGURE 1–10. Posterolateral corner of the knee joint. *A*) Popliteal hiatus. The popliteus tendon separates the deep posterolateral capsule from the lateral meniscus. The result is that the lateral meniscus is more mobile than the medial meniscus. *B*) The meniscofemoral ligament of Wrisberg. *C*) Posterior cruciate ligament. *D*) The meniscofemoral ligament of Humphry. (Illustration: Abby Drue, Inc. Adapted from Warren, FR, Arnoczyky, SP, and Wickiewicz, TL: Anatomy of the knee. In Nicholas, JA [ed]: The Lower Extremity and Spine in Sports Medicine. CV Mosby, St Louis, 1985, with permission.)

1–10). The anterior and posterior horns of both the medial and lateral menisci are anchored to the tibia along the intercondylar area.

The microvascular anatomy of the menisci was investigated by Arnoczky and Warren.[24] The menisci are supplied by branches of the lateral, medial, and middle genicular arteries. A perimeniscal capillary plexus in the capsular and synovial tissue supplies the peripheral 10 to 25 percent of the menisci. The exception is the posterolateral aspect of the lateral meniscus adjacent to the popliteus tendon, which is devoid of penetrating peripheral vessels. Additionally, the superior and inferior surfaces of the peripheral menisci are nourished by diffusion from the synovial fluid. Thus the central portions of the menisci are located farthest from the nutrient sources and are the site of predilection for early degenerative changes. The vascularization and ability of peripheral meniscal lesions to heal has resulted in a trend away from total meniscectomies to partial meniscectomies preserving the peripheral rim, or to peripheral meniscal repairs.[25]

Movement of the Menisci

The menisci move during flexion, extension, and rotation of the knee joint. The movement of the menisci during movement of the tibiofemoral joint, as shown in Figure 1–11, helps maintain a stable point of contact between the changing radii of curvature of the femoral condyles relative to the tibial plateaus. Therefore, the menisci help maintain joint congruity through knee joint range of motion. During extension of the knee joint, the femoral condyles push the menisci anteriorly. Additionally, the menisci

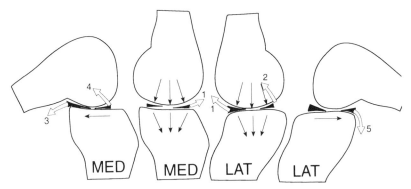

FIGURE 1–11. Movement of the menisci during flexion and extension of the knee joint. (From Kapandji,[1] p 99, with permission.)

are pulled forward due to contraction of the quadriceps femoris muscles and its attachment to the menisci through the meniscopatellar ligaments. During flexion of the knee joint, contraction of the semimembranosus muscle pulls the medial meniscus posteriorly. The lateral meniscus is pulled posteriorly by the popliteus muscle. Due to the more expansive capsular attachments of the medial meniscus compared with the lateral meniscus, the anteroposterior displacement of the lateral meniscus is twice that of the medial meniscus.

During rotation, meniscal movements follow the displacements of the femoral condyles and therefore can be seen to move in directions opposite the movement of the tibial plateaus. For example, during lateral tibial rotation the lateral meniscus moves toward the anterior portion of the tibial plateau while the medial meniscus moves posteriorly. Conversely, during medial tibial rotation the medial meniscus moves forward while the lateral meniscus recedes.

The movements of the menisci during tibiofemoral joint rotation are due to the passive displacement of the femoral condyles, as well as to the passive tension generated in the meniscopatellar ligaments. The menisci are injured if they fail to follow the movement of the femoral condyles along the tibial plateaus. The menisci can become trapped between the two joint surfaces in an abnormal position, resulting in a tear. A weight bearing, twisting injury in the knee joint involves lateral displacement and lateral rotation of the tibia on the femur. The medial meniscus is pulled toward the center of the knee joint under the convexity of the medial femoral condyle, resulting in a longitudinal buckethandle tear in the meniscus.

Functions of the Menisci

Several functions are attributed to the menisci. These functions include (1) joint stability, (2) lubrication and nutrition, and (3) shock absorption.

1. *Stability:* The triangular cross-sectional geometry of the menisci serves to deepen the fit between the relatively flat surfaces of the tibial plateaus and the convex surfaces of the femoral condyles. This observation is particularly important within the lateral compartment of the knee joint, where the lateral tibial plateau is slightly convex. Walker and Erkman[26] reported that the menisci transmit the majority of load from

the femur to the tibia in the weight bearing knee joint; 75 percent within the lateral compartment and 25 percent within the medial compartment. Therefore, the menisci form a trough for the bulbous femoral condyles. Tapper and Hoover[27] demonstrated a 14 percent increase in rotatory instability after meniscal resections in cadaveric knee joints. Levy and co-workers[28] demonstrated the affects of meniscectomy on the anteroposterior stability in knee joints. The authors performed anterior drawer tests on knee joints that had undergone meniscectomies and anterior cruciate ligament sectioning in different combinations. The findings indicated that the combination of meniscectomies and anterior cruciate ligament sectioning produced the greatest amount of anterior knee joint laxity. Isolated meniscectomies in the presence of intact anterior cruciate ligaments resulted in only minor levels of laxity. The results indicate that whereas the anterior cruciate ligament is the primary restraint to anterior laxity, the menisci provide a secondary stabilizing influence. Therefore, preservation of the menisci is imperative in the anterior cruciate ligament–deficient knee joint.

2. *Lubrication and nutrition:* According to MacConnaill,[29] the menisci act as buffers between the articulating surfaces of the tibia and femur and reduce the coefficient of friction between the joint surfaces. The coefficient of friction is the ratio between the force necessary to move one of any two surfaces horizontally over the other surface and the pressure between the two surfaces.[30] The standard coefficient of friction is 1.0, derived from rolling a rubber tire along a dry road. In joints the coefficient of friction is exceedingly low, reported as 0.005 in a bovine ankle joint. MacConnaill[29] reported a 20 percent increase in the coefficient of friction in the knee joint after a meniscectomy. Lufti[31] demonstrated increased contact between the femoral and tibial articulating surfaces in knee joints that had undergone meniscectomies. One can deduce that increased articulating surface contact during knee joint range of motion results in an increase of the coefficient of friction between the joint surfaces. Besides acting as a spacer between the tibiofemoral joint surfaces, the triangular-shaped menisci help to lubricate the knee joint surfaces by directing synovial fluid from the periphery to the central portion of the tibiofemoral joint.

3. *Shock absorption.* Several studies indicate the shock absorbing capabilities of the menisci. Fairbanks[32] noted radiographic changes in knee joints after meniscectomies, including narrowing of the joint spaces, flattening of the femoral condyles, and osteophytic formation. A study by Shrive and colleagues[33] demonstrated the weight bearing function in the tibiofemoral joint by placing a cadaveric knee joint in a compressive machine and measuring joint narrowing before and after meniscectomy. The authors demonstrated that the intact knee joint had a joint space of 1 mm at a pressure of two body weights. After a medial and lateral meniscectomy, the knee joint space was reduced by half. Kurosawa and associates[34] used pressure sensitive films to measure the contact stresses in the tibiofemoral joint. With increasing load in a normal knee joint, the contact area increased between the femoral and tibial joint surfaces. After meniscectomy, the overall contact area decreased with increasing loads. This decreased contact area between the joint surfaces results in increased stresses under increasing loads, per unit area. With time, increased stress patterns between articulating surfaces can result in accelerated breakdown in hyaline cartilage.

To understand the effects of partial meniscectomy and load transmission, it is necessary to understand the structural anatomy of the menisci. The majority of collagen fibers in the menisci are oriented circumferentially. Compressive forces between the weight bearing tibiofemoral joint tends to push the menisci outward between the two bones. This outward force is counteracted by the circumferentially oriented collagen fibers, which produce an opposing tensile force. These tensile forces, also referred to as *hoop forces,* are transmitted to the tibia through the strong anterior and posterior attachments of the menisci, including the meniscotibial and meniscofemoral ligaments. Therefore, compressive forces through the knee joint are partially converted into tensile forces by healthy menisci.[35] Shrive and colleagues[33] reported the loss of the hoop forces in a weight bearing knee joint in the presence of a single radial cut along the periphery of the meniscus. In the presence of a radial cut, the meniscus expands because of the loss of the restraining force offered by the peripheral collagen fibers. The result is increased compressive forces between the tibiofemoral joint surfaces. Ahmed and Burke[36] report that preservation of the meniscal rim can preserve the hoop tension mechanism. Therefore, the justification for a partial meniscectomy or a meniscal repair is to preserve the peripheral border of the meniscus and thereby retaining the hoop tension mechanism.

CRUCIATE LIGAMENTS

The cruciate ligaments include the anterior and posterior cruciate ligaments. A review of the cruciate ligaments should also include a discussion of the meniscofemoral ligaments. Several authorities have established the importance of the cruciate ligaments as major stabilizers of the knee joint.[37-43] This finding has led to the accepted practice amongst most orthopedic surgeons to reconstruct the acutely torn anterior cruciate ligament. Therefore, the physical therapist or athletic trainer must understand the anatomy and biomechanical functions of the cruciate ligaments to effectively develop and conduct a rehabilitation program.

Anterior Cruciate Ligament

Along with the menisci, the anterior cruciate ligament (ACL) begins to develop between the seventh and eighth week of fetal life.[44] The ACL attaches to the anteromedial area of the tibia, between the anterior insertions of the medial meniscus and lateral meniscus[45] (see Fig. 1–9F). From the tibial attachment, the ACL passes beneath the transverse meniscal ligament, where a few fascicles of the ACL blend with the anterior attachment of the lateral meniscus. Conversely, some fascicles along the posterior aspect of the tibial attachment of the ACL may blend with the posterior attachment of the lateral meniscus. Marshall and colleagues[46] studied 50 cadaveric knee joints and found that 100 percent of the ACLs attached to the anterior tibial origin of the lateral meniscus, and 20 percent reached posteriorly to attach to the posterior tibial origin of the lateral meniscus. This capsuloligamentous system formed between the ACL and menisci may partly explain the relatively high incidence of meniscal lesions that occur in the presence of acute ACL injuries.

The ACL courses posteriorly, laterally, and proximally across the tibiofemoral joint. As the ACL courses from the tibia to the femur, the ligament turns outward in a slight spiral. The ACL attaches to a fossa along the posterior aspect of the medial surface of the lateral femoral condyle. The femoral attachment is in the form of a segment of a circle, with the anterior border straight and the posterior border convex (Fig. 1–12). The long axis of the femoral attachment is tilted slightly forward from the vertical so that the ACL lies on a line forming a 40-degree angle with the long axis of the femur.

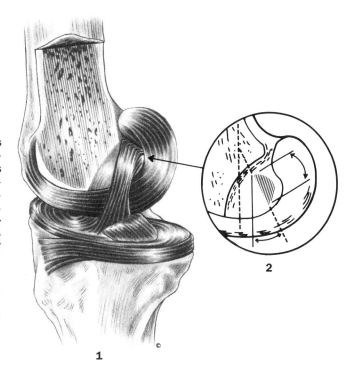

FIGURE 1–12. Attachments of the anterior cruciate ligament. 1) General attachments of the anterior cruciate ligament. 2) Cross section depicting the crescent-shaped attachment of the anterior cruciate ligament along the fossa of the medial aspect of the lateral femoral condyle. (Illustration: Abby Drue, Inc. Adapted from Girgis, FG, Marshall, JL, and Monajem, ARS: The cruciate ligaments of the knee joint. Clin Orthop 106:216, 1975, with permission.)

The ACL is a multifascicular structure that has a broad area of attachment along the tibia and the femur. Functionally, the ACL can be divided into an anteromedial band (AMB) and posterolateral band (PLB). An intermediate band divides the AMB and the PLB. These bands are named for their attachment sites along the tibial surface. When the knee joint is extended, the PLB is tight, whereas the AMB is moderately lax. As the knee joint is flexed, however, the femoral attachment of the ACL assumes a more horizontal orientation, causing the AMB to tighten and the PLB to relax (Fig. 1–13). The multifascicular nature of the ACL, in conjunction with its broad area of insertion on the

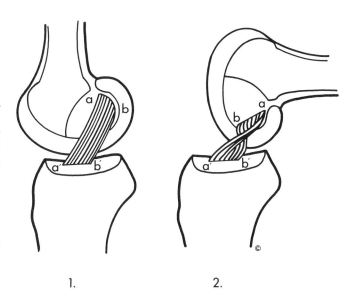

FIGURE 1–13. Tightening of the bands in the anterior cruciate ligament. 1) 0 degrees of knee joint extension the PLB is taut. 2) 90 degrees of knee joint flexion the AMB is taut. a − a′ = AMB. b − b′ = PLB. (Illustration: Abby Drue, Inc. Adapted from Girgis, FG, Marshall, JL, and Monajem, ARS: The cruciate ligaments of the knee joint. Clin Orthop 106:216, 1975, with permission.)

tibia and femur, makes replacement of the ligament during reconstructive surgery difficult. The surgeon must attempt to insert the graft tissue within the original attachment sites of the ACL. Relatively, isometric placement of the graft tissue that replicates the original attachment sites of the ACL insures the surgeon that the graft tissue will not undergo asymmetric loading during flexion and extension of the knee joint.

The major blood supply to the ACL arises from the ligamentous branches of the middle genicular artery, as well as from some terminal branches of the lateral and inferior genicular arteries.[47-48] The ACL is enveloped by synovial tissue, which is richly endowed with vessels primarily from the middle genicular artery. These vessels aborize and penetrate the ACL along with smaller vessels from the distal femoral and proximal tibial epiphyseal plates.

The ACL receives nerve fibers from the branches of the posterior tibial nerve. These fibers course along with periligamentous vessels surrounding the ACL and penetrate the ligament. These fibers have a vasomotor function as well as a proprioceptive function.[49-51] Schutte and associate[51] discovered that Ruffini, Golgi, and pacinian receptors comprise 1 percent of the total area of the ACL. Barrack and colleagues[52] examined proprioceptive deficits between the knee joints in patients with ACL deficiencies and matched control subjects with normal knee joints. The authors found that the ACL-deficient group showed a significantly higher threshold to detection of movement between their involved and uninvolved legs compared with the control group. The results demonstrated that proprioceptive deficits occur in the presence of ACL injuries. Loss of the ACL proprioceptive function may therefore contribute to functional instability through the loss of joint position sense and the dynamic stabilizing reflexes associated with the knee joint mechanoreceptors. Thus clinicians should include proprioceptive training, with closed kinetic chain balance board activities and agility drills as an integral component of their ACL rehabilitation program.

FUNCTION OF THE ANTERIOR CRUCIATE LIGAMENT

Because movement in the knee joint occurs in several dimensions,[53] the ligaments must function to protect the tibiofemoral joint in all planes of movement. The major ligaments in the knee joint, the cruciates, as well as the collaterals, provide primarily ligament-restraining force in a single plane but also act as secondary restraints in other planes. To thoroughly test the stability in the knee joint, the clinician must examine the function of each ligament as a primary and secondary restraint in each plane of movement. Previous in vitro biomechanical studies have correlated selective division of ligaments with changes in joint laxity in different planes of movement. These studies have provided clinicians with invaluable information concerning ligament function.

The functions of the ACL are to (1) restrain anterior tibial translation and prevent hyperextension of the knee joint, (2) limit tibial internal rotation, (3) provide a secondary restraint to varus and valgus stress at the knee joint, and (4) fine-tune the screw-home mechanism.[54-60]

1. The primary function of the ACL is to resist anterior translation of the tibia on the femur in knee joint flexion, as well as extension. Butler and associates[54] found that at both 30 degrees and 90 degrees of knee joint flexion, 85 percent of the restraining force to anterior tibial displacement was provided by the ACL. This resistance is mainly provided by the AMB of the ACL. The PLB is mainly tight from 20 degrees knee joint flexion to full extension. Furman and co-workers[55] found the greatest

amount of laxity in the entire ACL exists at approximately 40 degrees of knee joint flexion.

The ACL also prevents hyperextension of the knee joint. Tears of the ACL are produced when hyperextension forces are applied to cadaveric knee joints in an attempt to simulate total knee joint dislocations.[61]

2. A secondary function of the ACL is to limit tibial rotation. According to Lipke and colleagues,[59] internal rotation of the tibia in slight knee joint flexion is resisted by both the AMB and PLB of the ACL. Girgis and associates[45] showed that sectioning the ACL allows approximately 8 degrees of excessive internal tibial rotation at terminal knee joint extension. This finding is consistent with studies that find a high association of ACL injuries with histories of varus and internal rotation movements incurred after pivoting the torso to the side of the planted leg. The pivot shift phenomenon in the presence of a torn ACL with laxity of the secondary restraint offered by the iliotibial band results in subluxation of the anterolateral tibial plateau along the lateral femoral condyle. Interestingly, a recent study by Czernicki and Lippert[62] found no increase of tibial rotation during walking or running in individuals with ACL-deficient knee joints. The results of this study may indicate that the ACL functions only in a secondary role in preventing excessive tibal internal rotation in the weight bearing knee joint in the presence of healthy primary structures, such as the iliotibial band and lateral capsule.

3. Of less importance is the role of the ACL in resisting both valgus and varus stress in the knee joint in the presence of deficiency of the collateral ligaments.[60] Müller[4] notes that portions of each cruciate ligament, the ACL as well as the posterior cruciate ligament, are contained in the medial and lateral compartment of the tibiofemoral joint. The cruciates therefore act as collateral ligaments for their respective knee joint compartments. The ACL, in conjunction with the posterior cruciate ligament, offers greater resistance for varus and valgus stress at full knee joint extension compared with partial flexion.

4. Finally, the ACL fine-tunes the precision of the screw-home mechanism as the knee joint approaches terminal extension. The screw-home mechanism is primarily dictated by the osseous geometry of the tibia and femur. However, tension in the ACL as the knee joint approaches full extension is critical for the precision of the event. Rapid increase in the ACL tension as the knee joint reaches terminal extension results in the tibia rotating toward the direction of least resistance, which is external rotation. Loss of the ACL results in a tendency of the tibia to internally rotate, stretching the lateral knee joint capsule structures. This movement can result in a functional pivot shift or subluxation of the anterolateral tibial plateau.

Posterior Cruciate Ligament

The posterior cruciate ligament (PCL) is attached to a fossa on the posterior aspect of the lateral surface of the medial femoral condyle. The femoral attachment is in the form of a segment of a circle, with a straight anterior border and a convex posterior border (Fig. 1–14). The PCL passes posteriorly, laterally, and distally across the knee joint to attach to the tibia. The PCL is directed vertically in the frontal plane and angles forward 30 to 45 degrees in the sagittal plane. Therefore, the PCL is more vertical in knee joint extension and more horizontal in knee joint flexion.[63]

The PCL attaches to the tibia in a depression just posterior to the articular surface of the tibia (see Fig. 1–14). The tibial attachment extends for several millimeters on the

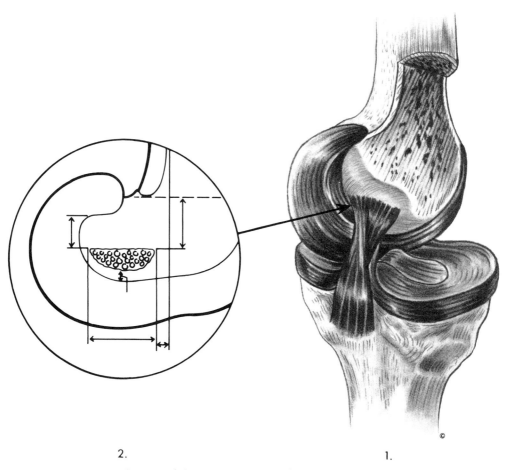

2.   1.

FIGURE 1–14. 1) Attachments of the posterior cruciate ligament. 2) Crescent-shaped attachment of the posterior cruciate ligament along the lateral aspect of the medial femoral condyle. (Illustration: Abby Drue, Inc. Adapted from Girgis, FG, Marshall, JL, and Monajem, ARS: The cruciate ligaments of the knee joint. Clin Orthop 106:216, 1975, with permission.)

posterior surface of the tibia. Proximally, a few of the fibers of the PCL extend laterally, where these fibers blend with the posterior horn of the lateral meniscus (see Fig. 1–9C).

As with the ACL, most authors identify two inseparable components of the PCL.[64] The anterior portion makes up the bulk of the ligament, whereas the posterior component is thinner. The posterior fibers, sometimes referred to as the oblique portion, originate on the medial femoral condyle and fan out to insert horizontally on the tibia. As with the ACL, flexion and extension of the tibiofemoral joint alter the relative tautness of these segments. The anterior component, which arises from the convex aspect of the femoral attachment, tightens with flexion, whereas the posterior oblique fibers tighten with knee joint extension.

The PCL is the most tear-resistant of all knee joint ligaments. According to Kennedy and associates, the ultimate force necessary to disrupt the PCL is 80 kg, twice as much as the force necessary to disrupt the ACL. Girgis and colleagues[45] found the PCL approximately 50 percent thicker than the ACL. Based on the relative strength of the PCL, it is not surprising that the reported incidence of injuries to the PCL is much less than that of injuries to the ACL. Recognition of these injuries is also somewhat difficult.

As with the ACL, the major blood supply to the PCL is through the synovial tissue surrounding and covering the ligament.[66] The middle genicular artery penetrates the posterior capsule of the knee joint and supplies blood through perisynovial capillaries to the PCL. The base of the PCL is also supplied by some of the capsular vessels arising from the popliteal and inferior genicular arteries.

The posterior articular nerve is the largest nerve supplying the knee joint and is a branch of the posterior tibial nerve. Branches of this nerve supply afferent sensation to the PCL. Schultz and colleagues[50] found that corpuscles in the cruciate ligaments resemble Golgi tendon organs. Therefore, as in the case of the ACL, injury to the PCL may result in varying degrees of proprioceptive deficit.

FUNCTION OF THE POSTERIOR CRUCIATE LIGAMENT

According to Butler and associates,[54] the PCL provides 90 to 95 percent of the total restraint to posterior displacement of the tibia on the femur. Although different portions of the PCL are taut in different degrees of knee joint flexion, tension is maximal in the PCL at full knee joint flexion.[67] Additionally, the tension in the PCL increases with internal rotation of the tibia. Hughston and co-workers[38] suggest that the PCL supports the posteromedial aspect of the knee joint, which prevents posteromedial tibiofemoral joint instability in the presence of an intact PCL. According to Wang and colleagues[67] during flexion of the knee joint the axis of rotation of the knee joint passes through the posterior part of the medial half of the tibiofemoral joint, close to or through the PCL. Thus, with flexion of the knee joint, the PCL is a major restraint for rotatory instability.

Meniscofemoral Ligaments

The meniscofemoral ligaments are accessory ligaments of the knee joint that extend from the posterior horn of the lateral meniscus to the lateral aspect of the medial femoral condyle[68] (see Fig. 1–10). Once described as the third cruciate ligament, the meniscofemoral ligaments are divided into anterior (ligament of Humphry) and posterior (ligament of Wrisberg) bands. The presence of the meniscofemoral ligaments in the knee joint are variable. Heller and Langman[68] found that either the anterior or the posterior meniscofemoral ligaments present in 71 percent of 140 dissected knee joints. The anterior meniscofemoral ligament was found in 50 knee joints (35 percent), the posterior meniscofemoral ligaments were present in 71 percent of 140 dissected knee joints, and both ligaments were found in only 8 knee joints (6 percent).

The action of the meniscofemoral ligaments is evident with flexion of the knee joint. As the weight bearing knee joint flexes, the femoral condyles slide forward along the tibial plateaus. This action results in increased tension in the meniscofemoral ligaments. The ligaments, by virtue of their attachments, pull the lateral meniscus forward. This action helps the lateral meniscus to maintain congruency with the lateral femoral condyle.

MEDIAL COMPARTMENT

The medial compartment structures of the knee joint are sometimes difficult to describe because of the large number of overlapping structures in a relatively small area. These structures include both contractile (muscle) and noncontractile (ligament) elements. However, a relatively concise but detailed description of the medial knee joint compartment is offered by Warren and Marshall,[69] and is presented in the following section.

Medial Compartment Anatomy

According to Warren and Marshall,[69] the medial compartment of the knee joint consists of three layers (Fig. 1–15). The superficial layer consists of the deep fascia that invests the sartorius, gracilis, and semitendinosus muscle tendons (pes anserinus tendons) and is continuous with the fascia that overlies the gastrocnemius muscle. The pes anserinus muscles function to flex and internally rotate the tibia on the femur, as well as to provide anteromedial stability to the knee joint.

The tibial collateral ligament (TCL) lies deep to the pes anserinus tendons and defines layer 2 of the medial compartment of the knee joint. The TCL is composed of two bundles of fibers, one vertical and one oblique. The vertical group originates from the femoral epicondyle and inserts posterior to the pes anserinus tendons on the proximal tibia. The fibers of the oblique bundle lie posterior to the vertical group of fibers and insert into the posteromedial aspect of the tibia. Hughston and Eilers[70] describe the oblique band of the TCL as the posterior oblique ligament (POL), a distinct thickening of the posteromedial capsule that is firmly attached to the medial meniscus. (Fig. 1–16). The POL is functionally independent of the TCL and is attached by a tendinous slip to the semimembranosus muscle (Fig. 1–17). Conversely, Müller[4] describes an attachment of the TCL with the vastus medialis muscle (see Fig. 1–17). Receptors similar to those found in the ACL, including Ruffini end organs, pacinian corpuscles, and Golgi tendon organs, have been found in the TCL.[71] These receptors

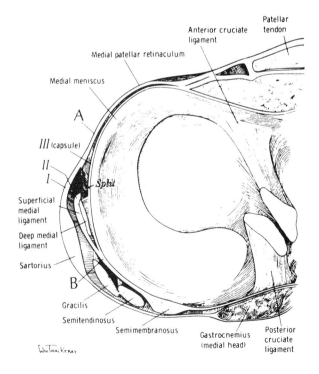

FIGURE 1–15. The medial compartment of the knee. I) Crural fascia. II) Tibial collateral ligament. III) Deep capsule. (From Warren and Marshall,[69] pp 56–62, with permission.)

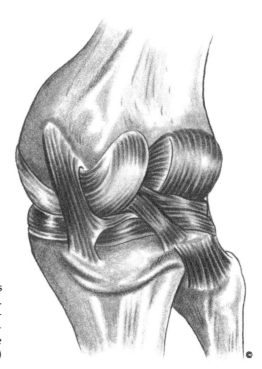

FIGURE 1–16. Posterior oblique ligament is also called the oblique tibial collateral ligament. The deep portion of the posterior oblique ligament contains meniscofemoral and meniscotibial attachments to the posterior aspect of the medial meniscus. (Illustration: Abby Drue, Inc.)

monitor joint position sense, as well as provide a protective reflex loop to the muscles attached to the ligament.

The semimembranosus-posteromedial complex of the knee joint is described by Fowler.[72] Figure 1–18 shows the five main insertions of the semimembranosus muscle. By virtue of its attachment, the semimembranosus muscle functions to flex and internally rotate the tibia on the femur, tighten the posteromedial capsuloligamentous structures of the knee joint, and pull the posterior horn of the medial meniscus posteriorly during flexion of the knee joint. The medial capsule of the knee joint makes up layer 3 of the medial compartment of the knee joint. Deep capsular fibers extend from the femur to the meniscus (meniscofemoral ligaments) and from the meniscus to the tibia (meniscotibial ligaments) (see Fig. 1–9).

Function of the Medial Capsular Structures

The relative contributions of the medial capsule to stability of the knee joint was studied by Grood and co-workers[73] in cadaveric knee joints. At 5 degrees and 25 degrees of knee joint flexion, the TCL was the primary restraint to valgus stress. At 5 degrees of knee joint flexion, the POL contributed 17.5 percent of the restraining force resisting valgus stress, compared with 57.4 percent contributed by the TCL. At 25 degrees of knee joint flexion, the POL contributed only 3.6 percent to the restraint of valgus stress, compared with 78.2 percent contributed by the TCL. However, observations made on surgical knee joints by Hughston and Barrett[74] indicated that repair of the POL compared with the TCL was more important in reestablishing medial stability to the knee joint. Whereas Grood and co-workers[73] performed their tests on cadavers, Hughston and Barrett[74] performed their examinations on living subjects. This difference alone may

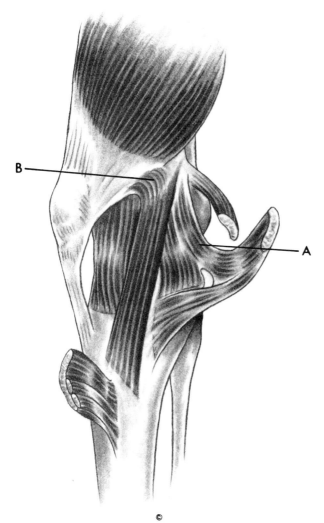

FIGURE 1-17. Interconnections between contractile and noncontractile tissues along the medial compartment of the knee joint. *A*) Semimembranosus muscle tendon attachment to the posterior oblique ligament. *B*) Vastus medialis muscle tendon attachment to the tibial collateral ligament. (Illustration: Abby Drue, Inc. Adapted from Indelicato, PA: Injury to the medial capsuloligamentous complex. In Feagin, JA [ed]: The Crucial Ligaments. Churchill Livingstone, New York, 1988, p 198, with permission.)

indicate the existence of a dynamic protective reflex arc from receptors in the POL to the semimembranosus muscle, which results in additional restraint to the POL to resist valgus stress to the knee joint.

LATERAL COMPARTMENT

Seebacher and colleagues[75] used a layered approach to describe the anatomy of the lateral knee joint compartment (Fig 1-19). This description, analogous to that of the medial knee joint compartment provided by Warren and Marshall,[69] is presented in the following section.

Anatomy of the Lateral Compartment

The most superficial layer (layer 1) of the lateral compartment of the knee joint is formed by the iliotibial tract anteriorly and the superficial portion of the biceps tendon and its expansion posteriorly. The iliotibial tract is firmly attached to both the lateral

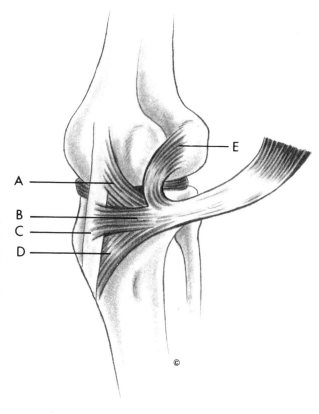

FIGURE 1–18. Semimembranous muscle attachments along the medial compartment of the knee joint. *A*) Attachment into the posterior oblique ligament. *B*) Primary posteromedial osseous insertion. *C*) Attachment to tibial collateral ligament. *D*) Osseous attachment underneath the tibial collateral ligament. *E*) Attachment into the oblique popliteal ligament. (Illustration: Abby Drue, Inc. Adapted from Fowler,[23] p 17, with permission.)

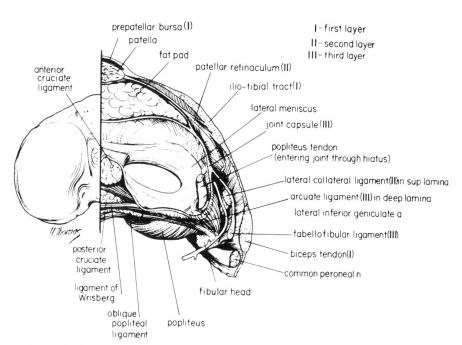

FIGURE 1–19. The lateral compartment of the knee. (From Seebacher, Inglis, and Marshall,[75] pp 536–541, with permission.)

supracondylar tubercle of the femur and the lateral tibial tubercle of Gerdy but remains independent of the deep lateral capsule. Cadaveric studies performed by Terry and associates[76] indicated that the iliotibial tract at the knee joint separates into two functional components, the iliopatellar band and iliotibial tract (Fig. 1–20). The iliopatellar band anatomically connects the anterior aspect of the iliotibial band and femur to the patella. The iliotibial tract is a multilayered structure consisting of aponeurotic, superficial, middle, and deep capsuloligamentous layers. The iliotibial tract therefore provides, along with the ACL, anterolateral stability to the knee joint. The iliopatellar band provides stabilization of the patella against a medially directed force and is dynamically influenced by the vastus lateralis muscle.

According to Fowler,[72] the biceps femoris muscle laminates into three layers proximal to the head of the fibula bone. The superficial lamina forms part of the lateral retinaculum, as well as the superficial fascia of the lateral gastrocnemius muscle. The middle lamina encompasses the fibular collateral ligament. The deep lamina inserts along the anterolateral tibia, the head of the fibula, and the posterolateral capsule of the lateral knee joint. Besides being a strong flexor and external rotator of the tibia on the femur, the biceps femoris muscle exerts influence on the fibular collateral ligament and the posterolateral capsule, tightening these structures during flexion of the knee joint.

The anterior aspect of layer 2 is formed by the lateral retinaculum of the quadriceps femoris muscles. The proximal and distal patellofemoral ligaments contribute to the posterior aspect of layer 2. The patellomeniscal ligament courses from the lateral border of the patella to the margin of the lateral meniscus and on to the tubercle of Gerdy.

Layer 3 includes the deep capsular ligament, which attaches to the articular margins of the tibia and femur. Seebacher and colleagues[75] divide the capsular ligament into deep and superficial laminae. The fibular collateral ligament, which attaches to the

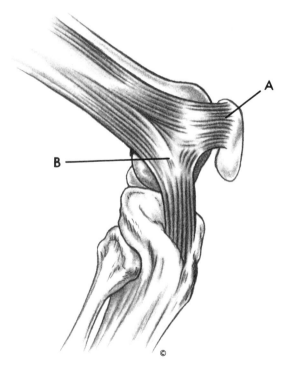

FIGURE 1–20. *A*) Iliotibial band. *B*) Iliotibial tract. (Illustration: Abby Drue, Inc. Adapted from Poole, RM and Blackburn, TA, Jr: Dysfunction, evaluation, and treatment of the knee. In Donatelli, R and Wooden, M (eds): Orthopaedic Physical Therapy. Churchill Livingstone, New York, 1988, p 497, with permission.)

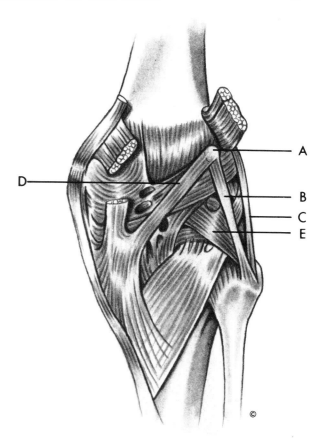

FIGURE 1-21. Posterior capsule of the knee joint. *A*) Fabella. *B*) Fabellofibular ligament. *C*) Fibular collateral ligament. *D*) Oblique popliteal ligament. *E*) Arcuate ligament. (Illustration: Abby Drue, Inc.)

lateral condylar tubercle of the femur and the lateral surface of the head of the fibula, lies between these two layers. The superficial lamina of the knee joint capsule continues posteriorly and terminates in the fabellofibular ligament (Fig. 1-21). The fabella is a sesamoid bone that lies in the tendon of the lateral gastrocnemius muscle. According to Müller,[4] the fabella, which is present in only about one fifth of the population, lies at the site of high intersecting tensile stresses along the posterolateral corner of the knee joint. The fabella acts like a pulley to redirect tensile forces and equalize stress along the posterolateral knee joint capsule. The fabellofibular ligament originates from the fabella and inserts on the head of the fibula.

The deep lamina of layer 3 is continuous with the lateral meniscus to form the meniscofemoral ligament and meniscotibial ligament. Along the posterolateral aspect of the knee joint, the deep lamina of the knee joint capsule forms a tunnel for passage of the tendon of the popliteus muscle (see Fig 1-10). The popliteus muscle crosses the back of the lateral side of the knee joint, passes through a hiatus in the deep lamina of the capsule, and inserts along the lateral femoral condyle, underneath the fibular collateral ligament. The popliteus tendon sends an expansion to the posterior horn of the lateral meniscus.[77] Contraction of the popliteus muscle assists with posterolateral knee joint stability and internally rotates the tibia on the femur to unlock the knee joint from the screw-home position at the beginning of knee joint flexion. Contraction of the popliteus muscle also helps to pull the posterior horn of the lateral meniscus posteriorly during flexion of the knee joint. This mechanism helps to maintain congruency between the lateral meniscus and the lateral femoral condyle as the femoral condyles roll posteriorly during knee joint flexion.

The deep lamina of the lateral knee joint capsule ultimately terminates as the lateral arch of the arcuate ligament. The arcuate ligament is a Y-shaped structure, which attaches distally on the fibula and fans over the posterior capsule to join the oblique popliteal ligament from the posteromedial aspect of the knee joint (see Fig. 1–21).

Function of the Lateral Capsular Structures

According to Grood and co-workers,[73] at 5 degrees of knee joint flexion the fibular collateral ligament contributed 54.8 percent of the restraining force to varus displacement. The posterolateral capsule, including the arcuate complex, contributed 13.2 percent. The iliotibial tract, popliteus, and biceps femoris tendons contributed 5.0 percent. At 25 degrees of knee joint flexion, the fibular collateral ligament contributed 69.2 percent of the restraint to varus displacement, while the posterolateral capsule contributed only 5.1 percent. According to operative and clinical findings by Hughston and associates,[39] the middle third of the deep lateral capsule and iliotibial tract are the major restraints to anterolateral knee joint instability. The arcuate complex, including the fibular collateral ligament, arcuate ligament, and popliteus tendon, is the major restraint to posterolateral instability in the knee joint.[78]

EXTENSOR MECHANISM

The extensor mechanism of the knee joint includes the quadriceps femoris muscles, patella, and related soft tissue attachments (Fig. 1–22). The quadriceps femoris muscles include the rectus femoris and three vasti muscles—the lateralis, intermedius, and medialis. The rectus femoris muscle is the only two-joint muscle, crossing both the hip and knee joints. Thus the position of the hip joint will influence the activity of the rectus femoris muscle during knee joint extension. Hip flexion greater than 90 degrees can result in active insufficiency of the rectus femoris muscle to extend the knee joint. Active insufficiency of a muscle basically occurs when there is too much overlapping between the actin and myosin filaments to form cross-bridging during muscle contraction. Therefore, during open kinetic chain knee joint extension exercises, the patient should be instructed to lean slightly back to reduce the amount of hip joint flexion.

The vasti muscles are one-joint muscles that extend the knee joint. During the stance phase of walking and running, the vasti muscles and rectus femoris muscle function eccentrically to decelerate the knee joint. Bennett and Stauber[79] emphasize the importance of eccentric function in anterior-knee-pain patients. Atrophy and dysfunction of the quadriceps femoris muscles have been associated with postsurgical immobilization of the knee joint[80–82] and knee joint effusion.[83] Specific changes have included selective atrophy of slow-twitch muscle fibers[82] and reflex inhibition of quadriceps femoris muscle contraction in the presence of knee joint effusion.[83] The clinician involved in rehabilitation of the knee joint should be aware of the effects of knee joint dysfunction on quadriceps femoris muscle function as an integral component of knee joint rehabilitation programs.

According to Lieb and Perry,[84] the vastus medialis muscle is composed of two components, the vastus medialis longus (VML) and the vastus medialis obliquus (VMO).

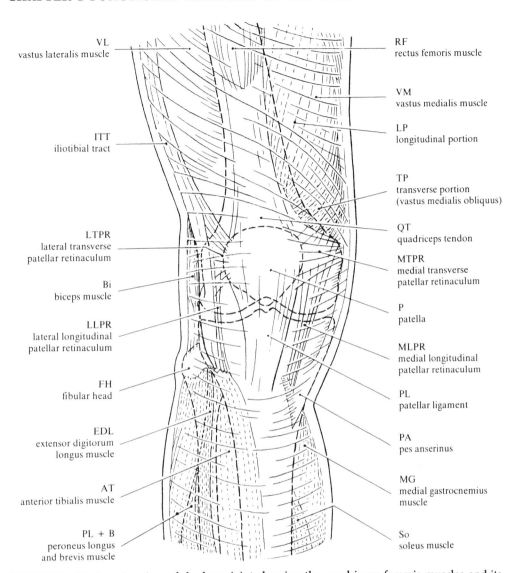

VL
vastus lateralis muscle

ITT
iliotibial tract

LTPR
lateral transverse
patellar retinaculum

Bi
biceps muscle

LLPR
lateral longitudinal
patellar retinaculum

FH
fibular head

EDL
extensor digitorum
longus muscle

AT
anterior tibialis muscle

PL + B
peroneus longus
and brevis muscle

RF
rectus femoris muscle

VM
vastus medialis muscle

LP
longitudinal portion

TP
transverse portion
(vastus medialis obliquus)

QT
quadriceps tendon

MTPR
medial transverse
patellar retinaculum

P
patella

MLPR
medial longitudinal
patellar retinaculum

PL
patellar ligament

PA
pes anserinus

MG
medial gastrocnemius
muscle

So
soleus muscle

FIGURE 1–22. Anterior view of the knee joint showing the quadriceps femoris muscles and its soft-tissue attachments to the patella. Not visible underneath the rectus femoris muscle are the vastus intermedius and articularis genu muscles. (From Müller,[4] p 3, with permission.)

The fibers of the VML are oriented 15 to 20 degrees to the longitudinal axis of the femur. The fibers of the VMO muscle are oriented 55 degrees to the longitudinal axis of the femur. Lieb and Perry[84] found a definite anatomic cleavage between the VML and VMO muscles. Electromyographic studies performed by Lieb and Perry[85] indicated that all the individual muscles of the quadriceps femoris muscle group were active throughout the range of knee joint extension. The authors found a 60 percent increase in all the muscles of the quadriceps femoris muscle group at terminal extension, and with no discrete onset and cessation of electromyographic activity of the VMO muscle. The authors point out that due to the orientation and lowness of attachment of the VMO along the medial aspect of the patella, the only reasonable function of the VMO muscle during extension of the knee joint is to help keep the patella centralized in the trochlear groove of the femur. Therefore, atrophy of the quadriceps femoris muscles, including the VMO muscle, can result in a loss of dynamic medial stabilization of the patella at terminal knee joint extension.

The vasti muscles, along with the rectus femoris muscle, conjoin to attach along the patella, centrally by a patella tendon, and medially and laterally by retinaculum. The medial retinaculum arises mainly from beneath the medial edge of the VMO muscle, the medial edge of the quadriceps femoris muscle and tendon, and the medial border of the patella to attach along the tibia, deep to the pes anserinus tendons.[86] The lateral retinaculum consists of longitudinal superficial fibers and a deep layer of transverse fibers. These fibers are an expansion of the vastus lateralis muscle and, according to Scheller and Martenson,[87] are tight in the presence of lateral tilt of the patella.

The articularis genu is a small muscle that lies underneath, but is distinct from, the vastus intermedius muscle. The articularis genu arises from the anterior surface of the femur and attaches to the superior knee joint capsule. The muscle functions to pull the synovial membrane of the knee joint upwards to prevent impingement of the suprapatellar pouch between the tibiofemoral joint during extension of the knee joint.

Patellofemoral ligaments form thickenings of the retinaculum from the midportion of the patella to the lateral and medial femoral condyles. The patellotibial ligaments extend from the inferior border of the patella, attach to the anterior margins of the tibia, and send a slip to their respective menisci. The patella has a thick distal ligamentous attachment to a tubercle on the anterior surface of the tibia.

PATELLOFEMORAL JOINT

The patellofemoral joint is formed between the articulations of the patella and trochlear groove of the femur. The patella is the largest sesamoid bone in the human body. It is shaped like an inverted triangle, with a proximal base and distal apex. The articular surface is divided into a medial and lateral facet by a central ridge giving the lateral facet a larger surface area.[88] An odd facet is situated along the extreme medial border of the medial facet. The articulating surface of the patella also contains a superior and inferior region (Fig. 1–23). The thickness of the articulating hyaline cartilage surface reaches 5 mm, which attests to the demanding function of the patellofemoral joint.

Six types of patellar facet configurations are described by Wiberg[89] and Baumgartl[90] (Fig. 1–24). Type I has equal facets, which are slightly concave. Type II has a smaller medial facet, which is still slightly concave, and type III has a smaller medial facet with a convex surface. Type II/III has a flatter medial facet. Type IV has a very small, steeply

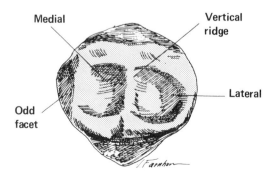

FIGURE 1–23. Articulating surface of the patella. (From Norkin, C and Levangie, P: Joint Structure and Function. A Comprehensive Analysis. FA Davis, Philadelphia, 1983, p 321.)

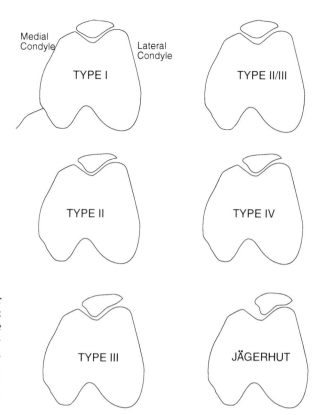

FIGURE 1-24. Six types of patellar configurations. (From Larson, RL: Fractures and dislocations of the knee, Part II. Dislocations and ligamentous injuries to the knee. In Rockwood, CA and Green, DP [eds]: Fractures. Vol 2. JB Lippincott, Philadelphia, 1975, p 1183, with permission.)

sloped facet with a medial ridge still present, and type V (Jägerhut) has no central ridge or medial facet. The type I and II patellae are those that are most stable with equal distributions of forces, whereas the other types of patellae are more prone to unequal stresses and to lateral subluxation or dislocation.

The lateral condyle of the trochlear groove of the femur is higher than the medial condyle and projects anteriorly at least 7 mm (see Fig. 1-4). The lateral projection of the lateral trochlear condyle affords osseous stability to prevent lateral dislocation of the patella. Brattstrom[91] defines the depth of the femoral groove by the femoral sulcus angle. The *sulcus angle* is the angle formed by a line drawn from the deepest point of the femoral groove or sulcus to the top of the lateral femoral condyle and a second line from the deepest point of the femoral sulcus to the medial femoral condyle. Larson and associates[92] measured the average sulcus angle in patients without patellofemoral pain to be 114 degrees. The average sulcus angle in a series of patients with recurrent lateral dislocating patellae measured 127 degrees. Therefore, the more acute the sulcus angle, the greater osseous stability is afforded to the patellofemoral joint during knee range of motion. Conversely, an obtuse angle or shallow femoral trochlear groove results in poor osseous stability and predisposes the patella to lateral subluxation or dislocation.

Function of the Patella

The primary function of the patella is to increase the perpendicular lever arm of resistance of the line of force of the quadriceps femoris muscles to the axis of rotation of the knee joint. Without the patella, there is an irreversible loss of knee joint extension torque. Kaufer[93] demonstrated that the force necessary to produce full knee joint extension after patellectomy was increased 15 to 30 percent. Second, the patella serves to centralize the attachment of the divergent muscles of the quadriceps femoris muscles. The centralization of the quadriceps femoris muscle force improves the efficiency of the muscle contraction to extend and control the knee joint. Third, the compressive forces from the femur are absorbed by the patella. Rather than the tibiofemoral joint forces being transferred directly as a compressive load, these forces are transformed into tension forces in the quadriceps femoris muscle tendon. This transformation allows the very powerful quadriceps femoris muscles to act as a retainer for the femur.[94] Fourth, the patella provides an osseous shield for the anterior aspect of the knee joint.

STRUCTURAL INTERRELATIONSHIPS

In discussions of the anatomy of the knee, structural interrelationships can be used to describe how some of the tissues interact during function. This process can perhaps establish a frame of reference of normal function from which one or more valuable conclusions might be drawn.

For example, the posterior slope of the tibial articulating surface is clinically signifi-cant when we consider that during normal standing, the tibial shaft is aligned in a vertical position with femoral loads to the tibia distributed along the tibial shaft. Therefore, the femur will tend to slide off the posterior side of the tibial surface. This tendency is negated primarily by the static resistance offered by the ACL and less so by the posterior horns of the menisci and the mensicotibial ligaments. The ACL is angled in a direction to help keep the femur from sliding back off the tibia. The posterior horns of the menisci curl around the femur, thereby providing a backstop, and the menisci are held very tightly in the tibial surface by the meniscotibial ligaments. In the presence of ACL deficiency, increased load to resist the posterior force of the femur on the tibia is placed on the menisci and its supporting ligaments, resulting in attenuation of the menisci and meniscotibial ligaments, and a functionally unstable knee joint.[95]

A simple knowledge of the shape of the articulating surfaces and loads imposed upon the knee joint allows the clinician to protect healing structures during rehabilita-tion. For example, based on the slope of the tibial surface, McLeod and Blackburn[96] found that to relieve stress on the ACL during stationary cycling, the seat height should be lowered and the patient should be instructed to pedal with the balls of his feet. The resultant knee joint flexion angle allows the femur to slide anteriorly into the patellofe-moral joint rather than posteriorly, thus diminishing the stress or the ACL and mensico-tibial ligaments.

The effect of muscle contraction on knee joint stability is considerable. Markolf and associates[97] studied the effects of maximum isometric contraction of the knee joint muscle on the overall stiffness of the tibiofemoral joint. Joint stiffness can be defined as the change in force per unit change in displacement of the joint. Subjects' knees were tested for anteroposterior and varus-valgus displacement. The authors found that on average the stiffness of the tibiofemoral joint was increased by a factor of 2.2 to 4.2 when the subjects made a maximal isometric contraction of the muscles, compared with when the muscles were relaxed.

In humans, the hamstring and quadriceps femoris muscles around the knee joint are activated simultaneously in a wide range of motor activities. Cocontraction of these muscles presses the articulating surfaces of the tibiofemoral joint together and contribute to increased, but equal, distribution of compressive loads within the joint.[98] The resulting increased stability of the joint underscores the importance of muscle coordination for functional activities.

The sensory role of ligaments to elicit protective muscle reflexes vis-à-vis a sensory feedback loop may be illustrated by examining the structural arrangement of muscles and ligaments within the medial and lateral knee compartment. The attachment of the TCL and the POL to the vastus medialis and semimembranosus muscles respectively, establishes a combination passive and dynamic restraint system. Ligamentous afferents when stimulated may activate muscles around the joint directly through a monosynaptic reflex arc to the muscle's alpha motoneuron.[99] Valgus force to the medial aspect of the knee, which stresses the TCL and POL, may stimulate ligamentous afferents and result in reflex contraction of the vastus medialis and semimembranosus muscles. The result is increased dynamic support to the medial compartment of the knee joint. Conversely, muscle contraction can assist in increasing the stiffness of ligaments around the knee joint. Hughston and Eilers[70] believe that contraction of the semimembranosus muscle during flexion of the knee joint, via its attachment to the POL, tightens the posteromedial capsule, thereby making that portion of the medial knee compartment the primary restraint to valgus stress. Because fibers of the biceps femoris muscle attach to the fibular collateral ligament, one may deduce that there is a protective reflex loop in the lateral knee compartment. Therefore, a varus force to the semiflexed weight bearing knee joint may result in reflex activation of the biceps femoris muscle to provide additional stability and protection to the lateral aspect of the knee joint.

BIOMECHANICAL PRINCIPLES

A review of the anatomy should, whenever possible, relate structures of the knee joint to a mechanical model. An understanding of some of the basic conceptual principles of mechanics facilitates an understanding of the functional anatomy of the knee joint.

Kinematics

Kinematics is the phase of mechanics that addresses the possible motion of a material body, irrespective of the forces that produce the motion.[30] When a body moves, it will do so in accordance with its kinematics, which in the human body includes principally the shape of the joints. In the human body, kinematics is divided into arthrokinematics and osteokinematics.[100] *Osteokinematics* describes the movement of the long bones relative to each other, for example, the movement of the tibia and femur bones during tibiofemoral joint flexion. *Arthrokinematics* describes the intimate mechanics of corresponding joint surfaces that occurs during osteokinematic movements. The arthrokinematic movements are described as roll, slide, and spin.[100] *Roll* occurs when points equidistant on one surface meet points equidistant on a corresponding surface. *Slide* occurs when one point contacts different points on the opposing surface. *Spin*, or rotation, occurs when a long bone rotates around its stationary mechanical axis. A knowledge of the normal combination of roll, slide, and spin in a joint allows the clinician to assess changes of the arthrokinematics in the presence of joint dysfunction.

The restoration of normal arthrokinematic movement is a primary goal in rehabilitation of the knee joint.

Open and Closed Kinetic Chains

Steindler[101] introduced the terms *open and closed kinetic chains* to describe how a joint or limb will be operating rather differently depending on whether or not the joint is operating against resistance. An open kinetic chain situation is one which the terminal joint is free, as in waving good-bye, or in extending the lower leg while sitting on a bench. Conversely, a closed kinetic chain situation is one which the terminal joint meets with some considerable external resistance which prohibits and restrains movement.

Significant differences occur in the internal dynamics of the knee joint performing weight bearing exercises (closed kinetic chain movements), and knee joint extension exercises over the side of an exercise bench (open kinetic chain movements). These differences include the compressive forces produced through the tibiofemoral and patellofemoral joints, and how we describe the arthrokinematic movement between the joint surfaces. The differences between closed and open kinetic chain situations during movements in the knee joint are therefore delineated in the following sections discussing tibiofemoral and patellofemoral joint mechanics.

BIOMECHANICS OF THE TIBIOFEMORAL JOINT

The traditional description of the tibiofemoral joint is that of a modified hinge joint with two degrees of freedom. These movements include flexion and extension around a mediolateral axis, and rotation around a superior-inferior axis. However, more recent analysis indicates that the tibiofemoral joint has six degrees of freedom, three rotational and three translational[102] (Fig. 1–25).

A description of the arthrokinematic movement of the tibiofemoral joint is based, in large part, on an analysis of the osseous anatomy and indicates that knee joint movements are coupled in a precise and predictable pattern. The possibility of a simple rolling movement of the femoral condyles is precluded by the fact that the lengths of the femoral condyles are twice as great as the lengths of the tibial plateaus. During flexion and extension of the knee joint, the femoral condyles roll and slide simultaneously along the tibial plateaus. The direction of the roll and slide is based on the shape of the corresponding articular surfaces. In an open kinetic chain situation, the concave articulating surfaces of the tibia move along the convex articulating surfaces of the femoral condyles. Roll and slide occur in the same direction. Under closed kinetic chain conditions, the convex articulating surfaces of the femoral condyles move along the concave articulating surfaces of the tibial plateaus. Roll and slide occur in opposite direction[100] (Fig. 1–26).

The ratio of rolling and sliding varies during flexion and extension of the tibiofemoral joint. For example, beginning from closed-kinetic-chain knee joint extension, the femoral condyles begin to roll without sliding, and then sliding becomes progressively more important. Ultimately, at the end of flexion, the femoral condyles slide without rolling. For the medial femoral condyle, pure rolling occurs during the initial 10 to 15 degrees of flexion, whereas the lateral femoral condyle continues to roll until 20 degrees of knee joint flexion. The ratio of roll to slide in early knee joint flexion is approximately $1:2$ and $1:4$ at the end range of knee joint flexion.[4]

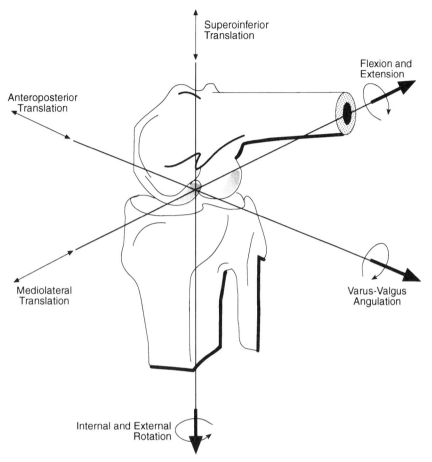

FIGURE 1-25. Six degrees of freedom of the tibiofemoral joint. The movements are flexion and extension with anteroposterior translation around a mediolateral axis, adduction and abduction (varus-valgus angulation) with mediolateral translation around an anteroposterior axis, and internal and external rotation with superoinferior translation around a superoinferior axis. (From Goodfellow and O'Connor,[102] p 358, with permission.)

During closed kinetic chain knee joint flexion, the femur initially spins or externally rotates on its long axis, approximately 15 degrees. The opposite movement of internal rotation of the femur occurs during the final 20 degrees of closed kinetic chain knee joint extension and is commonly referred to as the "screw-home" mechanism. The difference in the length and orientation between the two femoral condyles results in this helicoid or figure-eight motion between the tibia and femur. As the knee joint reaches full extension, the lateral femoral condyle will complete its slide along the lateral tibial plateau, while the annular sector of the medial femoral condyle continues to slide in place. As a result of the screwing home of the annular sector, the medial femoral condyle is forced into a medial oblique position on the tibia to check further extension. Therefore, the fully extended knee joint exhibits a moderate degree of osseous stability.

Along with the small amount of automatic rotation in the tibiofemoral joint there is a small amount of automatic abduction and adduction in the frontal plane. According to Kapandji,[1] the axis of the tibiofemoral joint is oriented inferiorly and medially relative to the transverse plane. The compressive forces acting through the tibiofemoral joint can

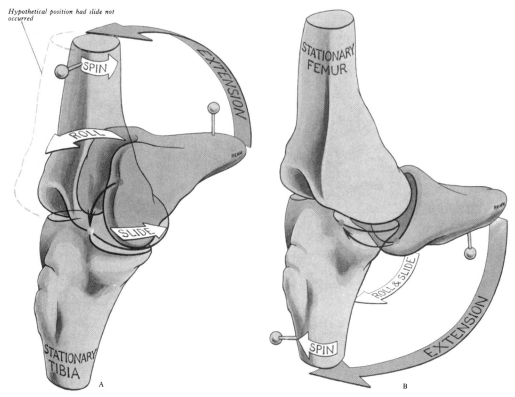

FIGURE 1–26. Arthrokinematic movement of the tibiofemoral joint under *A*) closed and *B*) open kinetic chain conditions. (From Warwick, R and Williams, PL: Gray's Anatomy. 35th British edition. Churchill Livingstone, New York, 1973, p 406, with permission.)

therefore be resolved into vertical and transverse components, which point horizontally and medially. The transverse component tends to tilt the tibiofemoral joint medially and move the tibia into abduction at full extension. Conversely, a small degree of automatic adduction of the tibia relative to the femur occurs during knee joint flexion.

In summary, active extension of the weight bearing knee joint is associated with posterior slide with anterior roll of the femoral condyles, internal rotation of the femur, and abduction of the tibia. Active weight bearing flexion is associated with anterior slide and posterior roll of the femoral condyles, external rotation of the femur, and adduction of the tibia. Of course, these movements are influenced and modified by surrounding capsular, ligamentous, and muscular structure.

Functional Kinematics

From a clinical standpoint, one should examine the kinematics of the knee joint under functional conditions. The range of motion in the tibiofemoral joint is greatest in the sagittal plane, where the range from full extension to complete flexion measures 0 degrees to approximately 140 degrees. The extent of active flexion varies with the position of the hip joint, attaining a maximal value of approximately 140 degrees with the hip flexed to 90 degrees, and a minimum value in the range of 120 degrees with the hip joint completely extended.

Data from Kettelkamp and associates[103] and Laubenthal and colleagues[104] established the range of tibiofemoral joint flexion and extension during common activities of daily living. The data establish that a minimum of 90 degrees of tibiofemoral joint flexion is necessary to perform normally the minimum levels of activities of daily living, such as descending stairs, with a maximum of 117 degrees of tibiofemoral joint flexion required for higher level activities, such as lifting an object.

Kinematics of the tibiofemoral joint during walking was investigated by Levens and colleagues[105] and Murray and associates.[106] Nearly complete extension of the tibiofemoral joint (5 degrees of flexion) was recorded both at the beginning and end of the stance phase, at heel strike, and just before toe-off. Maximal flexion of 75 degrees was observed during the middle portion of the swing phase of gait. In the transverse plane, Levens and colleagues,[105] observing serial photographs in 12 subjects, found that the total rotation of the tibia on the femur ranged from 4.1 to 13.1 degrees, or an average of 8.6 degrees. External rotation of the tibia on the femur occurred during the entire stance phase and at the end of the swing phase of gait.

In a related study, Kettelkamp and associates[103] studied tibiofemoral joint motion in the frontal plane in 22 subjects. The subjects were measured using an electric goniometer. Maximum abduction of the tibia was observed during knee joint extension, at heel strike, and at the beginning of the stance phase of gait. Whereas maximal adduction was observed as the knee joint flexed during the swing phase of gait, the total amount of abduction and adduction averaged 11 degrees.

Kinematic studies of normal knee joint function provides the clinician important normative data to make patient comparisons. A study by Czernicki and Lippert[62] described changes from normal tibiofemoral joint kinematics in the presence of knee joint pathology. Refinement in electrogoniometric measurement techniques and computer-assisted three-dimensional analysis will continue to provide additional data concerning knee joint kinematics in the presence of selected knee pathologies.

BIOMECHANICS OF THE PATELLOFEMORAL JOINT

The movement of the patella along the femoral trochlear groove is described by Hungerford and Barry.[107] Starting at full knee joint extension and proceeding to 20 degrees flexion, the patella glides from the lateral trochlear condyle deep into the trochlear groove, resulting in excellent osseous stability in the patellofemoral joint. Manual testing should produce very little lateral displacement of the patella at this point in the range of knee joint flexion. A clinician who is able to glide the patella an equal distance at full knee joint extension and at 20 degrees flexion should suspect a shallow trochlear groove. From 90 to approximately 135 degrees of knee joint flexion, the patella rotates along a vertical axis and the ridge between the medial and odd facet engages the lateral aspect of the medial femoral condyle. After 135 degrees of knee joint flexion, the patella slips into the intercondylar notch, rotates, and shifts laterally, thereby engaging the odd facet with the medial femoral condyle. The full course of patella movement, then, from full knee joint extension to full flexion, is one of a gentle "C" open laterally.

Patellofemoral Joint Reaction Forces

For our purposes, joint reaction forces may be defined as the internal forces produced between the articulating surfaces of two apposing joints during a specific activity, at any one point in a range of motion. The types or direction of joint reaction forces include compressive, shear, and tensile forces.[108] The type and magnitude of reaction forces produced within a joint may be beneficial or harmful, depending on what joint is being examined and under what circumstance we are examining that joint. For example, one of the primary goals for shoulder rehabilitation is to strengthen the rotator cuff muscles during elevation of the upper extremity so as to provide the necessary compressive forces within the glenohumeral joint to counteract the deleterious superior shear force created by the upward pull of the deltoid muscle.[109] Conversely, the goal of most knee joint rehabilitation programs is to strengthen the quadriceps femoris muscles while minimizing patellofemoral joint compressive forces. The patellofemoral joint sustains considerable compressive forces during movement. These compressive forces need to be calculated in order to understand which activities or positions provide the greatest compression and which the least.

For example, the magnitude of patellofemoral joint reaction forces (PFJRF) were examined by Reilly and associates,[110] who reported that PFJRFs ranged from 0.5 times body weight during normal walking, to 3.3 times body weight climbing stairs. Deep knee bends produced patellofemoral joint reaction forces to 7.8 times body weight. This information can be used for rehabilitation purposes.

Somewhat controversial is the most favorable range of motion to perform quadriceps femoris muscle strengthening exercises while minimizing PFJRFS. An examination taking into account PFJRFs, knee joint flexion angle, and functional activities requires a review of the relationship between PFJRFs and contact stresses.

Patellofemoral joint contact stresses are described by Goodfellow and associates.[7] Between 20 and 30 degrees of knee joint flexion, patellofemoral contact occurs between the medial and lateral patella facets and the trochlear groove of the femur. Between 30 and 90 degrees of knee joint flexion, the contact area increases to include the proximal patella and the ridge of the odd facet. After 90 degrees of knee joint flexion, the contact area includes the broad tendinous band of the quadriceps femoris muscles and the odd facet of the patella along the lateral margin of the medial femoral condyle. Ficat and Hungerford[111] delineated the patellofemoral contact areas in four cadaveric knee joints in different degrees of knee joint flexion. At 30 degrees of knee joint flexion, the total area of contact between the patellofemoral joint surfaces was 2.0 cm. At 60 degrees, the contact area increased to 3.1 cm. At 90 degrees of knee joint flexion, the total contact area between the patellofemoral joint surfaces was greatest, measuring 4.7 cm. Conversely, Ficat and Hungerford[111] examined the relationship between the PFJRFs as a function of the knee joint angle. The authors reported that the patellofemoral force was zero with the knee joint in full extension and increased linearly to 1.5 times the quadriceps femoris tendon force at 90 degrees of knee joint flexion.

What becomes obvious is that patellofemoral contact stresses and joint reaction forces increase and decrease together as the knee joint flexion angle changes. Increased contact stresses of the patellofemoral joint at 90 degrees of knee joint flexion provide a larger surface area to dissipate the joint reaction forces. The rationale for implementing a quadriceps femoris muscle strengthening program from 90 to 60 degrees of knee joint flexion, in a patient with patellofemoral dysfunction and retropatellar pain, is based on the larger patellofemoral contact area to dissipate joint reaction forces. Conversely, the reduced patellofemoral contact stresses toward terminal knee joint extension result in increased patellofemoral compressive forces per unit contact area. However, because there is a concomitant reduction in the patellofemoral joint reaction forces at terminal knee joint extension, many clinicians prefer to implement quadriceps femoris muscle strengthening toward full knee extension.

SUMMARY

A review of the anatomy of any single joint in the human body requires a description of various tissues and structures to enable the reader to gain insight as to their individual anatomy and function. At the same time, the reader needs to maintain an awareness of the functional integration of knee joint structures. The function of ligaments in a three-dimensional system as primary and secondary restraints to movement, the influence of meniscectomized knee joints on the tensile strength of the anterior cruciate ligament, and the effect of muscle function in providing dynamic stability to ligaments provide examples of the mutually supportive nature of knee joint structure and function. The clinician should understand the functional integration of knee joint structures to attain maximal rehabilitation goals.

REFERENCES

1. Kapandji, IA: The Physiology of the Joints, Vol 2. Churchill Livingstone, New York, 1970, pp 25, 74, 80, 92.
2. Kessler, RM and Hertling, D: Management of Common Musculoskeletal Disorders: Physical Therapy Principles and Methods. JB Lippincott, Philadelphia, 1983, pp 394, 402.
3. Frankel, VH and Nordin, M: Biomechanics of the knee. In Hunter, LY and Funk, JF, Jr (eds): Rehabilitation of the Injured Knee. CV Mosby, St Louis, 1984, p 34.
4. Müller, W: The Knee: Form, Function, and Ligament Reconstruction. Springer-Verlag, New York, 1983, pp 12, 13, 54, 65, 117, 192.
5. McLeod, WD, Moschi, A, and Andrews, JR: Tibial plateau topography. Am J Sports Med 5:13, 1977.
6. Kennedy, JC and Fowler, PJ: Medial and anterior instability of the knee: An anatomical and clinical study using stress machines. J Bone Joint Surg [Am] 53:1257, 1971.
7. Goodfellow, J, Hungerford, DS, and Zindel, M: Patellofemoral joint mechanics and pathology. I. Functional anatomy of the patellofemoral joint. J Bone Joint Surg [Br] 58:287, 1976.
8. Arnoczky, SP: Anatomy of the anterior cruciate ligament. Clin Orthop 172:19, 1983.
9. Patel, D: Arthroscopy of the plica-synovial folds and their significance. Am J Sports Med 6:5, 217, 1970.
10. Hughston, JD and Andrews, JR: The suprapatellar plica and internal derangement. Proceedings of the American Academy of Orthopedic Surgeons. J Bone Joint Surg [Am] 55:1318, 1973.
11. Sakakibara, J: Arthroscopic study of Iino's band (plica synovialis mediopatellaris). Journal of Japanese Orthopedic Association 50:513, 1976.
12. Iino, S: Normal arthroscopic findings in the knee joint in adult cadavers. Journal of Japanese Orthopedic Association 14:467, 1939.
13. Broom, MJ and Fulkerson, JP: The plica syndrome: A new perspective. Orthop Clin North Am 17:279, 1986.
14. Amatuzzi, MM, Fazzi, A, and Varella, MH: Pathologic synovial plica of the knee: Results of conservative treatment. Am J Sports Med 18:5, 466, 1990.
15. Paulos, L, et al: Infrapatellar contracture syndrome: An unrecognized cause of knee stiffness with patella entrapment and patella infera. Am J Sports Med 15:4, 331, 1987.
16. Krause, WR, et al: Mechanical changes in the knee after meniscectomy. J Bone Joint Surg [Am] 58:5, 599, 1976.
17. Moginty, JB, Geuss, LF, and Marvin, RA: Partial or total meniscectomy: A comparative analysis. J Bone Joint Surg [Am] 59:6, 763, 1977.
18. Jackson, JP: Degenerative changes in the knee after meniscectomy. BMJ 2:525, 1968.
19. Cox, JS and Cordell, LD: The degenerative effects of medial meniscus tears in dog knees. Clin Orthop 125:236, 1977.
20. Dandy, DJ and Jackson, RW: The diagnosis of problems after meniscectomy. J Bone Joint Surg [Br] 57:349, 1975
21. Radin, EL and Burr, DB: Meniscal function and the importance of meniscal regeneration in preventing late medial compartment osteoarthritis. Clin Orthop 171:121, 1982.
22. Kaplan, EB: The embryology of the knee joint. Bull Hosp J Dis Orthop Inst 16:111, 1955.
23. Fowler, PJ: Functional anatomy of the knee. In Hunter, LY and Funk, FJ, Jr (eds): Rehabilitation of the Injured Knee. CV Mosby, St Louis, 1984, p 13.
24. Arnoczky, SP and Warren, RF: Microvasculature of the human meniscus. Am J Sports Med 10:2, 90, 1982.
25. Hanks, GA, et al: Meniscus repair in the anterior cruciate deficient knee. Am J Sports Med 18:606, 1991.

26. Walker, PS and Erkman, MJ: The role of the menisci in force transmission across the knee. Clin Orthop 109:184, 1975.
27. Tapper, EM and Hoover, HW: Late results after meniscectomy. J Bone Joint Surg [Am] 51:517, 1969.
28. Levy, IM, Torzilli, PA, and Warren, RF: The effect of medial meniscectomy on the anterior-posterior motion of the knee. J Bone Joint Surg [Am] 64:883, 1982.
29. MacConnaill, MA: The function of the intraarticular cartilages with special reference to the knee and inferior radioulnar joints. J Anat 66:210, 1932.
30. Norkin, C and Levangie, P: Joint Structure and Function: A Comprehensive Analysis. FA Davis, Philadelphia, 1983, pp 4, 29.
31. Lufti, AM: Morphological changes in the articular cartilage after meniscectomy. J Bone Joint Surg [Br] 57:525, 1975.
32. Fairbanks, TJ: Knee joint changes after meniscectomy. J Bone Joint Surg [Br] 30:664, 1948.
33. Shrive, NG, O'Conner, JJ, and Goodfellow, JW: Loadbearing in the knee joint. Clin Orthop 131:279, 1978.
34. Kurosawa, H, Fukubayashi, T, and Nakajima, H: Load bearing mode of the knee joint. Clin Orthop 149:283, 1980.
35. Bullough, PB, et al: The strength of the menisci of the knee as it relates to their fine structures. J Bone Joint Surg [Br] 52:564, 1970.
36. Ahmed, AM and Burke, DL: In vivo measurements of static pressure distributions in synovial joints. I. Tibial surface of the knee. J Biomech Eng 105:201, 1983.
37. Abbot, LC, et al: Injuries to the ligaments of the knee joint. J Bone Joint Surg [Am] 26:503, 1944.
38. Hughston, JC, et al: Classification of knee ligament instabilities. I. The medial compartment and cruciate ligaments. J Bone Joint Surg [Am] 58:159, 1976.
39. Hughston, JC, et al: Classification of knee instabilities. II. The lateral compartment. J Bone Joint Surg [Am] 58:173, 1976.
40. Hughston, JC, et al: Acute tears of the posterior cruciate ligament. J Bone Joint Surg [Am] 62:438, 1980.
41. Kennedy, JC and Granger, RW: The posterior cruciate ligament. J Trauma 7:367, 1967.
42. Noyes, FR, et al: The three dimensional laxity of the anterior cruciate deficient knee as determined by clinical laxity tests. Iowa Orthopedic Journal 3:32, 44, 1983.
43. Feagin, JA and Walton, WC: Isolated tears of the anterior cruciate ligament: 5-year follow-up study. Am J Sports Med 4:95, 1976.
44. Gardner, E and Rahilly, R: The early development of the knee joint in staged human embryos. J Anat 102:289, 1968.
45. Girgis, FG, Marshall, JL, and Monajem, ARS: The cruciate ligaments of the knee joint: Anatomical, functional, and experimental analysis. Clin Orthop 106:216, 1975.
46. Marshall, JL, et al: The anterior drawer sign: What is it? Am J Sports Med 3:152, 1975.
47. Arnoczky, SP: Blood supply to the anterior cruciate ligament and supporting structures. Orthop Clin North Am 16:15, 1985.
48. Marshall, JL, et al: Microvasculature of the cruciate ligaments. The Physician and Sportsmedicine 7:87, 91, 1979.
49. Kennedy, JC, Weinberg, HW, and Wilson, AS: The anatomy and function of the anterior ligament as determined by clinical and morphological studies. J Bone Joint Surg [Am] 56:223, 1974.
50. Schultz, RA, et al: Mechanoreceptors in human cruciate ligaments. J Bone Joint Surg [Am] 66:1072, 1984.
51. Schutte, MJ, et al: Neural anatomy of the human anterior cruciate ligament. J Bone Joint Surg [Am] 69:243, 1987.
52. Barrack, RL, Skinner, HB, and Buckley, SL: Proprioception in the anterior deficient knee. Am J Sports Med 17:1, 1989.
53. Marans, EJ, et al: Anterior cruciate ligament insufficiency: A dynamic three dimensional motion analysis. Am J Sports Med 17:3, 325, 1989.
54. Butler, DL, Noyes, FR, and Grood, ES: Ligamentous restraints of anterior-posterior drawer in the human knee. J Bone Joint Surg [Am] 62:259, 1980.
55. Furman, W, Marshall, JL, and Girgis, FG: The anterior cruciate ligament: A functional analysis based on postmortem studies. J Bone Joint Surg [Am] 58:179, 1978
56. Robichon, J and Romero, C: The functional anatomy of the knee joint with special reference to the medial collateral and anterior cruciate ligaments. Can J Surg 11:36, 1968.
57. Cabaud, HE, Rodkey, WG, and Feagin, JA: Experimental studies of acute anterior ligament injury and repair. Am J Sports Med 7:22, 1979.
58. Hsieh, H and Walker, PS: Stabilizing mechanisms of the loaded and unloaded knee joint. J Bone Joint Surg [Am] 58:87, 1976.
59. Lipke, JM, et al: The role of incompetence of the anterior cruciate and lateral ligaments in anterolateral and anteromedial instability. J Bone Joint Surg [Am] 63:954, 1982.
60. Grood, ES, et al: Biomechanics of knee-extension exercises. J Bone Joint Surg [Am] 66:725, 1984.
61. Kennedy, JC: Complete dislocation of knee joint. J Bone Joint Surg [Am] 45:889, 1963.
62. Czernicki, JM and Lippert, F: A biomechanical evaluation of tibiofemoral rotation in anterior cruciate deficient knee during walking and running. Am J Sports Med 16:4, 327, 1988.

63. Van Dommelen, BA and Fowler, PJ: Anatomy of the posterior cruciate ligament: A review. Am J Sports Med 17:1, 1989.
64. Kennedy, JC, Roth, JH, and Walker, DM: Posterior cruciate ligament injuries. Orthopedic Digest 7:19, 1979.
65. Kennedy, JC, et al: Tension studies of human knee ligaments. J Bone Joint Surg [Am] 58:350, 1976.
66. Scapinelli, R: Studies of the vasculature of the human knee joint. Acta Anat (Basel) 70:305, 1968.
67. Wang, CJ, Walker, PS, and Wolf, B: Rotatory laxity of the human knee joint. J Bone Joint Surg [Am] 56:161, 1974.
68. Heller, L and Langman, J: The menisco-femoral ligaments of the human knee. J Bone Joint Surg [Br] 46:307, 1964.
69. Warren, LF and Marshall, JL: The supporting structures and layers on the medial side of the knee: An anatomical analysis. J Bone Joint Surg [Am] 61:56, 1979.
70. Hughston, JE and Eilers, AF: The role of the posterior oblique ligament in repairs of acute medial collateral ligament tears of the knee. J Bone Joint Surg [Am] 55:923, 1973.
71. Fetto, JF and Marshall, JL: Medial collateral ligament injuries of the knee: A rationale for treatment. Clin Orthop 132:206, 1978.
72. Fowler, PJ: Functional anatomy of the knee. In Hunter, LY and Funk, FJ, Jr (eds): Rehabilitation of the Injured Knee. CV Mosby, St Louis, 1984, pp 16–20.
73. Grood, ES, et al: Ligamentous and capsular restraints preventing straight medial and lateral laxity in intact human cadaver knee. J Bone Joint Surg [Am] 63:1257, 1981.
74. Hughston, JC and Barrett, GR: Acute anteromedial rotary instability: Long-term results of surgical repairs. J Bone Joint Surg [Am] 65A:145, 1983.
75. Seebacher, JR, Inglis, A, and Marshall, JL: The structure of the posterolateral aspect of the knee. J Bone Joint Surg [Am] 64:536, 1982.
76. Terry, SC, Hughston, JC, and Norwood, LA: The anatomy of the iliopatellar band and the iliotibial tract. Am J Sports Med 14:139, 1986.
77. Last, RJ: The popliteus muscle and the lateral meniscus. J Bone Joint Surg [Br] 32:93, 1950.
78. Hughston, JC and Norwood, LA: The posterolateral drawer test and external rotational recurvatum test for posterolateral rotatory instability of the knee. Clin Orthop 147:82, 1980.
79. Bennett, GB and Stauber, WT: Evaluation and treatment of anterior knee pain using eccentric exercise. Med Sci Sports Exerc 18:5, 1986.
80. Haggmark, T, Jannson, E, and Erikson, E: Fiber type, area, metabolic potential of the thigh muscle in man after knee surgery and immobilization. Int J Sports Med 2:17, 1981
81. Sargeant, AJ, et al: Functional and structural changes after disuse of human muscle. Clin Sci 52:337, 1977.
82. Edstrom, L: Selective atrophy in the quadriceps in long-standing knee-joint dysfunction: Injuries to the anterior cruciate ligament. J Neurol Sci 11:551, 1970.
83. de Andrade, JR, Grant, C, and Dixon, AB: Joint distension and reflex muscle inhibition in the knee joint. J Bone Joint Surg [Am] 47:313, 1965.
84. Lieb, FJ and Perry, J: Quadriceps function. An anatomical and mechanical study using amputated limbs. J Bone Joint Surg [Am] 50:1535, 1968.
85. Lieb, FJ and Perry, J: Quadriceps function: An electromyographic study under isometric conditions. J Bone Joint Surg [Am] 53:749, 1971.
86. Greenhill, BJ: The importance of the medial quadriceps expansion in medial ligament injury. Can J Surg 10:312, 1967.
87. Scheller, B and Martenson, L: Traumatic dislocation of the patella: A radiographic investigation. Acta Radiol Suppl (Stockh) 336A:6, 1974.
88. McMinn, RMH and Hutchings, RT: Color Atlas of Human Anatomy. Year Book Medical Publishers, Chicago, 1977, p 278.
89. Wiberg, B: Roentgenographic and anatomical studies of the femoropatellar joint, with special reference to chondromalacia patellae. Acta Orthop Scand 12:319, 1941.
90. Baumgartl, F: Das Knieglenk. Springer-Verlag, Berlin, 1944.
91. Brattström, H: Shape of the intercondylar groove normally and in recurrent dislocation of the patella. Acta Orthop Scand Suppl 68:5, 1964.
92. Larson, RL, et al: The patellar compression syndrome: Surgical treatment by lateral retinacular release. Clin Orthop 34:158, 1978.
93. Kaufer, H: Mechanical function of the patella. J Bone Joint Surg [Am] 53:1151, 1971.
94. McLeod, WD and Hunter, S: Biomechanical analysis of the knee: Primary functions as elucidated by anatomy. Phys Ther 60:1561, 1980.
95. Fetto, JF and Marshall, JL: The natural history and diagnosis of anterior cruciate ligament insufficiency. Clin Orthop 147:29, 1980.
96. McLeod, WD and Blackburn, TA: Biomechanics of knee rehabilitation with cycling. Am J Sports Med 8:175, 1980.
97. Markolf, KL, Graff-Radford, A, and Amstutz, HC; In vivo knee stability: A quantitative assessment using an instrumented clinical testing apparatus. J Bone Joint Surg [Am] 60:664, 1978.

98. Johansson, H, Sjolander, P, and Sojka, P: A sensory role for the cruciate ligaments. Clin Orthop 268:161, 1991.
99. Grillner, S, Hongo, T, and Lund, S: Descending monosynaptic and reflex control of y-motorneurones. Acta Physiol Scand 75:592, 1969.
100. Williams, PL and Warwick, R: Gray's Anatomy. 35th British Edition. WB Saunders, Philadelphia, 1973, pp 400–407.
101. Steindler, A: Kinesiology of the Human Body Under Normal and Pathological Conditions, ed 5. Charles C Thomas, Springfield, IL, 1977, pp 63–64.
102. Goodfellow, J and O'Connor, J: The mechanics of the knee and prosthesis design. J Bone Joint Surg [Br] 60:358, 1978.
103. Kettelkamp, DB, et al: An electrogoniometric study of knee motion in normal gait. J Bone Joint Surg [Am] 52:775, 1970.
104. Laubenthal, KN, Smidt, GL, and Kettelkamp, DB: A quantitative analysis of knee motion during ADLs. Phys Ther 52:34, 1972.
105. Levens, AB, Inman, VT, and Blosser, JA: Transverse rotation of the segments of the lower extremity in locomotion. J Bone Joint Surg [Am] 30:859, 1948.
106. Murray, MP, Drought, AB, and Kory, RC: Walking patterns of normal men. J Bone Joint Surg [Am] 46:335, 1964.
107. Hungerford, DS and Barry, M: Biomechanics of the patellofemoral joint. Clin Orthop 144:15, 1974.
108. Brunnstrom, S: Clinical Kinesiology, ed 3. FA Davis, Philadelphia, 1973, pp 14–15.
109. Inman, VT, Saunders, M, and Abbott, LC: Observations on the function of the shoulder joint. J Bone Joint Surg [Am] 26:1, 1946.
110. Reilly, DT and Martens, M: Experimental analysis of quadriceps muscle force and patello-femoral joint reaction force for various activities. Acta Orthop Scand 43:126, 1972.
111. Ficat, P and Hungerford, DS: Disorders of the Patello-Femoral Joint. Williams & Wilkins, Baltimore, 1977.

CHAPTER 2

Sequential Evaluation
of the Knee

Bruce H. Greenfield, MMSc, PT

A knee evaluation serves several purposes: identifying the primary and secondary tissues of injury or pathology; determining the current status and stage of reactivity of the joint structures; determining the prognosis for functional recovery and relative timetable for treatment; establishing baseline signs and symptoms to determine appropriate therapeutic measures and treatment goals; and identifying the underlying dysfunction that may have predisposed the patient to injury. Rehabilitation of the knee joint can only be initiated after a comprehensive evaluation is performed. The evaluation procedure should be based on knowledge of knee anatomy, biomechanics, and the natural history of orthopedic injury. Because the knee joint is complex, with numerous overlapping and contiguous contractile and noncontractile tissues in a relatively confined space, the evaluation of a patient with an injury to either the tibiofemoral or patellofemoral joints can be regarded as a challenge or a drudgery. The sequential approach to the knee joint evaluation described in this chapter is designed to clarify the picture; it is a systematic method to ascertain the nature and extent of the injury. The scope of this chapter does not include a review of all the available knee evaluation tests and techniques. Ten of the chapters in this text present special tests to evaluate specific pathologies or injuries. Additionally, the appendix to the book describes and illustrates special tests of the knee. The intent of this chapter is to present a guideline that provides the clinician with an expeditious but comprehensive blueprint to evaluate and establish a more specific treatment program.

Sequential evaluation of the knee is designed to provide a systems approach for assessing knee pathology and dysfunction. Figure 2–1 is an algorithm that outlines each step of the evaluation. The sequence of the evaluation is predicated on the previous findings. Based on the findings, the clinician may choose to bypass one or more steps.

The sequential evaluation is presented as a basic framework. Many experienced clinicians may choose to alter their evaluation sequence based on a particular finding. For instance, some clinicians will palpate structures earlier in the sequence, and many

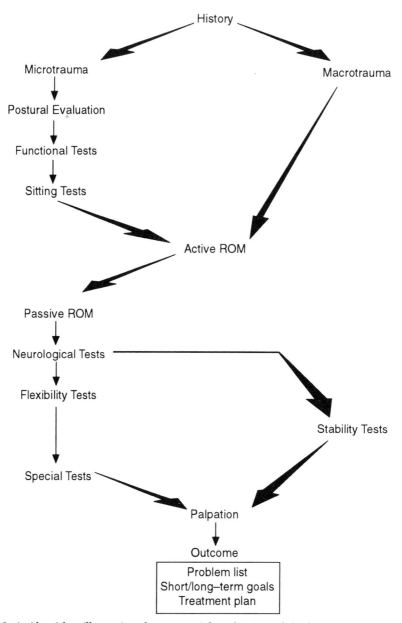

FIGURE 2-1. Algorithm illustrating the sequential evaluation of the knee joint.

clinicians will palpate continually throughout all portions of the evaluation. Therefore, some flexibility may be incorporated into the performance of the evaluation. This particular sequence reflects my own expertise and experience. Clinicians will undoubtedly want to modify this scheme based on their own experiences.

HISTORY

The first step in evaluation is to collect a complete history from the client, including subjective reports on the onset, nature, and location of pain and a medical screening.

Onset

A major goal of taking the subjective history is to ascertain whether the injury was caused by macrotrauma or microtrauma. This information is easily obtained by asking the patient the onset of the problem. *Macrotrauma* injuries result from specific trauma such as a ligamentous tear or dislocation of the patella.[1] Conversely, *microtrauma* is the persistent irritation of periarticular tissues, which initially provokes a local inflammatory response.[2] Examples of microtrauma injuries include tendinitis or bursitis and are detailed in Chapter 6. Whereas in the presence of macrotrauma, the patient invariably remembers the incident of injury, the microtrauma-injured patient will often report either a gradual onset of pain or an insidious onset.

The difference between a macrotrauma and a microtrauma injury will determine the line of questioning in the history, as well as the subsequent steps of the knee evaluation (see Fig. 2–1). As outlined in Table 2–1, microtrauma injuries result from predisposing intrinsic factors and precipitating extrinsic factors. *Extrinsic factors* are training errors, which may include overtraining, inadequate or inappropriate equipment, or faulty training mechanics. In the presence of suspected microtrauma injury, these extrinsic factors must be identified through the subjective history. Because the extrinsic factors are an integral part of the cause of the microtrauma injury, they must be corrected or modified if treatment is to be successful. Detailed strategies for identifying and resolving extrinsic factors in microtrauma are found in Chapter 6. Questions that should be asked of the patient relative to identifying extrinsic factors include: What is your occupation? What are your hobbies or vocational pursuits? In what sports or exercises do you participate? If the examiner finds that the problem is potentially related to a specific exercise regimen such as running, or to a specific sport, then training intensity, frequency, environment (e.g., hilly terrains for runners), and mechanics of the activity or sport need to be determined.

If the injury resulted from macrotrauma, then the examiner needs to ascertain the mechanism of injury. Injury to ligamentous tissues, menisci, and bone results from forces being applied in a specific direction with the knee joint in a particular position. Have the patient describe in detail the mechanism of injury. A precise prediction of the injured tissue or tissues may be made based on the clinician's knowledge of the complex anatomy and mechanics of the knee joint (see Chapter 1).

The majority of injuries originate in a valgus or varus angulation of the knee joint, with the foot fixed to the ground. Oftentimes, the tibia is moving into either external or internal rotation. Table 2–2 reviews the common mechanisms of injuries to the knee joint. Noyes and associates[3] demonstrated that approximately 70 percent of all severe knee joint ligamentous injuries result from noncontact at the time of injury. It is

TABLE 2–1 Etiologic Factors in Overuse Injuries

Predisposing (Intrinsic)	Precipitating (Extrinsic)	Perpetuating (Intrinsic and Extrinsic)
Malalignment syndromes	Training errors	The two types of factors
Leg length discrepancy	Running surfaces	in combination
Muscle dysfunction	Shoes and equipment	

Source: From Donatelli, R: The Biomechanics of the Foot and Ankle. FA Davis, Philadelphia, 1990, p 155.

TABLE 2–2 Common Mechanisms of Ligamentous and Meniscal Injuries to the Knee Joint

Structures	Mechanism of Injury
Medial compartment Tibial collateral ligament Deep medial capsule Medial meniscus (peripheral attachments)	Valgus force due to either (1) external blow to lateral aspects of the knee joint, or (2) fall to the opposite side with the involved leg firmly fixed on the ground Sidestep cutting
Lateral compartment Fibular collateral ligament Deep lateral capsule Lateral meniscus (peripheral attachments) Popliteus tendon Arcuate complex	Varus force due to either (1) external blow to medial aspect of the knee joint, or (2) fall away from the involved support leg with the foot fixed to the ground Cross-over cut
Anterior cruciate ligament (ACL)	Valgus force to the knee joint, with external rotation of the tibia Hyperextension of the knee joint Varus force to the knee joint, with internal rotation of the tibia Deceleration Cross-over cut
Posterior cruciate ligament (PCL)	Extreme rotation of the tibia, associated with a valgus or varus force to the knee joint Posterior displacement to a flexed knee joint, e.g., fall on a flexed knee joint Hyperextension of the knee joint with foot dorsiflexed
Menisci	Rotation injury on a semiflexed weight bearing knee joint

important to remember, while reviewing Table 2–2, that both the *magnitude* of force and the *direction* of force at the time of injury affect the extent of ligamentous damage. Therefore, even in the presence of a straight valgus force to the knee joint, sufficient force at the time of impact will disrupt the cruciate ligaments, as well as the medial or lateral meniscus. Additionally, a valgus or varus force, combined with rotation of the tibia at the time of injury, usually results in medial or lateral compartmental ligamentous damage, as well as damage to the cruciate ligaments. In the presence of an injury to the anterior cruciate ligament (ACL), the patient often reports the following: an audible pop at the time of injury, rapid swelling in the knee joint, loss of range of motion (ROM), and the inability to walk immediately after the injury.[3] In the presence of an acute meniscal injury, the patient often reports that his or her knee joint locks at a specific point in the ROM. Overnight swelling indicates a reactive synovitis due to a minor ligamentous tear or sprain, or a meniscal lesion.

Location and Nature of Pain

Additional questions are asked to determine the area, nature and behavior of pain, previous treatment, and associated health problems. Musculoskeletal injuries usually manifest by pain. Various tissues about the lower extremities and low back share the same segmental innervation as the tissues within and around the knee joint. These tissues or structures can therefore refer pain about the knee.[4,5] The clinician should delineate the boundaries of the patient's pain. The clinician should then be prepared to evaluate all the tissues and structures — that is, joints and muscles — that lie under or refer pain to the painful areas.[6] The depth and nature of the pain may indicate whether the injury occurred to a sclerotomic, myotomic, or dermatomic tissue. Generally, a deep dull ache that is poorly localized by the patient indicates injury to either myotomic or sclerotomic structures: joint capsule, ligament, bone, or muscle. A superficial, circumscribed, sharp or burning pain may indicate injury to a dermatomic or superficial tissue, such as skin, tendon, or bursa.[7] Complaints of paresthesia or anesthesia implicate a nerve injury. A throbbing pain may indicate a vascular injury. Temperature changes, especially coolness in and around the knee joint, with burning pain and hypersensitivity, should alert the clinician to possible sympathetic mediated pain.

Changes in the location and nature of pain over a 24-hour period should be ascertained.[6] Most musculoskeletal pain is not constant but will change in intensity or constancy due to changes in movement of the joint, activities, or body position.[8] Activities and positions that increase or relieve pain should be identified. Answers to the questions provide information concerning the stage of reactivity of the lesion, cues as to how aggressive to be during subsequent evaluation, and hints as to treatment strategies. For example, a patient with suspected chondromalacia patella reports a dull ache under her kneecap after driving a car for 20 minutes. This pain persists for approximately 2 hours after she removes herself from the car and lies down with her knee extended. Only after the application of ice for 20 minutes does the pain begin to subside. This information suggests to the clinician that the patient has a reactive lesion and to be relatively gentle with evaluation. Furthermore, effective initial strategies for treatment include avoiding positions where the patient's knee is maintained in a flexed position, and using ice to relieve pain.

Constant pain that is unaffected by movement and wakes the patient at night may indicate serious pathology, such as an osteosarcoma.

Medical Screening

The patient should also be questioned about current medication usage including nonsteroidal anti-inflammatory drugs (NSAIDs). The use of NSAIDs is an important medical adjunctive treatment to facilitate rehabilitation of reactive microtrauma injuries. The patient's general health is an important factor for rehabilitation. The clinician should ascertain any systemic problems—for example, rheumatoid arthritis, cardiac or pulmonary dysfunctions—that will affect the rehabilitation process. All information should be carefully recorded in the patient's chart or in a patient data base. Examples of data bases for recording patient history are illustrated in Figure 2–2.

POSTURAL EVALUATION

In the presence of suspected microtrauma injury to the knee, the next step of the sequential knee evaluation is a postural evaluation of the lower extremity alignment. Several studies[9-13] have correlated lower extremity malalignment with lower extremity microtrauma injuries. The goal of this evaluation step is to rule out any potential underlying malalignment problem that perpetuates the patient's microtrauma injury

```
                            KNEE HISTORY
Name _____
D.O.B. _____ ID Number _____ Sex _____
Referring Physician _____
Occupation _____ Date of Injury _____
Height _____ Weight _____
If an athlete, complete the following:
Athletic Event/Position Played _____
Chief Complaint _____
_____
History of Injury _____
_____
Swelling  _____ immediate        Motion:  _____ knee locked
          _____ late                      _____ motion lost quickly
          _____ degree                    _____ motion lost slowly
Knee Aspirated _____ Was fluid straw-colored or bloody? _____
Initial Diagnosis/Initial Treatment _____
_____
_____
Past History of Knee Trauma/Surgery (If surgery, please note dates,
surgeon's name, procedure performed) _____
_____
_____
```

A

FIGURE 2–2. Data bases for recording the history (A) and present status (B) of the patient's knee. (From Malone, T and Kegerreis, ST: Evaluation Process. In Mangine, RE [ed]: Physical Therapy of the Knee. Churchill Livingstone, New York, 1988, pp 77–78.)

PRESENT STATUS—KNEE HISTORY FORM

Has your knee bothered you just this one time? _____

On and off (intermittently)? _____ Constantly? _____

What makes the symptoms worse? _____
_____

What makes them better? _____

Where does it hurt? (Describe in relationship to your kneecap—does it hurt on the inside, the outside, above or below, in the front or in the back?)
_____
_____

What kind of pain do you have? (stabbing, sharp, etc.) _____
_____

How severe is the pain? (1 being not very severe, 5 being exquisite—very, very severe) _____

Does it hurt more in the night, in the morning, or all the time? (Circle one)

What makes the pain worse? _____

What decreases the pain? _____

Does the pain increase with (check all that apply): sitting? _____

stair climbing? _____ (going up? _____ coming down? _____)

climbing hills? _____ (going up? _____ coming down? _____)

standing _____ squatting? _____ kneeling? _____

sprinting? _____ jogging? _____ walking? _____

twisting? _____ cutting? _____

Does your knee lock? (Check all that apply.) _____ pop? _____

catch? _____ give way? _____ grind? _____ swell? _____

When your knee does swell, how long does the swelling last? _____

How severe is the swelling? (1 - little bit) _____ (2) _____

(3 - quite a bit) _____

Does your knee ever not allow you to completely straighten it? _____

Completely bend it? _____

Does your knee ever feel weak? _____

Does your knee ever slip? _____

Has your kneecap ever slipped out of place? _____ If yes, how many times? _____

Are there any medical problems that relate to this knee problem? _____

Are you an athlete? _____ If you are, at what level?

recreational _____ high school _____ collegiate _____

professional _____

What is your motivational level? (Check the one that applies.) highly motivated _____ motivated _____ somewhat motivated _____

not very interested in my fitness level _____

B

FIGURE 2-2. *Continued.*

(see Table 2–1). Intrinsic predisposing factors include frontal and transverse plane changes in the femur and tibia, as well as patellar and subtalar joint malalignment.

Table 2–3 outlines the structural evaluation of the lower extremities. Chapters 6 and 7 define and describe the specific components of the structural evaluation and methods of measurement, and they present examples of the relationship between lower extremity malalignment and microtrauma injuries to the knee.

TABLE 2–3 Evaluation of Common Lower Extremity Malalignment Problems

View	Landmark(s)/Structures	Biomechanical Correlate(s)
Anterior	Patellae	
	"Squinting"—inward-facing patella	Femoral anteversion
	"Grasshopper eyes"—outward-facing patella	Femoral retroversion
	Q-angle	Alignment of extensor mechanism
	Patella height relative to tibial tuberosity	Patella alta—"high-riding" patella
		Patella baja—"low-riding" patella
	Tibiofemoral joint alignment in frontal plane	Varus/valgus alignment
Lateral	Tibiofemoral joint alignment in sagittal plane	Genu recurvatum—hyperextension of the tibiofemoral joint; may indicate tibiofemoral joint ligamentous laxity and/or a shallow femoral trochlear groove, resulting in a hypermobile patella
Posterior	Side-side comparisons of PSIS*, greater trochanters, popliteus creases, fibular head	Leg length difference
	Tibial/floor alignment	Tibial varum
	Calcaneal/floor alignment	
	Subtalar joint valgus	Subtalar joint pronation
	Subtalar joint varus	Subtalar joint supination

*PSIS = posterior superior iliac spines.

FUNCTIONAL TESTS

Functional tests can be performed in patients with either macrotrauma and microtrauma injuries, although in the presence of acute macrotrauma this step is often skipped because of the patient's pain and loss of function (see Fig. 2–1). The functional tests are performed in closed kinetic chain situations (see description of closed kinetic chain in Chapter 1) and therefore require interaction between the contractile and noncontractile elements in the knee joint under compressive, shear, and tensile loading conditions.[14] The complexity of the functional tasks can vary widely between patients and should depend on the nature and extent of the pathology, as well as be individualized to the patient's general preinjury level of functioning. Therefore, the functional tests performed on a football player with suspected chronic ACL deficiency are quite different from those used with an elderly woman with an arthritic knee joint. Functional tests in the presence of patellofemoral joint microtrauma might include asking the patient to perform a simple squat maneuver or to ascend or descend stairs so as to ascertain the amount of retropatellar pain and crepitus (see Chapter 7). Chapter 8 reviews functional tests in patients with diagnosed tibiofemoral arthritis. Other functional tests, depending on the patient's activity level, may include jumping, running, lateral slides, and cutting and cross-over maneuvers including cariocas. An example of a functional test for ligamentous instability and suspected functional disability is the cross-over test[15] (Fig. 2–3).

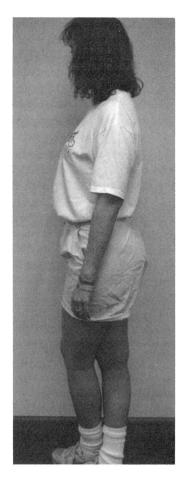

FIGURE 2–3. Cross-over test to assess for functional disability due to anterolateral instability. The patient crosses her free uninvolved lower extremity over the fixed foot of the involved extremity to face approximately 90 degrees in the opposite direction. In the presence of anterolateral instability, the patient will reproduce symptoms of a lateral pivot shift, including a sensation of "giving way" of the knee joint, pain, and discomfort.

Functional tests can also be used to assess the discharge status for a patient to return to the preinjury activity level or sport level, as well as to detect alterations in lower extremity function. The sensitivity of the single leg hop test, timed single leg hop test, triple single leg hop test, and cross-over single leg hop test (see Appendix) were studied by Noyes and associates[16] to detect alterations in lower extremity function in patients with diagnosed ACL-deficient knee joint compared with matched controls. The authors found that a sensitivity rating of 62 percent could be attained if at least two of these tests are used to detect lower extremity abnormalities in patients with ACL-deficient knee joints.

SITTING TESTS

With the patient in the sitting position, the clinician should reassess the Q angle (Fig. 2–4). Normally, sitting with the knee joint flexed to 90 degrees, the tibial tuberosity should either be in line with the patella or slightly medial. This alignment is due to the obligatory internal tibial rotation that occurs with knee joint flexion. Any abnormal findings would indicate that the tibial tuberosity is situated lateral to the midline of the

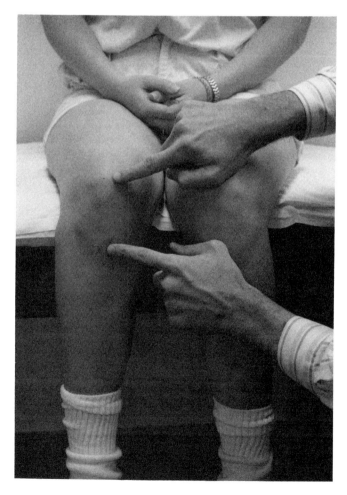

FIGURE 2–4. Assessment of the Q angle with the patient sitting.

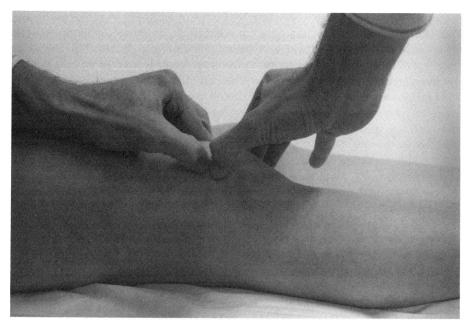

FIGURE 2–5. Eversion or medial tilt of the lateral border of the patella. The examiner's thumbs are "hooked" under the lateral patella facet. The lateral border of the patella is then everted or tilted medially in a transverse plane while the examiner's index fingers push down along the anterior aspect, the medial border of the patella.

patella. This finding can be correlated to an excessive Q angle that is measured with the knee joint in full extension (see Chapter 6). Mobility of the patella can also be assessed in the sitting position. First, with the patient's knee extended and relaxed, the patella should not glide more than one-half its total width in a lateral direction. Excessive patella gliding with the knee joint in full extension indicates a hypermobile patella. Next, the patellar gliding should be tested with the knee joint flexed from 20 to 30 degrees. In this position the patella should be seated snugly within the femoral trochlear groove.[17] Therefore, the total amount of lateral displacement of the patella at this point in the knee joint range of motion should be considerably reduced compared with full knee extension. If the clinician is able to glide the patella the same distance as when the knee joint was fully extended, the presence of a shallow femoral trochlear groove should be suspected. Finally, the amount of lateral patellar tilt should be assessed. With the patient's knee joint flexed 20 to 30 degrees, the clinician should attempt to evert the lateral border of the patella (Fig. 2–5). An inability by the clinician to evert the lateral border of the patella at least to the level of the frontal plane probably indicates tightness of the lateral retinaculum and iliopatellar band.

ACTIVE AND PASSIVE RANGE OF MOTION

Active range of motion (AROM) should be tested in both the macrotrauma and microtrauma patient. The major goals of assessing AROM include ascertaining the quality of movement, i.e., smoothness of the muscle contraction, the presence of a painful arc (which may reflect a "loose body," or meniscal flap tear in the knee joint), and the patient's willingness to perform that movement (pain). AROM can be assessed during functional testing, by having the patient squat, ambulate, or climb stairs. However, because of pain and effusion, these maneuvers may be difficult for the macrotrauma patient to perform. Furthermore, the interaction of weight bearing forces with active movements may fail to isolate the potential full AROM available in the knee joint. AROM may be assessed with the patient supine, prone, and sidelying, depending on the movement pattern that is being assessed. The usual movements tested are knee joint flexion and extension, as well as active movement in the hip joint and ankle joint. Limitations in the AROM in joints above and below the knee joint can result in altered stresses within the knee joint and can predispose or perpetuate the current injury. The clinician should always compare the ROM of each joint with that of the contralateral side, both for AROM and for passive range of motion (PROM). Evaluation should begin on the uninvolved extremity to ease the patient's apprehension and provide the clinician with baseline ROM measurements to make a bilateral assessment. What may appear as an aberrant movement or as limited motion in an injured joint, based on the clinician's knowledge of ROM normative values or on his or her own empirical knowledge, may be the normal variant for that particular patient.

PROM can be assessed immediately after AROM for each movement pattern. PROM for a particular movement can be immediately compared with the AROM. The difference between AROM and PROM within the knee joint reflects not only muscle strength but also the patient's willingness to move the knee joint. A greater amount of PROM than AROM probably indicates that the patient experiences pain during AROM. The evaluation of PROM has two functions: to assess the end feel of range of motion, and to assess the stage or level of reactivity. Cyriax[7] described end feels as (1) bony, (2) capsular, (3) springy block, (4) soft-tissue approximation, and (5) empty. Normal end feel for knee joint flexion is soft-tissue approximation of the hamstring muscles against the gastrocnemius-soleus muscles, and for extension, a capsular end feel. Cyriax[7] also described the pain-resistance sequence at end of range to assess for the level of reactivity. Pain before resistance indicates a reactive or acute lesion; pain and resistance that occur simultaneously indicate a subacute lesion; and resistance experienced before pain indicates a chronic or minimally reactive lesion. The assessment of reactivity will dictate, along with any soft-tissue healing constraints (see Chapter 4), the initial aggressiveness of treatment and the type of exercises that are implemented.

NEUROLOGIC ASSESSMENT

Neurologic assessment should be performed for both macrotrauma and microtrauma patients and include (1) sensory testing, (2) motor testing, and (3) proprioceptive testing.

Sensory Testing

The knee joint receives innervation from spinal segments L-3 through S-2. Branches of the tibial and peroneal nerves form the sural nerve, which supplies sensation along the posterior aspect of the knee joint. A branch of the common peroneal nerve and the lateral cutaneous nerve of the calf supply sensation along the lateral aspect of the knee joint, while cutaneous branches of the femoral and saphenous nerves provide sensation along the medial aspect of the knee joint.[18] In addition, the infrapatellar branch of the saphenous nerve supplies sensation along the medial aspect of the infrapatellar fat pad. Injuries to any of these nerves can result in paresthesia or anesthesia around the knee joint. Manual sensory tests for ascertaining the status of these nerves include sharp-dull differentiation and two-point discrimination. Because these nerves contain sympathetic nerve fibers,[19] injury to the knee joint or specifically to these nerves may result in reflex sympathetic dystrophy, or sympathetic mediated pain (SMP). In the presence of SMP, the patient will experience sudomotor and vasomotor changes, including blanching and mottled skin, and sweating along the distribution of the injured nerve. Other changes may include allodynia, or hypersensitivity to nonnoxious stimuli, and hypopathia, which is reduced threshold to pain. Long-term SMP may result in osteoporosis with potential stress fractures. Bone scans may indicate "hot spots" that reflect significant bone dimineralization, or possibly a stress fracture.[20]

Motor Testing

Several different methods assess the motor function of the muscles around the knee joint. These methods include manual testing with proper joint and muscle isolation[21]; isokinetic testing with comparisons of peak torque muscle values of the quadriceps femoris and hamstring muscles to age-, sex-, and weight-matched normative values[22]; and functional tests[9] that integrate muscle function with knee joint mechanics. In addition, because Nicholas and colleagues[23] demonstrated that knee joint dysfunction affects the motoric capabilities of most muscles in the lower extremity (see Chapter 5, Total Leg Strength), all the muscles in the lower extremity related to the side of the injured knee should be assessed.

A study by de Andrade and associates[24] demonstrated that effusion in the knee joint capsule results in inhibition of the quadriceps femoris muscle. Weakness of the quadriceps femoris muscle results in loss of stability of the knee joint during ambulation, as well as alteration in patellofemoral joint tracking. Altered patellar tracking may increase the potential for lateral subluxation of the patella from the femoral trochlear groove, during AROM of the knee joint. Bennett and Stauber[25] emphasized the importance of eccentric muscle control of the quadriceps femoris in patients with anterior knee pain. Furthermore, Edstrom[26] found selective atrophy of type I (slow-twitch) fibers in the quadriceps femoris muscles in patients with ACL-deficient knees. In a recent study, Voight and Weider[27] used electromyography to assess the reflex response times of the vastus medialis obliquus (VMO) muscle and the vastus lateralis (VL) muscle to a patellar tendon tap in patients with patellofemoral joint dysfunction and in matched control subjects. The authors found that normal subjects activated their VMO muscle significantly faster than their VL muscle, whereas in these patients the reverse occurred; the VL muscle was activated significantly faster than the VMO muscle. The results indicate that there is a reversal of the normal muscular activation orders between the two muscles in these patients. Patients with patellofemoral joint dysfunction may be demonstrating a neurophysiologic motor control imbalance that may account for or contribute to anterior knee pain. Therefore, in the presence of knee joint or patellofemoral joint dysfunction, the clinician should evaluate the motoric capability of the quadriceps femoris muscle, especially the VMO muscle. An assessment can be made of the recruitment pattern between the VMO muscle and VL muscle. This assessment is especially important in the presence of patellofemoral dysfunction, in that the major function of the oblique portion of the VM muscle is to provide dynamic medial stability to the patella.[28] The clinician can simply palpate the VMO and VL muscles while the patient performs a maximum voluntary quadriceps femoris muscle contraction (Fig. 2–6). Normally, the clinician should palpate an initial VMO muscle contraction immediately followed by a VL muscle contraction. If the difference is too subtle for the clinician to palpate, electromyography can be used to precisely measure the recruitment pattern.

Anthropometric measurements of thigh girth musculature can easily be performed using a tape measure. The clinician compares differences in thigh girth between the involved and uninvolved extremity. Usual measurements can be taken 7.5 and 15 cm above the medial and lateral joint line. Some controversy exists concerning the validity of anthropometric measurements to predict muscle strength. One study found no correlation between thigh girth and actual muscle strength in patients with ACL deficiencies.[29] Other studies found a positive correlation between thigh girth measurements and isokinetic quadriceps femoris muscle torque output in healthy subjects.[30–32] Because anthropometric measurements are a quick clinical assessment, many clinicians continue to use this method as an indicator for improvement of muscle strength.

Early in rehabilitation, the patient should perform a straight leg raise (SLR), and the amount of involuntary knee flexion that occurs during this maneuver should be mea-

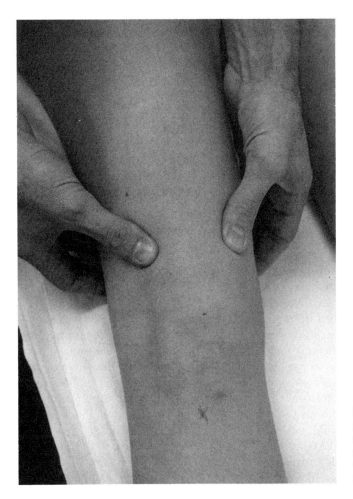

FIGURE 2–6. Palpation of the recruitment order during isometric contraction of the VMO and VL muscles in a patient with patellofemoral joint dysfunction.

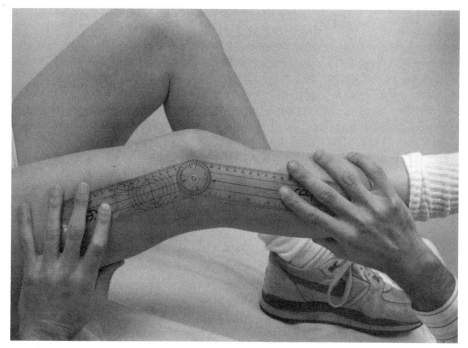

FIGURE 2-7. Measurement of a knee joint extensor lag in a patient with knee joint dysfunction.

sure (Fig. 2-7). The amount of involuntary knee flexion is known as the *quad or extensor lag* and is continually recorded in the patient's chart. Clinical experience indicates that after the patient eliminates an extensor lag and soft-tissue healing is complete, safe independent weight bearing can commence.

Proprioceptive Testing

Research[33] has shown the existence of joint mechanoreceptors within the major ligaments of the knee joint. As described in Chapter 1, these mechanoreceptors function to provide kinesthetic feedback and awareness of knee joint position and a protective reflex loop to the muscles attached to the ligaments. Barrack and associates[34] demonstrated the loss of kinesthetic awareness of knee joint position occurred in patients with ACL-deficient knee joints, compared with control subjects. Therefore, in the presence of both acute or chronic macrotrauma injury to major knee joint ligaments, or in the presence of certain microtrauma injuries such as degenerative joint disease, the clinician should assess the proprioceptive/kinesthetic status of the knee joint. Joint position sense can be assessed by placing the patient in a sitting position, with eyes closed. The clinician, with light hand contact to the patient's heel, moves the uninvolved knee joint to different points in the ROM and asks the patient to actively reproduce the position with the involved knee joint. The clinician can grossly estimate the degree of kinesthetic awareness by how well the patient can approximate the position of the involved knee joint to that of the uninvolved joint. Because the validity and reliability of this test has not been established, its degree of sensitivity as a true measure of kinesthetic ability is questionable. The clinician therefore should be circumspect about making definitive

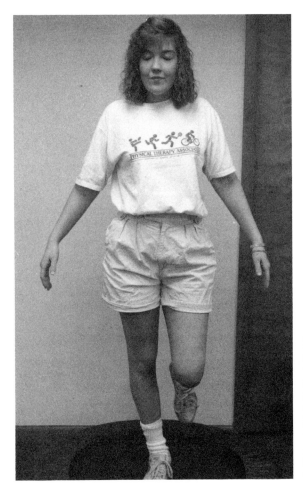

FIGURE 2-8. A patient performing a single leg stand on a mini trampoline with her eyes closed to eliminate visual feedback. The ability of the patient to successfully perform this maneuver without losing her balance is assessed by comparing her involved-to-uninvolved lower extremity. The clinician can use a preset time limit, for example, 30 seconds, as the criterion for the patient to successfully complete this test.

conclusions concerning the patient's kinesthetic status based on the results of this evaluation.

Several functional tests are used to assess proprioception and balance deficits in the injured knee joint. These tests are not precise measurement tools because they lack established validity and reliability. The patient can be asked to walk in tandem along a straight line or to perform a single leg stand either on a stable surface or unstable surface (mini-tramp) (Fig. 2-8). The degree of difficulty of these maneuvers may indicate underlying proprioceptive deficits.

FLEXIBILITY TESTS

As shown in the algorithm in Figure 2-1, testing the flexibility of the muscles and soft tissues around the knee joint and lower extremity can be omitted in patients with acute macrotrauma injuries. However, as shown in Table 2-1, muscle flexibility and its corollary, muscle imbalance, are primary intrinsic predisposing factors to microtrauma injuries. Janda[35] observed the effects of muscle imbalances around a joint: certain muscles tightened in dysfunction, while other muscles weakened. He also noted that a tight antagonist inhibited the strength of its weak agonist. Therefore, tight hamstring muscles may result in reflex inhibition to the corresponding quadriceps femoris muscles. The result may lead to increased retro patellofemoral joint compressive forces during extension of the knee joint. (For an overview of the relationship between muscle imbalances and microtrauma injuries to the knee, see Chapter 6.)

Additionally, decreased flexibility of the lateral retinaculum and the iliopatellar band of the iliotibial tract may lead to such conditions as lateral patellar compression syndrome, or iliotibial band friction syndrome (ITBFS). Flexibility testing should be performed for the hamstring muscles, the iliotibial band, the lateral retinaculum, the tensor fascia lata, and the gastrocnemius-soleus muscles. Various flexibility tests for these structures have been described elsewhere.[36,37]

SPECIAL TESTS

Special tests include the various patellar tests, including the patellar apprehension test, the patellar compression test, and the Noble test for ITBFS.[38] As shown in Figure 2–1, this step may be bypassed in patients with acute macrotrauma injuries.

STABILITY TESTS

Stability testing is primarily reserved for those patients with suspected macrotrauma to the knee joint (see Fig. 2–1). Of course, suspicion of this injury is based on the subjective history, where the patient is able to recall a specific trauma to the knee joint. Although Table 2–2 reviews the common mechanisms of injuries to selected knee ligaments and the menisci, these mechanisms of injury are sometimes difficult to determine, due in part to a majority of major traumatic knee injuries resulting from noncontact incidents (69 percent).[3] Compounding the problem of clearly establishing the mechanism of knee joint injury, and hence the tissues involved in the injury, are the complex mechanics within the tibiofemoral joint. As described by Goodfellow and associates[39] and depicted in Chapter 1, the tibiofemoral joint has six degrees of freedom, three rotational and three translational. Noyes and associates[40] concluded that injuries to the ligamentous structures of the tibiofemoral joint can occur by internal or external forces and varus or valgus forces being applied in any one of a possible six degrees of freedom. The authors also determined that each pattern of joint movement requires an understanding of the ligaments that restrict that movement. Through the process of selective tissue sectioning, the authors determined that for each degree of freedom, ligaments provide a primary and secondary stabilizing restraint to that movement. Therefore, to effectively isolate the primary and secondary ligamentous restraints involved in a suspected macrotrauma injury, the clinician may have to perform a series of stability tests in different planes of motion. In addition, the concept of rotational instabilities outlined by Hughston and co-workers[41,42] provides another classification system of tibiofemoral instabilities and further complicates the available ligamentous tests. Rotary instabilities of the knee joint occur around an axis that is close to the longitudinal axis of the tibia and are associated with increases in internal and external rotation of the tibia on the femur. For rotary instabilities to occur, the posterior cruciate ligament (PCL) must be intact. Hughston and co-workers[41] observed that the PCL is the primary ligament in the knee joint and thus acts as a central pivot between the tibia and femur. Therefore, all rotary instabilities in the knee joint occur around an intact PCL. Unless the PCL is absent, a pure straight instability cannot occur within the tibiofemoral joint.

Rotary instabilities are named by the respective direction of instability of the tibial condyle. There are four major rotary instabilities in the knee joint: anteromedial rotary instability (AMRI), anterolateral rotary instability (ALRI), posterolateral rotary instability (PLRI), and combined rotary instabilities. Table 2–4 summarizes the common ligamentous tests, the primary and secondary structures that are isolated with each test, and the type of instability associated with each test.

It is a good idea to assess the uninjured knee joint before performing stability tests. Doing so gives the clinician a baseline for comparison and eases the client's apprehension about the method and forces applied during the test. Make certain that the patient is as relaxed as possible, and that the tested lower extremity is well supported. Any muscle guarding by the patient because of pain will interfere with the outcome of the test and may produce a false-negative result. During testing, we have found it useful to oscillate the manual forces with increasing amplitude into the barrier. This approach seems to help relax the surrounding musculature, perhaps by stimulating type I and II joint mechanoreceptors, which by way of large, fast-conducting sensory fibers modulate concomitant nociceptive input propagated along slower-conducting sensory fibers within the dorsal horn of the spinal cord.[43]

The clinician should test for the amount of excursion and the end feel. Minimal excursion with a firm end point and minimal pain probably indicates a minor sprain (1+ instability); moderate excursion (5–10 mm) with a softer end point and pain may indicate a 2+ instability; significant opening (greater than 10 mm) with an empty end point indicates a 3+ instability, which could result in significant functional disability.[41] A number of stability tests are illustrated in the Appendix.

An alternative method for manual assessment of knee joint stability is instrument stability testing. There are several devices on the market, including the KT-1000 and KT-2000 arthrometers (Medmetric Inc., San Diego, CA), which measure primarily anteroposterior translation of the tibiofemoral joint; the Genucom (Faro Medical Analysis Systems, Faro Medical Inc., Montreal, Canada), which was designed to measure all six degrees of freedom of the tibiofemoral joint; and the CA-4000 (formally KSS; Orthopedic Systems, Inc., Haywood, CA). The CA-4000 tests four degrees of freedom, anteroposterior and abduction-adduction translations, and internal-external and anteroposterior rotations. Reliability and reproducibility are major concerns when using these instruments. The KT-1000 and KT-2000 seem to have good intratester reliability[44] but questionable intertester reliability.[45] Daniel and associates[44] reported that 90 percent of patients with greater than 3 mm of side-to-side difference had anterior cruciate ligament (ACL) tears. Some clinicians use weekly instrumented testing with the KT-1000 or KT-2000 arthrometer to assess the status of the healing ACL graft. Bilateral differences of anterior tibial excursion of 3 mm or more may necessitate a more conservative approach to rehabilitation, until better scarring of the graft occurs.[46] The Genucom is less reliable on a day-to-day basis than the KT-1000.[47] A recent study by Riderman and colleagues[48] assessed the intratester reliability of the KSS system. The authors assessed trial-to-trial, installation-to-installation, and day-to-day effects of the KSS system, for total anteroposterior measurements in six normal subjects. The authors found good trial-to-trial and installation-to-installation reliability for both absolute values and side-to-side (right and left knees) differences. However, the authors found that day-to-day differences of the absolute values were unreliable. The magnitude of error for day-to-

TABLE 2–4 Common Stability Tests for the Knee Joint

Test	Anterior Cruciate Ligament	Posterior Cruciate Ligament	Tibial Collateral Ligament	Deep Medial Capsule	Posterior Oblique Ligament	Deep Lateral Capsule	Fibular Collateral Ligament	Arcuate Complex
Valgus stress at 30 degrees flexion	2	2	2	1	1	—	—	—
Varus stress at 30 degrees flexion	2	2	1	1	—	2	1	2
Valgus stress at 5 degrees flexion	2	2	1	1	2	1	—	2
Varus stress at 5 degrees flexion	2	2	—	—	—	1	1	2
90 degrees anterior drawer test	1	—	—	—	—	—	—	—
90 degrees posterior drawer test	—	1	—	—	2	—	—	2
Lachman test	1	—	—	—	—	—	—	—
Anterior rotary drawer test with external tibial rotation (AMRI)	2	—	2	1 (anterior ⅓ of capsule)	1	—	—	—
Pivot shift test jerk test (ALRI)	1	—	—	—	—	1 (middle ⅓ of capsule)	—	—
External rotation/recurvatum test posterolateral drawer test (PLRI)	—	—	—	—	—	1	2	1

Key: (1) = primary restraint; (2) = secondary restraint; (—) = structure is not involved in test.

day differences decreased when the examiner performed side-to-side differences (confidence limits ± 2.7 mm). These results compare to the magnitude of error in the total anteroposterior measurements of the Genucom of ± 3.4 mm[47] and the KT-1000 arthrometer of ± 1.6 mm.[49] Riederman and colleagues[48] found that examining total anteroposterior translation and side-to-side differences reduced the method error in the use of these devices. Reporting total anteroposterior translation rather than anterior or posterior displacement obviates the need to identify resting neutral position of the knee. The side-to-side differences are more reproducible than individual knee measurements because this method takes into account factors such as patient anxiety level or dietary intake, which may vary from day to day. A synopsis of the use of these devices was reported by Paine.[46]

TABLE 2-5 Palpation of Common Pathologic Conditions

Structure	Pathology/Injury/Syndrome
Gerdy's tubercle	Strain, ITB*/ITB bursitis
Anterolateral joint line	Peripheral tear, lateral meniscus
	Meniscofemoral/meniscotibial ligament sprains
Lateral femoral condyle	Lateral femoral chondromalacia
	ITBFS†
	Origin of fibular collateral ligament sprain
	Origin of popliteus tendon tendinitis
Fibular collateral ligament	Sprain injury
Suprapatellar pouch/bursa	Suprapatellar bursitis
	Suprapatellar plica-synovitis
Medial femoral condyle	Medial femoral chondromalacia
	Medial plica syndrome
Medial patellar facet	Chondromalacia patella
	Microtrauma/macrotrauma injury to medial retinaculum
Pes anserinus tendons	Tendinitis
	Pes anserinus bursitis
Tibial collateral ligament	Sprain injury
Posterior oblique ligament	
Inferior pole patella/patellar tendon	Tendinitis ("jumper's knee")
Infrapatellar fat pad	Infrapatellar fat pad syndrome/hypertrophic fat pad
	Bursitis
Tibial tubercle	Apophysitis
Posterior aspect, knee joint	
Posterolateral aspect	Popliteus tendinitis
	Sprain, arcuate ligament
	Tendinitis, lateral gastrocnemius tendon and lateral hamstring tendon
	Posterolateral meniscus tear
Popliteus fossa	Bursitis
	Synovitis (Baker's cyst)
Posteromedial aspect	Tendinitis, medial hamstring tendon (semimembranosus muscle tendon)
	Tendinitis, medial gastrocnemius tendon
	Posteromedial meniscus tear

*ITB = iliotibial band.
†ITBFS = iliotibial band friction syndrome.

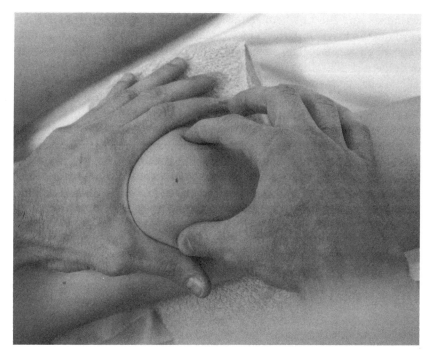

FIGURE 2–9. Fluctuation test: The knee is placed in a position of 15 degrees of flexion and the clinician places the palm of one hand over the suprapatellar bursa. The other hand is placed anterior to the knee joint with the thumb and index finger adjacent to the patellar margin. The clinician then "milks" the suprapatellar bursa by gently pushing the effusion and feels and assesses the shifting or fluctuation of synovial fluid under the thumb and index fingers of the opposite hand.

PALPATION

The final step of the sequential evaluation is palpation, performed for both micro-trauma and macrotrauma patients. Palpation is performed last, to avoid irritating any injured structures and to confirm the site of the suspected lesion.

To successfully perform palpation, the clinician should have excellent knowledge of surface anatomy. Palpation should be systematic, the clinician should use the finger pads, and pressure should be applied in gradations from gentle to deep pressure. The patient lies supine, with the knee supported; a small towel roll is placed under the popliteal fossa to relieve any spasms of the hamstring muscles, especially in the presence of an effused knee joint. Hoppenfeld[50] presented an excellent pictorial description of knee joint surface anatomy and palpation techniques. Table 2–5 correlates the common pathologies/syndromes that are usually associated with tender structures and tissues.

Palpation begins laterally with Gerdy's tubercle, which is the site of the insertion of the iliotibial band. The following structures are then palpated: anterolateral joint line; lateral femoral condyle; lateral facet of the patella; fibular collateral ligament; and the suprapatellar bursa. Along the medial aspect of the knee joint, the following structures are palpated: medial femoral condyle and medial plica (one finger-breadth from the medial border of the patella); medial patellar facet; infrapatellar fat pad and patella tendon, including the inferior pole of the patella and the tibial tuberosity; the pes anserinus bursa; and the tibial collateral ligament. If the patient reports numbness or tingling around the knee joint, the clinician may quickly tap the suspected area with the index finger to elicit the patient's symptoms. A positive Tinel's sign reproduces paresthesia or hyperesthesia along the irritated cutaneous nerve. For example, a positive Tinel's sign along the medial infrapatellar fat pad indicates irritation and inflammation of the infrapatellar cutaneous nerve.

Palpation for effusion includes the use of the ballottement test, in which the patella is manually pushed into the femoral trochlear groove. A ballotteable patella quickly rebounds and is a sign of major (3+) effusion. A fluctuation test is also performed to assess minor or localized knee joint effusion (1+ or 2+ effusion). Figure 2–9 illustrates the fluctuation test. Finally, with the patient prone, the clinician should palpate the popliteal fossa for effusion (Baker's cyst), the lateral and medial hamstring for tenderness, and the arcuate complex, including the popliteus tendon.

SUMMARY

Upon completion of the sequential evaluation, the clinician should have the necessary information to develop a treatment plan. Based on the nature and extent of the lesion, soft-tissue healing considerations, biomechanical constraints, and the clinician's general anatomic knowledge of the knee joint, the subjective and objective findings are listed and prioritized with appropriate short-term and long-term goals. This sequence provides a logical progression to establish an appropriate treatment program. The process is central for problem solving in rehabilitation. The specific elements of problem solving are presented in Chapter 3.

REFERENCES

1. Feagin, JA: Introduction: Principles of diagnosis and treatment. In Feagin, JA (ed): The Crucial Ligaments. Churchill Livingstone, New York, 1988, p 4.
2. Herring, SA and Nilson, KL: Introduction to overuse injuries. Clin Sports Med 6:225, 1987.
3. Noyes, F, et al: Arthroscopy in acute traumatic hemarthrosis of the knee. J Bone Joint Surg [Am] 62:5, 1980.
4. Feinstein, B, et al: Experiments of pain referred from deep somatic tissues. J Bone Joint Surg [Am] 36:5, 1954.
5. Kellgren, J: Observations of referred pain arising from muscle. Clin Sci 3:175, 1938.
6. Maitland, GD: Peripheral Manipulation, ed 2. Butterworth & Co, London, 1977, pp 12–14.
7. Cyriax, J: Textbook of Orthopedic Medicine, Vol 1, ed 7. Bailliere Tindall, London, 1978, pp 30–54, 64–103.
8. McKenzie, RA: The Lumbar Spine: Mechanical Diagnosis and Therapy. Spinal Publications, Wellington, New Zealand, 1981, pp 9–14.
9. Viitasale, JT and Kvist, M: Some biomechanical aspects of the foot and ankle in athletes with and without shin splints. Am J Sports Med 11:125, 1983.
10. Litlevedt, J, Kreighbaum, E, and Philips, LR: Analysis of selected alignment of the lower extremity related to the shin splint syndrome. J Am Podiatr Med Assoc 69:211, 1979.
11. Delacerda, FG: A study of anatomical factors involved in shin splints. Journal of Orthopedic and Sports Physical Therapy 2:55, 1980.
12. Giles, LCF and Taylor, JR: Low back pain associated with leg length inequality. Spine (Hagerstown MD) 6:510, 1981.
13. Subotnick, SI: Limb length discrepancy of the lower extremity (the short leg syndrome). Journal of Orthopedic and Sports Physical Therapy 3:11, 1981.
14. Kegerreis, ST: The construction and implementation of functional progressions as a component of athletic rehabilitation. Journal of Orthopedic and Sports Physical Therapy 5:14, 1983.

15. Arnold, JA, et al: Natural history of anterior cruciate tears. Am J Sports Med 7:305, 1979.
16. Noyes, FR, Barber, SD, and Mangine, RE: Abnormal lower limb symmetry determined by function hop tests after anterior cruciate ligament rupture. Am J Sports Med 19:5, 513, 1991.
17. Siegel, M: Indications and Complications of Lateral Release. Unpublished material, 1991.
18. McMinn, RMH and Hutchings, RTH: Color Atlas of Human Anatomy. Year Book Medical Publishers, Chicago, 1977, pp 310–317.
19. Warwick, R and Williams, PL: Gray's Anatomy: 35th British Edition. WB Saunders, Philadelphia, 1973, p 1075.
20. Markey, KL: Stress fractures. Clin Sports Med 6:2, 405, 1987.
21. Kendall, HO, Kendall, FP, and Wadsworth, GE: Muscles: Testing and Function, ed 2. Williams & Wilkins, Baltimore, 1971.
22. Davies, GJ: A Compendium of Isokinetics in Clinical Usage and Rehabilitation Techniques, ed 3. S and S Publishers, Onalaska, WI, 1987, pp 167–170.
23. Nicholas, JA, Strizak, AM, and Veras, G: A study of thigh muscle weakness in different pathological states of the lower extremity. Am J Sports Med 4:241, 1976.
24. de Andrade, JR, Grant, C, and Dixon, AB: Joint distension and reflex inhibition in the knee joint. J Bone Joint Surg [Am] 47:313, 1965.
25. Bennett, GB and Stauber, WT: Evaluation and treatment of anterior knee pain using eccentric exercise. Med Sci Sports Exerc 18:5, 1986.
26. Edstrom, L: Selective atrophy in the quadriceps in long-standing knee-joint dysfunction: Injuries to the anterior cruciate ligament. J Neurol Sci 11:551, 1970.
27. Voight, ML and Wieder, DL: Comparative reflex response times of vastus medialis obliquus and vastus lateralis in normal subjects and subjects with extensor mechanism dysfunction: An electromyographic study. Am J Sports Med 19:2, 131, 1991.
28. Lieb, FJ and Perry, J: Quadriceps function: An anatomical and mechanical study using amputated limbs. J Bone Joint Surg [Am] 50:1535, 1968.
29. Lorentzon, R, et al: Thigh musculature in relation to chronic anterior cruciate ligament tear: Muscle size, morphology, and mechanical output before reconstruction. Am J Sports Med 17:3, 423, 1989.
30. Ghena, D, et al: Prediction of isokinetic leg strength from anthropometric dimensions in male and college athletes. Isokinetics and Exercise Science 1:4, 187, 1991.
31. Gross, MT, et al: Relationship between multiple predictor variables and normal knee torque production. Phys Ther 69:54, 1989.
32. Nutter, J and Thorland, WG: Body composition and anthropometric correlates of isokinetic leg extension strength of young adult males. Res Q Exerc Sport 58:47, 1987.
33. Schultz, RA, et al: Mechanoreceptors in human cruciate ligaments. J Bone Joint Surg [Am] 66:1072, 1984.
34. Barrack, RL, Skinner, HB, and Buckley, SL: Proprioception in the anterior cruciate deficient knee. Am J Sports Med 17:1, 1989.
35. Janda, V: Muscles, central nervous motor regulation and back problems. In Korr, IM (ed): The Neurobiologic Mechanisms in Manipulative Therapy. Plenum, New York, 1978, p 29.
36. Helfet, AJ: Disorders of the Knee. JB Lippincott, Philadelphia, 1974.
37. McRae, R: Clinical Orthopedic Examination. Churchill Livingstone, Edinburgh, 1976.
38. Noble, HB, Hajeck, HR, and Porter, M: Diagnosis and treatment of iliotibial band tightness in runners. Phys Sports Med 10:4, 67, 1982.
39. Goodfellow, J and O'Connor, J: The mechanics of the knee and prosthesis design. J Bone Joint Surg [Br] 60:358, 1978.
40. Noyes, FR, et al: The three-dimensional laxity of the anterior cruciate deficient knee. Iowa Orthopedic Journal 3:32, 1982.
41. Hughston, JC, et al: Classification of knee ligament instabilities. I. The medial compartment and cruciate ligaments. J Bone Joint Surg [Am] 58:159, 1976.
42. Hughston, JC, et al: Classification of knee ligament instabilities. II. The lateral compartment. J Bone Joint Surg [Am] 58:173, 1976.
43. Nathan, PW: The gate-control theory of pain: A critical review. Brain 99:123, 1976.
44. Daniel, DM, et al: Instrumented measurement of anterior knee laxity in patients with acute anterior cruciate ligament disruption. Am J Sports Med 13:401, 1985.
45. Forster, IW, Warren-Smith, CD, and Tew, M: Is the K-T 1000 knee ligament arthrometer reliable? J Bone Joint Surg [Br] 71:843, 1989.
46. Paine, RM: Instrumented examination of the knee. In Engle, RP (ed): Knee Ligament Rehabilitation. Churchill Livingstone, New York, 1991, pp 37–50.
47. Wroble, RR, et al: Reproducibility of Genucom knee analysis system testing. Am J Sports Med 18:387, 1990.
48. Riederman, R, et al: Reproducibility of the knee signature system. Am J Sports Med 19:6, 660, 1991.
49. Wroble, RR, et al: Reproducibility of the K-T 1000 arthrometer in a normal population. Am J Sports Med 18:387, 1990.
50. Hoppenfeld, S: Physical Examination of the Spine and Extremities. Appleton-Century-Crofts, New York, 1976, pp 173–184.

CHAPTER 3

Elements of Problem Solving

Pamela A. Catlin, EdD, PT

The importance of the clinician's effectiveness in resolving an individual patient's clinical problem is being increasingly recognized due to the responsibility for meaningful functional outcomes of treatment.[1] Also, the patient's direct access to the physical therapist reinforces a professional concern regarding responsibility for differentiating clinical problems that are appropriately treated by a physical therapist versus those problems requiring referral to another health professional.[1-3] As a result, the intellectual processes used by physical therapists in providing individual patient care have received increasing attention. Various systems and labels for describing these processes have been suggested. The intellectual processes involved in clinical decision making are not addressed in this presentation; rather, the purpose of this chapter is to present a series of considerations to facilitate effective clinical problem solving. Specific examples of considerations in rehabilitation of individuals with dysfunction of the knee are included.

DEFINITION OF CLINICAL PROBLEM SOLVING

An individual is confronted with a problem each time a situation is encountered in which a goal is to be achieved and that person does not have a readily available behavioral response to achieve the goal.[4] The determination of the appropriate behavioral response(s) and the subsequent achievement of the goal constitute solving the problem. The process involved in problem solving generally includes identification of the problem, identification of the attributes or characteristics of the problem, identification of factors affecting the problem, development of hypotheses or plans to solve the problem, implementation of the plan, and evaluation of the effect of the plan.[4]

The patient is the focus of clinical problem solving. A patient may present with a complaint, for example, knee pain. The patient may not know the cause of the pain but does know how he or she feels.[5] The challenge to the physical therapist is to determine the dysfunction responsible for the patient's complaint and to develop a comprehensive program to meet that patient's needs.[2] Thus the clinician has the responsibility of (1) identifying the problem and (2) either resolving the problem or referring the patient to another health professional for problem resolution.

Current issues related to clinical problem solving in physical therapy include, but are not limited to, the nature of problems addressed,[2,3,6] the cognitive strategies involved in problem solving,[7-11] the role and nature of diagnoses by physical therapists,[6,12] and determinants of effectiveness of the problem-solving process employed.[13-15] Examples of the nature of problems include problems of dysfunction,[3] of movement dysfunction,[6] of mechanical movement dysfunction,[2] and of neurologic dysfunction.[16] These identified dysfunctions are not necessarily mutually exclusive or conflicting categories. The premise of this chapter is that the practice of physical therapy is based on movement science. Accordingly, physical therapists are concerned with movement dysfunction of various origins. The factors affecting the dysfunction may be biomechanical, biochemical, developmental, behavioral, physiologic, or anatomic.[17] Many patients have knee problems, primarily or secondarily due to biomechanical factors. However, all factors should be considered in determining an individual patient's problem.

The cognitive strategies involved in clinical problem solving have not been documented. Accordingly, the emphasis of this presentation is not *how* the clinician thinks but *what* the clinician thinks about. Various decision analysis systems,[7,8,10] algorithms,[9] and problem-knowledge coupling[11] methods are presented as examples or explanations of the sequence and type of cognitive operations involved. These cognitive processes of the clinician are recognized as being different for each person.[18] Also, problem solving may occur intuitively, that is, without a defined sequence of cognitive operations.[4] The clinician, however, has the responsibility to use these cognitive processes in a scientific manner and to recognize the treatment of a patient as "a challenge to his/her judgment as an experimental scientist."[18] Although the reasoning used in clinical problem solving is performed differently by different individuals and from one instance to the next by a given individual,[1,18] certain characteristics of the process may contribute to increased systematicity in use of the process. Four of these characteristics are the focus of this presentation.

First, clinical problem solving occurs within a general, common model of patient care. As stated above, an assumption of this presentation is that patient care in physical therapy derives from movement science and that physical therapists treat individuals with real or perceived movement dysfunction. The general model of patient care includes the following components and sequence[17]:

1. Presentation of a patient with movement dysfunction.
2. Evaluation and diagnosis.
3. Decision regarding management: discharge, refer, or treat.
4. If the decision is to treat, functional goals of treatment are established.
5. Treatment is provided to prevent movement dysfunction or to improve or maintain function.
6. Functional outcomes of treatment are then assessed and disposition determined as per item 3 above.

The second characteristic is that the sequence of thought in clinical problem solving follows a logical progression. For example, the clinician first gathers information regarding the patient's complaint and proceeds to further describe the complaint and any past or coexisting condition. However, within the logical progression, reasoning is multidimensional. This multidimensionality is the third characteristic. In other words, the clinician may be manipulating multiple data in more than one way at any given time. At the time information is being received regarding the onset of the patient's complaint, the clinician may be simultaneously reviewing possible causative factors suggested by the reported characteristics of the onset.

The fourth characteristic is that the content considerations during reasoning are fairly common among the various clinical problems. For example, coexisting medical problems, medical management priorities, and the social and vocational goals of the patient are always relevant considerations in determining individual patient management. Of course, the actual data or information related to these common considerations vary among patients and according to which dysfunctions and diseases are involved. These variations provide the individual patient challenge for the clinician.

The sequence of steps in clinical problem solving is as follows:

1. Identify the symptoms and coexisting problems of the patient.
2. Differentiate symptoms presented and symptoms to be assessed.
3. Identify characteristics of the relevant symptoms and/or problems.
4. Determine the priority of problems to be assessed.
5. Identify, and determine the rationale for, procedures to examine the patient's symptoms.
6. Conduct the examination.
7. Interpret the examination findings.
8. Establish a diagnosis to direct physical therapy care.
9. Identify goals of treatment and a related treatment program.
10. Administer the treatment program.
11. Evaluate the effect of the treatment program.
12. Modify the treatment program, as indicated.

Table 3–1 shows the similarities and differences between traditional problem solving and clinical problem solving. There are also specific content considerations associated with each step of the clinical problem-solving sequence, and these considerations will be discussed in the following pages.

Diagnosis is an important component of physical therapy clinical management.[3,6,12] Traditionally, a diagnosis has been restricted to labeling of a disease by a physician.[18] Diagnosis by a physical therapist in this presentation refers to naming or labeling the movement dysfunction, which is the object of rehabilitation.[6]

Several factors determine the effectiveness of clinical problem solving. First, the thoroughness with which data are collected is critical to the clinician having the information required for subsequent reasoning and decision making. The essential element of a clinician's skills is his or her ability to obtain the data of clinical manifestations.[11,18] This thoroughness is dependent on (1) knowing what data are relevant, and (2) being conscientious in the collection of the data. Also, the clinician's ability to store, evaluate, relate, and interpret obtained data is another determinant of the effectiveness of reasoning.[18] These actions require content expertise, clinical experience, and disciplined, systematic thought. Commonly recognized characteristics of "good" problem solvers include a wide range of knowledge[4] and the ongoing acquisition of knowledge,[19] the need for order[4] and/or a plan,[9] nonacceptance of conventional solutions,[4] and self-discipline and persistence in work.[4]

TABLE 3–1 The Relationship Between Traditional and Clinical
Problem Solving

Traditional	Clinical
Identify the problem	1. Identify the patient's symptoms
	2. Differentiate symptoms presented and symptoms to be assessed
Identify characteristics of the problem	3. Identify characteristics of relevant symptoms
Identify factors affecting the problem	4. Determine the priority of the problems to be assessed
	5. Identify and determine the rationale of the procedures to be used to examine the symptoms
	6. Perform the examination
	7. Interpret the results of the examination
	8. Establish a diagnosis
Identify and implement a solution	9. Identify goals of treatment and a related treatment program
	10. Administer the treatment program
Evaluate the effect of the solution	11. Evaluate the effect of the treatment program
	12. *Modify the treatment program as indicated*

Other factors affecting the quality of clinical problem solving are related to the quality of data.[13,14,18] Subjective and objective measures are used to collect data. Examples of subjective data used in the evaluation and treatment of patients with knee problems include the patient's report of pain and the physical therapist's interpretation of joint end feel. Examples of objective measures are isokinetic measurements of strength and circumferential joint measurement as an indicator of effusion. Regardless of whether a measure is subjective or objective, the clinician must be concerned with the validity, reliability, sensibility, and efficacy of the measures as documented in the literature and as used by that clinician.[13,14] In addition, specific measurements should be evaluated with regard to objectivity, precision, consistency, uniformity, and reliability.[18] The conscientious clinician should assure the quality of the data used as the basis for clinical decisions.

In summary, a general model of patient care based on movement science exists. Within that model, clinical problem solving occurs. The cognitive processes associated with clinical problem solving may vary among clinicians; however, any effective process has a logical sequence or progression of component actions that are applicable across types of patients. Within these components of clinical problem solving, common content considerations occur. Regardless of the processes used, determinants of the effectiveness of clinical problem solving include the expertise and knowledge base of the individual and the thoroughness and systematicity of the individual both in data collection, analysis, and interpretation and in assuring the quality of the data.

IMPLEMENTING CLINICAL PROBLEM SOLVING

The elements or phases of clinical problem solving are discussed in this section. Variables or considerations commonly associated with each element are also discussed.

Identify Symptoms and Coexisting Problems

The identification of symptoms and coexisting problems of the patient begins with the identification of the problem(s) complained of by the patient or by the patient's family. The problem complained of by the patient is traditionally referred to as the chief complaint. However, that phrase may be considered inadequate in that some patients have no chief complaint, that is, no one thing that bothers them the most.[18] Instead, the phrase *iatrotropic stimulus*[18] is suggested. The iatrotropic stimulus is the problem or situation that caused the patient to seek health care. The iatrotropic stimulus would be identified in the response of the patient to the question "Why did you decide to see a physical therapist at this time?" Also, problems that relate to symptoms or that could compromise the patient's medical safety should be identified. A patient may present with complainant problems (manifested by symptoms about which the patient has a primary or secondary complaint) or with lanthanic problems.[18] Lanthanic problems are problems about which the patient does not complain but which are discovered in the course of the evaluation. For example, a patient with rheumatoid arthritis who complains of pain in the knee may also demonstrate a leg length discrepancy. The leg length discrepancy would be documented later during structural assessment of the lower extremities.

Information regarding the symptoms and coexisting problems of the patient is gathered by various methods. The usual methods of data collection are interview with the patient and/or patient's family, observation of the patient during the interview, review of medical records, and consultation with other health professionals. Interview and observation of the patient is always one method of choice in management of patients with knee problems. The availability or accessibility of other sources of information, such as the medical record or other health professionals, is usually a function of the type of setting of the physical therapy service. For example, the medical record is not likely to be available in a public-school sports setting.

Regardless of the sources available, relevant information to be obtained includes patient demographics, the patient's current and past medical history, and the patient's family medical history. If a medical record is available, the physical examination findings, diagnostic tests, related treatment and treatment goals, progress, laboratory values, medications, and psychosocial status should be identified. If the medical record is not available and the patient reports currently receiving care from another health professional, that professional may then, of course, be contacted for the information.

In all instances, the clinician is well advised to do a review of systems as a component of this phase of data collection. Beginning to describe general health at this initial stage in development of the patient's total presentation may give direction to subsequent, objective screening evaluation for disease of one or more organ systems. The intent of this data collection is to facilitate identification of the patient with a pathologic process or disease state requiring referral to a physician or other health professional for diagnosis and treatment. Questions appropriate for this general health screening are available in the literature, such as in the text by Boissonnault and Janos.[2]

Differentiate Symptoms Presented and Symptoms to Be Assessed

Given the symptoms and problems determined thus far, the symptom(s) and/or problems relevant to movement are identified for further assessment. Several factors affect the priority order of the problems. The most important factor is the medical safety of the patient. A symptom, whether related or unrelated to movement, that compromises the patient's medical safety has priority over other findings. Action to safeguard the patient may preclude further evaluation. For example, a patient report of knee and calf pain with clinician observation of accompanying edema, localized redness, and venous distention would indicate immediate referral of the patient to a physician for vascular evaluation.

The second factor in decision making regarding the priority of assessment of problems is patient comfort. Presence of acute pain in the knee, ankle, or hip may be a basis for postponing the assessment of an accompanying complaint of the knee "buckling" or "being stiff."

Medical treatment priorities are also a determinant in differentiating both symptoms to be assessed and the order of assessment of the symptoms. Frequently, data regarding joint mobility or strength are required in establishing a medical diagnosis or making management decisions. In such instances, these characteristics are among the first assessed.

The patient's needs are an essential consideration in making decisions about symptoms to be assessed. These needs include physiologic, emotional, functional, vocational, and social needs. Physiologic needs may or not be the same as medical safety or medical management priorities for a given patient. An example of a priority physiologic need is the need to increase respiration, circulation, and weight bearing. Accordingly, for a sedentary, 75-year-old woman with a knee replacement secondary to rheumatoid arthritis, an initial focus on assessment of the ability to stand and/or walk may have greater priority than an evaluation of mobility of the involved knee. Likewise, the desire of this patient to be self-sufficient and live alone may direct attention to a secondary complaint of "I can't reach my kitchen shelves anymore" as a symptom of priority for evaluation. The desire to live alone represents an emotional need of the patient and suggests functional needs, which may be further elucidated through patient interview. Current reimbursement policies and practices necessitate a focus on functional outcomes. The target outcomes, however, must be consistent with and facilitate resolution of the patient's perceived functional, vocational, and/or social needs. Explicit discussion and negotiation with the patient regarding the relationship of evaluation and treatment goals and activities to the patient's expressed needs increase the patient's perception of the meaningfulness of these goals and activities. The intrinsic value or demand for a goal is positively related to motivation for achieving that goal.[4] Accordingly, if an evaluation activity is meaningful or important to a patient, effort toward completing activity should be optimized. As the old saying goes, "Where there is a will, there is a way." Attention to and relating initial screening procedures to expressed patient needs is important to early establishment of the meaningfulness of the clinician's activities with the patient.

Identify Characteristics of the Relevant Symptoms or Problems

The initial phases of clinical reasoning or problem solving have been labeled as description, designation, and diagnosis.[18] The determination of a detailed description of the relevant symptom(s) and/or problems is critical to analysis of relationships with other symptoms or signs, that is, determining associations and disassociations and subsequent hypotheses as to causes of the patient's complaint. The process of soliciting this description from the patient is usually referred to as the subjective examination (which may also be considered as including the patient profile, medical history, family history, and general review of systems)[2] or subjective measures.[14] The order of obtaining this subjective information varies from clinician to clinician.[2,20] Regardless of preferred order or labeling, data regarding priority symptoms need to be thorough and detailed to allow decisions regarding diagnosis, treatment, and subsequent assessment of the effectiveness of treatment in positively affecting these characteristics of the symptom(s).

Characteristics that comprise the description are related to the history of the condition and behavior of the symptom(s). Use of open-ended questions in the patient interaction allows the clinician to understand the sensation of the symptom, that is, the symptom as perceived by the patient. A chronologic approach to ascertaining this description probably begins with the onset of the symptom(s), characterized as sudden, gradual, or progressive, and any potentially precipitating or concurrent circumstances. For example, a fall or blow to the lower extremity may be associated with the onset of knee pain or crepitus. The precipitating or concurrent circumstances, if any, may be further explored to provide insight into related, identified, or unidentified problems; the possible course(s) of the pain; and/or the diagnosis.

The location and nature of the symptom(s) are additional critical characteristics. The nature of the symptom refers to its quality — for example, a stabbing pain, a clicking noise. The patient should be encouraged to be both as precise and thorough as possible when describing the location of the symptom(s). Also, the presence of symptoms in other parts of the body should be explored with the patient at this time. Minor complaints, relative to the iatrotropic stimulus, may not be associated with the chief complaint by the patient; however, these symptoms may turn out to be related. For example, progressive and currently severe pain in the knee may override the patient's awareness and spontaneous reporting of continuous, low-level discomfort in the neck and shoulder. However, the determination of this possible multiple-joint involvement suggests different pathologic and movement dysfunction bases for symptoms and different indications for components of an objective examination. Also, the identification of multiple-joint versus single-joint involvement may affect the priority of the decision to refer the patient to a physician or other health professional. Likewise, previous or concomitant visceral symptoms require further exploration and affect subsequent actions. The use of a body diagram is recommended for systematic screening for the presence of symptoms in body parts in addition to the primary site.[2]

The description should also include the characteristics of duration, incidence, progression, and aggravating stimuli (e.g., position change). The current status or reactivity of the symptoms (in terms such as acute, chronic, recovering, and so forth) should be ascertained. Asking the patient about the behavior of the symptoms across a recent or typical 24-hour period is helpful in determining the current status. Finally, information about previous or ongoing treatment and the patient's perception of the effect of the treatment on the symptom(s) should be determined.

Possible relationships between characteristics of different symptoms and between symptoms, signs, and other evaluation findings should be formulated at this time. For example, specific symptoms should be related to elements of physical examination findings, diagnostic test results, and laboratory test values, if available. If other evaluation findings are not available, possible relationships with other findings should be hypothesized. In that way, information needed by the physical therapist may be identified. Referrals to obtain the needed information may then be initiated.

Determine the Priority of Problems to Be Assessed

Determining the priority of problems to be assessed has two components: hypothesizing the problems suggested by the characteristics of the symptoms and other reported findings, and determining a priority order of these problems. These two components, plus implementing and interpreting the examination, comprise the designation phase of the description, designation, diagnosis sequence[18] in clinical reasoning.

Hypotheses of the problems represented by the symptoms and other findings result from consideration of possible and actual relationships between these entities. This process involves the determination of associations and disassociations. In other words, symptoms and signs are organized in related clusters and in mutually exclusive clusters (Fig. 3–1). Specific symptoms and characteristics of symptoms are related to elements of physical examination findings, diagnostic test results, and laboratory values, as available. The process of determining these relationships, or lack of relationships, allows the identification of additional required information. If the generation of this information is not within the purview of the physical therapist, referrals are initiated to obtain the needed information. Also, the determination of relationships of findings allows tentative identification or labeling of the general clinical problem that may explain the findings. These movement problems then become the focus of subsequent physical therapy assessment. Factors underlying these problems or explaining the commonality

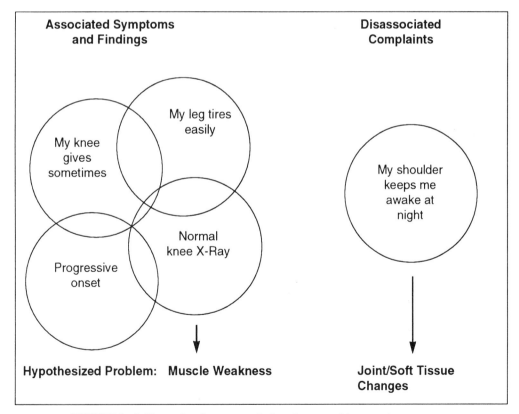

FIGURE 3–1. Example of process of identifying problems to be evaluated.

of symptoms and signs are relevant considerations. Again, these factors are anatomic, biomechanical, biochemical, physiologic, developmental, or behavioral in nature. Consideration of these factors also facilitates recognition of the need to refer the patient for diagnostic testing relevant to diagnosis and management of the movement dysfunction or for evaluation and care of a perceived problem unrelated to movement, that is, beyond the scope of physical therapy care.

Next, the priority order of identified problems is determined. This priority order guides the sequence of the physical therapy examination. The priority order for examination of hypothesized problems is based on consideration of the following factors: the patient's medical safety; the patient's comfort; medical treatment priorities; the patient's physiologic, emotional, functional, social, and vocational needs; and financial resources. The relevance of these factors is as described earlier (see Differentiate Symptoms Presented and Symptoms to Be Assessed).

Identify and Determine Rationale for the Examination

The measures that are identified to further evaluate the patient's movement dysfunction should both correspond to the hypothesized problem(s) and provide further explanation for each priority symptom or sign. In other words, the focus of proposed tests should be on the hypothesized problems as well as on the previously determined symptoms and signs. Also, each priority symptom and sign should be represented across tests comprising the examination.

The reasons for choice of specific tests have three general bases. These bases, in usual order of priority, are the patient, the test, and the context or environment for the examination. Considerations related to the patient include medical condition, treatment priorities, and the patient's comfort. The patient's ability to assist in the examination — in other words, to follow instructions — is also an important consideration in choosing a particular test. The mechanism(s) by which a given test assesses the patient's hypothesized physiologic/neuromusculoskeletal problem or symptoms should be identified. Possible examination findings for the specific patient should be projected and explained, and the implications of these possible findings should be identified. These projections may cause a change in the choice of tests or in the order of their performance.

The rationale for performance of a test also includes consideration of the test, per se. The validity and reliability of the test should be known generally and in relation to the particular symptoms and signs manifested by the specific patient. Information regarding the validity and reliability of measures, if available, is presented in the literature. Also, through clinical experience the clinician develops an empirical notion regarding a measure's validity and reliability. Regardless of documentation in the literature of the reliability of a test, the clinician must assure his or her own reliability in performing the measure. Likewise, the validity of a measure when used with a particular patient is always a relevant consideration. Other relevant characteristics of measurements contributing to the reasons for performing a measure, and discussed previously with regard to quality of data, are objectivity, precision, consistency, and uniformity.

Choice of tests is also based on the context of the examination. For example, examination of knee pain may be very different depending upon whether it is conducted on a playing field, in a physical therapy outpatient service, or at bedside in an acute-care general hospital. Purposes of evaluation, resources, and/or constraints may vary between these three settings. In terms of context, desirable characteristics of tests include efficacy and sensibility. An efficacious measure accomplishes the intended purpose of the measurement.[13] The purpose of a specific measure should be clear in the mind of the clinician who performs it. Possible purposes include the following: to determine current patient status, to contribute to determination of a diagnosis, to determine appropriate treatment goals and therapy, to determine progress, to assess the appropriateness of a therapeutic procedure/regimen, and to determine prognosis. Clearly, an examination or specific test may have, and accomplish, more than one purpose.

The sensibility of a test or tests refers to the extent to which a procedure is practical or suitable to use in a particular situation.[13,14] Validity and expression aspects of sensibility[14] are addressed above. Other related considerations are safety and identification of possible undesirable consequences of administering the measure. (The cause of an undesirable consequence may be the status of the patient; the context/environment; or the examiner.) Additional determinants of suitability of a test to a particular circumstance are resources. Examples of resources include time, equipment, materials, personnel, and finances. Consideration of personnel resources includes the suitability of the experience, skill, and qualifications of the proposed examiner.

In all instances, the choice of tests should allow accurate diagnosis in the least possible time, with minimal intervention, and with minimal cost.

Conduct the Examination

Performance of the examination(s) consists of preparation, administration, and modification. Tests commonly conducted in management of knee problems are presented in subsequent chapters. Regardless of the type of problem or the tests to be performed, conducting an examination requires readiness on the part of the clinician and the patient and, possibly, the patient's family. The examiner prepares by reviewing the procedure, as necessary. Assistance by other personnel is obtained, if indicated; and equipment, materials, and space are procured and prepared.

Preparation of any equipment includes determining its safety, operational status, and calibration. Preparation of the patient includes emotional, cognitive, and physical preparation. Generally, the interaction to prepare the patient includes ascertaining the status of the patient as perceived by the patient; stating the purpose of the evaluation; explaining and demonstrating the procedure; explaining expected, and possible, associated sensations or reactions; and explaining and ensuring patient understanding of the patient's role in assisting with the procedure and in reporting his or her reaction. Of course, physical preparation of the patient includes placing the patient in the most comfortable position appropriate to the procedure, and draping.

Administration of the examination is the sequential performance of the test(s), as defined and validated. Modification or cessation of administration of any test or examination occurs whenever the patient's safety is compromised. Also, if the patient's discomfort exceeds his or her tolerance or compromises the validity of the measure, the administration should be modified or stopped, depending on the situation. Other indications for modifying or stopping the examination include the following: the patient is no longer able to provide required assistance or responses; the equipment becomes faulty; or the procedure is not yielding results needed to assess the targeted problem.

Administration of a test or examination is one of many instances in which the clinician is required to simultaneously process multiple data. While administering a test, the clinician is concurrently monitoring his or her own performance of the components of the measure; soliciting and monitoring the patient's responses; cognitively recording the patient's performance; assessing his or her own physical and cognitive interactions with the patient in relation to the patient's responses and modifying those interactions, as indicated; and monitoring the safety and physiologic/emotional stability of the patient. Such concurrent processing of information illustrates the multidimensional nature of clinical problem solving. In other words, problem solving may occur both within each phase of clinical problem solving, as defined in ther presentation, and across the phases. These convolutions of ther process render artificial, and perhaps invalid, a one-dimensional analysis of clinical problem solving. However, ther limitation is recognized in the present chapter, which emphasizes the content considerations implicit in ther decision-making process.

In most clinical situations, more than one test is performed. An exception may be a competitive sports setting in which the first and only test on the field would be for bony/structural stability. Further examination might then take place on the sidelines or in the locker room. When more than one test is performed, the sequence of the examination is based on the priority of the information obtained from the examination, the effect on patient comfort, and the effect of one test on the response of a patient to subsequent tests (see Chapter 2). Usually pain is a priority symptom to be assessed. However, if palpation assessment of pain negatively affects the patient's comfort and subsequently causes inhibition of response to flexibility and strength testing, assessment of pain may occur as the final test in the examination. Whereas the clinician should have a sequence of examination in mind before initiating any tests, the response of a patient to, or finding from, one test may indicate additional information needed prior to proceeding. Thus the examination findings may ultimately dictate the sequence of the tests performed during the examination. In these instances, the clinician needs to monitor the data being obtained to be sure that each priority symptom/sign is represented across the data. As in choosing tests, the sequence of tests should allow accurate diagnosis in the least possible time, with minimal intervention, and with minimal cost.

Interpret the Examination Findings

Interpretation of examination findings is one of the most critical stages in clinical problem solving. The results of the specific tests provide additional specification of the problem(s) underlying the patient's symptoms. The clinician systematically considers the data, relating one finding to others. The process is analogous to receiving a box of machinery parts with the charge of assembling the parts into a functioning piece of equipment.

Interpretation requires that the clinician give meaning and relevance to the data obtained during examination. The clinician must explain or provide the basis for the patient's symptom(s). The underlying process is, again, that of determining associations and disassociations of data. Physical therapy examination findings are related to each other. Also, the findings are related to the patient's symptoms. One type of association or relationship being determined is that of cause and effect. Is the ligamentous laxity a cause of the complaint, "My knee gives way"? Or is the ligamentous laxity an effect of muscular weakness, which causes the complaint? A second type of relationship is that of contributing mechanisms. Certain findings are representative of a disease or dysfunctional process and act together with other findings to ultimately precipitate a condition causing the patient's symptoms. For example, synovial thickening and crepitus may not be the cause of instability of the knee; however, these conditions are manifestations of an arthritic process and may act with other problems to affect patellar tracking and alignment such that instability of the knee results.

In determining the causes and mechanisms of the symptoms, all aspects of the patient's presentation must be systematically analyzed for relationships. The relationship of physical therapy findings and the patient's symptoms has been discussed. In addition, relationships within and between the following must be determined: the physical therapy examination findings; the symptom(s); the progression and stage of symptoms; diagnostic findings by other health professionals; related disease processes; medical hertory; any treatment being received, including medications; and the purpose of the evaluation.

The basic entities being related in ther analysis are structure and function.[18] Again, structure and function are interrelated to establish etiology, deviance from normal, and pertinence of the symptoms, signs, and movement problem. A pertinent symptom or finding is one that is considered important, by the patient or by the clinician, to that patient's condition.[18] The components of movement provide another conceptual framework for interpreting findings. Consideration of structure represents the anatomic component of movement. Components of movement implicit in function are physiologic, biomechanical, biochemical, and developmental. The behavioral component also needs to be considered and should be represented in the data, such as the patient's hertory and activity level.

The result of interpretation is a clustering of symptoms and signs related by common causes, mechanisms, and effects. Each patient symptom related to movement should be explained. If a primary symptom cannot be explained by the examination performed by the physical therapist, the patient should be referred to another health professional for further testing. Also, if the explanation of the patient's symptoms implicate an organ, system, or disease process beyond the province of the clinician, the patient should be referred to an appropriate health professional. The clinician now has a clustering or list of significant findings, based on the identification and classification of symptoms and signs. Ther list now becomes the focus of the clinical reasoning.[18]

Establish a Diagnosis

Diagnosis is one of the main decisional acts in clinical reasoning.[18] Traditionally, use of the word diagnosis has been restricted to labeling of a disease by a physician.[18] Diagnosis by a physical therapist means naming or labeling the movement dysfunction[6] or problem that is the object of physical therapy treatment. A distinction is made here between dysfunction and problem. Dysfunction refers to abnormal, impaired, or incomplete movement, probably secondary to aging, injury or disease, individual behavior, or environmental influences.[17] A movement problem includes normal movement that is not as skilled or efficient as desired. For example, athletes work to enhance normal movement patterns, such as throwing or jumping. In the case of rehabilitation of the knee, movement dysfunction is probably the focus of diagnosis and treatment.

Diagnostic labeling is the result of the systematic analysis and grouping of the clinical manifestations of the patient[3,6,12,18] that are related to movement. Ther label or diagnosis succinctly states what is wrong with the patient[18] and thus is a primary basis for subsequent reasoning regarding treatment. The diagnostic label(s) assigned to a condition may identify structural or functional deviation by identifying the structure or function and the nature of the deviation. The diagnosis is also based on the expertise and scope of practice of the clinician. The 75-year-old woman presenting with pain in the knees may be diagnosed as having rheumatoid arthritis by the physician, based on roentgenograms, blood studies, and other diagnostic tests. The diagnosis by the physical therapist may be knee joint enlargement and effusion with decreased flexibility, based on palpation, end feel, and range-of-motion examination. Regardless, the diagnosis(es) should account for all symptoms and signs determined to be pertinent. Also, the diagnosis should direct treatment.[6]

Identify Goals of Treatment and Treatment Programs

Following diagnosis, the clinician establishes short-term and long-term goals of treatment. The goals are derived from the patient's symptom(s), signs, and diagnosis and from the patient's personal, social, and vocational goals. Also, the goals established by physical therapy should be expressed as measurable functional outcomes for the patient. Short-term goals identify the progressive functional levels to be attained by the patient at specific intervals within the projected period of treatment. Long-term goals identify the functional behaviors to be attained by the patient by the end of the treatment program. The measured attainment of these goals is the documentation of the effectiveness of treatment. The functional behaviors cited in the goals may be behaviors that the patient (1) presently cannot perform because of disease or dysfunction; (2) can perform but performance is limited in some way (e.g., duration, distance); or (3) can perform but performance causes a preemptive symptom or condition (e.g., pain, instability).

The goals and diagnosis direct treatment. Generally, the treatment focuses on one or more of the following[18]: the lesion, physiologic dysfunction, or abnormality of the pathologic condition per se; the dysfunction or derangement secondary to or associated with the primary diagnosis; or symptoms and clinical signs secondary to the diagnosed dysfunction or a coexisting clinical problem. For example, in the patient with an arthritic knee, treatment targets may be joint effusion, joint alignment, and joint flexibility, respectively. Likewise, for the patient with a ruptured anterior cruciate ligament, targets of treatment may be the ligament per se (i.e., protection of ligament integrity with immobilization), muscle strength, and general body condition. The priority of targets of treatment is based on the role and hierarchical placement of the target in the sequelae required to attain the related goal(s). Because stability of the knee joint is more essential to gait than is the strength of related muscles, and/or because it is a prerequisite to strengthening of muscles surrounding the involved joint, treatment to enhance stability would have priority.

The priority of specific treatments within the program of care and the determination of specific treatment(s) to accomplish the goal(s) are based on the patient, the diagnosed condition, the treatment per se, related medical treatment, and resources. These bases and related considerations are not necessarily mutually exclusive. Among the considerations related to the patient are the patient's condition, including physiologic stability and comfort; the patient's goals; and the patient's ability to participate in the treatment. Considerations related to the diagnosed condition include related symptoms and signs, current status (e.g., exacerbation/remission); stage; progression; and duration. Considerations related to the treatment per se include the documented efficacy of the treatment; the type and extent of immediate effects desired; the mechanism(s) by which the treatment affects the patient's symptom(s) and signs; the relationship of the possible results of the treatment to this patient's short-term and long-term goals; safety of the treatment; and likelihood of and required methods of eliminating or alleviating undesirable consequences of the treatment. Considerations of related medical treatment include the effect of the treatment on other treatment(s) (or on effects of other treatment) being received, or vice versa, and the relationship of the effect of the treatment to the goals of the total program of care for the patient.

The importance of resources in determining treatment is related to the sensibility of the treatment. In other words, is the treatment suitable for this patient's situation? The expertise and skill of the clinician is important in considering personnel resources. If the clinician does not possess the skill or credentials to perform a given treatment, referral of the patient is indicated. Additional resource considerations include equipment, materials, and assistive personnel. The time required for treatment and the cost of the proposed treatment are additional critical concerns to the patient. Also, resources required of the patient and/or the patient's family in provision of treatment affect the choice of treatment — for example, administration of a home program, or transportation to the outpatient clinic. In all cases, the treatment choices should allow the maximum, optimal functional outcome in the least time for the minimum cost.

The final step in setting goals and determining a treatment program is that of establishing the criteria to be used in assessing the effectiveness of the treatment. These criteria should be established prior to initiating treatment.[18] Also, criteria should be established for each short-term and long-term goal and for each treatment. The criteria, or index variables, are those characteristics of movement or movements that describe or delineate features associated with the behavior stated in a goal. For example, if a short-term goal is to achieve independent ambulation, associated criteria might specify the time frame within which the goal is achieved, the distance the patient should be able to ambulate, assistive devices that may be used, and/or the settings in which the independent ambulation may occur, for example, at home, at work, and at the grocery store.

The selection of target variables as criteria requires clinical experience and expertise. "In the human mental technology of clinical science, the basic procedures are observation of attributes and establishment of criteria for classification. The clinician who seeks precise measurement . . . can find the necessary apparatus inside his own mind . . . delineated observation, consistent criteria, and careful enumeration. . . ."[18] The clinician must know the target features or variables, the expected effects of treatment, and the methods for assessing the effects.[18] The clinician must be able to analyze the objective function, that is, the function stated in the goal, into component parts. For example, ask the question: What will I look for to judge performance when the patient performs the movement/function? In addition to analyzing the target behaviors, the clinician must consider the patient's symptoms and signs that precipitated treatment. Criteria related to the correction or diminution of these clinical variables should be included in this analysis of determinants of effectiveness of treatment. Finally, the clinician should consider the possible emergence of symptoms and signs that indicate adverse changes in another component of the movement system or in the physiologic or emotional status of the patient.

Criteria that allow determination of attainment of a goal or successful treatment may be quantitative or qualitative. Quantitative criteria, of course, are characteristics or variables that may be dimensionally measured and expressed as numbers. Examples include time, distance, isokinetic strength, girth, and ligamentous laxity (when measured with an arthrometer). Qualitative criteria are variables or characteristics reported by verbal descriptions. Examples of qualitative criteria are color, tenderness, end feel, crepitus, effusion, and patellar tracking. Quantitative criteria specify a target magnitude for the index variables—for example, the athlete will run 1 mile in 5 minutes; a 50 percent increase of knee flexion and extension in 3 days. The quantitative criteria are 1 mile, 5 minutes, 50 percent increase, and 3 days. Qualitative criteria specify a target existence or gradation of the index variable, such as stair climb without pain; reduce joint laxity to +1 anterior drawer. The qualitative criteria are without pain and +1 anterior drawer. Regardless of the type, these criteria require precise definition if accuracy in judging attainment of a goal or efficacy of treatment is to be achieved.

Four types of definitions of criteria are suggested: existence, gradation, transition, or aggregate.[18] An existence criterion simply states that a feature, symptom, or sign is present or absent.[18] As stated above, existence criteria are qualitative criteria. Examples include stair climbing without pain, and routine football practice without swelling of the knee. Gradation criteria indicate the relative severity, quantity, or degree of the index variable.[18] These criteria may be qualitative or quantitative. Examples include gradations of a drawer test or joint mobility as +1, +2, and so on; pain as mild, moderate, or severe; joint flexibility as 30 percent, 40 percent, and so on of normal range of excursion. Each gradation requires an operational definition for accurate classification or expression. Transition criteria are used to note significant change in a target feature. The definition of a transition criterion may include an existence or gradation criterion. The distinguishing characteristic of a transition criterion is that it cites the change or lack of change in a feature considered to be clinically significant in judging recovery from, or progression of, the dysfunction and/or any underlying pathologic condition. If designation of a feature as appearing or disappearing is more important than designation as an existence criterion, that is, present or absent, the feature is defined as a transition criterion. Another example is the definition of pain. Defining pain as mild, moderate, or severe indicates a gradation of the entity. However, defining pain as better or worse indicates a significant clinical change in this index variable. Again, the transitional levels require operational definitions. Aggregate criteria are a cluster of individual variable changes that represent a total effect.[18] Definitional levels of an aggregate criterion may be success and failure; or excellent, good, or fair response to treatment. Success in treatment or excellent results may be determined if all target symptoms and signs have disappeared; good results might be the judgment if all the symptoms have disappeared, but not all the signs. As always, the labels indicating the level of total effect require definition in terms of the individual signs and symptoms comprising the aggregate.

In summary, the diagnosis directs goal setting and treatment. Criteria for assessing goal attainment and treatment outcomes need to be established prior to initiating treatment. Establishing these criteria requires careful analysis and definition of components of the desired outcomes.

Administer the Treatment Program

Implementation of the solution to the patient's clinical problem begins with the initiation of treatment. Administration of the treatment program includes preparation, provision, and modification. Readiness for treatment is required of the clinician, the patient, and, in some instances, the patient's family. The clinician prepares by establishing a schedule, reviewing procedures, and reviewing the sequence of components of the treatment program. Assistance by other personnel is obtained, as indicated. Equipment, materials, and space are procured and prepared. Preparation of any equipment includes determining the safety, operational status, and calibration of equipment. Preparation of the patient includes emotional, cognitive, and physical preparation. Generally, the interaction to prepare the patient for any treatment includes ascertaining the status of the patient from the patient; providing an overview of the treatment program; and relating the elements of the treatment program to the negotiated short-term and long-term goals. The treatment is explained and demonstrated and the purpose of the treatment stated. Expected and possible reactions to treatment are identified, and the patient's role in assisting with the procedure and reporting reactions is determined and explained. Physical preparation of the patient includes appropriate dress or draping, and placing the patient in the most comfortable position appropriate to the procedure. Proper and careful preparation is important to realizing optimal effects of the treatment.

Treatment is then sequentially administered as defined and validated. When the program includes more than one treatment, the sequence of treatments is based on the effect of any one treatment on patient comfort and the effect of one treatment on the response of the patient to subsequent treatments. For example, treatment to alleviate pain may occur first and/or last depending on other treatment objectives. Treatment, such as heat, that positively affects tissue mobility may occur prior to joint mobilization or proprioceptive neuromuscular facilitation techniques to increase range of motion. The priority of the change effected by a given treatment is a third consideration in determining sequence of treatment.

Just as in conducting an examination, the clinician must simultaneously process multiple data and respond in a way that promotes the effectiveness of the treatment intervention. When administering a treatment, the clinician is concurrently doing the following: monitoring his or her own performance of treatment; soliciting and monitoring the patient's participation or performance, cognitively and physically receiving information on the patient's performance; cognitively and physically responding based on the patient's performance; assessing the physical and cognitive interactions with the patient in relation to the patient's responses and modifying those interactions as indicated; and monitoring the safety and the physiologic and emotional stability of the patient. Again, this concurrent processing of information represents an example of problem solving occurring within one phase of a related problem-solving context, that is, total management of the patient. The ability to receive these data and respond appropriately is critical to the success of treatment.

Frequently in rehabilitation of the knee, exercise and adjunct therapy (e.g., ice, heat) are performed by the patient at home as one component of the total treatment program. Monitoring of both the patient's performance and the results of the home program occur on an ongoing basis. The bases for deciding on use of a home program and the components of that program are the same bases discussed previously in identifying a treatment program.

Modification of a given treatment may occur at any point in the administration of treatment. Modification or cessation of treatment occurs whenever the patient's safety may be compromised. Also, if the patient's discomfort exceeds his or her tolerance or compromises the validity of the treatment, the treatment should be modified or stopped, depending on the situation. Additional indications for modifying or stopping a treatment: (1) the patient is not able to provide required assistance or responses; (2) the equipment becomes faulty; or (3) the procedure is not yielding the desired immediate effects.

Evaluate the Effects of the Treatment Program

> Although a clinician can be both a healer and a scientist, he cannot be an effective therapist if he merely joins these two roles in tandem by oscillating between them, adding laboratory science to bedside art. A clinician's objective in therapy is not just a conjunction, but a true synthesis, of art and science, fusing the parts into a whole that unifies his work and makes his two roles one: a scientific healer. A clinician is always a healer; the healing function is basic to his care of sick people. The 'scientific' performance of that function, however, is what distinguishes a well-trained . . . clinician from other healers whose aid and comfort is given without the rational support of valid evidence, logical analysis, and demonstrable proofs.[18]

Evaluation of the effect of the treatment program involves (1) assessment of the previously identified index variables related to the criteria for the goals of treatment and (2) interpretation of the findings of this reassessment. Evaluation of change in certain signs and symptoms (e.g., pain, flexibility, swelling) may occur on an ongoing basis. However, at specific times in the course of treatment, a formal assessment should be made. The timing of this assessment is based on the time frames specified in the short-term and long-term goals, the patient's progress or lack of progress, and related medical care.

In conducting this evaluation, each symptom and significant clinical finding should be reassessed. During the examination, the clinician should also be looking for any undesired effects of treatment. Most importantly, each symptom and sign determined on the initial (and any previous) examination must be accounted for. The data are gathered and organized according to the criteria that were previously established as the bases for determining progress and attainment of goals.

These results are then explained and related to the various aspects of the patient's presentation. The explanation addresses how and why the treatment program accounts for the observed change or lack of change. Additional considerations in explaining the obtained outcomes include the progression and stage of symptoms; other diagnostic findings; the disease process; the patient's medical history; the feasibility of the short-term and long-term goals; other treatment programs, such as medications; and patient compliance.

The result of this analysis is again a clustering of signs and symptoms related by common causes, mechanisms, and effects. The extent to which this clustering and resultant diagnostic label is the same as or different from previous clustering and diagnosis dictates subsequent continuation, modification, or cessation of treatment. If progress toward attainment of functional goals is satisfactory and according to the time frame specified in the criteria, the decision of choice may be to continue treatment. Additional short-term goals and/or criteria may or not be established. If goals have been met, the decision may be to stop treatment. Also, if no progress has been made or the patient is judged as not responding to treatment as expected, treatment may be stopped. The failure of the patient to progress toward attainment of valid short-term goals is an important indicator of a clinical problem beyond the purview of that particular clinician. In this instance, the patient should be referred to another health professional for evaluation.

Implement Modifications of the Treatment Program

Modification of treatment is based on patient status and rate of progress. If patient status reflects positive movement toward attainment of goals, treatment is usually continued. However, components of treatment may be changed based on the rate of progress or change in any one or more index symptoms or signs. The decision to modify the treatment program necessitates a concomitant reconsideration and probable modification of short-term goals.

Modification of a treatment is based on the following considerations related to patient status and rate of progress: medical safety of the patient; patient comfort relative to demands of a treatment procedure; the patient's ability to provide required assistance; the effect of the measure on the target symptom or sign; indications for the treatment; priorities of treatment; related treatment by other health professionals; and patient resources. Patient change may be positive or negative with regard to any one of the above considerations. For example, a patient with a ligament reconstruction or total knee replacement may have progressed to the point of being able to independently perform exercises. In that instance, exercise may become only a component of the patient's home program. Conversely, a patient with arthritis may have degenerated or experienced an exacerbation such that exercise, previously done at home, can now only be performed with clinician assistance and following adjunct treatment.

In determining and implementing revised goals, related treatment, and criteria, the clinician is again at the problem-solving stages of determining and administering treatment. The difference is that the clinician now has additional data on which to base treatment and judge the effectiveness of treatment in achieving desired functional outcomes. This recycling through the problem-solving process continues until the decision to stop treatment is reached.

SUMMARY

Clinical problem solving is a multidimensional process that has a logical sequence. The goal of the clinician is to resolve the patient's problem(s) and facilitate the patient's attainment of desired functional goals. Achievement of the clinician's goal and the patient's goal requires systematic and thorough data collection as a basis for diagnosis and related goal setting, and for treatment planning and implementation. The clinician's expertise, experience, and discipline are the determinants of success in clinical problem solving.

REFERENCES

1. Magistro, CM: Clinical decision making in physical therapy: A practitioner's perspective. Phys Ther 69:7, 1989.
2. Boissonault, WG and Janos, SC: Screening for medical disease: Physical therapy assessment and treatment principles. In Boissonault, WG (ed): Examination in Physical Therapy Practice: Screening for Medical Disease. Churchill Livingstone, New York, 1991.
3. Rose, SJ: Physical therapy diagnosis: Role and function. Phys Ther 69:7, 1989.
4. Travers, RMW: Essentials of Learning. Macmillan, New York, 1977.
5. Hislop, HJ: Clinical decision making: Educational, data, and risk factors. In Wolf, SL (ed): Clinical Decision Making in Physical Therapy. FA Davis, Philadelphia, 1985.
6. Sahrmann, S: Diagnosis by the physical therapist: A prerequisite for treatment. Phys Ther 68:11, 1988.
7. Watts, NT: Decision Analysis: A tool for improving physical therapy practice and education. In Wolf, SL (ed): Clinical Decision Making in Physical Therapy. FA Davis, Philadelphia, 1985.
8. Watts, NT: Clinical decision analysis. Phys Ther 69:7, 1989.
9. Echternach, JL and Rothstein, JM: Hypothesis-oriented algorithms. Phys Ther 69:7, 1989.
10. Shervchuk, RM and Francis, KT: Principles of clinical decision-making: An introduction to decision analysis. Phys Ther 68:3, 1988.
11. Zimmy, NJ and Tandy, CJ: Problem-knowledge coupling: A tool for physical therapy clinical practice. Phys Ther 69:2, 1989.

12. Jette, AM: Diagnosis and classification by physical therapists: A special communication. Phys Ther 69:11, 1989.
13. Jette, AM: Measuring subjective clinical outcomes. Phys Ther 69:7, 1989.
14. Delitto, A: Subjective measures and clinical decision making. Phys Ther 69:7, 1989.
15. Bohannon, RW: Objective measures. Phys Ther 69:7, 1989.
16. Schenkman, M and Butler, R: A model for multisystem evaluation, interpretation, and treatment of individuals with neurologic dysfunction. Phys Ther 69:7, 1989.
17. Rose Garden: The Clinical Practice of Physical Therapy in the 21st Century. Executive Communications, Inc., Pittsburgh, 1992.
18. Feinstein, AR: Clinical Judgment. Robert E. Kreiger Publishing, Malabar, FL, 1967.
19. Wolf, SL: Summation: Identification of principles underlying clinical decisions. In Wolf, SL (ed): Clinical Decision Making in Physical Therapy. FA Davis, Philadelphia, 1985.
20. Kessler, RM and Hertling, D: Assessment of musculoskeletal disorders. In Kessler, R and Hertling, D: Management of Common Musculoskeletal Disorders. JB Lippincott, Philadelphia, 1990.

CHAPTER **4**

Physiology of Soft-Tissue Healing

Holly R. Ford, MSEd, PT

Soft-tissue injury results in a series of time-phased events that are chemically mediated and influenced by external factors. These external factors include the application of therapeutic exercise. In the presence of protective or soft-tissue injuries, the goal of treatment is to balance the application of exercise with the phases of healing. This approach entails the integration of the time constraints of soft-tissue healing with the return of function. Successful rehabilitation is predicated upon understanding the biomechanics of joint function, the effects of immobilization, the time constraints associated with the phases of healing, and the effects of exercise on soft tissue.[1] The process of healing may slightly differ between kinds of tissue but generally follows a similar basic sequence of events.

Most macrotrauma injuries to the knee involve disruption of ligaments. Therefore, this chapter focuses primarily on the healing phases of ligaments in the knee, with subsections that briefly review the healing of other commonly injured tissues. Specific information includes the causes of cell death, the biomechanics of ligaments, factors influencing the healing rate, the stages of healing, and the effects of immobilization on the healing ligament. Also presented is a discussion of the healing of biologic and synthetic graft materials.

CAUSES OF CELL DEATH

The many causes of cell death include anoxia; excessive use of physical, chemical, or biologic agents; trauma; excessive radiant energy; derangements of the immune system; and genetic defects.[2] Cell injury results in the dramatic process of necrosis within the cell. This process includes cloudy swelling of the cytoplasm, hydropic or vacuolar degenerations, mucoid degeneration, fading of the nuclear chromatin, hyaline degeneration, and fatty metamorphosis.[2]

Trauma

Macrotrauma to the knee often results in ligamentous injury with necrosis of the fibrocyte cells.[2,3] Ligaments provide medial, lateral, and rotational stability to the knee joint through the tibial and fibular collateral ligaments and joint capsule, respectively. Anterior and posterior stability is provided by the anterior and posterior cruciate ligaments.[4] These ligaments are particularly prone to trauma because the knee has minimal osseous stability.[4] Trauma to ligament results in a microscopic rupture of the cell membrane with intracellular dislocation.[2,3]

The tibial collateral ligament (TCL) is the ligament most frequently involved in injury, but all ligaments are subject to rupture or failure.[3,5] Ligament injuries may result from contact or noncontact activities.[3] The most common mechanism of contact injury results from a blow to the lateral aspect of the knee, resulting in external rotation, valgus, and possibly hyperextension.[3] The most common noncontact injury is that of deceleration, as seen with cutting in football.[3] Chapter 2 reviews the common mechanisms of ligamentous and meniscal injuries to the knee.

BIOMECHANICS OF LIGAMENTS

Ligaments contain a large cross section of collagen fibers and are able to withstand great force, or stress.[6] Stress may be defined as the internal force per unit of cross-sectional area in response to external force.[6] Many models have been developed to represent the response of a ligament to stress.[7-10] Stresses may be placed on a ligament perpendicular to the cross section of fibers (tensile stress), parallel to the cross section of fibers (shear stress), or as a shortening or squeezing force to the fiber cross section (compression stress).[11] Each of these stresses affects the ligament in a different manner. Tensile stress will cause stretching or elongation, shearing stress will elicit a shape change perpendicular to the parallel arrangement of the collagen fibers, and compressive stress will result in a contraction or shortening of the ligament. Ligaments are best able to resist tensile stresses.

Ligaments respond to tensile stresses in a consistent manner. This response is graphically illustrated by a stress-strain model (Fig. 4–1). Stress, as previously mentioned, is force per unit area. Strain is defined as elongation per unit length.

Initially the tissue elongates with minimal stress. This elongation is referred to as the toe region on the stress-strain curve. Most researchers agree that this response is a result of the wavy pattern of helically arranged collagen fibers in the ligament straightening into a parallel formation.[11,12] Ligament is composed primarily of collagen fibers, interspersed with small amounts of elastic and reticular fibers.[22,23] As a greater force is applied to a ligament, the ligament will elastically stretch. Eventually the ligament will reach the limits of its elasticity; further tension will result in microscopic tears. The amount of force required to further stretch the ligament will decrease, resulting in less stress per unit strain. As the increase in tensile force is continued, more collagen fibers are disrupted, and the stress per unit strain ratio will significantly diminish until a point is reached where the ligament is permanently elongated.[6] Tensile failure can occur within the midsubstance of the ligament, at a bony avulsion, or at the tenoperiosteal insertion site.[4,6]

Failure in the midsubstance of the ligament is likely if the injury occurs quickly, not allowing time for protective response by the muscles.[4,5] Rapid loading does not allow

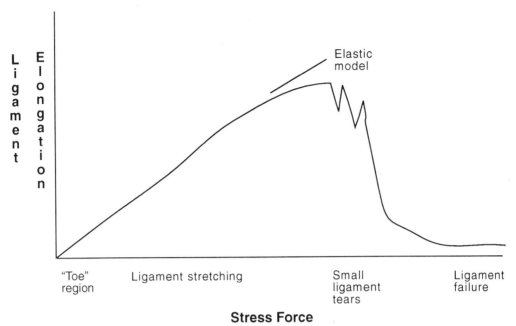

FIGURE 4–1. Graph illustrating how a ligament responds to stress, with the initial toe region resulting from an unwinding of the wavy pattern of collagen fibers followed by the elastic response of the ligament. Small dips are noted when tears or ruptures occur in the ligament. Eventually, as more ligament fibers are compromised, the ligament becomes permanently elongated.

the stimulation of ligamentous mechanoreceptors to reflexively recruit muscular protection around the knee joint.[5,22] Conversely, a slower rate of loading is likely to result in insertional site failure.[22] The insertional site is where the ligament inserts into the bone. Therefore, insertional site failure occurs at the ligament-bone interface. Other factors influencing the failure rate of a ligament include age, weight, gender, endocrine status, physical activity level, pH (the degree of acidity or alkalinity of the blood and tissue), and previous immobility.[6,18,24-37]

In the presence of midsubstance ligament injury, fibers at the injury site will appear frayed, similar to a mop end.[6] This type of tear or failure is most common in the adult population.[6,24] Unfortunately, if the midsubstance of the ligament is poorly vascularized, as is the case with the anterior cruciate ligament (ACL), and nutrition through the synovium is not available, the result is rapid degeneration of the ligament.[6,24-27]

A bony avulsion usually occurs through the cancellous bone beneath the insertion site.[6] This lesion is most prevalent in children and adolescents and usually occurs at the tibial insertion site. An additional complication in a child or adolescent is an epiphyseal plate fracture.[5]

The insertion site contains several zones in which the failure may occur.[6,38-40] These zone are transitions of ligament to fibrocartilage, fibrocartilage to mineralized fibrocartilage, and mineralized fibrocartilage to cortical bone.[6,22] Each zone differs in its histologic components and provides a gradual progression from the flexible ligament to the firm bone.[6,22] Failure may occur within any of these zones, but the transition zone between mineralized fibrocartilage and bone is particularly prone to injury.[2] Laros and associates[41] found that immobilization of dog knees weakened the tibial insertion site more than the femoral insertion site. Immobilization was characterized by resorption of Haversian bone and weakening of the bone cortex, which resulted in weakening of the ligament as well as bony avulsions.[41] According to some authorities,[5,22,24] the TCL insertion sites are the weakest, compared with other ligaments, which could partially explain the high occurrence of TCL injury. Nevertheless, the close proximity of the TCL insertion sites with the synovium provides a vascular and protective sheath to the ligament. Therefore, TCL failures do not degenerate to the same degree as do other ligamentous failures.[5,22,24]

FACTORS INFLUENCING HEALING RATE

The degree of trauma will influence the rate of healing.[42] A ligament may be sprained even if complete failure of the ligament does not occur.[4,6] Sprains are usually classified by grade according to their severity, with grade I being a mild sprain with no increased joint laxity, grade II a moderate sprain with minimal laxity, and grade III a severe, complete disruption with significant laxity.[3] The majority of ligamentous injuries consist of partial tears (grades I and II).[5] Most partial tears and some complete grade III tears do not require surgical intervention, although treatment approaches vary based on the injured ligament. For example, the treatment choice for complete tears to the ACL is repair or reconstruction (see Chapter 9), whereas isolated grade III TCL tears usually are treated nonsurgically with aggressive rehabilitation (see Chapter 12).

The severity of trauma will dictate the amount of cell death and tissue necrosis. Chronic ligamentous injury can result in knee joint instability and may lead to damage of other structures such as the menisci, articulating surfaces, and tendons.

A multitude of environmental conditions can influence the rate and quality of healing. Some of these factors or conditions are infection; diabetes; oxygen gradient; nutritional deficiencies (especially vitamin A, vitamin C, or protein); cortisone/steroid therapy; radiation; suturing techniques; dressings; age; anemia; blood and tissue pH; heparin; nicotine; electromagnetic fields; and even stress factors such as heat, cold, or noise.[43-49] These factors can have a significant effect on normal cellular activities, and their importance is accentuated in the case of ligament injury, which makes their role crucial to the result of the healing process.[46] The significance of these factors varies according to the stage of healing.

STAGES OF HEALING

Ligamentous healing progresses through a series of events and stages. These stages are labeled inflammatory, granulation, fibroblastic, and maturation.[45,50] A synopsis of the stages of healing, relative time frames, characteristics of healing, and therapeutic considerations is presented in Table 4–1.

Inflammatory Stage

Inflammation is an immediate protective response to a cell injury and lasts for approximately 72 hours.[3] The inflammatory response destroys, dilutes, or isolates the injurious agent, and/or the cells, which may have been injured.[17] Five signs that characterize the inflammatory stage are calor, rubor, tumor, dolor, and functio laesa.[2,3,45]

TABLE 4–1 Stages of Ligament Healing

	Inflammatory	Granulation	Fibroblastic	Maturation
Time frame	1–72 hr	24–72 hr	18 hr–6 wk	12–18 mo
Characteristics	Increased vascularity, edema, pain, decreased function, PMNs begin phagocytosis	Progressive development of capillary buds, loops, and networks	Fibroblasts attracted and begin collagen synthesis Collagenase begins lysis	Collagen fibers mature and become more dense
Therapeutic considerations	Rest, ice, compression, elevation, TENS, and CPM Avoid aspirin	Avoid heat and excess movement Ingest protein	Avoid cortisone, initiate controlled exercise, and mobilization of soft tissues Ingest vitamin C	Progressively advanced with exercises

Calor and rubor are, respectively, an increase in temperature and a reddening of the injured area that results from increased vascularity.[2] The latter may be difficult to observe with an injury to internal structures, such as the cruciate ligaments. Injured blood vessels allow blood to enter the injured area, filling in any potential space in the ligament.[3] For optimal healing to occur, the torn fibers must remain continuous or in a well-vascularized area. An initial vasoconstriction is regulated by histamine, which prevents excessive leakage of blood and fluid from the surrounding blood vessels.[44,51,52] This response lasts from 5 to 10 minutes and allows for the aggregation and coagulation of platelet cells to seal off the injured blood vessel(s) and lymphatic channels.[44-46,51] Platelet cells adhere to injured collagen fibers in the presence of midsubstance ligament tears.[6,46] The platelets also release constituents such as histamine, serotonin, and brady-kinins, which increase vascular permeability.[3,44,45,51] This response is reinforced by chemicals such as prostaglandins, which are released by the injured tissues and initiate vasodilation in noninjured blood vessels. Use of steroids or aspirin inhibits the release of prostaglandin.[51]

The increased permeability and vasodilation of nearby blood vessels result in the third cardinal sign of inflammation: tumor. Tumor, or the inflammatory edema that is derived from the blood, fills all the spaces in the injured area and surrounds all damaged structures.[44,50,53,57] Joint effusion results from injury to the synovial membrane of the knee.[5] Mast cells then release hyaluronic acid and other proteoglycans into the injured area; these, in turn, bind with the watery, edematous fluid and create a gel.[51] This gel is in contact with all injured structures and binds them together as one wound.[54]

Edema is a normal and important process within healing.[5,51] Too little edema can slow the healing process. Excessive edema in the injured area can stimulate excessive scar formation, cause pain, limit motion, and reflexively limit quadriceps femoris and hamstring muscle activity, leading to muscle atrophy.[1,5,51] Joint effusion of 20 to 30 ml can reflexively inhibit the quadriceps femoris muscle; effusion of 30 to 40 ml can reduce both quadriceps femoris and hamstring muscle activity.[55]

The effusion may influence the positioning of the joint. Activation of joint mechanoreceptors in the presence of effusion facilitates muscle action to position a joint in its "loosely packed" position to lessen the joint pressure.[55] For the injured knee, this position is in approximately 30 degrees of flexion[5] and is maintained in the presence of joint effusion. An effused knee joint results in reflex inhibition of the quadriceps femoris muscle, a flexion contracture, and an inability to walk normally.[2,45] Decreased function may be related to dolor, which is pain resulting from physical pressure or chemical irritation of the nerve fibers.[2,5,45,56,57] Dolor may also elicit muscle spasm in the adjacent area.[5] Rest is advised during first 24 to 48 hours postinjury. Joint movement could possibly reopen sealed blood vessels and lymph channels, leading to an excessive inflammatory response and possibly a hematoma.[50,51] The ligament must not be exposed to harmful stresses during this period so as to allow normal healing to progress.[58] The classic regimen of RICE (rest, ice, compression, and elevation) is recommended.[59,60] An epidural block or the use of a transcutaneous electrical nerve stimulation (TENS) may be employed to decrease pain (dolor).[56,57,61-66]

During this phase, the patient initially is non–weight bearing or weight bearing as tolerated and may be immobilized by a cast or brace.[67] In most cases, strict immobilization is detrimental and should be avoided. Partial immobilization is usually accompanied by isometric muscle contractions, to prevent muscle atrophy and to facilitate dynamic stabilization of the knee joint.

The patient may be placed on a continuous passive motion (CPM) machine to provide movement to the joint. This activity allows tissues in the knee to gain nutrition through a pumping mechanism, while not disrupting the healing structures.[67-69] Thus the CPM serves as a means to stimulate healing, particularly of articular cartilage.[70] The use of CPM results in continuous proprioceptive impulses that override sensations of pain, thus allowing for increased motion.[71,72] Additionally, CPM may reduce hemarthrosis following surgery.[71]

Simultaneously, as the five signs of inflammation begin to develop, polymorphonuclear cells (PMNs), which exist in large numbers in the peripheral blood, migrate to the injured site minutes after the injury[2,3,44,52,73] (Fig. 4-2). The PMNs are chemically attracted to the injured site by C3a and C5a, which are generated by complement activation in the formation of the platelet seal, and by anaphylotoxins. Complements are a series of plasma proteins that are released at the site of injury due to an antibody-antigen reaction. Anaphylotoxin is a substance composed of small polypeptides split from C3a and C4a, which are enzymatic components of complements. These components of the complement are involved in a great number of immune defense mechanisms, including chemotaxis and phagocytosis. Polymorphonuclear cells are followed by the accumulation of monocyte, histocyte, and macrophage cells, the latter of which will dominate the site in 24 to 36 hours postinjury.[2,44,45,51] Steroids interfere with the healing process by inhibiting the amount and mobility of PMNs and monocytes.[45,46,51]

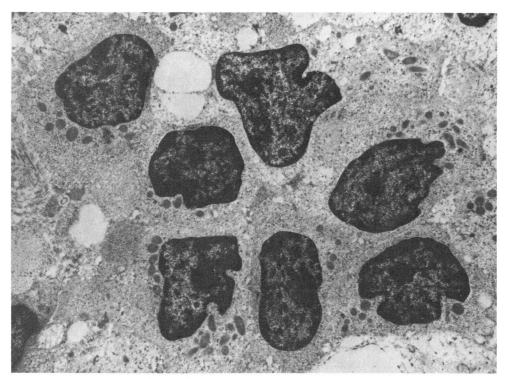

FIGURE 4-2. A group of polymorphonuclear cells (PMNs) magnified 8,300 times as seen in the inflammatory stage. (Courtesy of George Price, electron microscopist, Orlando Regional Medical Center.)

The macrophages and PMNs begin the process of phagocytosis, or the engulfing and subsequent destruction of debris and any foreign matter. Mast cells may assist in this process as well, by liberating polysaccharides and enzymes.[44,45] The latter, which include heparin, histamine, and a variety of other hydrolytic enzymes, assist in the breakdown and absorption of debris and also of collagen.[44,45] This process is one of cleaning the injured area of bacteria, foreign objects, and necrotic tissue to prevent or lessen infection.[43,44,50,51] Macrophages and PMNs are assisted in phagocytosis by C3b, an enzymatic component of complement, which binds to particles and objects and promotes their recognition as necrotic debris.[52]

Macrophage cells continue to migrate to the injured area and serve as the primary agent in the destruction of tissue debris. Macrophages produce amino acids, simple sugars, ascorbic acid, lactic acid, and hydrogen peroxide as a by-product of phagocytosis.[45,51] The amino acids and simple sugars are used later in repair processes.[45] Ascorbic and lactic acids signal the extent of damage and the need for more phagocytic cells in the injured area.[51] Hydrogen peroxide aids in the control of anaerobic microbial growth. Macrophages also produce interleukin 1 (IL-1) which enhances lymphocyte proliferation and processes; fibronectin, which is chemotactic to fibroblasts; and MDGF (macrophage-derived growth factor), a substance that stimulates neovascularization.[51,52,73]

The use of steroids inhibits the macrophage cells, resulting in decreased debridement and a delay in the healing process.[5,26,46,51] The use of low-dosage pulsed ultrasound during this phase can significantly reduce the chance of infection.[60] Ultrasound agitation may disintegrate some macrophages, which, in turn, will stimulate an even greater number of phagocytic cells into the area.[51] However, macrophages that are chronically activated may result in chronic inflammation.

THERAPEUTIC CONSIDERATIONS DURING THE INFLAMMATORY STAGE

In the inflammatory stage, or the first 72 hours following an injury, aspirin or steroids should not be administered.[6,45,46,51] The classic regimen of rest, ice, compression, and elevation is recommended during this stage.[58-60] CPM may be applied to reduce pain, provide joint nutrition, and reduce hemarthrosis.[69-72] Immoblization is discouraged but, if necessary, should be accompanied by isometric exercises. A patient should be non–weight bearing, or weight bearing as tolerated.[67] Low-dosage pulsed ultrasound may be utilized if a chance of infection exists[51] (see Table 4–1).

Granulation Stage

The granulation stage begins within the first 24 hours after injury and overlaps the inflammatory stage. The granulation stage is named for the small red granules that begin to appear within the injured area.[50] These granules are actually capillary buds or sprouts, which grow from the incised or injured area or from the periphery of the injured area.[50,51] Capillary buds are stimulated by angiogenesis factors released by macrophage cells.[3] Angiogenesis factors are a group of polypeptides that act in one of two ways: to stimulate vascular endothelial cells to move or divide; or to act indirectly by mobilizing macrophages to release endothelial growth factors. As capillary buds develop, they join to form capillary loops, and eventually capillary networks.[50,51]

In the capillary bud stage, the healing tissue is very delicate and easily injured. Immobilization is recommended to prevent damage to these fragile vessels and thus promote vascular regrowth.[51] Early motion may result in microhemorrhaging and increase the likelihood of infection.[74] Heat is contraindicated during this phase because of the risk of injury to the delicate vessels, and consequent blood loss.[75] Diabetes and protein deficiency have been found to impair the development of these vessels.[45] Patients who are involved in preinjury aerobic exercise programs usually have increased tissue capillarization, which may facilitate blood flow and oxygenation to the healing ligaments.[6,23,64] The healing process is expedited with a constant supply of oxygen and nourishment to the injured tissues through a functioning circulatory system.

THERAPEUTIC CONSIDERATIONS DURING THE GRANULATION STAGE

During granulation, 24 to 72 hours after injury, motion should be limited.[52] Heat is contraindicated.[75] Patients should ingest a sufficient amount of protein to facilitate the development of blood vessels during this phase[45] (see Table 4–1).

Fibroblastic Stage

During the fibroblastic stage the vascularization process reaches maturity (48 to 72 hours).[3] *Fibrinolysin*, produced from blood vessels, acts to dissolve clots and reopen the lymphatic channels, promoting resorption of exudate. Later in the fibroblastic stage, some of the capillary loops will cease functioning and retract, which makes the injured area, if visible, no longer appear reddened but actually white.[51]

Because the MDGF reaches an optimal level in 6 to 8 hours, the fibroblasts begin to respond and are attracted to the injured site within the next 18 hours.[6,45,56,76] Fibroblast migration results from platelet-derived growth factor (PDGF) released from platelets during clotting.[51] A topical application of PDGF may be used to stimulate fibroplasia in chronic, nonhealing open wounds.

The fibrin strands composing the clot and dispersed throughout the coagulated wound gel provide the passageway for fibroblasts to enter the injured area at all tissue levels.[45,50,52] Fibroblasts may develop from pericyte cells, which are a form of mesenchymal cells; from perivascular connective tissue adjacent to the injured area; or from large mononuclear cells in the blood.[43–45,50,51,77] Characteristics of the fibroblasts include a large number of mitochondria and an extensive, highly developed, rough endoplasmic recticulum, which is used to synthesize and secrete protein for the ultimate production of collagen[44,45,50,78] (Fig. 4–3). Fibroblasts produce extracellular scar matrix as well as collagen.[2,77] Various factors in the environment of the injured area influence the synthesis and secretion of collagen from the fibroblast. Those factors include diabetes, cortisone, lactic acid, blood and tissue pH, oxygen, protein, uremia, ascorbic acid, zinc, iron, copper, and the presence of synovial fluid.[3,43–45,50,79] Collagen is an amino acid containing large amounts of glycine, proline, hydroxyproline, and hydroxylysine.[6,44,53,80–82] Hydroxyproline cannot be ingested but must be synthesized by hydroxylation of proline.[44,53,83] A deficiency in vitamin C (ascorbic acid), iron, or oxygen decreases the conversion of proline to hydroxyproline, and cortisone completely halts the conversion.[45,46,53,83]

The fibroblast cells (see Fig. 4–3) initially produce three polypeptide chains, which form a right-handed helix called procollagen.[6,44,51,80–82,84] Weak electrostatic forces aid in the bonding of these three chains. During this phase, salt water application, vibration,

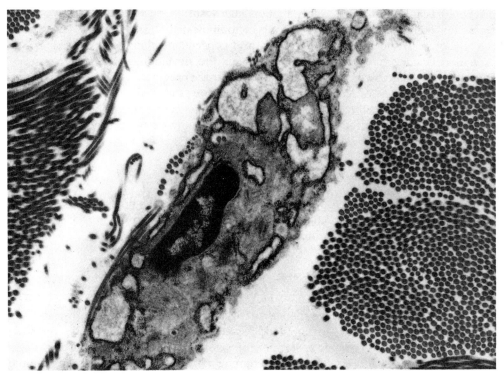

FIGURE 4-3. A fibroblast magnified 17,300 times with an extensive, highly developed rough endoplasmic recticulum which is used during synthesis and secretion of protein for the production of collagen. (Courtesy of George Price, electron microscopist, Orlando Regional Medical Center.)

heat, and enzymes can denature and/or separate these chains. Once exocytosed, the procollagen forms intramolecular bonds or cross-links at specific terminal sites and is then labeled tropocollagen.[44,51,81] The intramolecular cross-links are covalent bonds, which produce a stable molecule.[85,86] Tropocollagen molecules form intermolecular cross-links with each other and result in collagen fibrils[44] (Fig. 4-4). Hydroxylysine is essential for the formation of intermolecular cross-links.[6] Cross-links allow the healing ligament to tolerate early controlled motion without disruption.[51]

Collagen fibers are surrounded by a ground substance of water, hyaluronic acid, chondroitin sulfate, mucopolysaccharides, and glycosaminoglycans (GAG), which are produced by fibroblasts.[6,9,22] The ground substance provides lubrication between moving collagen fibers and assists with the maintenance of the collagen fibril molecular arrangement.[22,51,87,88] Decreased ground substance may occur as a result of immobilization.[89]

Because the fibrin strands on which the fibroblasts traveled are randomly dispersed throughout the injured area, collagen produced by the fibroblast cells is also randomly aligned[73,90] (Fig. 4-5). A thin cytoplasmic extension that exists between adjacent fibroblast cells may assist in providing some structural integrity to developing ligaments and tendons.[87]

The collagen fiber network develops and forms layers of tissue. The development of a collagen network was examined by Frank and colleagues,[91] in untreated healing defects of TCLs in dogs. Figure 4-6 demonstrates the appearance of the healing TCLs 10 through 40 weeks after experimental injury. A transparent scar gradually bridged the

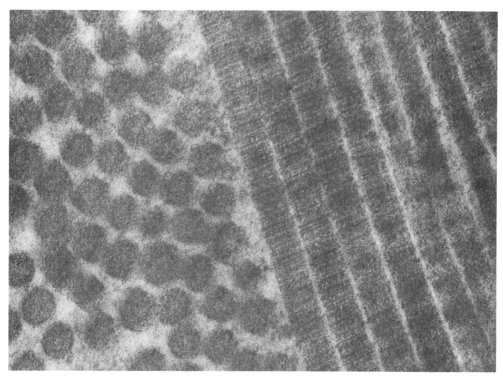

FIGURE 4–4. Collagen fibers magnified 91,700 times shown in cross-sectional and longitudinal views. (Courtesy of George Price, electron microscopist, Orlando Regional Medical Center.)

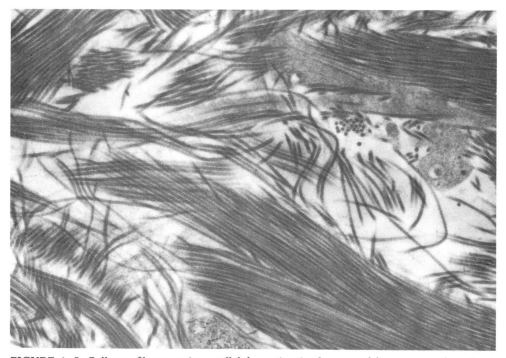

FIGURE 4–5. Collagen fibers are in parallel formation in the normal ligaments and randomly dispersed in areas in which newly formed fibers are not yet stressed into parallel alignment. Magnification 17,300 times. (Courtesy of George Price, electron microscopist, Orlando Regional Medical Center.)

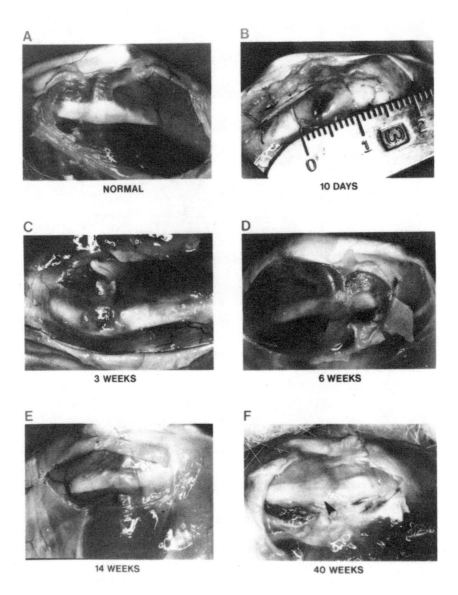

FIGURE 4-6. The "gap" between the ends of an experimentally injured TCL in a canine at 10 days through 40 weeks. *A*) A normal TCL taken from the contralateral control limb of a canine. *B*) Macroscopic appearance of the experimentally torn TCL at 10 days. Note the bloody appearance within the injured tissue. This appearance characterizes the late inflammatory stage of healing. *C*) At 3 weeks, the torn ends were beginning to scar, although the injured area appeared edematous and hemorrhagic. *D*) At 6 weeks, the "gap" between the injured end of the TCL had bridged with scar, which contained a combination of type I and type III collagen fibers. This stage coincides with late fibroplasia. *E*) At 14 weeks the edema and hemorrhage in the "gap" reduced considerably. *F*) The TCL at 40 weeks postinjury had healed significantly; the injured area appeared similar to the normal ligament in *A*. This stage of healing represents late maturation. (From Frank et al,[91] p 383, with permission.)

dense, dull white ends of the original ligament[3,6,91] (see Fig. 4 – 6). Histologic examination indicated that collagen fibers continued to develop in diameter, number, and alignment throughout the fibroblastic stage (up to 6 weeks) and into the maturation stage[91] (Fig. 4 – 7).

A carefully supervised exercise program increases collagen and proteoglycan biosynthesis in ligaments and in tendons. Early exercises are performed in such a way that the repair is not disrupted and gentle stresses are provided to the remodeling scar.[1,2] The frequency of exercise should be slowly and progressively increased.[10] Stress from controlled exercise causes the collagen fibers to move from a random position and align parallel to the direction of stress. Ligament collagen fiber bundles may be aligned in parallel, oblique, or spiral arrangements adapting to the particular ligament's function of restraining and controlling joint displacement.[6] Secondary effects of early exercise are to prevent muscle atrophy and joint adhesions and to maintain joint nutrition.[22,71,72]

The type of collagen formed during this stage is primarily type III with a smaller portion of type I.[3,73,80,91,92] Type III collagen provides stabilization to the extracellular collagen meshwork.[3] As the scar matures and remodels, type III is replaced by type I.[73,82,92] This change may take up to 15 months.[73]

Collagen is responsible for the strength of the ligament.[44,45,73] This strength, usually referred to as tensile strength, is not dependent on the amount of collagen produced or the number of fibers, but rather on the number of microscopic intermolecular and intramolecular cross-links.[89] Radiation will decrease tensile strength, though a dose less than 100 rad (radiation absorbed dose) (1 Gy) has little effect on the formation and number of intermolecular and intramolecular cross-links.[43] X-rays have little effect because their radiation is usually 1 rad (0.01 Gy) or less. Tensile strength is also influenced by resuturing, which increases the rate of cross-linking, although this mechanism is not fully understood.[44]

Scar should possess extensibility as well as tensile strength. The extensibility of scar is derived from the structure of a loose network of fibers with redundant folds.[45] These folds (which some refer to as waves) allow the scar mobility, much like a spring composed of nonelastic metal.

A wave pattern exists in the collagen fibers to allow for greater extensibility and to permit the fibers to align themselves in the direction of any imposed stress.[45,50,73] Elastic fibers, which constitute a small portion of the intercellular matrix of tendons and ligaments, may contribute to this wavy collagen-fiber formation.[78,93] The elastic properties of ligaments and tendons can be modified by the ratio of soluble to insoluble collagen, the water content, and by changes in the intramolecular and intermolecular bonding of collagen.[23,33,94-96]

In an open wound the epithelial cells at the edge of the injured site begin to undergo hypertrophy and hyperplasia.[43,45,73] This division of cells varies with age, activity, and menstruation.[43] The increase in mitotic rate of epidermal cells cannot be explained by an increase of blood supply or release of mitotic hormones, in that the rate only increases in those cells adjacent to the injured area.[43] The theory is that a mitotic inhibitor, chalone, is temporarily lost with the break in the epidermis from the injury.[73,89,90,97]

If the injured area is viable and has a good blood supply, migration of epithelial cells moves along the bioelectrical gradient that has developed between the junctions of normal and injured tissues.[43,52,73] This delicate layer of cells will prevent loss of fluid, act as a barrier to infection, and serve as a protective covering.[45] Epithelial cells that contact eschar (necrotic tissue), foreign material, sutures, or blood clots will migrate down-

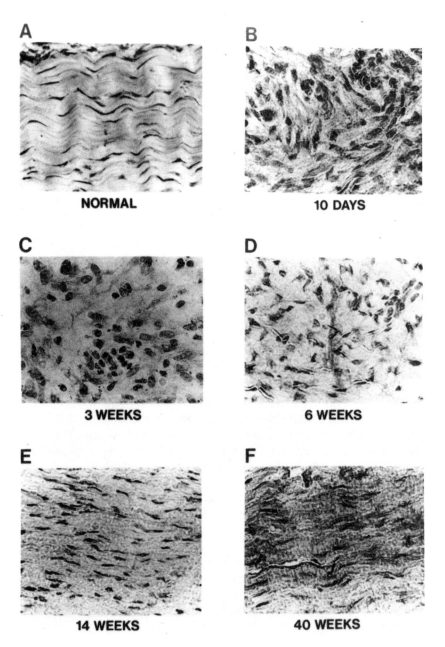

FIGURE 4-7. Histological analysis of tissue from experimental untreated midsubstance tears of TCLs in canines taken during intervals of healing. From the initial injury to 10 days, the ligament healing site is infiltrated with large oval inflammatory cells which represented the inflammatory stage of healing. From 10 days to 3 weeks thin, long fibrocyte cells were seen within the healing site along with deposition of collagen fibers. According to Frank et al, maximum collagenization occurred at approximately 3 weeks postinjury. However, many of these collagen fibers were of the type III variety, as opposed to type I collagen fibers which predominate in normal ligament. In addition, the collagen fibers at 3 weeks were randomly oriented and provided very little tensile strength. The photograph at 6 weeks shows that the collagen fibers have begun to orient along the lines of stress. Biomechanical analysis indicated that the TCL was developing tensile strength, although the tensile strength was well below that of the normal contralateral TCL in the canine limb that served as a control. The stage of healing at 6 weeks represented late fibroplasia and the beginning of maturation. From 6 weeks to 40 weeks, the collagen fibers continued to orient along the lines of stress, increase the number of intermolecular cross links, and convert from type III to type I fibers. However, biomechanical analysis indicated that at 14 weeks postinjury, the tensile strength of the healing TCL was approximately 40 percent of the normal control ligament. The restoration of full tensile strength of the healing ligament remains below the normal ligament at 40 weeks postinjury. (From Frank et al,[91] p 384, with permission.)

ward.[43,90] This leads to the destruction of living tissue and collagenous ground substance by the lytic enzymes produced by the epithelial cells.[73] Various factors can influence epithelization. Epithelization is decreased by hypothermia, scab formation or necrotic tissue, poor oxygenation, protein deficiency, or cortisone (although the effect of cortisone may be reversed by vitamin A), increased by moderate hyperthermia (up to 40° C), and facilitated by moist dressings.[43-45,73,90,98-100]

Epithelial cells maintain contact with their parent cell and subsequently may exert a pull on the normal skin around the wound edge. Contact between epithelial cells results in a cessation of movement.[101] Several weeks are then required for the delicate covering to become multilayered.[46] Necrotic tissue and dry exudate form the scab, which will slough off after the multilayered epithelium is formed.[73]

Epithelial cells, as well as PMNs, eosinophil leukocytes, and the granulation bed, produce the potent enzyme *collagenase*.[46,102] Collagenase requires zinc and calcium for its activities.[81] Collagenase is capable of breaking the bonds between tropocollagen fibers, thus making the molecule soluble.[46,81] This soluble collagen molecule will then be excreted as waste.[103] Thus, while collagen synthesis continues at a high rate, the lysis of collagen by collagenase holds the scar in balance.

There are cases, such as those of the hypertrophic scar or keloid, where the genetic inhibition of lysis offsets scar balance. Balance may be restored by the application of pressure (greater than 22 mm Hg) to the scar.[98] Prolonged pressure leads to an ischemic condition with decreased oxygen tension. Collagen synthesis, which is oxygen dependent, is therefore suppressed by the lack of oxygen.[100] However, the lysis of collagen is not oxygen dependent; thus collagen continues to break down into a soluble material.[100] Balance between scar lysis and synthesis is achieved when the scar is level with adjacent tissue, but pressure should not be removed until remodeling is completed and the rate of collagen synthesis has returned to normal. As long as the scar exhibits a pinkish coloring, remodeling is likely underway.

Wound closure usually occurs within 5 days in a small, clean wound, whereas larger wounds may require from 8 days to 3 weeks.[45,50] Incision sites begin to contract, decreasing the surface area, while the surrounding tissue is thinned and stretched under the tension.[45,51] If closure does not occur within 3 weeks, contraction usually ceases due to the resistance of the stretched tissues. Fibroblasts play an important role at this stage. Some fibroblasts contain *myofibrils*, which are similar to actomyosin contractile units and are thus highly contractile.[44,45,54,73] These *myofibroblasts*, as they are called, are activated by kinins and prostaglandins and attach along the margins of the incision. Myofibroblasts pull the layers of the incision inward.[50,73,90,104] Incision contraction is diminished or alleviated by irradiation, skin grafts, and cortisone.

Internal and external forces such as muscle tension, joint movement, passive gliding, fascial planes, soft-tissue loading and unloading, splinting, temperature changes, and mobilization provide stress and strain that influence the remodeling of collagen.[62] As stress is applied to the ligament, a small direct current is produced.[50] This piezoelectric current may facilitate alignment of collagen fibers. Fibroblasts and collagen fibers begin to migrate and realign themselves parallel to the lines of tension.[44,45]

The application of stress or tension is directly related to an increase in tensile strength of the ligament.[99,105-111] Exercises that promote muscle tension and joint mobility as well as patellar mobilization also facilitate scar tensile strength. Various tissues, including fascia, skin, tendon, ligament, cartilage, bone, and capsule, lose tensile strength when deprived of stress or when they have been immobilized.[99,105-109,112,113] Vitamin C deficiency inhibits tensile strength gain in ligament.[44,45] Controlled movement including long-duration, low-load stress is beneficial during scar remodeling.[3,50] Dynamic splints, serial casting, positional heat and stretching techniques, functional electrical stimulation, and selective exercises can provide the stress necessary to influence the scar.[51] The most significant gain in tensile strength occurs between 15 and 20 days, but gains in tensile strength continue to develop for up to 18 months.[43,46,50,51]

EFFECTS OF IMMOBILIZATION DURING THE FIBROBLASTIC STAGE

In general, immobilization reduces scar quantity and quality.[3] A joint that has been immobilized may be stiff from intra-articular adhesions. There is also evidence that the ligament itself can shorten and limit joint mobility.[3] This shortening of the ligament is due to alterations of collagen cross-linking, synthesis, and degradation and to changes of water and proteoglycan content of tissues surrounding the ligament.[89] Adhesions may occur as a result of newly produced collagen fibers forming interfibrillar contacts at strategic sites. Administration of hyaluronic acid can aid in limiting cross-linking or fusion of newly deposited collagen fibers, through its water-binding and lubricating abilities. Both ultrasound, which weakens polypeptide bonds, and transverse friction massage can be used to treat adhesions.[79,114]

Immobilization also prevents the normal pumping action that results from intermittent stretching of tissues. Immobilization subsequently influences the nutritional status of the knee, particularly of the hyaline cartilage. Atrophy of the thigh muscles results from immobilization.[115,116] Type I fibers appear to be especially sensitive to immobilization.[117-119] Electrical stimulation has been shown to prevent the reduction of enzyme activity in muscle that occurs with immobilization, especially in type I fibers.[120] Upper-body and contralateral extremity exercises should be initiated for maintenance and possible cross-over strengthening.[121]

THERAPEUTIC CONSIDERATIONS DURING THE FIBROBLASTIC STAGE

Nutrition plays a significant role during the fibroblastic stage, which lasts from 18 hours to 6 weeks.* Ingestion of vitamin C (ascorbic acid), iron, protein, zinc, calcium, and copper should be encouraged.[3,42-44,50,78,80] The use of cortisone is not recommended during this stage.[44,45,53,81] Salt water application, vibration, and heat are also discouraged because of their weakening effect on procollagen.[51] A controlled exercise program is continued during this phase, with the intent of providing gentle stress.[1,22] Mobilization of soft tissue, such as patellar mobilization and scar massage, dynamic splints, serial casting, stretching, and functional electrical stimulation may also be used to provide needed stress to the healing structures.[51,62] Radiation of greater than 100 rad (1 Gy) should be avoided[51] (x-rays are about 1 rad, or 0.01 Gy) (see Table 4-1).

Maturation Stage

As the scar continues to mature, the collagen fibers become dense, their diameter increases, vascularity decreases, ground substance composition changes, and the scar becomes smaller and less sensitive.[91] Specialized or complex structures at the surgical or

---

*References 3, 6, 42–44, 50, 55, 56, 76, 78.

traumatic site, such as hair follicles or sweat glands, usually either do not regenerate or heal with some deformity.[46,52] Maturation occurs in 12 to 18 months after injury.[91] This time frame may vary between individuals, and even between ligaments[3] (see Table 4–1).

A continued progression of resisted exercises should be pursued through this stage of healing. In addition, the patient should be progressively guided through functional activities such as two-leg hopping, one-leg hopping, partial squat to vertical jump, trampoline, sliding board, and a walk-jog progression. Sprints, backward running, agility drills (such as figure-eights, carioca, cutting, cross-over stepping, and shuffling), plyometrics, and sports-specific skills can be progressively performed (see Chapter 5). Return to sport is generally permitted after 80 to 90 percent isokinetic scores are achieved.[22,67]

INTRA-ARTICULAR RECONSTRUCTION

In some cases of ligamentous injury—most commonly in the case of ACL injury— reconstructive surgery is indicated. Reconstruction involves substitution of the damaged ligament. The most contemporary surgical technique is a reconstruction using the patellar tendon, as described by Clancy.[122] This procedure involves routing the midsection of the patellar tendon through the tibia to the femur to substitute for the ACL (see Chapter 9). The surgery can be lengthy and difficult, requiring precise placement and necessitating extensive rehabilitation. Reconstructive surgery requires special consideration. The tendon graft must be protected from injury and allowed time to develop its own blood supply. Several studies have demonstrated that patellar tendon grafts used to replace the ACL are essentially avascular at the time of transplantation.[123–125] Experimental studies have shown that following transplantation, patellar tendon autografts are initially enveloped with a vascular synovial tissue that originated from the infrapatellar fat pad and synovium.[124] During the first 4 to 6 weeks after transplantation, vascular buds from the surrounding soft tissues penetrate to revascularize the patellar tendon autograft. During that time the central portion of the graft is ischemic and undergoing necrosis (Fig. 4–8). At 6 weeks there is evidence of revascularization of the patellar tendon graft (Fig. 4–9). Therefore, during the initial few weeks after autograft implementation, the clinician must control stresses to the knee to protect the healing graft. Revascularization can take up to 20 weeks postreconstruction. Fibroplasia occurs during that time, but remodeling of the graft to regain the structural and mechanical characteristics of the ACL takes from 12 to 18 months.[124,125]

Vascularized Patellar Tendon Autografts

Vascularized patellar tendon (VPT) autografts were developed to reduce the period of avascular necrosis that occurs with detached patellar tendon autograft reconstructions.[126,127] The reconstruction is performed using a central one-third patellar tendon attached to its infrapatellar fat pad blood supply, or with a medial one-third patellar tendon strip attached to its medial retinaculum blood supply (Fig. 4–10). However, experimental evidence indicates that with respect to biomechanical or structural properties, the use of the VPT autograft shows no advantages compared with the detached patellar tendon autograft.

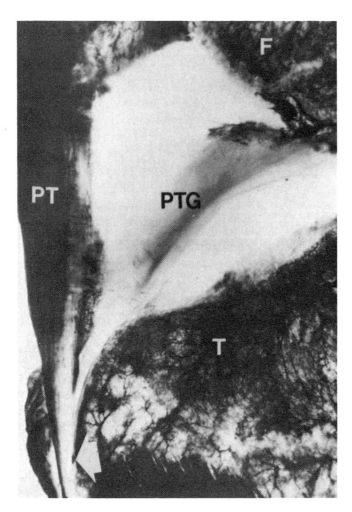

FIGURE 4-8. A 5-mm thick sagittal section of a dog knee 2 weeks after replacement of the ACL with a patellar tendon graft (PTG). The arrow indicates that the tibial attachment of the PTG shows no evidence of perfused vessels. F = femur. T = tibia. PT = patella tendon. (From Arnoczky, Tarvin, and Marshall,[124] p 218, with permission.)

Allografts

The revascularization process of allograft material undergoes the same relative periods of revascularization as the autograft material,[128,129] despite the preservation techniques, including freeze-drying or deep freezing. The vascular tissues of the infrapatellar fat pad and synovium provide a vascular envelope around the graft resulting in intrinsic revascularization and fibroplasia. This process takes from 6 to 12 months. Therefore, rehabilitation for a patient with a patellar tendon allograft may proceed similarly to that for a patient with autogenous reconstruction.

Synthetics

Chapter 9 describes the different classification of synthetic materials that are used for intra-articular reconstruction for ACL deficiency. True prosthetic devices such as the Gore-tex (W. L. Gore and Co., Flagstaff, AZ) do not require a period of revascularization. Therefore, soft-tissue healing of the graft is not a major concern, and rapid, aggressive rehabilitation is possible. Scaffold devices are designed to allow connective

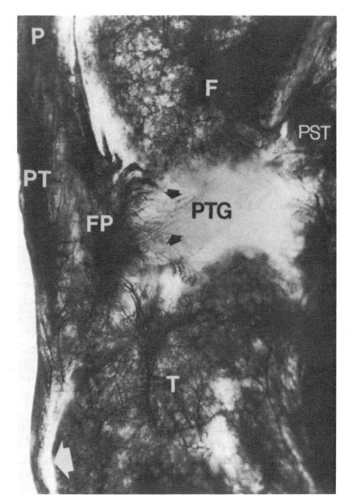

FIGURE 4-9. A 5-mm sagittal section of a dog knee 6 weeks after replacement of the ACL with a PTG. The white arrow indicates the nonvascularized tibial attachment of the PTG. Note the vascular response of the infrapatellar fat pad (FP) (*black arrows*), tibia (T), and posterior soft tissue (PST). F = femur. P = patella. PT = patella tendon. (From Arnoczky, Tarvin, and Marshall,[124] p 218, with permission.)

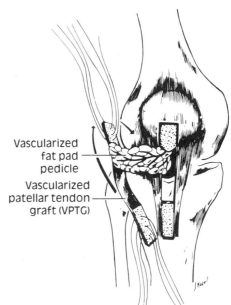

FIGURE 4-10. Illustration of the knee showing the central third of the patella with its vascular supply intact harvested as an ACL replacement. (From Clancy, WG: Anterior cruciate ligament functional instability: A static intra-articular and dynamic extra-articular procedure. Clin Orthop 172:104, 1983, with permission.)

tissue to proliferate and form a neoalignment.[130,131] The neoalignment occurs through revascularization of the scaffold by surrounding soft tissues, that is, the infrapatellar fat pad, and synovium. The success of neoalignment of connective tissue through and around the scaffold is dependent upon the material used for the scaffold, as well as the mechanical materials placed around the healing graft. The most common scaffold device is made of carbon fiber. Collagen typing has been done on neoaligned tissue in the carbon fiber. The ratio of collagen fiber types was 60 percent type I to 40 percent type II, compared with normal ACL, which is composed of 85 percent type I and 15 percent type II collagen fibers.[132]

OTHER STRUCTURES

Muscle

As noted earlier in the chapter, different tissue types may heal at different rates.[43,51] Muscle undergoes degeneration and regeneration after injury. Cell death in muscle is characterized by membrane damage, Z-band sarcomere disruption, nuclear pyknosis, and mitochondrial swelling, all of which is followed by muscle fragmentation.[133] If vascular integrity remains, macrophages appear within 12 hours. In the presence of a muscle graft, blood vessels must penetrate into the healing sites.[3,44] This revascularization can take weeks to complete. As macrophages are "cleaning" the area, activated spindle-shaped myogenic cells appear beneath the basal lamina of the original muscle fibers. These cells produce myoblasts, which fuse into long syncytial myotubes that eventually become a muscle fiber.

Results from biomechanical studies have found faster recovery occurring when the muscles are mobilized.[134] The time frames of the healing processes of muscle vary significantly depending on the type of muscle, its vascularity, and the severity of injury. Muscle regeneration may be completed in 5 days to 6 months.[133]

Meniscus

The meniscus has a vascular zone comprising the peripheral 10 to 30 percent of its total area.[135] Blood supply in this zone is from perimeniscal capillaries, which arise as branches from the medial and lateral genicular arteries. The area where healing does not occur is the avascular zone, which comprises the inner two thirds of the meniscus. This area is where 15 to 20 percent of meniscal tears occur.[3] In the peripheral, vascular zone, total or subtotal healing is reported.[136] The normal healing response to a peripheral tear occurs with a fibrin clot. The clot allows blood vessels from the capillary plexus to proliferate along this fibrous scaffold. The fibrin clot is filled with inflammatory cells. Eventually, the tear is filled with a cellular fibrovascular scar. This entire process can take as long as 10 weeks after injury.[136] Too-early knee range of motion, that is, within the initial 4 to 6 weeks, can result in a low-level release of lysosomal enzymes from the inflammatory cells, which inhibits the fibrin clot formation. The patient should remain non–weight bearing to partial weight bearing during this period. Complete remodeling of the scar to normal fibrocartilage can take several months. A complete review of rehabilitation for meniscal injuries is presented in Chapter 14.

Blood Vessels

Injuries to blood vessels are usually self-limiting. Endothelial tissue undergoes the cellular proliferative responses with time frames of healing similar to those for ligaments. In severe cases, such as the rupture of all four ligaments and knee dislocation, the popliteal artery may be injured.[4] Immediate reduction is required to minimize the arterial injury and prevent distal gangrene. If the blood vessel is severely injured or severed, surgical repair may be necessary. Depending on the severity and the type of surgery conducted, the duration of the healing response may vary. Occasionally, a functionally insignificant internal thickening of the vessel may occur, or the lumen may be completely occluded.

Nerves

In severe injuries to the knee, the medial popliteal nerve may be injured.[4] Immediate reduction of the knee should minimize nerve injury. The regeneration of nerves entails a short inflammation stage, and a fibroblastic stage within 48 hours.[3,44] The nerve is a specialized connective tissue and requires specific molecules to maintain the growth capacities of the damaged neuron, stimulate the growth and elongation of axons, guide the axon, reconnect the axon with the target cell, and stimulate the Schwann cell to resheath and remyelinate the new axon. Low-load, long-duration stress is beneficial in the regeneration of the nerve.[51] The average rate of nerve regeneration is, at most, 1 to 2 mm per day. The extent of injury and other extraneous variables will influence the rate of healing. Excessive scar formation may completely obstruct the regenerating nerve.[52]

Tendons

Tendons pass through the same stages of healing as ligaments. Inflammation occurs in the first 72 hours, and collagen synthesis occurs within the first week. Fibroplasia occurs from intrinsic (from adjacent cells) or extrinsic (arriving via blood vessels) sources.[3,44,51] Fibroblastic activity occurs in the first 4 weeks following injury. Immobilization is advised for the initial 2 to 3 days following tendon repair to prevent disruption.[99,105] Afterward, controlled motion in the form of exercise or CPM should be initiated.[99] Controlled motion furnishes nutrients to the tendon. Although tensile strength of injured tendons occurs after physiologic loading, it is unlikely that full tensile strength is ever regained.[3,44] Healing should be complete by 4 months post injury.

SUMMARY

A large body of scientific and clinical research has been conducted to clarify the physiology and duration of healing. This chapter has described the general stages of healing, with corresponding time frames. The assumption is that foremost, in the presence of soft-tissue injuries, clinicians should understand the physiology of soft-tissue healing to conduct rehabilitation effectively and safely. Nutritional, mechanical, and anatomic factors that affect healing should be manipulated to promote maximum healing in minimal time. Immobilization and its effects must be considered with each patient. Measures should be taken to minimize the deleterious effects of immobilization on surrounding tissues. Clinicians should maintain a level of scientific knowledge commensurate with their clinical and experiental skills.

REFERENCES

1. Davies, GJ (ed): Rehabilitation of the Surgical Knee. CyPress, Ronkonkoma, NY, 1984.
2. Robbins, RM, et al: Pathological Basis of Disease. WB Saunders, Philadelphia, 1971, p 1.
3. Woo, S L-Y and Buckwalter, JA (ed): Injury and Repair of the Musculoskeletal Soft Tissues. American Academy of Orthopedic Surgeons, Savannah, GA, 1987.
4. Salter, RB: The Musculoskeletal System. Williams & Wilkins, Baltimore, 1984, p 418.
5. Smillie, IS: Injuries of the Knee Joint. Williams & Wilkins, Baltimore, 1970, p 130.
6. Butler, DL, Grood, ES, and Noyes, FR: Biomechanics of ligaments and tendons. Exerc Sport Sci Rev 6:125, 1975.
7. Fung, YCB: Biomechanics: Its Foundations and Objectives. Prentice Hall, Englewood Cliffs, NJ, 1972, p 1.
8. Dale, WC and Baer, E: Fibre-buckling in composite systems: A model for the ultrastructure of uncalcified collagen tissues. Journal of Material Science 9:369, 1974.
9. Torp, S, Baer, E, and Friedman, B: Effects of aging and of mechanical deformation on the ultrastructure of tendon. Proceedings of 1974 Colston Conference. Department of Physics, University of Bristol, United Kingdom, 1974, p 223.
10. Malvern, L: Introduction to the Mechanics of a Continuous Medium. Prentice Hall, Englewood Cliffs, NJ, 1969, p 1.
11. Gustavson, KH: The Chemistry and Reactivity of Collagen. Academic Press, NY, 1956, p 1.
12. Shah, JS, Jayson, MI, and Hampson, WG: Low tension studies of collagen fibers from ligaments of the human spine. Ann Rheum Dis 36:139, 1977.
13. Hirsch, G: Tensile properties during tendon healing. Acta Orthop Scand Suppl 153:13, 1974.
14. Partington, FR and Wood, GC: The role of non-collagen components in the mechanical behavior of tendon fibres. Biochimica et Biophysica Acta 69:489, 1963.
15. Rigby, BJ, Hirai, N, Spikes, JD, and Eyring, H: The mechanical properties of rat tail tendon. J Gen Physiol 43:265, 1959.
16. Stromberg, DD and Widerheilm, CA: Viscoelastic description of a collagenous tissue in simple elongation. J Appl Physiol 26:857, 1969.
17. Tkaczuk, H: Tensile properties of human lumbar longitudinal ligaments. Acta Orthop Scand Suppl 115:2, 1968.
18. Trent, PS, Walker, PS, and Wolf, B: Ligament length patterns, strength, and rotation axes of the knee joint. Clin Orthop 117:263, 1976.
19. Viidik, A: Studies on the Anatomy and Function of Bones and Joints. Springer, Berlin, 1966, p 17.
20. Viidik, A: The effect of training on the tensile strength of isolated rabbit tendons. Scand J Plast Reconstr Surg Hand Surg 1, 1967.
21. Viidik, A: Functional properties of collagenous tissues. International Review of Connective Tissue Research 6:127, 1973.
22. Jenkins, DH (ed): Ligament Injuries and Their Treatment. Aspen Publications, Rockville, MD, 1985, p 3.
23. Tipton, CM, et al: The influence of physical activity on ligaments and tendons. Med Sci Sports Exerc 7(3):165, 1976.
24. Nachemson, AL and Evans, JH: Some mechanical properties of the third human lumbar interlaminar ligament (ligamentum flavum). J Biomech 1:211, 1968.
25. Noyes, FR and Grood, ES: The strength of the anterior cruciate ligament in humans and rhesus monkeys. Age-related and species-related changes. J Bone Joint Surg [Am] 58:1074, 1976.
26. Booth, FW and Tipton, CM: Ligamentous strength measurements in prepubescent and pubescent rats. Growth 34:177, 1970.
27. Akeson, WH, Ameil, P, and La Violette, D: The connective tissue response to immobility: An accelerated aging response. Exp Gerontol 3:239, 1968.
28. Noyes, FR, DeLucas, JL, and Torvik, PJ: Biomechanics of anterior cruciate ligament failure: An analysis of strain-rate sensitivity and mechanisms of failure in primates. J Bone Joint Surg [Am] 56:236, 1974.
29. Tipton, CM, Barnard, RJ, and Terjung, RL: Response of thyroidectomized rats to training. Am J Physiol 215:1137, 1968.
30. Tipton, CM, et al: Response of adrenalectomized rats to exercise. Endocrinology 91:573, 1972.
31. Tipton, CM, Tcheng, TK, and Mergner, W: Influence of immobilization, training, exogenous hormones, and surgical repair on knee ligaments from hypophysectomized rats. Am J Physiol 221:1144, 1971.

32. McGraw, WT: The effect of tension on collagen remodeling by fibroblasts: A stereological ultrastructural study. Connect Tissue Res 14:229, 1986.
33. Viidik, A: Elasticity and tensile strength of the anterior cruciate ligament in rabbits as influenced by training. Acta Physiol Scand 74:372, 1968.
34. Zuckerman, J and Stull, GA: Effects of exercise on knee ligament separation force in rats. J Appl Physiol 26:716, 1969.
35. Tipton, CM, et al: Influence of exercise on the strength of the medial collateral knee ligament of dogs. Am J Physiol 218:894, 1970.
36. Tipton, CM, et al: Hydroxyproline concentration in ligaments from trained and non-trained rats. Presented at Second International Symposium on Biochemistry of Exercise, Philadelphia, 1976.
37. Tipton, CM, Matthes, RD, and Sandage, DS: In situ measurement of junction strength and ligament elongation in rats. J Appl Physiol 37:758, 1974.
38. Allman, FL: A program of injury prevention for high schools. Med Sci Sports Exerc 3(2):1, 1963.
39. Hughston, JC, Whatley, GS, and Dodelin, RA: The athlete and his knees. South Med J 554:1372, 1961.
40. Thorndike, A: Athletic Injuries. Lea & Febiger, Philadelphia, 1950, p 64.
41. Laros, GS, Tipton, CM, and Cooper, RR: Influence of physical activity on ligament insertions in the knees of dogs. J Bone Joint Surg [Am] 53:275, 1971.
42. Miltner, LJ, Hu, CH, and Fang, HC: Experimental joint sprain, pathologic study. Arch Surg 35:234, 1937.
43. Wilson, JN (ed): Fractures and Joint Injuries. Churchill Livingstone, New York, 1982, p 1.
44. Dunphy, JE (ed): Wound Healing. Medcom Press, New York, 1974, p 1.
45. Hotter, AN: Physiologic aspects and clinical implications of wound healing. Heart Lung 11(6):522, 1982.
46. Shoshan, S: Wound Healing. Hebrew University of Jerusalem, Jerusalem, 1980, p 1.
47. Clayton, ML and Weir, GJ: Experimental investigations of ligamentous healing. Am J Surg 98:27, 1959.
48. Clayton, ML, Miles, JS, and Abdulla, M: Experimental investigations of ligamentous healing. Clin Orthop 61:373, 1968.
49. O'Donoghue, DH, et al: Repair of knee ligaments in dogs. J Bone Joint Surg [Am] 43:112, 1961.
50. Cummings, GS, Crutchfield, CA, and Barnes, MR: Soft Tissue Changes in Contractures. Stokesville Publishing, Atlanta, 1985, p 1.
51. Hardy, MA: The biology of scar formation. Phys Ther 69:12, 1989.
52. Gidlof, JD, et al: Induced Skeletal Muscle Ischemia in Man. Kargel, Basel, 1982.
53. Levenson, SM, Stein, J, and Grossblatt, N (ed): Wound Healing: Proceedings of a Workshop. National Academy of Sciences—National Research Council, Washington, DC, 1966.
54. Cocke, WM, et al: Wound Care. Churchill Livingstone, New York, 1986, p 1.
55. Young, A, Stokes, M, and Iles, JF: Effects of joint pathology on muscle. Clin Orthop 219:21, 1987.
56. Arvidsson, I, et al: Reduction of pain inhibition on voluntary muscle activation by epidural analgesia. Orthopedics 9:1415, 1986.
57. Arvidsson, I and Eriksson, E: Postoperative TENS pain relief after knee surgery: Objective evaluation. Orthopedics 9:1346, 1986.
58. Jack, EA: Experimental rupture of the medial collateral ligament of the knee. J Bone Joint Surg [Br] 32:14, 1950.
59. Barcroft, H and Edholm, K: The effects of temperature on blood flow and deep temperature on the human forearm. J Physiol (Lond) 102:5, 1943.
60. Waylonis, GW: The physiological effects of ice massage. Arch Phys Med Rehabil 48:47, 1967.
61. Smith, MJ: Electrical stimulation for relief of musculoskeletal pain. The Physician and Sportsmedicine 11:47, 1983.
62. Jensen, JE, et al: The use of transcutaneous neural stimulation and isokinetic testing in arthroscopic knee surgery. Am J Sports Med 13:27, 1985.
63. Massey, BH, et al: Effects of high frequency electrical stimulation on the size and strength of skeletal muscle. J Sports Med Phys Fitness 11:136, 1965.
64. Serrato, JC: Pain control by transcutaneous nerve stimulation. South Med J 72:67, 1979.
65. Melzack, R and Wall, PD: Pain mechanisms: A new theory. Science 150:971, 1965.
66. Melzack, R and Wall, PD: Prolonged relief of pain by brief, intense transcutaneous somatic stimulation. Pain 1:357, 1975.
67. McCarroll, JR, Shelbourne, KD, and Rettig, AC: Athletes and their ACL injury. Surgical Rounds in Orthopedics 7:39, 1989.
68. Henning, CE, Lynch, MA, and Glick, KR: An in vivo strain gauge study of elongation of the anterior cruciate ligament. Am J Sports Med 13:22, 1985.
69. Paulos, L, et al: Knee rehabilitation after ACL reconstruction and repair. Am J Sports Med 9:140, 1981.
70. Salter, RB, et al: Clinical application of basic research on continuous passive motion for disorders and injuries to the synovial joints: A preliminary report of a feasibility study. J Orthop Res 1:325, 1984.
71. Tomaro, JE: Prevention and treatment of patellar entrapment following intra-articular ACL reconstruction. Athletic Training 26:11, 1991.
72. Feagin, JA: The Crucial Ligaments. Churchill Livingstone, New York, 1988, p 341.
73. Silver, IA: The physiology of wound healing. Schweiz Rundsch Med Prax 73(30):942, 1984.
74. Lotz, M, Duncan, M, and Gerber, L: Early versus delayed shoulder motion following axillary dissection. Ann Surg 193:72, 1981.

75. Paletta, FX, Shehadi, SI, and Mudd, JG: Hypothermia and tourniquet ischemia. Plast Reconstr Surg 29:19, 1962.
76. Arms, SW, et al: The biomechanics of anterior cruciate ligament rehabilitation and reconstruction. Am J Sports Med 12:8, 1984.
77. Langman, J: Medical Embryology. Williams & Wilkins, Baltimore, 1969, p 1.
78. Greenlee, TK and Ross, R: The development of the rat flexor digital tendon, a fine structure study. Journal of Ultrastructure Research 18:354, 1967.
79. Griffen, JE and Karselis, TC: Physical Agents for Physical Therapists. Charles C Thomas, Springfield, MA, 1982, p 290.
80. Ramirez, F, Sangiorgi, FO, and Tsipouras, P: Human collagens: Biochemical, molecular and genetic features in normal and diseased states. Horiz Biochem Biophys 86(8):27, 1986.
81. Robins, SP: Functional properties of collagen and elastin. Bailliere's Clin Rheumatol 2(1):1, 1988.
82. Zernicke, RF: Biomechanical and biochemical synthesis. Med Sci Sports Exerc 15(1):6, 1983.
83. Steeten, MR: Some aspects of the metabolism of hydroxyproline, studied with the aid of isotopic nitrogen. J Biol Chem 181:4, 1949.
84. Burgeson, RE: The collagens of skin. Curr Probl Dermatol 17:1, 1987.
85. Peacock, EE and Van Winkle, W (ed): Wound Repair. WB Saunders, Philadelphia, 1976, p 1.
86. Rojkind, M: Chemistry and biosynthesis of collagen. Bull Rheum Dis 30(1):1006, 1980.
87. Fitton-Jackson, S: Treatise on Collagen. Academic Press, London, 1968, p 1.
88. Flint, M: Interrelationships of mucopolysaccharide and collagen in connective tissue remodeling. Journal of Embryology and Experimental Morphology 27:481, 1972.
89. Akeson, WH, et al: Collagen cross-linking alterations in joint contractures: Changes in the reducible cross-links in periarticular connective tissue collagen after nine weeks of immobilization. Connect Tissue Res 5:95, 1977.
90. Kloth, LC, McCulloch, JM, and Feedar, JA: Wound Healing: Alternatives in Management. FA Davis, Philadelphia, 1990, p 18.
91. Frank, C, et al: Medial collateral ligament healing. Am J Sports Med 11:380, 1983.
92. Miller, EJ: The collagens: An overview and update. Methods Enzymol 144:3, 1987.
93. Minns, RJ, Soden, PD, and Jackson, DS: The role of the fibrous components and ground substance in the mechanical properties of biological tissues: A preliminary investigation. J Biomech 6:1, 1973.
94. Frisen, M, et al: Rheological analysis of soft collagenous tissue. I. Theoretical considerations. J Biomech 1:13, 1968.
95. Viidik, A: Functional properties of collagenous tissues. International Review of Connective Tissue Research 6:127, 1973.
96. Viidik, A: A rheological model for uncalcified parallel-fibred collagenous tissue. J Biomech 1:3, 1968.
97. Carter, SB: Principles in cell motility: The directional control of cell movement. Nature 208:12, 1965.
98. Riley, WB: Wound healing. Annals of Family Practice 24(5):107, 1981.
99. Gelberman, RH, et al: Effects of early intermittent passive mobilization on healing canine flexor tendons. J Hand Surg [Am] 7:78, 1982.
100. Hunt, TK and Van Winkle, W: Wound Healing: Normal Repair—Fundamentals of Wound Management Surgery. Chirurgecom, South Plainfield, NJ, 1976, p 1.
101. Flynn, ME and Rovee, DT: Wound healing mechanisms. Am J Nurs 11:1544, 1982.
102. Riley, WB and Peacock, EE: Identification, distribution and significance of all collagenealytic enzyme in human tissues. Proc Soc Exp Biol Med 124:7, 1967.
103. Peacock, EE: Collagenolysis: The other side of the equation. World J Surg 4:43, 1980.
104. Watts, GT, Grillo, HC, and Gross, J: Studies in wound healing. II. The role of granulation tissue in contraction. Ann Surg 148:187, 1958.
105. Noyes, FR: Functional properties of knee ligaments and alterations induced by immobilization. Clin Orthop 123:210, 1977.
106. Videman, T: Connective tissue and immobilization. Clin Orthop 123:212, 1977.
107. Thorngate, S and Ferguson, DJ: Effect of tension on healing aponeurotic wounds. Surgery 44:29, 1958.
108. Finsterbush, A and Friedman, B: Reversibility of joint changes produced by immobilization in rabbits. Clin Orthop 111:38, 1975.
109. Akeson, WH, et al: Effects of immobilization on joints. Clin Orthop 219:421, 1986.
110. Sussman, MD: Effect of increased tissue traction upon tensile strength of cutaneous incisions in rats. Proc Soc Exp Biol Med 123:91, 1966.
111. Vailas, AC, et al: Physical activity and its influence on the repair process of medial collateral ligaments. Connect Tissue Res 9:113, 1981.
112. Akeson, WH, Amiel, D, and Woo, SL-Y: Immobility effects on synovial joints: The pathomechanics of joint contracture. Biorheology 17:95, 1980.
113. Peacock, EE: Some biochemical and biophysical aspects of joint stiffness: Role of collagen synthesis as opposed to altered molecular bonding. Ann Surg 164:17, 1966.
114. Andrish, J and Holmes, R: Effects of synovial fluid on fibroblasts in tissue culture. Clin Orthop 138:279, 1979.
115. Nicholas, JA, Strizak, AM, and Veras, G: A study of thigh weakness in different pathological states of the lower extremity. Am J Sports Med 6:241, 1976.

116. Watson-Jones, R: Fractures and Joint Injuries, ed 5. Churchill Livingstone, Edinburgh, 1976, p 1.
117. Halkjaer-Kristrensen, J and Ingemann-Hansen, T: Effect of immobilization on fiber composition in the human quadriceps muscle. Scand J Rheumatol 7:62, 1978.
118. Haggmark, T, Jansson, E, and Svane, B: Cross-sectional areas of the thigh muscle in man measured by computed tomography. Scand J Clin Lab Invest 38:355, 1978.
119. Haggmark, T and Eriksson, E: Hypotrophy of the soleus muscle in man after Achilles tendon rupture. Am J Sports Med 7:121, 1979.
120. Eriksson, E and Haggmark, T: Comparison of isometric muscle training and electrical stimulation supplementing isometric muscle training in the recovery after major knee ligament surgery. Am J Sports Med 7:169, 1979.
121. Stanish, WD, et al: The effects of immobilization and of electrical stimulation on muscle glycogen and myofibrillar ATPase. Can J Sports Sci 7:267, 1982.
122. Clancy, WG, Nelson, PA, and Reider, B: Anterior cruciate ligament reconstructions using one-third of the patellar ligament augmented by extra-articular tendon transfers. J Bone Joint Surg [Am] 64:352, 1982.
123. Alm, A, Liljedahl, SO, and Stromberg, B: Clinical and experimental experience in reconstruction of the anterior cruciate ligament. Orthop Clin North Am 7:181, 1976.
124. Arnoczky, SP, Tarvin, GB, and Marshall, JL: Anterior cruciate ligament replacement using patella tendon: An evaluation of graft revascularization in the dog. J Bone Joint Surg [Am] 64:217, 1982.
125. Clancy, WG, et al: Anterior and posterior cruciate ligament reconstruction in rhesus monkeys: A histologic, microangiographic, and biomechanical analysis. J Bone Joint Surg [Am] 63:1270, 1981.
126. Clancy, WG: Anterior cruciate ligament functional instability: A static intra-articular and dynamic extra-articular procedure. Clin Orthop 172:102, 1983.
127. Paulos, LE, et al: Intra-articular reconstruction II replacement with vascularized patellar tendon. Clin Orthop 172:78, 1983.
128. Arnoczky, SP, Warren, RF, and Ashlock, MA: Anterior cruciate ligament replacement using a patellar tendon allograft: An experimental study in the dog. J Bone Joint Surg [Am] 68:376, 1986.
129. Shino, K, et al: Replacement of the anterior cruciate ligament by an allogenic tendon graft: An experimental study in the dog. J Bone Joint Surg [Br] 66:672, 1984.
130. Arnoczky, SP, Warren, RF, and Minei, JP: Replacement of the anterior cruciate ligament using synthetic prosthesis: An evaluation of graft biology in the dog. Am J Sports Med 14:1, 1986.
131. Forster, IW, et al: Biological reation to carbon fiber implants: The formation and structure of carbon-induced "neotendon". Clin Orthop 131:299, 1978.
132. Bonnarens, FO and Drez, D, Jr: Biomechanics of artificial ligaments and associated problems. In Jackson, DW and Drez, D, Jr (eds): The Anterior Cruciate Deficient Knee: New Concepts in Ligament Repair. CV Mosby, St. Louis, 1987, p. 251.
133. Cooper, RR: Alterations during immobilization and regeneration of skeletal muscle in cats. J Bone Joint Surg [Am] 54:919, 1972.
134. Tabary, JC, et al: Experimental rapid sarcomere loss with concomitant hypoextensibility. Muscle Nerve 4:198, 1981.
135. Arnoczky, SP and Warren, RF: Microvasculature of the human meniscus. Am J Sports Med 10:90, 1982.
136. Arnoczky, SP and Warren, RF: The microvasculature of the meniscus and its response to injury: An experimental study in the dog. Am J Sports Med 11:131, 1983.

CHAPTER 5

Principles of Exercise Progression

Mark S. Albert, MEd, PT, ATC, SCS

Rehabilitation, for the purposes of this chapter, may be described as a progressive sequence of therapeutic exercises complemented by electric and thermal modalities, external support devices, and specific joint mobilizations. Rehabilitation is individualized to restore preinjury levels of skill and performance and remediate abnormal postural problems or physiologic conditions. Rehabilitation has evolved as an integral part of comprehensive care for knee problems. Supported by advances in technology, rehabilitation will continue to maintain its importance and undergo changes, as physical therapy techniques and knowledge attain increased sophistication.

Individual clinicians' educational and experiential background and preferences produce many diverse approaches to rehabilitation. Nearly all rehabilitation programs emphasize resistive exercise training applied with assorted machines, devices, and systems. Manual resistance, as outlined by Knott and Voss,[1] is also a highly effective and efficient means of exercise training, but it is not the focus of this discussion.

Protocols (defined as preset time limits for activity progressions) may be useful as general introductory guidelines, but they are limited by the variability of clinical facilities and equipment, patient characteristics, past history of dysfunction, injury mechanisms, clinician preferences, diagnosis, and surgical techniques.

Consequently, the focus of this chapter will be to highlight benefits of resistive exercise training, investigate program design, and describe rationale for clinical decision making with various types of exercise and other supplemental techniques.

REHABILITATION RATIONALE

The multiple benefits of structured, supervised, and biomechanically designed rehabilitation programs resemble those of a medicine. Mindful of this analogy, clinicians should carefully utilize the appropriate "dosage" that is applied to clients, expressed in terms of frequency, duration, intensity, and type (or mode) of exercise. The "dosage" of exercise programs is based on selective changes and supportive documentation, which entails continual reassessment in order to avoid an allergic response (or outright injury) of the affected body tissues. The concept of exercise dosage empowers the clinician to responsibly plan and skillfully manipulate each component exercise and phase within an entire rehabilitation progression. Houglum[2] describes an important perspective of rehabilitation, whereby therapeutic exercise is in itself an effective modality. Primary goals of modalities are to increase blood flow to healing tissues and to relieve pain and stiffness, both of which are effectively and economically accomplished with appropriate exercise applications.

Structured knee rehabilitation for mixed diagnoses in 5,381 knee patients was demonstrated as effective in 40 to 90 percent of cases in a 5-year follow-up study; by contrast, a home program by itself produced a 100 percent failure rate for functional activities.[3] Synovial joints (diarthrodial) such as the knee depend on the integrity of both static and dynamic stabilizers (muscles). The inherently poor articular congruence of the knee joint complex causes an increased reliance of joint protection from muscular forces and control. Overall, dynamic stabilization forces of the knee are from the quadriceps femoris muscles at slow joint speeds (under 180 degrees per second) and from the hamstring muscles at high speeds.[4]

HIP AND KNEE INTERACTION

Several of the muscles acting on the knee are two-joint (biarticular) structures that provide efficiency for locomotion and, due to a combination of longitudinal and bipennate architecture, provide a balance between strength and mobility.[5] A biomechanical trade-off exists, however, because two-joint muscles are subject to both active and passive insufficiency. Hence, the two-joint configuration cannot allow the muscles to stretch fully across the hip and knee simultaneously (passive), nor can the muscles contract simultaneously at the hip and knee with functional forces (active).[5] Consequently, muscle strengthening is a critical element of recovery of normal knee function, with emphasis required for both hip and knee contractile units. Empirical or clinical experience of the importance of hip muscle strength to the integrity of the knee was demonstrated by a poll of sports physical therapists/clinical facilities, in which 98 percent of 73 respondents felt that specific hip rehabilitation was a critical element in knee rehabilitation.[6] In addition, this survey also demonstrated that 90 percent of the respondents believed in the importance of total leg strength (TLS), a concept developed by Nicholas and Gleim.[7-9] Total leg strength incorporates a summation of hip, knee, and ankle muscle force measures from isokinetic testing into a predictive measure of discharge readiness when compared with the noninjured side.

PHILOSOPHY

An important concept within the rehabilitation process involves enlisting and motivating patients to achieve goals through lengthy, demanding treatment sessions that may last for weeks or months. Patient education includes the use of simple written descriptions of the array of benefits from multiple types of exercises (Table 5–1). The recruitment and retention of patient compliance is a multifactorial behavioral issue and

TABLE 5–1 Why Exercise?

Exercise has many beneficial and healing properties.
Exercise . . .
1. decreases muscle soreness, tension, and spasms.
2. enhances general venous and arterial tone for improved circulation.
3. increases efficiency of the cardiovascular system, with resulting resistance to fatigue and decreased risk of degenerative disease.
4. maintains/improves strength of bone, ligament, and joint structures.
5. improves muscular strength, flexibility, and efficiency.
6. improves balance and postural control.
7. improves the body's neurochemical system, which relieves pain and reduces stress.
8. decreases/controls body fat percentage.
9. helps with normal bowel regularity and function.
10. helps protect and stabilize injured body areas.
11. maintains normal breathing mechanics.
12. maintains healthy, pliable skin.
13. increases efficiency of the body's thermoregulation system.

is best approached with a combination of modeling, written instructions, physical repetition, intermittent positive reinforcement, specific goal setting, and other related psychological techniques. Throughout the rehabilitation program, professional rapport is necessary to facilitate the tremendous effort required from the patient, and as Shelton[10] suggests, the rehabilitation specialist must fulfill the diverse roles of coach, teacher, and counselor.

The importance of skilled rehabilitation after joint trauma, overuse microtrauma, surgery, or disuse from inactivity or immobilization cannot be overstressed. A staunch supporter of musculoskeletal rehabilitation from the orthopedic community, Dr. Jack Hughston, stated that rehabilitation contributed at least 50 percent of the eventual functional recovery after surgery or injury to joints.[11] Inadequate rehabilitation will produce physiologically weak tissue, which will often lead to reinjury and/or failure in the capacity to return to effective participation in vigorous activities.

Several important indications for the use of resistive-type exercise rehabilitation for the knee are outlined in Table 5–2. To ensure a comprehensive knee rehabilitation program, each of the physical parameters of muscular strength, power and endurance, flexibility, and balance and coordination, as well as cardiovascular endurance, should be addressed. Resistive exercises applied in the rehabilitation setting need not be of a maximal effort nature, and in many instances, maximal effort is strictly contraindicated (i.e., acute patellofemoral joint arthosis or early postoperative intra-articular ligament repair). The use of submaximal resistive exercises, as advocated by Davies,[12] may incorporate distinct physiologic benefits such as pain relief/reduction through stimula-

TABLE 5–2 Indications for Resistive Exercise

Reverse muscular atrophy
Control joint instability
Reverse reflex inhibition of muscle
Improve functional skills
Improve physical parameters: strength, power, and muscular endurance
Facilitate joint lubrication and arthrokinematics
Decrease pain
Improve neuromuscular control and proprioception

TABLE 5–3 Davies Exercise Progression Continuum

Multiple-angle isometrics (submaximal effort)
Multiple-angle isometrics (maximal), inertial
Short-arc concentric isokinetics (submaximal), inertial
Short-arc isotonics
Short-arc concentric isokinetics (maximal)
Full ROM* concentric isokinetics (submaximal)
Full ROM* isotonics
Full ROM* concentric isokinetics (maximal)

*ROM = range-of-motion.
Source: Adapted from Davies,[12] p 74.

tion of appropriate nerve afference; increased muscular endurance; joint lubrication in synovial joints; and improved joint stability. Most types of resistive exercise types (modes) are best applied in gradually more stressful hierarchies, in which each stage provides a trial and preparation for the next successive level as outlined by Davies[12] (Table 5–3). A gradual application of exercise stresses allows natural adaptations to soft tissue (Davis's law) and bone (Wolff's law) to occur.[13] Tissue maturation is, of course, a biologic, time-based process (see Chapter 4), in which collagen scar tissue assumes a configuration dictated by applied stresses and gradually gains tensile strength following the initial 3 to 6 weeks after disruption.[14]

PROGRAM DESIGN CONCEPTS

Each rehabilitation plan must consider the variable effects of both type and duration of immobilization on articular cartilage stiffness, soft-tissue healing, decreased bone stiffness/density, and joint contracture.[11] Today even the most disabling and serious knee problems (ligament ruptures, fractures, dislocations) are managed by limiting strict immobilization to less than 3 weeks, and by the use of early protected motion with cast braces or functional-type braces. The universally devastating effects of stress deprivation on human tissues, or "immobilization disease," are extensively documented in the scientific literature.[15-21] The negative effects of immobilization on both biochemical and mechanical properties of human tissue are rapid and dramatic, following an exponential pattern. With early restitution of appropriate exercise on the immobilized part, recovery is still exceedingly slow, following a more linear return of function. For example, injury to ligamentous tissue may require a full year[22] to regain normal tensile strength. Muscle tissue is also inherently slow to recover normal function, with inordinately prolonged recovery time manifested by the quadriceps femoris muscles (see the following section, A Common Deficit Profile). After 4 weeks of immobilization, normal joint structures begin to resemble those of degenerative joints,[23] a process that is especially relevant in the clinical management of the patellofemoral joint secondary to all knee injuries. Continuous passive motion, avoidance of slow-speed shearing forces, range of motion restrictions, and avoidance of steady-state compression loads (such as prolonged standing) or impact loads are important guidelines in the early stages after knee injury, in order to spare the softened articular cartilage.

Despite modern surgical advances; improved preoperative education and training; and early, aggressive postoperative measures, most serious knee injuries share common problems of pain, effusion, limited joint mobility, and muscular incoordination and

TABLE 5–4 Key Parameters of Rehabilitation Structure and Discharge

Strength relative to body weight
Right vs. left comparisons
Muscular endurance measures
Proprioceptive testing
Eccentric/concentric force ratios
Joint stability tests
Girth measurements
Agonist/antagonist ratios
Total leg strength
Functional tests
Total work values
Pain descriptors
Flexibility measures
Active/passive mobility

imbalance.[11] Even in the absence of these common problems restoration of normal muscular function remains a difficult rehabilitation challenge. Table 5–4 reviews key parameters used to assess normal muscle function and performance. Pain-free muscle training in the form of active motion within allowed ranges and isometric contractions for all dynamic stabilizers adjacent to an injured or postsurgical joint are important guidelines in early rehabilitation. Both joint pain and immobilization produce selective atrophy of slow-twitch or type I muscle fibers.[21] Consequently, submaximal effort isometrics are ideally suited to early muscle strengthening because they effectively train type I muscle fibers and can be used safely when joint motion is painful or contraindicated. A primary, safe exercise for knee dysfunction of all varieties is the straight leg raise (SLR), which produces a combined isometric-isotonic type of muscle loading. Clinical experience dictates that the SLR be performed without so-called quad lag (Fig. 5–1) and in a repetitive, multiple-daily-session format. In addition, SLRs performed

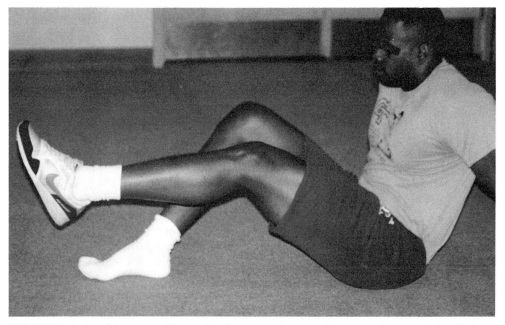

FIGURE 5–1. Quadriceps lag. The goal is for the patient to fully extend the knee joint during a straight leg raise.

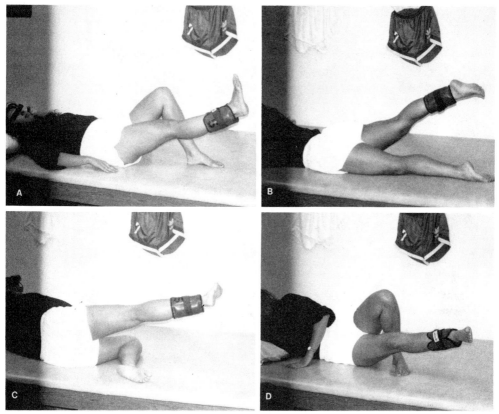

FIGURE 5-2. Four hip position straight leg raises. *A*) Hip flexion. *B*) Hip extension. *C*) Hip abduction. *D*) Hip adduction.

with four different hip motions (Figs. 5-2A, B, C, D) will recruit all hip-knee musculature but may be contraindicated for some pathologies (e.g., posterolateral instabilities due to increased varus stress/stretch on lateral ligaments).

A Common Deficit Profile

Most knee injuries beyond a mild degree of severity demonstrate a consistent, predictable profile of physical findings independent of specific diagnoses. The primary deficit is a weak, atrophic, and neuromuscularly inhibited quadriceps femoris muscle with the most significant loss in the vastus medialis obliquus (VMO) (Fig. 5-3). The patient will demonstrate difficulty or inability to actively recruit a strong, stable, and firm contraction of the VMO muscle which is readily verified by surface or needle electromyography (EMG). Occasionally, a maximal effort to recruit the muscle will prove uncomfortable or painful in the area of the patellofemoral joint or suprapatellar bursa and capsule.

LoPresti and associates[24] accurately described this dysfunctional component of muscle as quadriceps muscle suppression and found significant quadriceps femoris deficits with anterior cruciate ligament (ACL) patients for 13 months after injury. Quadriceps muscle suppression is usually coupled with unilateral hamstring muscle tightness, defined here as inability to achieve at least 70 degrees on the active straight leg raise test. In addition, the hip joint on the side of dysfunction will also demonstrate

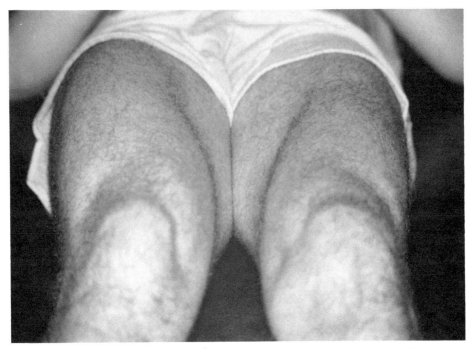

FIGURE 5–3. VMO muscle hypertrophy in the right quadriceps femoris muscle and VMO muscle atrophy in the left.

unilateral hip flexion weakness, as assessed by Kendall and Worthingham's[25] manual muscle test position and techniques. To a lesser extent, unilateral hip abductor and hip extensor muscle weakness may also exist. Clinical observations have revealed the importance of complete strengthening of these hip muscles and flexibility training of the hamstring muscles. Consequently, strengthening of the quadriceps femoris and hip flexor, extensor, and abductor muscles and flexibility of the hamstring muscle are the generic cornerstones of knee injury rehabilitation.

FEATURES OF REHABILITATION

Rehabilitation programs are administered either presurgically, postsurgically, or on a conservative basis. The postsurgical rehabilitation program is universal for a host of orthopedic, sports medicine, and industrial medicine procedures.

Conservative rehabilitation programs are applied when surgery is clearly not indicated (for example, with muscle strains, tendonitis, contusions, and many types of retropatellar pain) or may be too risky in light of the patient's general health; when economic issues interfere; or in those instances when the patient decides against surgical intervention. Selection for conservative rehabilitation as an alternative to surgery is a growing occurrence for a selected number of patient pathologies, especially in the case of the medial (tibial) collateral ligament. Knee joint laxity associated with moderate or grade III ligament tears is successfully managed without surgery, or even casting (see Chapter 12). Classic stages shared by rehabilitation programs are reviewed in Table 5–5.

TABLE 5–5 Stages of Rehabilitation

Acute	Maximal joint protection (or) immobilization
	Modalities
	Rest from activities
Subacute	Moderate protection
	Early exercise stresses
	Aerobic, endurance training
	Modalities
Settled (resolved)	Minimal protection
	Braces or supports
	Progressive exercise intensity
	Graded functional progression

In the early 1970s, a pioneering approach by orthopedists, physical therapists, and athletic trainers (most of whom worked closely with major college football programs) developed principles to provide athletes with the earliest possible return to activity consistent with safe tissue function and necessary performance levels. The so-called aggressive approach is currently used with many nonathletic orthopedic patients and has evolved into the standard for rehabilitation of knee injuries.

Program Design versus Protocols

Clinical program design is based on a thorough initial evaluation and continual reassessment (see Chapters 2 and 3). Treatment goals, timetable for progression, and discharge readiness are based on the patient's response and tolerance. Conversely, the concept of protocols is suspect because protocols fail to account for individual differences in physiology, posture, kinematics, and personality. Hence, protocols serve only to combine important milestones with phased physical skills, rather than as a "prescription" of appropriate rehabilitation techniques. The model rehabilitation program is subject to variation but combines several important, decisive principles. First, rehabilitation strengthening should be practiced according to the rule that pain equals no gain, in contrast to stereotypic attitudes associated with weight training for the healthy individual. Pain provides a useful warning that should be respected during exercise applications. Avoidance of strict immobilization, provision of early protected motion, control of early stresses in a time-phased manner,[11] and vigorous substitute aerobic conditioning activities are all key principles for complete and effective rehabilitation programs. In addition, muscle strengthening should be used for all key dynamic stabilizers at the knee and hip. Positive reinforcement through ongoing achievement of preset rehabilitation goals is paramount for success. The allowance for periodic rests (both physical and psychologic benefits) from the routine schedule are particularly beneficial.[26]

Specificity Issues

The principle of specificity dictates that the human system will perform most effectively and efficiently when trained with movements that closely approximate the actual functional skill required. During early rehabilitation stages, it is often impossible (due to healing constraints and physical capacity) to exactly replicate movement demands. Therefore, a key challenge in program design is the selection of appropriate movements and exercises that are safe and well tolerated by the patient, and relevant to their motoric needs.

Thorough assessment of the patient's functional movement with respect to (1) biomechanical complexities; (2) appropriate energy systems (e.g., adenosine triphosphate–phosphocreatine [ATP-PC], aerobic); (3) types of muscle contraction (e.g., isometric, eccentric); (4) neuromuscular control demands; and (5) the type of kinetic chain pattern used (open versus closed) should be performed as a basis for program design. Closed kinetic chain training should be instituted as soon as muscular responses and joint reactions will allow. Thorough understanding of and reliance on exercise physiology principles is the keystone of successful and expedient rehabilitation.

MULTIMODAL TRAINING

Based on the tremendous sophistication of the human muscular system, many studies advocate the importance of multimodal resistive exercise training.[3,12,27–31] Multimodal training incorporates exercises from each of the major available resistive modes: isometric, isotonic (with eccentrics)[32]; isodynamic; isokinetic (with the important subset of robotics)[32]; and inertial exercise. Elftman's proposal[33] describes the relationship of peak available muscle force between respective exercise modes as follows: eccentric > isometric > concentric. This principle has been consistently verified without exception for all upper and lower extremity muscle groups as well as for trunk/spine musculature. Table 5–6 illustrates the differences between contraction modes for the quadriceps femoris muscle at selected knee position angles and further supports the role of multimodal resistive exercises. Furthermore, multimodal training influences variables that produce daily fluctuations of strength values (Table 5–7). Skillful integration of varied exercise modes can minimize such daily fluctuations.

Although it is not the purpose of this chapter to analyze the differential effects and clinical rationale for each major resistive mode, sources by Davies,[12] Kisner and Colby,[34] Essel,[35] and Albert[32] examine these areas for rehabilitation applications. Table 5–8 outlines comparative advantages and disadvantages of various exercise modes.

SPEED SPECIFICITY

Primary variables in resistance training programs are the speed of movement and the load of resistance.[36] The speed of a given training exercise or selected functional activity has great impact on injury prevention, neuromuscular control, muscle-fiber–type recruitment, and preferred mode of contraction, as well as achievable range of

TABLE 5–6 Quadriceps Femoris Muscle Contraction Modes with the Knee Joint in Selected Positions

0 degrees	Peak EMG activity for isometric contraction, all muscles except rectus femoris
0–15 degrees	Biomechanics and muscle tension cause difficulty with eccentric responses
0–30 degrees	Muscular length-tension relationships cause this to be the most difficult arc to achieve concentrically
30 degrees	Most efficient position for isometric tension
30–60 degrees	"Power" zone for concentric force
	55° of flexion angle for peak tension
90 degrees	Peak tension capacity for eccentric loading
	3 × greater force than concentrics

TABLE 5–7 Factors That May Affect Strength Values

1. Weight of the tested part
2. Relationship of the tested part with the horizontal
3. Angle of the joint if analyzing a one-joint muscle
4. Angle of joints if analyzing a two-joint muscle
5. Angle of applied resistance
6. Distance of point of application of resistance from the joint
7. Stabilization of adjacent body parts
8. Type of contraction
9. Speed of contraction
10. Duration of contraction
11. Number of warm-ups and learning trials
12. Motivation of subject
13. Rest between trials
14. Age of subject
15. Gender of subject
16. Control of cocontraction
17. Joint limitations
    a. Friction
    b. Bony mechanical block
    c. Soft-tissue tightness
    d. Pain

motion. In the human articular system, speed variability is enormous, ranging from 0 degrees per second (isometric state) to over 10,000 degrees per second in some athletic, open kinetic chain activities such as baseball pitching.[37] Clinical observations indicate that the more distal joints in a kinetic chain have correspondingly lower speed potential. For example, in the upper-extremity chain, the shoulder can generate much higher speeds from voluntary muscle activation than can the wrist.

NONRESISTIVE EXERCISE COMPONENTS

Comprehensive rehabilitation programs include the nonstrength factors, such as flexibility, muscular endurance, kinesthesia, and skill in the activity. Each component is important to the final outcome of the rehabilitation program. *Flexibility* is the capacity of the soft tissues to elongate safely under tensile loads and is critical to both injury prevention and optimal performance. Musculotendinous prestretch allows a given cross-sectional area of muscle tissue to produce increased forces. Functional flexibility demands a combination of both static and dynamic characteristics.[38] However, static stretching methods are the safest initially to avoid stimulation of the stretch reflex and should be used as preparatory phases to any dynamic (ballistic) stretches. *Kinesthesia*, or a combination of balance, coordination, and proprioceptive capacities, is paramount to normal function of the knee joint under weight-bearing compressive, rotational, and tensile loads, and acceleration/deceleration demands. A multitude of simple kinesthetic exercises exist, such as one-legged standing with eyes open or closed, walking on a curved line, and step-ups. Many commercially available devices, such as the mini-tramp, sliding boards, tilt or balance boards, balance beams, and Sand Dune (Universal Gym Corp Co., P.O. Box 1270, Cedar Rapids, IA 52406), are useful during rehabilitation programs. Besides sports-specific skills, the ultimate late-stage kinematic training is plyometrics, which are useful for some types of ground-based athletics.[32]

TABLE 5-8 Resistive Exercise Modes: Differential Features

Type	Advantages	Disadvantages
Isometric	Prevents decrease of ligament, bone, and muscle strength	Peak effort can be injurious
	Retards atrophy and reflex dissociation	Limited functional transfer
	Strengthening with no joint motion	Vascular bed collapse
	Can be applied during immobilization	Increase blood pressure
Isotonic	Ready accessibility	Physiologic "stick point"
	Functional proprioceptive, eccentric, and stabilization patterns	Technique vs. safety considerations
	Versatile applications	Post-exercise soreness
Isokinetic	Synovial joint lubrication	Expense considerations
	Accommodating resistance features	Questionable functional transfer
	Objective quantification	Joint axis alignment problems
	Safety with fast training speeds	Impact load potential
	Fiber type conversion: type IIa to IIb	
	Medico-legal support	
Inertial	High-speed, functional eccentrics	Short arc of motion at high speeds
	Safety	Minimal research base
	Versatile patterns	
	Neuromuscular training effects	
Open chain training	Single joint axis	Potential for joint shear
	Single joint plane	Limited functional applications
	Concentrics dominate	Limited eccentrics and proprioception
	Stable proximal segment	
Closed chain training	Translatory, multiple joint axes	Potential for loss of control of the target joint
	Spiral, diagonal movement patterns	Summation of forces may produce excessive momentum loads
	Facilitates postural and stabilization mechanics	
	Proprioceptive input	

Ongoing, progressive endurance training (of both muscular and cardiovascular emphasis) is beneficial to the knee patient by facilitating blood flow and oxygenation of the healing tissues; reduction of physiologic and psychologic stressors associated with inactivity, disability, and pain; and prevention of general physical deconditioning and associated weight gain due to inactivity. In addition, endurance training offers a localized continuous passive motion (CPM) effect for the injured knee and a substitute physical outlet for the obligatory exerciser. Effective training principles advocated and tested by Cooper[39] and the American College of Sports Medicine[40] include a minimum of three weekly training sessions for 20 minutes, with a target heart rate of 80 percent of age-adjusted maximum. Modern technology has introduced many novel training alternatives, which include pool training, upper-extremity-only, lower-extremity-only, and full-body training on selected machines (Table 5-9).

TABLE 5–9 Equipment Alternatives for Cardiorespiratory/Aerobic Training (Sample Listing Only)

Full Body	Upper Body	Lower Body
Rowing machines	Upper body ergometer	Treadmills
Schwinn Airdyne	Upper cycle	Bicycles
Swimming	BTE (Baltimore Therapeutic	Stairclimber
Stationary ski track	Equipment Co., Hanover, MD)	Running in water
Running in deep water (wet vest)		Running
		Underwater treadmills

Selection of the appropriate exercise mode depends on the specific demands of the patient's functional activities; patient preference variables; and the appropriate healing stage of the injured knee tissue.

BICYCLING CONCEPTS

Key considerations in selecting the bicycle for training are pedal sequence (forward versus backward) and knee flexion range. Individual patient limb length variations usually require 95 to 105 degrees of active knee flexion to smoothly rotate a full pedal revolution. Inadequate knee flexion results in compensatory hip hiking and trunk lean. In the patient without sufficient knee flexion, the bicycle still provides a beneficial means for mobilizing knee joint flexion. This is accomplished through repeated reversal of forward and backward pedaling at the extreme of tolerable flexion. Such an application incorporates advantages of CPM on the patellofemoral articular cartilage, as well as the positive benefits of improved synovial fluid dispersal and reduced joint frictional forces.[41,42] Patients with knee flexion restrictions are able to complete initial full pedal revolutions in the backward direction before they will tolerate the forward direction. McLeod and Blackburn[43] explain this concept by means of the angulation of the tibia that reduces ligamentous tension during the backward stroke. Raising the seat height or pedaling with heel-only contact assists clearance of a full pedal stroke. However, these mechanical changes produce limited increases of knee flexion. Febey[44] offers a biomechanical solution for bicycling with limited knee flexion using a device that attaches to the pedal to allow for completion of a full crank cycle (Fig. 5–4). Bicycling produces lower-extremity mechanics similar to those observed in running. The acceleration or propulsion phase of cycling (when quadriceps femoris muscles are maximally active) resembles the midstance phase of running, with compressive loads producing subtalar joint pronation and corresponding closed-chain internal tibial rotation (Fig. 5–5).

Bicycling depends on quadriceps femoris dominant activity, with minimal recruitment of other important lower-extremity muscle groups. Careful orientation of the patient and the use of toe clips may increase recruitment of the hamstrings, hip flexors, and ankle dorsiflexor muscles. Stationary bicycling requires minimal gluteal muscle response, whereas street cycling recruits gluteal muscles, especially on hilly terrain. Hill climbing requires high concentric muscle force, generated by antigravity muscle groups; it is optimally performed in the standing position. In addition, bicycling is a functional application of isokinetic-type (fixed-speed, variable-resistance) muscle loading, provided that it is applied with a stationary bicycle, or in the form of continuous-level-surface street pedaling. An inherent disadvantage of stationary bicycling is the absence of

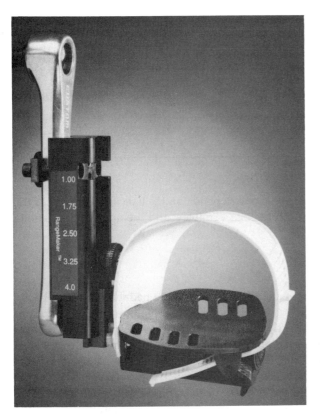

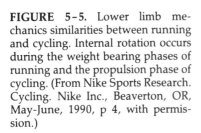

FIGURE 5–4. Bicycle pedal adjustment for limited knee flexion. The radius of the pedal may be adjusted between 1 to approximately 7 inches. (Rangemaker-Rainbow Rehabilitation and Fitness, PO Box 49, 100 Ottawa St, Grayling, MI, 49738.)

FIGURE 5–5. Lower limb mechanics similarities between running and cycling. Internal rotation occurs during the weight bearing phases of running and the propulsion phase of cycling. (From Nike Sports Research. Cycling. Nike Inc., Beaverton, OR, May-June, 1990, p 4, with permission.)

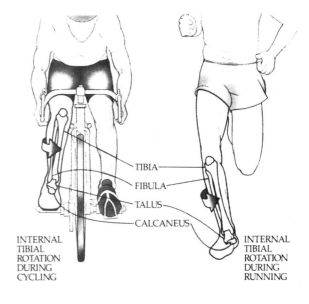

eccentric muscle control. Disadvantages of street bicycling include inclement weather; risks of crashes (with high incidence of head injuries unless helmets are used); hasty dismounts that produce instantaneous rotational, compressive loads on the knee; mistimed gear shifts that cause sudden impulse loads with associated risks on the retropatellar articular cartilage; and the tendency of the patient to coast when fatigued.

Progressions

Judicious implementation and monitoring of graded exercise intensity is crucial to knee rehabilitation programs. Despite cautious program design, the introduction of new exercises may cause muscular soreness or joint irritability. Negative muscle and joint reactions to exercise can be termed exercise "overdose," and the associated signs and symptoms of overdose are reviewed in Table 5–10. Overuse reactions require immediate and appropriate alteration in the treatment program and treatment techniques. In more serious episodes of overdose, time is required for recovery of previous functional levels. Exercise overdose is often psychologically debilitating to even the most motivated, disciplined patient.

Table 5–3 provides one useful guideline for safe and efficient exercise progression from the earliest, most protective phase after injury or surgery to the highest level of stress training. However, the final, critical test of patient tolerance is the actual functional demand that is required of each patient. Consequently, each rehabilitation program must evolve into functional training progressions. Functional training principles for the upper and lower extremity and spine are commonly applied in sport and industrial rehabilitation settings. Functional progressions are based on time-phased, symptom/sign-guided increases in activities that simulate the true movement and incorporate sequentially increased joint speeds, shear, and compression forces with greater skill requirements. Functional progressions result in increased demands on the muscular/articular system and recruit eccentric muscle responses, with resultant alterations in the neuromuscular system.[32,45] For example, in the lower extremity, functional progressions graduate from two-legged movement to single/injured-leg-only movements, from non–weight bearing to weight bearing, and from slow to fast speeds. The clinician should provide a rehabilitation environment with mixed or multimodal training to ensure both functional specificity and the greatest degree of injury prevention.[46] Although isokinetic training offers several important clinical benefits (Table 5–11), only robotic dynamometers, for example, the KinCom (Chattanooga Corp., P.O. Box 489, Hixson, TN 37343), can provide eccentric muscle loading. However, eccentric isokinetic loads, specifically the eccentric/eccentric variety, are nonphysiologic and therefore

TABLE 5–10 Signs/Symptoms of Resistive Exercise Overdose

Increased pain
Effusion/swelling
Continued burning in muscle
Headache
Persistent stiffness
Dizziness
Hyperventilation
Onset/change of crepitus
Decrease in strength or plateau
Fasciculation/cramps

TABLE 5–11 Advantages of Isokinetic Training

High-speed training
Safety
Fiber type conversion (type IIa to type IIb)
Pain relief
Physiologic overflow with respect to speed
Effects resistant to detraining
Submaximal exercise
Accommodative resistance
Joint lubrication
Neuromuscular control

should be supplemented by other forms of training. Isokinetic torque of the quadriceps femoris muscles has higher functional predictability at higher speeds (at or above 240 degrees per second),[47,48] illustrated by the fact that even basic human activities of daily living, such as walking, produce joint speeds of the knee at 240 degrees per second.[49]

Free weight use during advanced rehabilitation stages will recruit eccentric muscle control and promote muscular hypertrophy, as well as prepare the knee for ballistic loads and plyometric exercises. Plyometrics are series of functional movements designed to maximize speed and performance that utilize the stretch-shorten cycle outlined by Cavagna.[50] Plyometrics selectively recruit the series elastic, or noncontractile, component of muscle to provide facilitated muscle power through the use of potential kinetic energy.[32] Free-weight resistive training may begin with multiple joint training, gravity eliminated (e.g., leg press), and advance to higher stress movements and antigravity movements (e.g., the squat). The squat performed with power lifting techniques does not resemble the biomechanics of deep knee bends and therefore is not inherently risky to the knee articular cartilage or ligaments. The squat biomechanics closely resemble those of many daily tasks, such as climbing, stooping, lifting from below knee level, jumping, sitting, and using the toilet. A critical issue with the use of free weights during rehabilitation is that of the instruction and practice of correct techniques (Figs. 5–6 and 5–7).

Modalities and Supplemental Care

Relief of pain and the resolution or control of joint effusion is preliminary to exercise considerations. Documented as early as 1965 by deAndrade and associates,[51] the presence of knee joint effusion produces significant neuromuscular inhibition of the quadriceps femoris muscles with attendant weakness and atrophy.[52–54]

Optimal performance of the quadriceps femoris muscles is achieved only when the patient is pain-free with no effusion in the knee.[55,56] Consequently, mechanically induced pain must be treated prior to, or in conjunction with, the earliest modes of exercise and motion.

Whereas a host of treatment options are available to decrease or control pain, including various types of anti-inflammatory medications, the use of varied types of electrical stimulation is both a common and effective clinical measure for the relief of knee pain. Multiple approaches for the treatment of pain with transcutaneous electrical nerve stimulation (TENS) are described by Mannheimer[57] and may decrease or obviate the need for medications. Other types of electrical stimulation for the relief of pain

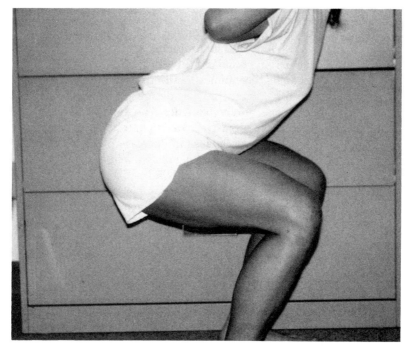

FIGURE 5-6. Squat mechanics—pelvic position. The pelvis is positioned in an anterior tilt to maintain the lumbar spine lordosis. The anterior pelvic tilt requires cocontraction of the abdominal, lumbar paraspinal, and latissimus dorsi muscles as the knees flex to stabilize an erect position of the trunk.

FIGURE 5-7. Squat mechanics—knee/tibial position. The knees should not pass over the toes in a sagittal plane. With the knees in this position, the alignment of the tibial bones relative to the supporting surface is nearly vertical, which results in minimal strain to both the patellofemoral joints and the ACLs.

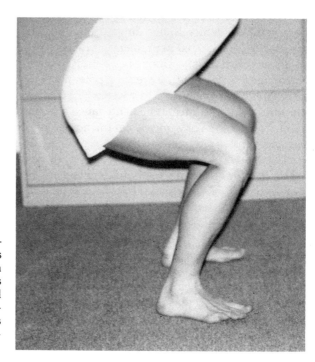

include microcurrent electrical nerve stimulation (MENS), which is described by Wallace[58] and Becker[59]; high-volt galvanic stimulation, which has an additional reported effectiveness in decreasing swelling; and interferential spiked-wave types of alternating current, and the so-called Russian stimulation.

Perhaps the most accessible, economical, and effective modality for knee inflammation and pain is cryotherapy. Cryotherapy is administered in many forms, including whirlpools, ice packs, ice massage, and cryokinetics. The multiple beneficial physiologic effects of cold therapy have been extensively documented[60-63] to include pain relief; decrease of edema, effusion, and muscle spasm; decrease of metabolism and oxygen requirement in injured tissues; and slowing of nerve conduction velocity. In conjunction with cryotherapy, the well-known acronym of RICE (*rest, ice, compression,* and *elevation*) principles are effective methods for immediate and early knee treatment, as well as for postrehabilitation sessions and functional lower extremity progressions, and for continued use during the patient's initial return to work, sports, or recreational pursuits.

Selected Manual/Mechanical Techniques

Patients with injured or diseased knee joints may benefit from many manual techniques. Healing soft tissues must be stimulated with an appropriate degree of stresses and with appropriate timing to produce effective remodeling and the restoration of a normal tensile stress-bearing scar. During early rehabilitation phases when full-active range of motion is limited by pain or restricted by functional braces, passive motion with skilled manual contacts, directed in appropriate joint planes or in arthrokinematic patterns, will assist in restoration of normal active motion of the knee joint, or in other instances help prevent joint adhesions and soft-tissue contractures.

Restoration of normal passive glide to the patellofemoral joint should precede full flexion exercises, resisted exercises, and bicycling. Of equal importance is the restoration of normal tibiofemoral joint range of motion. Postsurgical knee joint contractures are frequently encountered in problems as diverse as intra-articular ACL reconstruction and total knee arthroplasty. Timing is a critical concern for effective and safe tissue remodeling about the knee, with increasing potential for contractures encountered if full range of motion is not gained in 3 to 4 weeks.[64,65] Contractures are also common sequelae with fractures about the knee. When end-range knee movements are met with resistance that cannot be overcome by muscle contraction alone, the use of external stretching forces is required. Prolonged low-load stretches provide the most effective response[66-68] with the goal of 1 hour of sustained stretch daily at or near end-range of the restricted motion. Heating tissues prior to stretch is advantageous from both physiologic and psychologic perspectives.[69] Heating tissue improves extensibility (through visco elastic properties), which, in turn, improves patient comfort during the stretch. Moist heat packs and ultrasound are ready sources applied prior to, or simultaneous with, stretching. Patient comfort and tolerance during the stretch can be improved by the use of TENS and periodic brief breaks (no more than 1 minute) of external stress unloading. Some patients also benefit from distractions such as reading.

Stretching forces may be applied through prolonged manual contacts, cuff weights, machine weights from isotonic weight stacks, or weights combined with pulley set-ups to produce a prolonged stretching stimulus. Pulleys can also impart proper arthrokinematic forces[70] (Figs. 5–8 and 5–9). External forces may also be applied by physical contacts from the exercise specialist and the use of commercially available, spring-loaded brace devices such as Dynasplints (Dynasplints, 6655 Amberton Dr., Ste. A,

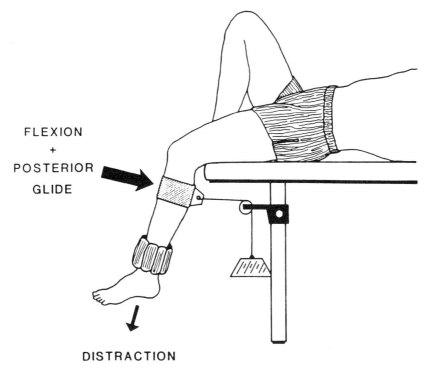

FIGURE 5-8. Stretch position to gain knee flexion. Low-load passive forces are applied via traction cuffs to increase knee flexion. (From Sapega, A and Rogan, LK: Optimizing the nonsurgical treatment of joint contractures. In Engle, RP [ed]: Knee Ligament Rehabilitation. Churchill Livingstone, New York, 1991, p 195, with permission.)

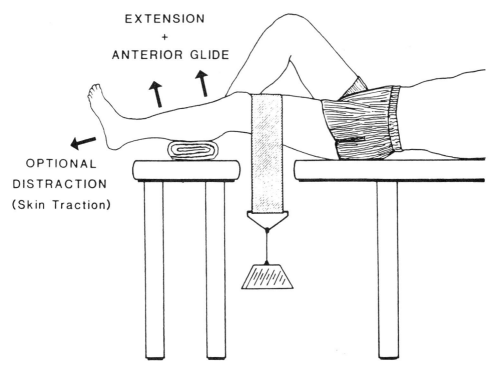

FIGURE 5-9. Stretch position to gain extension. Low-load forces are created by hanging weights directly to increase knee extension. (From Sapega, A and Rogan, LK: Optimizing the nonsurgical treatment of joint contractures. In Engle, RP [ed]: Knee Ligament Rehabilitation. Churchill Livingstone, New York, 1991, p 194, with permission.)

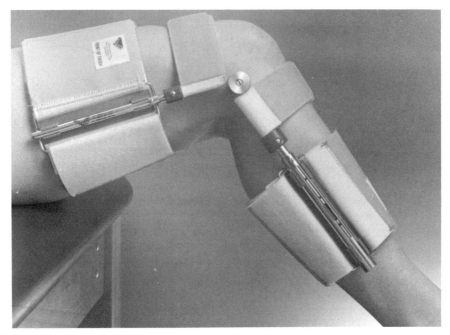

FIGURE 5–10. Dynasplint is used to gain either knee flexion or extension due to a knee joint contracture. The splint should be worn approximately 8 to 10 hours daily using a low-load force. (Dynasplint is a trademark of Dynasplint Systems, Inc., 6655 Amberton Dr., Ste. A, Baltimore, MD 21227.)

Baltimore, MD 21227) (Fig. 5–10). Dynasplints are made to restore either lost extension or lost flexion, but not both movements in the same brace.

SELECTED REHABILITATION PRINCIPLES

Effective quadriceps femoris muscle training is the foundation of resistive exercise training for the knee. The initial goal is to recruit the VMO portion of the quadriceps femoris muscle group because of its dynamic medial displacing action on the patella. Activation of the VMO is achieved throughout the range of motion, with strong quadriceps muscle activation occurring at both terminal knee extension (30 to 0 degrees) and at 0 degrees of extension (the training position for quadriceps muscle sets and SLRs).[71]

Electrical stimulation is strongly supported as an adjunctive method for strengthening and facilitating appropriate neuromuscular control of the quadriceps femoris muscle.[71–78] However, controversy exists as to which electrical parameters produce the most effective methods for strengthening. Recommendations for optimizing strength effects include the use of a flexed knee position with fixed distal tibia, and use of high- or medium-frequency stimulation with intensity sufficient to recruit 33 to 91 percent of the maximal voluntary isometric contraction.[76–78] My preference is to use the Electrostim 180 (Promatek Medical, 1851 Black Rd., Joilet, IL 60435), based on successful clinical results with patient tolerance to intensity levels sufficient to produce strong visible and palpable tetanic contractions. The use of amplified biofeedback with surface electrodes placed on the VMO facilitates rapid control of the quadriceps femoris muscles, especially of the VMO muscle. The author uses the Davicon (Biomedical Instrument Co.,

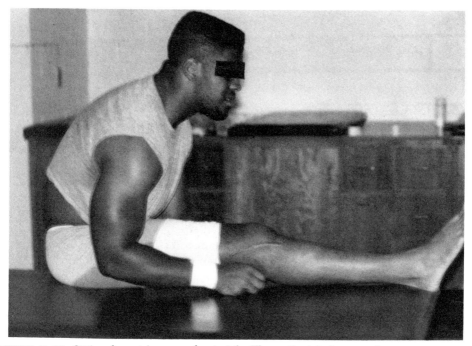

FIGURE 5–11. Sitting hamstring muscle stretch. The patient is instructed to try to maintain lumbar spine lordosis and flex from the waist. A low-load, prolonged stretch, 30 sec to 1 min, is most effective to increase soft tissue extensibility.

Inc., 2387 E. Eight Mile Rd., Warren, MI 48091-2403) for this biofeedback-facilitated quadriceps training.

Hamstring muscle inflexibility (which is very common when assessed by the active SLR test) produces a net resistance force to the extension force of the quadriceps femoris muscles. This resistance is most detrimental to the final 30 degrees of extension concentrically and also increases retropatellar compressive loads.[79] Hence the routine use of presession and postsession hamstring muscle stretches with static, prolonged holds (30 seconds to 1 minute) and home program stretches is instrumental. If retropatellar complaints are increased by the supine active SLR stretching position, the alternative of a sitting stretch is employed (Fig. 5–11).

Closed kinetic chain-type strengthening exercises are integrated early in the rehabilitation progression. Closed kinetic chain exercises incorporate joint proprioceptive input and eccentric muscle control; facilitate stable patellar positions in the femoral trochlear groove; and produce a synchronous activity from antigravity musculature in the hip and ankle in conjunction with the quadriceps femoris muscle group, which in essence shares compressive and tensile loads that the patellofemoral joint must bear.

Rehabilitation Scheme

Provided that optimal intervention with various knee dysfunction is possible, rehabilitation begins soon after injury has occurred and for the first 3 days focuses on symptom control with appropriate medications; modalities such as ice and electrical stimulation; activity modification; and use of long leg immobilizer, patellar brace, or crutches as indicated by patient weight bearing tolerance and joint control. The principal exercise during this phase is the quadriceps femoris muscle set, *performed in a pain-free manner!*

SUBACUTE PHASE

The subacute phase is instituted when minimal pain with movement; active flexion to at least 90 degrees; ability to initiate a quadriceps femoris muscle set; and minimal peripatellar effusion are present. Activity status in this period includes partial weight bearing or full weight bearing for ambulation, with strict avoidance of all ballistic movements such as jumping or running, squatting, use of stairs, street cycling, and prolonged sitting with the knee hyperextended or in flexion greater than 40 degrees. This phase corresponds to the use of graduated strengthening exercises for all lower extremity muscles; flexibility exercises for the hamstring, iliotibial band, and gastrocnemius-soleus muscle groups; and electric stimulation for the quadriceps femoris muscles. These exercises are performed twice daily with progressive additions of weight for (SLRs) up to 15 lb (unless the patient has extremely long legs).[80] Multiple angle isometrics are used to prepare the muscle and joint structures for increased-intensity resistive exercises and are effective for remediating painful extension arcs or points in the range of motion with insufficient arthrokinematic control. Eccentric training is also effective in remediating painful arcs and dysfunctional positions in the range of motion.

In addition, submaximal isometric contractions also prevent atrophy and reflex dissociation of the quadriceps femoris muscle. Physiologic overflow of position has been demonstrated by Davies,[12] which supports the use of multiple angle isometrics applied at 20-degree increments throughout the desired range of motion. As quadriceps femoris muscle strength and control develops, resistance exercises are performed on isotonic or cam/pulley type machines. Isokinetic training may be instituted in this phase as dictated by patient symptoms and muscular control. Several special considerations allow for safer and less stressful isokinetic muscle training. First, the use of terminal knee extensions (0 to 35 degrees) affords training with decreased demand on patellar tracking and moderate retropatellar compression forces. The use of intermediate speeds (120 to 180 degrees per second) allows the patient sufficient capacity to "catch" the machine speed with minimal risk of harmful impact loads.

In the case of eccentric isokinetics, suggested guidelines include patient experience and tolerance of concentric isokinetics; strict maintenance of appropriate patellar tracking through the use of both visual and palpation methods; use of training speeds of 60, 90, and 120 degrees per second with repetitions from 30 in initial sessions to 90 in advanced sessions. Despite cautious and graduated exercise progressions, some patients will develop peripatellar pain that is exacerbated or caused by remedial strengthening exercises, such as quadriceps femoris muscle sets, terminal extensions, and to a lesser extent, SLRs. Antich and Brewster[81] review several effective and simple modifications of exercises that can prevent or relieve exercise-induced pain (Table 5–12). In addition, eccentric, submaximal knee-extension contractions can be effective in ameliorating pain problems in patients who do not demonstrate retropatellar pain produced by the patellofemoral grinding test (see Appendix).

Persistent quadriceps femoris muscle suppression in patients with long-standing dysfunction may also respond to an interesting physiologic phenomenon described by Caiozzo.[82] Caiozzo demonstrated an instantaneous 25 percent increase of quadriceps

TABLE 5–12 Modification of Quad Sets/Straight Leg Raises
to Prevent or Reduce Patellofemoral Joint Strain

Ankle dorsiflexion during quad sets
Use of small wedge in popliteal fossa
Hamstring cocontraction
Ankle dorsiflexion with inversion
Quad set augmented by electrical stimulation
Isometric hip adduction (prior to quad sets)
Ice application after exercise

Source: Adapted from Antich and Brewster.[81]

femoris muscle torque when augmented by a preceding forceful isometric contraction of the hamstring muscles.

Adjunctive techniques for strengthening include proprioceptive neuromuscular facilitation of lower extremity patterns, such as a hip flexion, abduction, and external rotation diagonal pattern, and indirect strength techniques as described by Black and Alten for patellar tendonitis[83] (Fig. 5–12).

FUNCTIONAL PHASE (PROGRESSING TO DISCHARGE)

The final phase is a continuum of joint and muscular stresses that have been initiated in the previous phase with increasing emphasis and time spent on actual functional training with certain restrictions. Quadriceps femoris muscle strengthening should continue on a minimal twice-per-week basis, as should regular aerobic training. The total aerobic training time may be adjusted to allow for the time involved in the functional activity. Patient tolerance is monitored and the patient's psychologic response is also observed. Beyond physical readiness, the patient should also demonstrate confidence and enthusiasm for each new functional level. Isokinetic test parameters (such as peak torque or total work levels) are important guidelines about patient progress. It may be impossible to achieve bilateral equality of isokinetic torque levels with certain patients or pathologies. In my experience, reasonable minimal goals include 70 percent quadriceps femoris muscle torque comparisons prior to running, and 90 percent peak torque and total work for discharge. For patients requiring ballistic movements in their preferred activities, a plyometric progression should be provided.[32] In all other patients a phased, symptom-guided functional progression should be administered (Table 5–13). As healing constraints have passed and all functional progression tasks have been mastered, the patient returns to normal function and is discharged from formal rehabilitation sessions. The patient may need to continue use of patellar or other knee braces, but this is an individual matter based on the preferences of physician, therapist or trainer, and patient. A 6-month follow-up visit for isokinetic assessment with special emphasis on quadriceps femoris muscle status is advisable. Unfortunately, this may not be feasible due to patient unavailability and/or cost considerations.

SUMMARY

Rehabilitation for the knee is an integral part of conservative and postsurgical management plans. Maximum effectiveness dictates a comprehensive, biomechanically based design, individualized progression, and skillful application of the art of patient

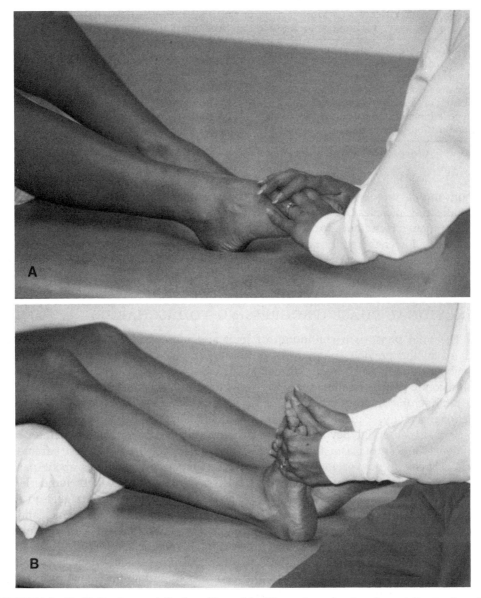

FIGURE 5-12. *A*) Starting and final position of facilitory strengthening for patellar tendon. *B*) Midposition of facilitory stengthening for patellar tendon.

interaction and motivation. Knowledge of time constraints on healing, immobilization effects, specialized anatomy, exercise physiology benefits and indications, and available equipment and technology are all vital for the rehabilitation specialist. However, the cornerstone of rehabilitation is therapeutic resistive exercises that are applied in a multimodal fashion to ensure specificity. Although impressively large research bases exist for knee biomechanics and selected pathophysiologies (such as ACL rupture), continued research into clinical interventions and outcome assessments will guide future programs toward optimal patient success.

TABLE 5-13 Sample 8-Week Reconditioning Program

General guidelines	6 days per week—Sunday off
	Alternate running days with cycling/step machines (3 days each)
	Progress cycling 2 minutes per week starting at 10 minutes
Week 1	Easy pace, straight ahead running—4 × 100-yard repeats
	Run upstairs (30–60 steps), walk down, balance board
Week 2	Stairs, medium-speed running (approx. 8 minutes per mile
	2–4 repeats of ¼ mile, balance board
Week 3	Repeat week 2
	Lateral slide board movements (10–20 times on 6–8-ft board)
Week 4	1 mile medium-speed run
	2 build-up sprints (50 yards)
	"S" running—¼ total
	Skipping rope—10 minutes
Week 5	Repeat week 4 with increase of "S" runs to ½ mile
	1½-mile runs at medium speed
	Backward runs—10 times, 10 yards
	Hopping
Week 6	¼ mile of "Z" running
	¼ mile of carioca or crossover running
	2 mile medium-speed running
	Vertical and linear jumping, 3–5 minute total
Week 7	Repeat week 6
	Increase to ½ mile "Z" running and ½ mile of cariocas
	Add figure-eight skill runs
	Early depth (box) jumping
Week 8	Figure-eight sprinting
	40-yard sprints—6–8 times
	Plyometrics

REFERENCES

1. Knott, M and Voss, DE: Proprioceptive Neuro-muscular Facilitation: Patterns and Techniques, ed 2. Harper & Row, New York, 1968.
2. Houglum, P: The modality of therapeutic exercise: Objectives and principles. Athletic Training 12:42, 1977.
3. Timm, KE: Postsurgical knee rehabilitation: A five year study of four methods and 5,381 patients. Am J Sports Med 16(5):463, 1988.
4. Stafford, MG and Grana, WA: Hamstring/quadriceps ratios in college football players: A high velocity evaluation. Am J Sports Med 12(3):209, 1984
5. Kreighbaum, E and Barthels, KM: Biomechanics: A Qualitative Approach for Studying Human Movement, ed 2. MacMillan, New York, 1985, p 228.
6. Wallace, L: Isokinetic testing survey. Unpublished survey, Sports Physical Therapy Section, American Physical Therapy Association, 1988.
7. Nicholas, JA, Strizak, AM, and Veras, G: A study of thigh muscle weakness in different pathological states of the lower extremity. Am J Sports Med 4(6):241, 1976.
8. Gleim, GW, Nicholas, JA, and Webb, JN: Isokinetic evaluation following leg injuries. The Physician and Sportsmedicine 6(8):74, 1978.
9. Nicholas, JA and Marino, M: The relationship of injuries of the leg, foot and ankle to proximal thigh strength in athletes. Foot Ankle 7(4):218, 1987.
10. Shelton, GL: Principles of musculo-skeletal rehabilitation. In Mellion, MB: Office Management of Sports Injuries and Athletic Problems. Hanley & Belfus, Philadelphia, 1988.
11. Davies, GJ (ed): Rehabilitation of the Surgical Knee. Cypress, Ronkonkoma, NY, 1984.
12. Davies, GJ: A Compendium of Isokinetics in Clinical Usage, ed 3. S & S Publishers, Onalaska, WI, 1987.
13. Frankel, V and Nordin, M: Basic Biomechanics of the Skeletal System. Lea & Febiger, Philadelphia, 1980.
14. Hardy, MA: The biology of scar formation. Phys Ther 69(12):1014, 1989.
15. Troyer, H: The effect of short term immobilization on the rabbit knee joint cartilage: A histochemical study. Clin Orthop 107:249, 1975.
16. Evans, EB: Experimental immobilization and remobilization of rat knee joints. J Bone Joint Surg [Am] 42:757, 1960.
17. Akeson, WH, Amiel, D, and Woo, SLY: Immobility effects on synovial joints: The pathomechanics of joint contractures. Biorheology 17:95, 1980.
18. Akeson, WH, Amiel, D, and Woo, SLY: The connective tissue response to immobility: Biochemical changes in periarticular connective tissue of the immobilized rabbit knee. Clin Orthop 93:356, 1973.
19. Woo, SLY: Mechanical properties of tendons and ligaments. II. The relationship of immobilization and exercise on tissue remodeling. Biorheology 19:385, 1982.
20. Tipton, CM: The influence of physical activity on ligaments and tendons. Med Sci Sports Exerc 7(3):165, 1970.
21. Haggmark, T and Erickson, T: Fiber-type area and metabolic potential of the thigh muscle in man after knee surgery and immobilization. Int J Sports Med 2(1):12, 1981.
22. Lysholm, J and Gilquist, J: Evaluation of knee ligament surgery results with special emphasis on use of scoring scale. Am J Sports Med 10:150, 1982.
23. Ginsberg, JM: Continuous compression of rabbit articular cartilage producing loss of hydroxyproline before loss of hexosamine. J Bone Joint Surg [Am] 51:467, 1969.
24. LoPresti, C, et al: Quadriceps insufficiency following repair of the anterior cruciate ligament. Journal of Orthopedic and Sports Physical Therapy 9(7):248, 1988.
25. Daniels, L and Worthingham, C: Muscle Testing: Techniques of Manual Examination, ed 5. WB Saunders, Philadelphia, 1986.
26. DePalma, BF and Zelko, RR: Knee rehabilitation following anterior cruciate ligament injury or surgery. Athletic Training 21(3):200, 1986.
27. Costill, DL, Fink, WJ, and Habansky, AJ: Muscle rehabilitation after knee surgery. The Physician and Sportsmedicine 5:71, 1971.
28. Lieb, FJ and Perry, J: Quadriceps function: An anatomical and mechanical study using amputated limbs. J Bone Joint Surg [Am] 50:1535, 1968.
29. Steadman, JR: Rehabilitation of athletic injuries. Am J Sports Med 7(2):147, 1979.
30. Hakkinen, K and Komi, PV: Effect of different combined concentric and eccentric muscle work regimens on maximal strength development. Journal of Human Movement Studies 7:33, 1981.
31. Belka, D: Comparison of dynamic, static and combination training on dominant wrist flexor muscles. Research Quarterly 39:244, 1968.
32. Albert, M: Eccentric Muscle Training in Sports and Orthopedics. Churchill Livingstone, New York, 1991.
33. Elftman, H: Biomechanics of muscle. J Bone Joint Surg [Am] 48:363, 1966.
34. Kisner, C and Colby, LA: Therapeutic Exercise: Foundation and Techniques. FA Davis, Philadelphia, 1985.

35. Essel, D: Pumping rubber: Resistance with elasticized bands. SportsCare Fitness, March/April, 1989.
36. McDonagh, MJ and Davies, CT: Adaptive response of mammalian skeletal muscle with high loads. Eur J Appl Physiol 52(2):136, 1984.
37. McLeod, W: Biomechanics of throwing. Unpublished study, Columbus, GA, 1986.
38. Zachazewski, J: Changes in muscle flexibility: Pathophysiology and management. Paper presented at the American Physical Therapy Association National Conference, San Antonio, TX, 1988.
39. Cooper, K: Aerobics: A Way of Life. Bantam Books, New York, 1983.
40. American College of Sports Medicine: The recommended quantity and quality of exercise for developing and maintaining cardiorespiratory and muscular fitness in healthy adults. Med Sci Sports Exerc 22(2):265, 1990.
41. Barham, JN: Mechanical Kinesiology. CV Mosby, St Louis, MO, 1978.
42. Packard, B: Refuting the myth of quadriceps function: Implications in treatment of chondromalacia patellae. Paper presented at the Cybex Isokinetic Seminar, Las Vegas, 1981.
43. McLeod, W and Blackburn, TA: Biomechanics of knee rehabilitation with cycling. Am J Sports Med 8(3):175, 1980.
44. Febey, R: PT creates bike device to aid range-of-motion. P.T. Bulletin, Nov 15, 1989.
45. Stanton, P and Purdam, C: Hamstring injuries in sprinting: The role of eccentric exercise. Journal of Orthopedic and Sports Physical Therapy 11(3):343, 1989.
46. Stauber, WT: Eccentric action of muscles: Physiology, injury and adaptation. Exerc Sports Sci Rev 19:157, 1989.
47. Kannus, P: Peak torque and total work relationship in the thigh muscles after anterior cruciate ligament injury. Journal of Orthopedic and Sports Physical Therapy 10(3):97, 1988.
48. Johansson, C, et al: Sprinters and marathon runners. Does isokinetic knee extensor performance reflect muscle size and structure? Acta Physiol Scand 130:663, 1987.
49. Wyatt, MP and Edwards, AM: Comparison of quadriceps and hamstring torque values during isokinetic exercises. Journal of Orthopedic and Sports Physical Therapy 3(2):48, 1981.
50. Cavagna, GA, Saibene, FP, and Margaria, R: Effect of negative work on the amount of positive work performed by an isolated muscle. J Appl Physiol 20:157, 1965.
51. deAndrade, JR, Grant, C, and Dixon, AS: Joint distention and reflex muscle inhibition in the knee. J Bone Joint Surg [Am] 47:313, 1965.
52. Spencer, J, Hayes, K, and Alexander, I: Knee joint effusion and quadriceps reflex inhibition in man. Arch Phys Med Rehabil 65:171, 1984.
53. Wood, L, Ferrell, WR, and Boxendale, RH: Pressures in normal and acutely distended human knee joint and effects of quadriceps maximal voluntary contractions. Exp Physiol 73:305, 1988.
54. Stokes, M and Young, A: The contribution of reflex inhibition to arthrogenous muscle weakness. Clin Sci 67:7, 1984.
55. James, SL: Extensor mechanism—anatomy. In Kennedy, JC (ed): The Injured Adolescent Knee. Williams & Wilkins, Baltimore, 1979, p 205.
56. Jensen, K and DiFabio, RP: Evaluation of eccentric exercise in the treatment of patellar tendonitis. Phys Ther 69(3):211, 1989.
57. Mannheimer, JS and Lampe, GN: Clinical Transcutaneous Electrical Nerve Stimulation. FA Davis, Philadelphia, 1984.
58. Wallace, L: Mens Therapy: An Introduction. Unpublished manual, Lyndhurst, OH 1986.
59. Becker, RO and Selden, G: The Body Electric: Electromagnetism and the Foundation of Life. William Morrow, New York, 1985.
60. Knight, KL: Cryotherapy: Theory, Technique and Physiology. Chattanooga Corp, Chattanooga, TN, 1986.
61. McMaster, W: Cryotherapy. The Physician and Sportsmedicine 10:112, 1982.
62. Prentice, WE: An electromyographic analysis of the effectiveness of heat, cold, and stretching for inducing relaxation in injured muscle. Journal of Orthopedic and Sports Physical Therapy 3:132, 1982.
63. Olson, JE and Stravino, VD: A review of cryotherapy. Phys Ther 52(8):840, 1972.
64. Riddle, D: Case Study: A treatment approach for a resistant knee extension contracture. Journal of Orthopedic and Sports Physical Therapy 7:162, 1986.
65. Shelbourne, KD and Nitz, P: Accelerated rehabilitation after anterior cruciate ligament reconstruction. Am J Sports Med 18(3):292, 1990.
66. Light, KE, et al: Low load prolonged stretch versus high load brief stretch in treating knee contractures. Phys Ther 64(4):330, 1984.
67. Bohannon, RW, et al: Effectiveness of repeated prolonged loading for increasing flexion in knees demonstrating postoperative stiffness. Phys Ther 65(4):494, 1985.
68. Warren, C, Lehmann, J, and Koblanski, J: Heat and stretch procedures: In evaluation using the rat tail tendon. Arch Phys Med Rehabil 57:122, 1976.
69. Lehman, JF: Effect of therapeutic temperatures on tendon extensibility. Arch Phys Med Rehabil 51:487, 1970.
70. Sapega, A and Rogan, LK: Optimizing the nonsurgical treatment of joint contractures. In Engle, RP (ed): Churchill Livingstone, New York, 1991.

71. Woodall, W and Welsh, J: A biomechanical basis for rehabilitation programs involving the patello-femoral joint. Journal of Orthopedic and Sports Physical Therapy 11(11):535, 1990.
72. Soderberg, GL, et al: Electro-myographic analysis of knee exercises in healthy subjects and in patients with knee pathologies. Phys Ther 67(11):1691, 1987.
73. Snyder-Mackler, L, Garrett, M, and Roberti, M: A comparison of torque generating capabilities of three different electrical stimulating currents. Journal of Orthopedic and Sports Physical Therapy 11:297, 1989.
74. Steadman, JR: Non-operative measures for patello-femoral problems. Am J Sports Med 7(6):344, 1979.
75. Morrissey, MC, et al: The effects of electrical stimulation on the quadriceps during post-op knee immobilization. Am J Sports Med 13(1):1330, 1985.
76. Currier, DP and Mann, R: Muscular strength development by electric stimulation in healthy individuals. Phys Ther 63(6):915, 1983.
77. Selkowitz, DM: Improvement in isometric strength of the quadriceps femoris muscle after training with electric stimulation. Phys Ther 65(2):186, 1985.
78. Johnson, DH, Thurston, P, and Ashcrof, PJ: The Russian technique of faradism in the treatment of chondromalacia patella. Physiotherapy Canada 29:266, 1977.
79. Amatuzzi, MM, Fazzi, A, and Varella, MH: Pathologic synovial plica of the knee: Results of conservative treatment. Am J Sports Med 18(5):468, 1991.
80. DeHaven, KE, Dolan, WA, and Mayer, PJ: Chondromalacia patellae in athletes. Am J Sports Med 7(1):5, 1979.
81. Antich, TJ and Brewster, CE: Modification of quadriceps femoris muscle exercises during knee rehabilitation. Phys Ther 66(8):1248, 1986.
82. Caiozzo, VJ, et al: The affect of isometric precontraction on the slow velocity-high force region of the in-vivo force velocity relationship. Med Sci Sports Exerc 13:128, 1981.
83. Black, JE and Alten, SR: How I manage infrapatellar tendonitis. The Physician and Sportsmedicine 12(10):86, 1984.

Nonprotective Injuries to the Knee

CHAPTER 6

Rehabilitation of Microtrauma Injuries

Marie A. Johanson, MS, PT
Robert Donatelli, MA, PT, OCS
Bruce H. Greenfield, MMSc, PT

Microtrauma injuries, or *overuse* injuries, are musculoskeletal injuries that result from repetitive stress to tissues. The result of repetitive stress is microtrauma to tissue that extends beyond the ability of the tissue to repair itself.[1] Whereas many different tissues may be involved, the common denominator is inflammation, degeneration, or both at the site of microtrauma. In response to an increase in the popularity of aerobic exercise regimens and increased interest in work-related medical costs, attention has been directed to the cause and treatment of these injuries. This chapter reviews the incidence of microtrauma injuries, etiologic factors in microtrauma injuries, and common microtrauma injuries at the knee. Case studies illustrate the basic principles for evaluation and treatment of common microtrauma injuries at the knee.

Whenever mechanical trauma in the form of tension, compression, or shearing forces occurs, the initial response is frequently an inflammatory process.[2] Microtrauma injuries consist of structural disruption of tissue that often triggers the inflammatory process.[1] Stages of healing after tissue damage are the inflammatory stage, the granulation stage, the fibroblastic stage, and the maturation stage.[3] As well as being reviewed in Chapter 4, the characteristics and relative duration of the stages of healing are described in several works.[2-11] The reader should refer to these sources for thorough coverage of inflammation and the healing process.

DEGENERATION AND INFLAMMATION IN MICROTRAUMA INJURIES

Signs of classic inflammation cannot be found in all microtrauma injuries.[12,13] The relationship between tissue damage and inflammation is unclear. Leadbetter[12] suggests that the classic inflammatory response only occurs after a sufficient degree of structural and microvascular damage is reached.

Cell atrophy results in degeneration of tissue. Causes of cell atrophy include chronic inflammation, immobilization, decreased nutrition, and aging.[12] Degenerated tissue is more vulnerable to repetitive stress and can result in mechanical fatigue or failure. Mechanical disruption of tissue increases the likelihood of recurrent inflammation.[12]

Because chronic inflammation can result in degeneration of tissue, and degenerated tissue is vulnerable to recurrent inflammation when repetitively stressed, both are likely to occur in microtrauma injuries.

INCIDENCE OF MICROTRAUMA INJURIES AT THE KNEE

Aerobic exercise has grown in popularity as participants pursue goals of cardiovascular fitness, increased calorie consumption, and stress reduction. The increased popularity of running has brought to the clinics of health professionals a host of injuries that differ from the macrotraumatic injuries associated with team sports.[14] The "running boom" of the 1970s and 1980s captivated 15 percent of Americans (about 30 million). Cycling and swimming have also attracted the amateur sports enthusiast, with a reported 10 to 20 million and 75 million American participants, respectively.[1] Almost 1 million people completed triathlons in 1984.[11] With the aerobic exercise boom, it is not surprising that an estimated 30 to 50 percent of all sports injuries are due to microtrauma.[16]

Microtrauma injuries at the knee joint commonly occur in the running population.[17] In a study of 4,358 runners and joggers, 45.8 percent were found to have suffered at least one jogging injury.[18] Seventy percent of this group suffered from microtrauma injuries, and knee joint injuries constituted the largest single group. A study of 171 injuries in 121 runners found roughly one third of the injuries were at the knee.[19] Yet another retrospective study of microtrauma injuries at the knee found that 75 percent of the patients were amateur sports enthusiasts. James and associates[20] reported the most common complaint of the runner was knee pain. However, microtrauma injuries of the knee joint are not confined to runners. Weiss[21] reported complaints of nontraumatic knee pain in 20.7 percent of 132 cyclists participating in an 8-day, 500-mile bike tour.

Health professionals involved in the evaluation and treatment of musculoskeletal injuries should familiarize themselves with the common microtrauma injuries of the knee joint. When treating microtrauma injuries of the knee joint, all etiologic factors must be considered to ensure the patient the most rapid progress possible and to prevent recurrence. Therefore, the following sections review the etiologic factors involved with microtrauma injuries at the knee joint.

ETIOLOGY OF MICROTRAUMA INJURIES AT THE KNEE

Successful treatment of microtrauma injuries of the knee joint includes the identification and correction of all contributing etiologic factors to injury. Etiologic factors are of two basic types: extrinsic or intrinsic.[16] *Extrinsic factors* are related to the external conditions under which the activity is performed (Table 6–1) and are reviewed in the following section.

TABLE 6-1 Etiologic Factors in Microtrauma Injuries

Extrinsic Factors	Intrinsic Factors
Training errors	Lower extremity alignment
Terrain	Leg length discrepancy
Temperature	Muscle imbalance
Footwear	

Extrinsic Factors

Extrinsic factors are the most common cause of microtrauma injuries[17,22,23] and include training errors, terrain, shoes, and temperature (see Table 6-1). James and associates[20] state that 60 percent of injuries to runners can be attributed to training errors. Training errors may render body tissues unable to recover from accumulated fatigue and microtrauma.[22] Marti and colleagues[18] found a statistically significant correlation between jogging injuries and higher weekly mileages.

TRAINING ERRORS

Training errors usually involve a change in either distance or speed. Increasing distance and speed of exercise may induce muscular fatigue. Muscle fatigue is characterized by a decrease in the ability of the muscle to sustain its normal strength and endurance levels at increased activity levels.[24] James and associates[20] reported that 29 percent of training errors in a group of 180 runners were due to excessive mileage.

As the speed of walking or running increases, the lower extremities must absorb the shock produced by ground reaction forces in a shorter time. One gait cycle occurs in 1 second at a 5.0-km-per-hour walking speed, but occurs in only 0.6 seconds during 20-km-per-hour running.[25] The stance phase consists of 62 percent of the walking gait cycle, but only 31 percent of the running cycle. The foot is on the ground for only 0.2 seconds when running 3 to 4 m per second.[14] Generally, sagittal joint motion increases as speed increases. The knee joint flexes to approximately 10 degrees immediately following heelstrike in walking, but increases to about 35 degrees when running in response to greater vertical forces. Vertical force at midstance of running is reported to be 250 to 300 percent of body weight.[26] Subtalar joint pronation reaches its maximal level in 0.15 seconds during walking, but in only 0.03 seconds during running.[26]

To accommodate for accelerated lower extremity joint movements in running compared with walking, muscles demonstrate longer relative periods of electrical activity.[25] The quadriceps femoris muscles are active from the last 10 percent of swing phase to the first 15 percent of stance phase in walking. The contraction time of the quadriceps muscles increases from the last 20 percent of swing phase to the first 50 percent of stance phase in running. The hamstring muscles are active through 80 percent of the stance phase in running, compared with only 10 percent for walking. Presumably, hamstring muscle activity increases to help modulate the more rapid extension of the knee joint required in running during the swing phase of gait.

Neuromuscular control is often sacrificed to accommodate speed, potentially resulting in greater stress to joints, muscles, and connective tissues.[24] Increased rapidity of movement results in decreased activity of the antagonistic muscle groups and can lead to knee joint hyperextension as well as overstretching of the musculotendinous unit.[24]

TRAINING SURFACES

Running surfaces are also important possible precursors to microtrauma injuries of the knee. Factors that may influence microtrauma injuries are hills, road camber, track running, and rigidity of surface. The ideal terrain is flat, smooth, resilient, and reasonably soft.[27] Running downhill is associated with patellofemoral joint microtrauma injuries, due to increased eccentric contraction of the quadriceps muscles to decelerate the downward motion of the body.[17,27] Most authors report that downhill running can instigate iliotibial band friction syndrome (ITBFS),[23,28-31] though this observation has not always been supported.[17]

New streets and sidewalks are constructed with transverse grades of 2 degrees. Gutters have a 4-to-5-degree grade, and roadway shoulders vary.[27] Running on these unlevel surfaces results in greater subtalar joint pronation of the uphill foot and greater subtalar joint supination of the downhill foot. Repetitive excessive pronation or supination can create excessive stresses in the knee joint. Messier and Pittala[31] reported that 20 percent more runners suffering from ITBFS ran on crowned roads compared with a control group of noninjured runners. Running on transverse grades has also been implicated in pes anserine musculotendinous strain and patellofemoral joint problems.[17,27] Similar problems can develop from running on a track. While on the curved portion of the track, the inside foot must pronate to a greater degree than when running on the straightaways, creating the same potential problems to the knee joint and patellofemoral joint as running on crowned roads.[27]

The final factor related to the effects of terrain on microtrauma injuries is the rigidity of the surface. Hard running surfaces, such as cement sidewalks, are also thought to cause knee injuries by increasing joint reaction forces.[20,27] However, one retrospective study found no correlation between injury and the rigidity of running surface.[18]

SHOES

Because foot and ankle mechanics affect the mechanics and stresses in the knee joint, the runner should wear a shoe appropriate for hisor her foot type and running style. Shoe characteristics such as cushioning, proper heel width, proper heel counter support, firm midsole, and straighter lasting are all important factors influencing the mechanics of the subtalar joint.[32,33] The sole of the heel should include a lift of approximately 1.8 centimeters.[34] Shock absorption capability can be provided both by material and by design of the sole of the heel and forefoot. The outsole of the shoe should be constructed with tough but flexible rubber for force attenuation.[35] A "wheelbarrow" heel and the "doughnut" or "waffle-iron" sole is thought to aid in the distribution of stress. Wedge-shaped cutouts in the heel also assist with shock absorption. Commonly, shoes will erode on the outside of the heel. Care should be taken to periodically fill this area with the appropriate patching material. A rigid heel counter stabilizes the calcaneus and prevents breakdown of this portion of the shoe. A flare in the heel of the shoe dissipates forces over a broader area. If, however, the flare is too wide (over 7.5 cm), pronation may occur more rapidly and may result in increased strain in the knee.

The midsole should be constructed of a highly resilient material to provide additional shock absorption. Some shoes are fabricated with channels of pressurized gas within the heel and midsoles to reduce impact forces. These shoes are ideal for runners with rigid feet, or for training on hard, even surfaces.[35] Conversely, these shoes are less suited for obese runners or overpronators.

The flexibility of the forefoot portion of the shoe can be grossly ascertained by bending this portion upwards. It should not bend back into a "U" position but should not feel rigid either, so that the metatarsalphalangeal joints are allowed to dorsiflex during the push-off phase. A rounded toe box prevents crowding of the toes. The shoe length should exceed the longest toe by about ½ inch when the foot is bearing weight.

Straight-lasted shoes are those with symmetry around the long axis of the midsole and toe box. Because they provide more support to the medial aspect of the shoe, they are recommended for slower runners who are classified rearfoot strikers, and for runners who overpronate.[35] Curve-lasted shoes are designed to provide more support to the lateral portion of the foot and are more suited to faster runners.

Cleated shoes pose additional problems. Whereas long cleats increase traction, danger of locking the foot onto the surface increases. Hence, shoes with a relatively large number of lower but wider cleats (approximately 9 mm high and 12 mm wide) are recommended.[34]

TEMPERATURE

Microtrauma injuries can also be precipitated by temperature-related events, such as exercise without proper warm-up activities or exercise in a cold environment.[24] The warm-up period is thought to reduce incidence of muscle strains by increasing the efficiency of the muscles.[36]

Warm-up activities stimulate an increase in blood circulation, which increases the temperature of muscles. Increased blood circulation to the muscle improves the supply of oxygen and other nutrients to the muscle.[24] The increase in muscle temperature following warm-up activities also reduces the viscosity of muscle and connective tissue, and therefore reduces friction during muscle contraction.[24]

Generally, submaximal exercise performed to the point of perspiration is ideal under normal climatic conditions. Since type I endurance muscle fibers utilize oxygen-dependent energy sources provided by circulating blood, middle- and long-distance runners may benefit from longer warm-up periods than sprinters.

Intrinsic Factors

Intrinsic factors are physical characteristics that predispose an individual to microtrauma injuries (see Table 6-1). Many authors incriminate intrinsic factors in microtrauma injuries of the knee.[17,19,20,22,31,37-44] Insall[41] found patella malalignment problems in the majority of 105 patients diagnosed with chondromalacia patellae. Thirty-eight percent of these patients had a quadriceps angle (Q angle) of 20 degrees or greater, and 23 percent demonstrated patella alta. In a retrospective study of 213 runners with knee injuries, 77 percent were found to have abnormal foot position: 43 percent with pronation, and 34 percent with cavus feet.[43] Lutter[19] asserts that abnormal foot pronation is the single most important factor in production of injuries in the lower extremity. Lutter performed a retrospective study of 171 injuries in 121 runners and found that 54 percent of knee injuries in this group were related to abnormal foot pronation. Taunton and associates[17] found excessive Q angles or leg length discrepancies (LLDs) in 15 of 42 runners diagnosed with patellofemoral pain syndrome. Grana and Coniglione[44] reported genu varum deformities in 10 of 16 knee joints diagnosed with ITBFS.

We prefer to group intrinsic factors according to lower extremity malalignment, leg length discrepancy, and muscle imbalance problems. These factors are described in the following sections.

LOWER EXTREMITY MALALIGNMENT

Common lower extremity malalignment problems include abnormal pronation, excessive Q angle, "miserable malalignment," malpositioning of the patella, and cavus feet. Lower extremity malalignment can adversely affect the normal mechanics of gait and potentially contribute to onset of microtrauma injuries.

Abnormal Pronation

The etiology of abnormal pronation can be classified into three basic categories: congenital, acquired, or neurologic.[45] Congenital deformities that result in abnormal pronation are further classified as rigid or flexible. Common congenital rigid deformities include convex pes valgus (congenital vertical talus), tarsal coalition, and congenital metatarsus varus; the most common congenital flexible deformity is talipes calcaneo-valgus.[46,47] Acquired abnormalities that result in abnormal pronation are a result of factors intrinsic to the foot and ankle, factors extrinsic to the foot and ankle, or a combination of intrinsic and extrinsic factors.[45] Intrinsic factors of acquired abnormal pronation are trauma, ligament laxity, bony abnormalities of the subtalar joint, forefoot varus, forefoot supinatus, rearfoot varus, and ankle joint equinus. Extrinsic factors of acquired abnormal pronation are rotational deformities of the lower extremity and leg length discrepancies. Abnormal pronation can also result from neuromuscular diseases such as cerebral palsy.

Forefoot varus is the most common factor intrinsic to the foot that results in abnormal pronation.[48] Forefoot varus is defined as inversion of the forefoot on the rearfoot with the subtalar joint in neutral.[48,49] Forefoot varus is measured in the non-weight bearing position (Fig. 6–1). Hlavac[49] believes the etiology of forefoot varus is a delay in the normal ontogenic development of the foot. The talus does not migrate as far superiorly to the calcaneus from its original medial position. Additionally, the normal 35 to 40 degrees of valgus torsion of the talar head and neck on the trochlea does not advance as far from its initial parallel position. Normal valgus torsion allows the metatarsal heads to lie parallel to the transverse weight bearing plane and perpendicular to the rearfoot.

Root and colleagues[48] define normal anatomic forefoot position as zero degrees of varus or valgus relative to the rearfoot with the subtalar joint in neutral. Taunton and associates[50] define a mild forefoot varus deformity as 4 to 6 degrees, a moderate deformity as 7 to 10 degrees, and a severe deformity as greater than 10 degrees. However, a study measuring forefoot position of 240 feet on 120 normal subjects found an average angle of 7.18 degrees varus.[51] These results call into question prior assumptions regarding normal forefoot position.

Forefoot varus does not, in and of itself, result in significant pathology. Theoretically, a forefoot varus deformity creates an abnormal gait pattern with weight bearing under the lateral metatarsal heads during propulsion. The inverted position of the forefoot keeps the medial metatarsal heads off the weight bearing surface during stance (Fig. 6–2). Pathologies seen clinically are most often related to the compensatory mechanisms that allow weight bearing under the medial metatarsal heads.[14,26,49,52] The most common compensatory mechanism that allows the medial metatarsals contact with the weight bearing surface is subtalar joint pronation (Fig. 6–3). The result is abnormal pronation during the gait cycle.

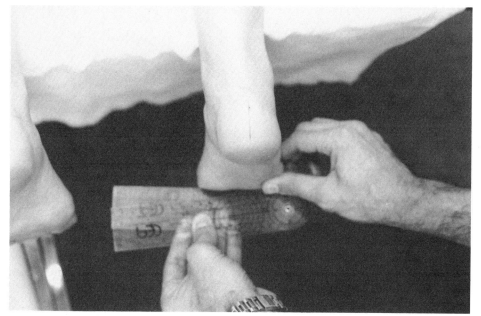

FIGURE 6-1. Forefoot varus measurement is obtained with the subtalar joint held in neutral. One arm of the goniometer is aligned in the plane of the metatarsal heads, and the other arm is held perpendicular to a line bisecting the calcaneus.

Abnormal pronation of the foot has been implicated in many pathologies of the foot, ankle, knee, and more infrequently, the hip and lumbar spine.[20,37,53-56] Normally, subtalar joint pronation provides a mechanism for shock absorption and adaptation to uneven terrain early in the stance phase of gait.[26,57] The subtalar joint is in neutral or slight supination at heelstrike. Rapid pronation occurs for two reasons. First, the center of gravity falls medial to the subtalar joint axis, resulting in calcaneal eversion. Second,

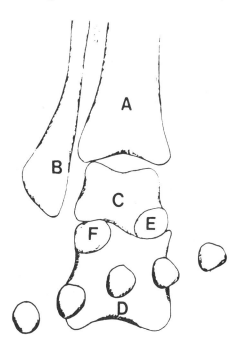

FIGURE 6-2. Forefoot varus deformity. If there is no compensation for the deformity, the medial metatarsals do not contact the weight bearing surface due to the inverted position of the forefoot relative to the rearfoot. A) Tibia. B) Fibula. C) Talus. D) Calcaneus. E) Talonavicular articulation. F) Calcaneal-cuboid articulation. (From Donatelli,[45] p 44.)

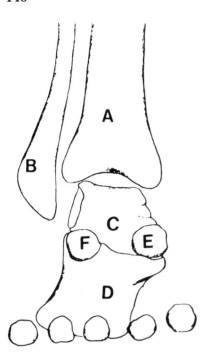

FIGURE 6-3. Compensatory subtalar joint pronation allows the medial metatarsals contact with the weight bearing surface during gait. A) Tibia. B) Fibula. C) Talus. D) Calcaneus. E) Talonavicular articulation. F) Calcaneal-cuboid articulation. (From Donatelli,[45] p 44.)

the talus follows the action of the tibia in the transverse plane during weight bearing movements. Therefore, when the tibia internally rotates during initial stance, the talus adducts and plantar flexes.[48] Pronation during weight bearing consists of these concurrent motions of calcaneal eversion, talar adduction, and talar plantar flexion (Fig. 6-4A and B). Maximal pronation occurs at 20 to 35 percent of the stance phase of gait.[48,49,59,60] Resupination then commences in preparation for pushoff. Maximal subtalar pronation measures approximately 4 to 8 degrees for normal subjects ambulating,[26,48,57,60] and 7 to 10 degrees for subjects running.[26,61-64]

Abnormal pronation during the gait cycle is pronation that occurs out of its normal phase. Commonly, abnormal pronation continues beyond 20 to 35 percent of stance phase when supination normally occurs.[49] Excessive pronation is pronation that is of greater magnitude than normal. Excessive pronation is difficult to define; a literature review reveals no study indicating the degree of subtalar joint pronation in a large number of normal subjects.

Effects of Abnormal Pronation on the Knee. The subtalar joint (STJ) serves as a torque converter for the series of segmental rotations occurring during human locomotion.[65,66] The interaction between rotation of the tibia and supination and pronation of the subtalar joint behaves as a mitered hinge.[65,66] The STJ axis is about 45 degrees inclined to the horizontal.[65,66] Rotation of the proximal segment, represented by the tibia bone, causes the STJ to rotate around the transverse axis with resultant calcaneal eversion with tibial internal rotation, and calcaneal inversion with tibial external rotation (Fig. 6-5).[67-70] Prolonged or excessive STJ pronation may result in prolonged or excessive tibial internal rotation. The increased rotational force of the tibia is transmitted up the lower leg to the knee joint. The biomechanical consequences of increased tibial internal rotation due to abnormal or excessive STJ pronation may include microtrauma injuries to the knee.[19-21,26,37,39,40,42,43]

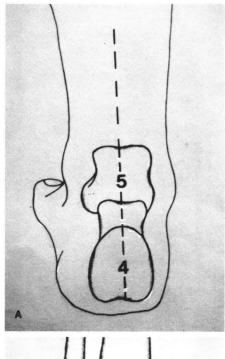

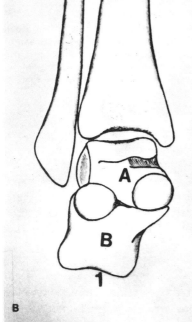

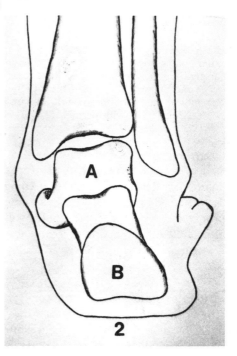

FIGURE 6-4. *A*) Neutral position of the subtalar joint. 4 = calcaneus. 5 = talus. *B*) Anterior (1) and posterior (2) views of subtalar joint pronation during gait. A = talus. B = calcaneus. (From Donatelli,[45] pp 15 and 17.)

Abnormal tibial internal rotation related to prolonged or excessive STJ pronation can affect patellofemoral joint mechanics. Prolonged or excessive tibial internal rotation occurs during midstance. The knee joint needs to extend in midstance, which requires external rotation of the tibia.[39] The compensatory mechanism is hypothesized to be internal rotation of the femur.[39,43] While this compensatory femoral internal rotation is occurring, the patella is articulating with the femoral trochlea groove, and the quadri-

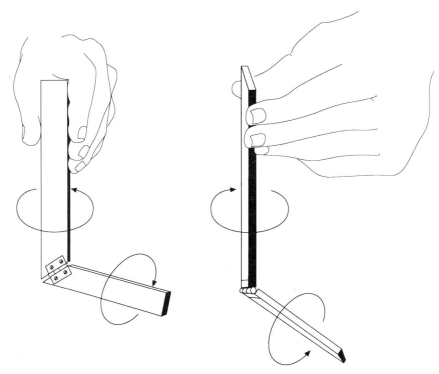

FIGURE 6–5. The axis of the subtalar joint is approximately 45 degrees to the vertical (leg) and horizontal (foot) planes, and thus, acts as a mitered hinge. Due to this orientation of the axis of the subtalar joint, external rotation of the tibia results in supination at the subtalar joint, and internal rotation of the tibia results in pronation at the subtalar joint. (From Inman, VT and Mann, R: Biomechanics of the foot and ankle. In Inman, VT [ed]: DuVries' Surgery of the Foot, ed 3. CV Mosby, St. Louis, 1973, with permission.)

ceps muscles are still contracting. As a result of lateral patella tracking, compression occurs between the lateral articular surface of the patella and the lateral femoral condyle and may precipitate a lateral patellar compression syndrome.[39]

Excessive STJ pronation is also an intrinsic predisposing factor in ITBFS. Excessive STJ pronation causes the insertion of the iliotibial band to be pulled anteromedially, so that the iliotibial band is drawn tightly across the lateral femoral epicondyle.[30,70,71] The result is excessive friction forces between the iliotibial band and the lateral femoral condyle.

Increased Q Angle

The Q angle (quadriceps angle) can be measured by placing a goniometer over the center of the patella with the patient standing. One arm of the goniometer is aligned with the ASIS and the other arm is aligned with the tibial tuberosity (Fig. 6–6A). A gross assessment of the Q angle can also be ascertained with the patient in a sitting position (Fig. 6–6B). Normal Q angles measure 10 degrees or less for men, and 15 degrees or less for women.[40] The Q angle is intended to represent the force vector of the quadriceps femoris muscle. Any biomechanical problem that increases the Q angle potentially results in lateral patellar compression syndrome or subluxation of the patella. Lower extremity malalignments that tend to increase the Q angle include femoral anteversion, genu recurvatum, foot pronation, and external tibial torsion.[40,72]

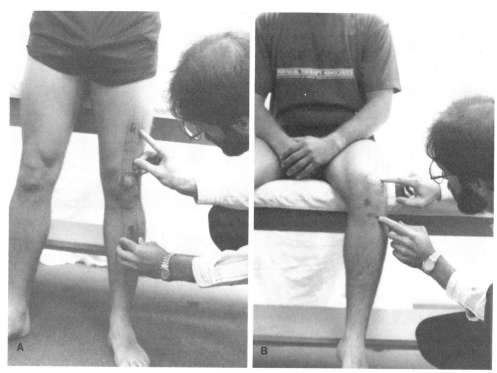

FIGURE 6–6. *A*) Quadriceps-angle (Q-angle) measurement. The axis of the angle is the midpoint of the patella. One arm of the goniometer is aligned with the ASIS and the other arm is aligned with the tibial tuberosity. *B*) An indication of the Q-angle can also be obtained by palpating the midpoint of the patella and the tibial tuberosity, with the patient seated on the examining table. A tibial tuberosity lateral to the midpoint of the patella, suggests an excessive Q-angle.

"Miserable Malalignment"

Many malalignment problems of the lower extremities are due to compensatory mechanisms that occur in response to developmental anomalies. James[40] describes "miserable malalignment" as a pattern of compensatory torsional and frontal plane changes in the lower extremities, in response to femoral anteversion. *Femoral anteversion* is defined as the angle of anterior rotation of the proximal head and neck of the femur to the transcondylar axis of the femur.[45] Normal femoral anteversion angles range from 8 to 15 degrees in the adult.[47] Compensatory torsional and frontal plane changes that may occur in response to excessive femoral anteversion include proximal tibial external torsion, tibial varum, and STJ pronation (Fig. 6–7). Miserable malalignment increases the Q angle due to the increase in proximal external tibial torsion and may predispose the individual to patellofemoral dysfunctions such as subluxation of the patella or lateral patellar compression syndrome.

Malposition or Soft-Tissue Abnormalities of the Patella

Lateral patella tilt, patella alta, and hypermobility of the patella are also factors in microtrauma patellofemoral problems (see Chapter 7).[40,41,72,73] Malpositioning of the patella results in abnormal contact patterns of the patella within the femoral trochlea and increases the patellofemoral joint reaction forces. A tight lateral retinaculum or a deficient vastus medialis muscle may result in lateral tracking of the patella and lead to increased patellofemoral joint reaction forces.[74]

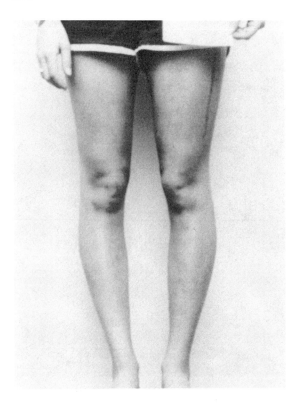

FIGURE 6-7. "Miserable malalignment". The patient pictured demonstrates compensatory changes in response to femoral anteversion, with proximal tibial external rotation, tibial varum, and subtalar joint pronation. Note the "squinting patellae," which reflect the internal femoral rotation associated with femoral anteversion.

Cavus Feet

The term *pes cavus* is used to describe deformities of the forefoot and rearfoot in the sagittal and/or frontal plane.[45] *Pes cavovarus* is defined as plantar flexion of the medial column of the forefoot with compensatory rearfoot varus when the foot is bearing weight. The etiology of pes cavus feet is classified into three groups: neurologic, contracture of soft tissue structures, and idiopathic.[45] At heelstrike, cavovarus feet tend to maintain the rearfoot in varus.[75] Reduction in normal STJ pronation decreases attenuation of forces at the foot and ankle, passing increased forces up to the knee. Most frequently, cavovarus feet are associated with iliotibial band pain, lateral knee pain, and less frequently, chondromalacia patellae.[75]

LEG LENGTH DISCREPANCY

Leg length discrepancies of varying degrees are common in the normal population.[76] Subotnick[77] reported some degree of leg length difference in 40 percent of more than 4,000 athletes. Discrepancies of up to 1.1 cm are considered normal.[76] LLDs are generally classified according to structural or functional etiologies.[78] Structural LLDs. represent true anatomic differences in length of the tibia or femur. Functional LLDs are compensatory lengthening or shortening of a limb in response to joint contractures or muscle imbalances.

The knee may be subjected to abnormal stress on both the long-limb and short-limb sides. If an individual attempts to compensate on the short-limb side by externally rotating the lower extremity, an increased valgus force will be imparted to the knee joint, resulting in predisposition to patellofemoral joint microtrauma syndromes.[79] Another possible compensatory mechanism on the short-limb side is excessive or pro-longed STJ supination.[45,78] Excessive STJ supination may create a "functional cavovarus foot" with resultant increased forces to the lateral knee joint (as noted in the Cavus Feet section above). Conversely, the STJ on the long-limb side may attempt to reduce the vertical height of the lower extremity by eversion of the calcaneus, resulting in excessive pronation.[45,78] The long-limb side may also maintain a longer stance phase of gait, subjecting the limb to greater ground reaction forces.[78] Increased ground reaction forces combined with excessive pronation predisposes the knee joint on the long-limb side to the same types of microtrauma syndromes discussed in the Abnormal Pronation section.

The importance of leg length discrepancies in onset of ITBFS remains controversial.[30,71] Supporters of a correlation between LLDs and ITBFS contend that excessive lateral pelvic tilting occurring on the long-limb side produces abnormal tension in the iliotibial band, predisposing the individual to ITBFS. Environmental functional LLDs can result from running on transverse grades and reportedly predispose the runner to ITBFS on the downhill, or "long-limb" side.[27,30,31]

MUSCLE IMBALANCE

Muscle imbalances result from either a weak agonist, a tight antagonist, or a combination of the two. According to Janda and Schmid,[80] and Jull and Janda,[81] muscles respond to an altered state of mechanics of the musculoskeletal system in a distinct and consistent pattern. Altered mechanical states can result from a skeletal malalignment such as "miserable malalignment," described by James,[40] or a leg length discrepancy. Jull and Janda[81] classify muscles by their response to dysfunction. Muscles that shorten and tighten in dysfunction are classified as postural muscles. Examples of postural muscles in the lower extremity include the hip adductor muscles, the hamstring muscles, the hip flexor muscles, the rectus femoris muscle, and the gastrocnemius-soleus muscle group. Conversely, muscles that lengthen and weaken in dysfunction are classified as phasic muscles. Examples of phasic muscles include the gluteal muscles, the vastus medialis, intermedius, and lateralis muscles, and the pretibial or ankle dorsiflexor muscle group.

Muscle imbalance may be a significant factor in both the onset and the perpetuation of musculoskeletal dysfunction.[81] Jull and Janda[81] cite two theories to explain development of muscle imbalances. First, pain and pathology in a motion segment may initiate weakness in phasic muscles and tightness in postural muscles. If the muscle responses persist, patterns of motion are disturbed and may subject the motion segment to further strain. Second, muscle imbalances may develop in response to impairment of the motor control mechanisms of the central nervous system. Impairment of motor control may alter normal movement patterns, imposing abnormal strain on the motion segment.

Muscle imbalances may contribute to the onset of patellofemoral joint dysfunction or may perpetuate an existing dysfunction. The patella is anatomically stabilized from lateral displacement primarily by the vastus medialis obliquus muscle, and secondarily by the medial patella retinaculum and anterior prominence of the lateral femoral condyle.[17,40] The medial pull of the vastus medialis obliquus muscle fibers is balanced by the counterpull of the vastus lateralis muscle, iliotibial band, and lateral patella retinaculum, so as to afford normal patella tracking in the femoral trochlea. Insufficient contractile force of the vastus medialis obliquus muscle may result in lateral subluxation of the patella during quadriceps femoris muscle contraction, leading to irritation of the lateral patellar facet.[17,40,72] Tightness of the vastus lateralis muscle, iliopatellar band of the iliotibial tract, or lateral patella retinaculum can produce a lateral patellar tilt or lateral subluxation of the patella.

Quadriceps femoris muscle weakness predisposes the knee to microtrauma injuries. Bennett and Stauber[82] have theorized that loss of eccentric quadriceps femoris muscle strength results in altered patellofemoral joint reaction forces. Eccentric muscle contraction of the quadriceps femoris muscle group at heelstrike controls knee joint flexion during early stance. Knee joint flexion in early stance assists with attenuation of ground reaction forces.[14,25] Altered joint reaction forces in the patellofemoral joint as a result of impaired eccentric quadriceps femoris muscle function may result in microtrauma to the retropatellar hyaline cartilage or patella tendon.[20]

Leg length discrepancies may also affect muscle function of the lower extremities. The long-limb side may exhibit shortening and tightening of the hip adductor muscles, the hip flexor muscles (especially the iliopsoas muscle), and the gastrocnemius-soleus muscles; and lengthening and weakening of the gluteus medius and maximus muscles, the vastus medialis and lateralis muscles, and the pretibial muscles (anterior tibialis, extensor hallucis longus, and extensor digitorus longus muscles).[79,80] The resultant muscle imbalance during both walking and running can produce dynamic instability in both the hip and knee joints, as well as in the patellofemoral joint.

The counterrotatory pulls of the semimembranosus muscle and the pes anserinus muscle group medially, and the biceps femoris muscle laterally, contribute to the functional stability of the knee and dynamic control of tibial rotation.[17] A weakness in the medial hamstring muscle group in early stance phase of gait may permit excessive lateral rotation of the tibia. The result of excessive lateral tibial rotation as the knee joint flexes during midstance is a functional increase in the Q angle.

Hamstring muscle tightness and quadriceps femoris muscle weakness are common clinical findings in the presence of knee joint pathology. Antich and colleagues[38] reported significant hamstring muscle tightness on the involved side in a group of 112 patients diagnosed with microtrauma injuries of the knee. Janda[80,81] reported shortness and tightness of the hamstring muscles, and lengthening and weakness of the quadriceps femoris muscles, in postural dysfunctions of the trunk and lower extremities including the "pelvic crossed syndrome." According to Janda's[81] electromyographic data, a tight muscle will result in reflex inhibition of its antagonist muscles. For example, activation of weak quadriceps femoris muscles in the presence of tight hamstring muscles will increase activity in the hamstring muscles. However, stretching of the tight hamstring muscles immediately followed by knee joint extension will facilitate activity of the quadriceps femoris muscles. Hamstring muscle tightness combined with quadriceps femoris weakness is often associated with microtrauma patellofemoral joint syndromes, presumably due to increased strain on the extensor mechanism as it contracts against greater resistance when extending the knee joint in preparation for heelstrike.[17,23,83]

Ten degrees of ankle joint dorsiflexion is necessary for normal ambulation,[40,48,84] whereas running requires 15 degrees. Tightness of the gastrocnemius-soleus muscles limits the normal excursion of ankle joint dorsiflexion during walking and running. Increased subtalar and midtarsal joint pronation may compensate for tight plantarflexor muscles of the ankle joint.[40] Effects of abnormal pronation on the knee were discussed above, in the section on extrinsic factors in microtrauma injuries at the knee.

In accordance with Janda's[80,81] principles of postural and phasic muscle groups, runners are prone to developing tightness of the posterior muscle groups of the lower extremities and weakness of the anterior muscle groups.[19] Therefore, appropriate stretching and strengthening exercises are advisable as a preventive measure.

TABLE 6-2 Structures Commonly Involved
in Microtrauma Injuries at the Knee

Bursa	Musculotendinous	Cartilage
Prepatellar Pes anserinus	Patella tendon Iliotibial band Popliteal tendon Semimembranosus tendon Skeletal muscle	Retropatellar cartilage

COMMON MICROTRAUMA INJURIES AT THE KNEE

Structures commonly involved in microtrauma injuries at the knee are listed in Table 6-2 and include the bursae, musculotendinous unit, and articular cartilage. The common microtrauma syndromes affecting these structures at the knee are discussed below.

Bursae and Microtrauma Injuries

Bursae are cavities usually found in continuity with a joint, but not usually in communication with the joint (see Chapter 1). They are loosely attached to the joint capsule, tendons, ligaments, or overlying skin, so they are intimately involved with these structures.[85] Bursae are formed by two layers of synovial membrane and can be found at sites of friction between tendon and bone (e.g., pes anserinus bursa) or between skin and bone (e.g., prepatellar bursa).[1] Normally the bursae produce a small amount of fluid that acts as a lubricant between the two bursal surfaces. The function of bursae is to reduce friction between two adjacent structures, therefore improving gliding motion. Bursae may be injured with acute trauma, such as a blow to the anterior patella, but often they become inflamed with repetitive microtrauma. Inflammation of bursae leads to effusion and often results in thickening or fibrosis of the bursal tissue.

The knee joint has many associated bursae (see Chapter 1). The three anterior bursae are the prepatellar bursa, which lies between the skin and the patella; the deep infrapatellar bursa, between the patellar tendon and the tibia; and the superficial infrapatellar bursa, between the patellar tendon and the overlying skin.[85] The suprapatellar pouch is part of the joint cavity but serves as a bursa as well and thus may also be called the suprapatellar bursa. This structure can be found between the quadriceps femoris muscle tendon and femur.[86] Posteriorly, a bursa that sometimes communicates with the joint is located between the semimembranosus muscle tendon and the medial origin of the gastrocnemius muscle. Medially, the pes anserinus bursa may be found between the medial collateral ligament and the pes anserinus group of tendons (sartorius, gracilis, and semitendinosus tendons).[85] Laterally, bursae may be found between the lateral collateral ligament and both the biceps femoris tendon and the popliteus tendon.[85] Another bursa is located between the popliteus tendon and the lateral femoral condyle. Several other bursae can be found, but these are not commonly associated with microtrauma injuries.

The most common bursitis at the knee in sports is prepatellar bursitis,[85] which can also occur with excessive kneeling ("housemaid's knee").[87] The patient will complain of anterior knee pain of insidious onset. Flexion will be full or nearly full. An antalgic gait is common, and moderate effusion may be observed. Muscle response typically follows Janda's[80,81] principles, resulting in quadriceps femoris muscle atrophy and tightness of the hamstring muscle and gastrocnemius-soleus muscles.

With running sports, the pes anserinus bursa can become inflamed. Pain will be reported along the anteromedial portion of the proximal tibia, over or just posterior to the medial collateral ligament,[85] and may extend superiorly to the medial joint line. Runners may report increasing pain with increased mileage. Intrinsic factors associated with pes anserinus bursitis are femoral anteversion, hamstring muscle tightness, genu valgus alignment, and external tibial torsion.[85] Extrinsic factors may be excessive hill running, excessive mileage, and inadequate stretching of the hamstring muscle group.

The Musculotendinous Unit and Microtrauma Injuries

The musculotendinous unit is the most commonly involved structure in microtrauma injuries. Tendons are composed of collagen and elastin. Staggered fibrils of collagen and elastin are organized into fibers, which form larger bundles of fascicles.[1] Tendons join muscle to bone and are subjected to tensile stresses. The blood supply to tendons is usually sparse,[88] rendering tendons vulnerable to injury and compromising their healing potential. Injuries to tendons can occur when (1) tension is applied suddenly or obliquely, (2) the tendon is under tension before additional loading occurs, (3) the muscle attached to the tendon has a high motoneuron-to-muscle-fiber innervation ratio, (4) external stretch is applied to the muscle group, or (5) the tendon is weak in relation to the muscle.[89] The most common types of tendinitis at the knee are patella tendinitis ("jumper's knee") and ITBFS. Popliteal tendinitis and semimembranosus tendinitis are also frequently reported.[23]

PATELLAR TENDINITIS

Patellar tendinitis occurs with repeated stress to the insertion of the quadriceps femoris tendon, or to the insertion of the patellar tendon on the inferior pole of the patella.[90,91] Microruptures and local tendon degeneration at the insertion site of the quadriceps or patellar tendon ensues. The condition is common in individuals who engage in athletic activities that demand repetitive extensor mechanism activity, such as jumping, climbing, kicking, or running. The extensor mechanism includes the quadriceps femoris muscle group, the quadriceps femoris tendon, the patella tendon, and the patellofemoral joint. Athletes in volleyball, basketball, soccer, or high jumping may succumb to this microtrauma syndrome. Intrinsic factors that predispose an individual to patellar tendinitis are patella hypermobility, patella alta, increased Q angle, and excessive pronation.[17,22,91,92] Tenderness is most common at the inferior pole of the patella but may also occur at the tibial insertion of the patella tendon or at the insertion of the quadriceps tendon along the superior pole of the patella.[92] Retropatellar crepitus, patella hypermobility, and quadriceps muscle atrophy may be present in individuals suffering from patellar tendon tendinitis. Occasionally, swelling is seen over the patellar tendon insertion. Typically, roentgenographic findings are negative. Symptoms usually begin insidiously, with pain or aching around the infrapatellar or suprapatellar region after activity,[90,92] and progress to pain during and after activity that disables the patient from participation in the activity. The end-stage of patellar tendinitis is rupture of the patellar tendon.

ILIOTIBIAL BAND FRICTION SYNDROME (ITBFS)

Iliotibial band friction syndrome (ITBFS), common among the running population, was first described in 1975 by Renne[28] in a group of military men engaged in vigorous physical training. More recently, Noble[29] reported ITBFS in 52 percent of 200 consecutive patients with knee injuries associated with running. Taunton and colleagues[17] found ITBFS constituted 14 percent of knee problems in runners. ITBFS accounted for 17 percent of knee injuries in a study by James and associates.[20]

The iliotibial band connects the ilium with the tibia.[70] This thick fascial band receives part of the insertions of the tensor facia latae muscle anteriorly and gluteus maximus muscle posteriorly, and courses down the lateral aspect of the thigh to insert onto Gerdy's tubercle.[88] When the knee joint is in the terminal portion of extension, the iliotibial band lies anterior to the axis of the knee joint, but at 30 degrees of flexion it passes posterior to the knee joint axis.[28,70] Being free of bony attachment between the lateral femoral condyle and the tibial tuberosity, the band moves anteriorly and posteriorly with extension and flexion of the knee joint. Thus repetitive flexion and extension motions of the knee joint may subject the iliotibial band to increased stress, and excessive friction may develop between the iliotibial band and the femoral condyle, resulting in irritation and inflammation within the iliotibial band, the bursa underneath, or the periosteum of the lateral femoral epicondyle.[70] Intrinsic factors involved with this condition are an anatomically prominent lateral epicondyle, tight iliotibial band, excessive genu varum, and excessive STJ pronation.[17,29-31,44,71] Prolonged internal rotation of the tibia that occurs during abnormal pronation results in anteromedial traction of the insertion of the iliotibial band. The result is to draw the iliotibial band more tightly across the lateral femoral condyle so that excessive friction is more likely.[71]

Extrinsic factors play a large role in production of ITBFS. Noble[25] found 84 percent of a group of 100 patients with ITBFS guilty of training errors, and Grana and Coniglione[44] found that 6 of 16 patients with the syndrome committed training errors. Training errors included sudden increases in mileage, training on transverse grades (affecting the leg on the downhill side), excessive downhill running, running on hard surfaces, and running in shoes with excessive lateral heel wear.[27,29-31]

Pain will be reported diffusely over the lateral aspect of the knee and can extend below the joint line.[29] In cases with more severe pain, the patient will walk stiff-legged to avoid knee joint flexion. The pain is usually provoked with running, although sometimes it appears early in the run and then decreases as the runner warms up. Pain is worse during downhill running. Occasionally, swelling can be seen over the lateral femoral epicondyle, and there is tenderness to palpation over the lateral epicondyle.

Three tests are commonly performed to assist in the identification of ITBFS. First, full weight bearing on the involved knee with the knee in 30 degrees of flexion will generally reproduce the pain. Second, with the patient supine and the knee flexed to 90 degrees, pressure can be applied to the iliotibial band over the lateral epicondyle while moving the knee joint into extension. At 30 degrees of flexion, pain will be elicited. Third, Ober's test ascertains flexibility of the iliotibial band (Fig. 6–8).[87] With the patient lying on the uninvolved side, the hip is abducted and extended and the knee is flexed to 90 degrees. With the hip in 0 degrees of extension, the thigh is dropped. In an individual with normal flexibility, the thigh will drop into adduction.

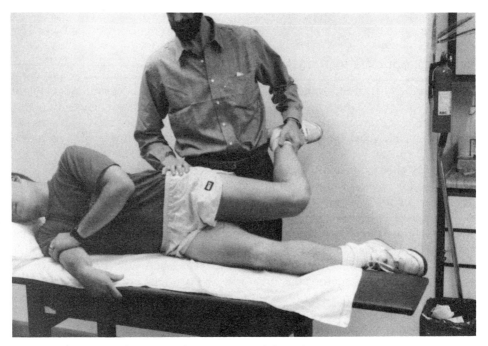

FIGURE 6-8. Positive Ober's test. The examiner stabilizes the pelvis and moves the hip into the anatomically neutral position with the knee flexed to 90 degrees. The examiner attempts to passively adduct the thigh. In an individual with normal flexibility, the thigh drops into adduction and approaches the table.

POPLITEAL TENDINITIS

Popliteal tendinitis results in pain along the lateral knee joint.[23] The popliteus muscle is an internal rotator of the tibia on the femur,[90] and functions during knee joint flexion from the fully extended position to about 20 degrees of flexion to "unlock" the knee. Ability of the tibia to rotate freely is limited during weight bearing activities, and is dependent on the actions of the STJ. The femur rotates more freely when the lower extremity is bearing weight, so the action of the popliteus muscle during weight bearing activities is that of external rotation of the femur on the tibia. Popliteal tendinitis can occur in runners. Extrinsic factors related to this syndrome are excessive downhill running and excessive STJ pronation.[23,83] Excessive pronation produces prolonged tibial internal rotation. Compensatory internal rotation of the femur potentially produces abnormal tensile forces in the politeus tendon.[39] The popliteus tendon is stressed in downhill running as the muscle attempts to stabilize the knee joint against increased posterolateral rotary forces. In running downhill, pronation in early stance phase occurs concomitantly with greater knee joint extension than when running on level surfaces. The popliteal tendon may be overstressed as the popliteus muscle contracts to counter-act the external rotation of the tibia that occurs in response to increased knee joint extension during downhill running. Pain can be elicited with palpation of the tendon in the "figure 4" position, just anterior and distal to the femoral attachment of the lateral collateral ligament (Fig. 6-9).

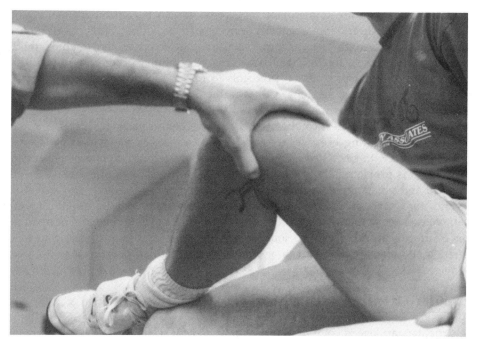

FIGURE 6–9. "Figure 4" position for palpation of popliteal tendon. The popliteal tendon courses beneath the lateral collateral ligament (LCL) near its origin on the lateral femoral condyle, but may be palpated just anterior and distal to the LCL.

SEMIMEMBRANOSUS TENDINITIS

Runners also can suffer from semimembranosus tendinitis. The semimembranosus tendon functions synergistically with the popliteus muscle to control excessive external rotation of the tibia.[83] Consequently, excessive STJ pronation can predispose the runner to semimembranosus tendinitis in the same manner as that described for popliteal tendinitis. Medial knee joint pain near the joint line is due to microtears of the tendon.[23] The pain is usually described as a vague, aching pain over the posteromedial aspect of the knee joint. Intrinsic factors that predispose the runner to semimembranosus tendinitis are excessive STJ pronation, poor hamstring muscle flexibility, and weakness of the hamstring muscles. The hamstring muscle group functions eccentrically in the swing phase of gait to control knee joint extension, and impairment in eccentric strength may predispose the semimembranosus tendon to microtrauma.

MUSCLE MICROTRAUMA INJURIES

Three types of muscle soreness are related to muscular contraction against high loads for prolonged periods.[24] The first and most common is "delayed-onset muscle soreness" (DOMS) that appears 12 to 48 hours after exercise. Characteristically, diffuse soreness is reported in the muscle, with tenderness to palpation of the muscle belly, muscular stiffness, and decreased active range of motion. Symptoms can continue for 4 to 12 days but gradually decrease. DOMS is common when the athlete is a novice, when activities are resumed after a period of inactivity, or when sudden increases in loads or repetitions of activity are undertaken. The soreness can be attributed to mechanical damage to the muscle and its associated connective tissue. DOMS is also associated with eccentric muscle strength training programs or other activities that require unaccustomed eccentric muscle forces.[93] Eccentric strength training programs use a different schedule and different progression protocols to prevent DOMS, including longer rest periods between exercise sessions. Curwin and Stanish[94] have outlined an eccentric strengthening protocol for rehabilitation.

Second, muscle soreness can be of the "acute" soreness variety. This type of muscle soreness appears during exercise, resolves with cessation of the activity, and is most often associated with sustained isometric contractions of multiple muscle groups in an extremity. This problem is linked to ischemia of the muscle, when excessive levels of lactic acid and potassium stimulate pain fibers.

The third type of soreness is muscle pain incurred with injury during rapid, repetitive exercise at high speeds and loads. These injuries are due to loss of neuromuscular control of an activity, with joint and muscle hyperextension leading to tendon stretching and tears, joint subluxation, and ligament injuries.

Articular Cartilage and Microtrauma Injuries

Articular cartilage is composed of 60 to 80 percent water, collagen, a proteoglycan gel, and a few chondrocytes.[1] Cartilage is generally considered avascular and aneural.[87] Articular cartilage is lubricated by a hydrostatic mechanism. Interstitial fluid is forced out of the cartilage in response to joint reaction forces, and the fluid bears load between the two opposing articular surfaces. The hydrostatic mechanism is most prominent at high speeds and high loads.[1] At lower speeds and lower loads, the *boundary surface phenomenon* is the predominant mechanism that lubricates and protects the articular cartilage.[1] Proteoglycan lubricants preferentially bind to opposing articular surfaces, and function to keep them separate. The underlying cancellous bone also deforms with stress and helps to protect the cartilage. The most common microtrauma to articular cartilage at the knee joint occurs in the patellofemoral joint.

CHONDROMALACIA PATELLAE

The pathology of chondromalacia begins with softening of the retropatellar hyaline cartilage, initially involving the noncontact areas and progressing to include the entire articular surface.[95] Fissuring generally develops first over the odd facet and then extends to other areas. James and associates[20] reported 25 percent of knee problems in runners was due to chondromalacia. Lutter[19] also reported that chondromalacia patellae was the single most common diagnosis of knee pain in runners. Intrinsic factors associated with chondromalacia patellae are increased Q angle, patella alta, lateral tilt or lateral tracking patella, excessive femoral or tibial torsion, a prominent medial femoral condylar ridge, internal derangement of the knee joint, quadriceps femoris muscle insufficiency or imbalance, and excessive STJ pronation.[40,41,43,90]

Symptoms include diffuse aching or pain, usually intermittent, over the anterior or anteromedial knee.[40,41,43,95] Distance runners often report retropatellar pain. Pain increases with stair climbing, hill climbing, squatting, prolonged ambulation or running, and prolonged sitting with the knee flexed (cinema sign). Complaints of retropatellar grating, locking, stiffness, swelling, and buckling are also common. Objectively, knee joint range of motion is full with no appreciable effusion. Retropatellar crepitus can be palpated with passive and active knee motion. Retropatellar tenderness is provoked by patellofemoral joint compression, with the knee joint flexed to approximately 30 degrees so that the patella is in contact with the femoral groove. Tenderness may be palpated over the medial or lateral patellar facet or about the peripatellar area. Gross quadriceps femoris muscle atrophy or specific vastus medialis muscle atrophy is usually seen or palpated. The lateral retinaculum may be tight and tender.[74]

CASE STUDIES

The following case studies illustrate the problem-solving approach to the evaluation and treatment of microtrauma injuries of the knee joint. The elements of problem solving for clinical decision making are extrapolated from Chapter 3 and include identification of the patient's problem; characteristics of the problem (symptoms); factors affecting the problem (evaluative findings, extrinsic factors, intrinsic factors); determination of a method to resolve the problem; treatment program; evaluation of effectiveness of the treatment program; and modification of the treatment program.

CASE STUDY 1

I. IDENTIFYING THE PATIENT'S PROBLEM

The patient is a 23-year-old male who states he developed left lateral knee pain over a 2-month period. His activities include participation on a recreational soccer team, and jogging 4 to 7 miles four or five times weekly for the past 5 years. His goal is participation in a 10-km race in 6 months.

II. IDENTIFYING CHARACTERISTICS OF THE PROBLEM

1. The pain is intermittent and appears during both jogging and soccer play, but is worse with running.
2. Occasionally, mild discomfort is felt when ascending or descending stairs.
3. Pain resolves with cessation of the activities in about 3 to 4 hours.

III. IDENTIFYING FACTORS AFFECTING THE PROBLEM

Evaluation

Palpation elicited tenderness over the lateral femoral condyle. Ober's test was positive for tightness of the iliotibial band (see Fig. 6–8). Range of motion of the knee joint was full. Compression of the iliotibial tract during flexion of the knee reproduced the patient's pain at 30 degrees of flexion (Noble's sign). Ligamentous stability tests were negative. Forefoot varus measurements were 4 degrees on the right and 5 degrees on the left. Normal pronation patterns were observed with the patient walking and jogging on a treadmill. Left hip abduction demonstrated less flexibility with the hip and knee in the extended position compared with the right side, indicating tightness of the gracilis muscle. No quadriceps femoris muscle atrophy was observed or palpated.

Extrinsic Factors

1. The patient moved to a new location 3 months ago. At that time, he began jogging on his neighborhood streets rather than jogging along a dirt trail where he had been training. He also initiated some interval training to improve his speed. He runs against traffic for safety purposes. As a result, his left lower extremity is always on the downhill side of the transverse grade of the road, resulting in functional supination and functional genu varum, thus increasing stress to the lateral side of the left knee joint.
2. The patient had begun increased hill training 4 months ago in preparation for a race on a hilly course.

Intrinsic Factors

1. Excessive genu varum bilaterally.
2. Tightness of the gracilis muscle, worse on the left.
3. Tight iliotibial band on the left.

IV. DETERMINING A METHOD TO RESOLVE THE PROBLEM

Assessment

ITBFS in a subacute phase. The patient is predisposed to this injury due to genu varum alignment. However, the syndrome was precipitated by running on crowned roads, initiation of hill running, and increased stride length during interval training. A tight gracilis muscle may have developed as a result of the increased stride length. Increased stride length results in decreased stride width and theoretically increases tension on the lateral knee structures.

Program of Treatment

1. Iontophoresis was applied at 5.0 milliamperes (mA) for 20 minutes using dexamethasone and 4 percent xylocaine every other day for three treatments. Glass and co-workers[96] demonstrated that this dosage produced higher local tissue concentration of these agents in monkeys than did systemic administration of the same medications. Clinical research also indicates that iontophoresis is effective in the treatment of tendinitis, both for subjective pain levels and for range of motion and function.[97,98]
2. The patient was advised to return to level running for 2 weeks and then gradually to return to roads and hills. He was instructed to alternate running with and against traffic whenever possible to distribute these stresses more equally. The goal is to prevent an environmentally induced leg length discrep-

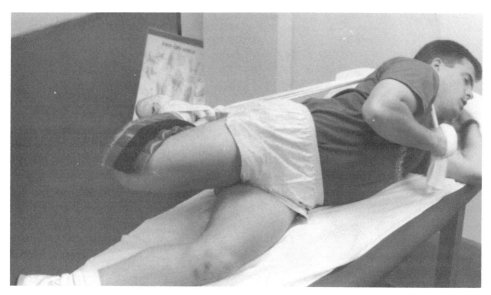

FIGURE 6-10. Stretching of the tensor fasciae latae muscle and the iliotibial band. A similar position to that used for Ober's test can be employed. The patient holds the hip in extension and the knee in flexion, with a sheet or other device strapped to the ankle. A light weight of approximately 5 lbs is applied over the lateral, distal thigh to provide an adduction stretch. The weight applies a low-load prolonged stretch of the hip directly into adduction. The stretch may be held up to 20-30 minutes.

ancy, and to temporarily avoid hill running that is associated with increased stress to the iliotibial band.[29,30,70]

3. The patient was instructed to ice the knee after running for 15 to 20 minutes. Ice is used following activity to reduce tissue inflammation. Ice acts as a vasoconstrictor and slows cell metabolism, thereby preventing or reducing swelling that results from inflammation.[99]

4. The patient was instructed in stretching the tensor fasciae latae muscle and iliotibial band for 10 minutes 3 times per day (Fig. 6-10) and the hip adductor muscles with the knee joint in the extended position, for 10 repetitions of 10 seconds 10 times per day (Fig. 6-11). Because Ober's test was positive for tightness of the iliotibial band, increased extensibility of the iliotibial band is an important treatment goal. Increased extensibility of the iliotibial band is hypothesized to decrease symptoms and prevent recurrence of ITBFS.[70,100]

V. EVALUATING EFFECTIVENESS OF THE METHOD OF RESOLUTION

The patient followed up by telephone 2 weeks after the final clinic treatment and was seen 1 month later in the clinic. Subjective symptoms had decreased 90 percent from the initial evaluation (based on a subjective improvement scale of 0 to 10). Ober's test was negative for tightness, although the test position produced some discomfort at end range of stretch of the iliotibial band. Hip adductor muscle flexibility was equal to that of the uninvolved side. Mild tenderness was palpable over the lateral femoral condyle. Range of motion was full without a painful arc at 30 degrees flexion.

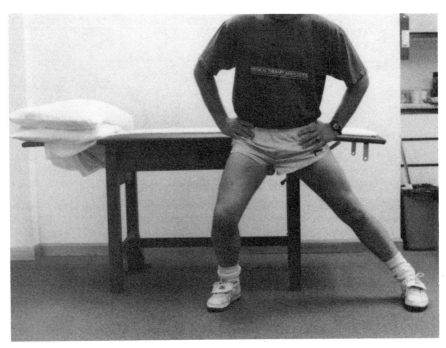

FIGURE 6–11. Stretching of hip joint adductors, including the gracilis muscle. The patient maintains the leg on the affected side in a neutral position with respect to rotation and the knee extended. In this case, the patient is stretching the adductors along his left lower extremity.

Reassessment

The present preventive program is effective. No modifications were necessary. The patient was instructed to return to the clinic if the symptoms did not fully resolve within another month.

CASE STUDY 2

I. IDENTIFYING THE PATIENT'S PROBLEM

The patient is a 43-year-old woman who reported bilateral anterior knee pain, worse on the right. She recently joined her church volleyball team and is practicing with the team one or two times weekly. She is an administrative assistant by occupation. Her usual exercise routine is working on a stairclimbing machine at a moderate intensity level for 20 minutes at a YWCA, three times weekly. Her goals are continued participation on the volleyball team without pain, as well as pain-free activities of daily living.

II. IDENTIFYING CHARACTERISTICS OF THE PROBLEM

1. Pain begins with the practice sessions but decreases as the activities continue.
2. In the evening, after practice, she experiences aching in the anterior knee, and pain with stair climbing or stooping.

III. IDENTIFYING FACTORS AFFECTING THE PROBLEM

Evaluation

Range of motion of the knee joint was full, with mild anterior knee pain at end range of flexion. Rectus femoris muscle tightness was noted with the Modified Thomas test (Fig. 6–12). Ankle dorsiflexion with the subtalar joint held in neutral was 5 degrees with the knee joint extended, and 8 degrees with the knee joint flexed on the right; and 10 degrees and 15 degrees, respectively, on the left. Knee joint flexion in weight bearing was painful on the right. Resisted eccentric quadriceps femoris muscle contractions were painful bilaterally. The patient demonstrated moderate forefoot varus deformities bilaterally, of 8 degrees on the right and 10 degrees on the left (see Fig. 6–1). The patient was observed to pronate excessively on the right during gait (Fig. 6–13). There was tenderness to palpation over the inferior pole of the patella with the knee extended and the quadriceps muscles relaxed.

Extrinsic Factor

Inadequate preparation for high-impact plyometric exercise.

Intrinsic Factors

1. Tightness of the gastrocnemius-soleus muscle group.

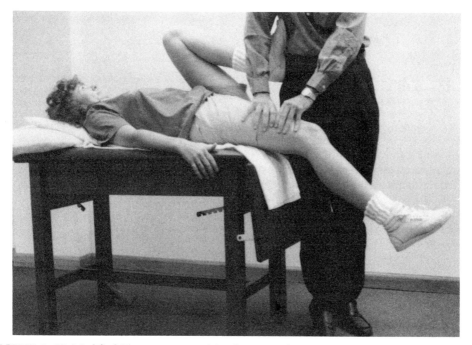

FIGURE 6–12. Modified Thomas test, positive for rectus femoris tightness. The test assesses the flexibility of the iliopsoas, rectus femoris, hip adductor, and hip abductor muscles. Tightness of the rectus femoris muscle is detected when the hip is extended to a neutral position and the knee cannot be flexed to 90 degrees. A pillow under the trunk may be used to ensure that increased lumbar lordosis does not substitute for hip extension.

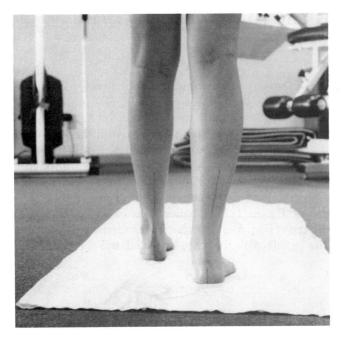

FIGURE 6-13. With lines applied bisecting the calf and the calcaneus, the calf-to-calcaneal angle can be grossly assessed during gait to indicate abnormal or excessive pronation.

2. Isokinetic strength testing at 90 degrees per second showed a 40 percent deficit of the quadriceps muscle for peak torque at 20 degrees of flexion on the right, compared with the left. Peak torque-to-body-weight ratios of the quadriceps muscle were approximately 40 percent bilaterally. Quadriceps-to-hamstring-muscle ratio was approximately 45 percent.
3. LLD of 9 mm, longer on the right side.

IV. DETERMINING A METHOD TO RESOLVE THE PROBLEM

Assessment

Phase 2 Patellar Tendinitis (Table 6-3). The patient's previously performed concentric quadriceps muscle contractions were of long duration/low intensity, and the patellar tendon was unable to tolerate a sudden demand for more forceful quadriceps muscle contractions of short-duration/high intensity, especially with the increased tensile forces of eccentric loading when landing after jumps. The

TABLE 6-3 Classification of Patella Tendinitis According to Symptoms

Phase 1	Pain at the infrapatellar or suprapatellar region after practice or after an event.
Phase 2	Pain at the beginning of the activity, disappearing after "warming up" and reappearing after completion of activity.
Phase 3	The pain remains during and after activity, and the patient is unable to participate in sports.
Phase 4	Represents a complete rupture of the tendon.

Source: From Roels et al,[92] p 363, with permission.

isokinetic strength test identified significant concentric muscle weakness of the quadriceps femoris muscle group.[101] Weakness of the quadriceps muscle results in greater tensile strain within the patellar tendon during functional activities. Additionally, the tightness of the Achilles tendon and the longer lower extremity on the right may necessitate greater compensatory pronation on that side during jumping activities.

Program of Treatment

1. Phonophoresis using 10 percent hydrocortisone ointment for 6 minutes at 1.0 W per cm^2 over six visits. Phonophoresis introduces hydrocortisone into tissue, thereby decreasing inflammation, providing pain alleviation, and increasing range of motion for a variety of inflammatory problems.[102,103] A 10 percent solution has been reported as more effective than a 1 percent solution.[103]

2. Instruction in a progressive resistive exercise (PRE) program for the quadriceps muscles. Exercise began with terminal knee joint extension and SLR exercises, and progressed to one-quarter squats and leg extensions (knee joint extension performed from 90 degrees flexion to full extension) as symptoms decreased. The patient began performing 3 sets of 10 repetitions slowly, with 90-second rest periods. She progressed by increasing the speed of the eccentric phase of the exercise to a moderate, and then fast, speed. Speed of the eccentric phase of the exercise was determined in seconds, using the second hand of a watch. She then increased the resistance by 1 lb while returning to a slow speed during the eccentric phase, and then resumed the same cycle. Eccentric muscle contractions allow higher musculotendinous tension levels than concentric contractions, and unlike concentric contractions, the tension level rises with increases in angular joint velocity.[104] Specific eccentric muscle weakness has been associated with tendinitis conditions.[82,94] The PRE program outlined by Curwin and Stanish[94] uses both resistance and velocity, at different times, to gradually increase tendon strength.

3. The patient was instructed to warm up by light jogging to the point of light perspiration before volleyball practice, and to apply ice to the knee for 20 minutes immediately following practice. Warm-up activities prior to exercise increase circulation within the muscle and tendon, thereby increasing cellular metabolism, and are thought to decrease incidence of muscle soreness.[35,99]

4. The patient was instructed in stretching of the gastrocnemius and soleus muscles. Increased extensibility of the gastrocnemius-soleus muscle group results in increased dorsiflexion range of motion at the ankle joint, and the need for compensatory STJ pronation is reduced.[40]

5. Temporary orthoses were fabricated with a 3-mm heel lift on the left, forefoot varus posts of 4 degrees on the right and 5 degrees on the left, and rearfoot varus posts of 4 degrees bilaterally. Abnormal STJ pronation increases tibial internal rotation, resulting in increased transverse plane forces at the knee joint.[19-21,26,37,39,40,42,43] Orthoses with varus posting have been found to decrease STJ pronation in the frontal plane,[50,105-107] resulting in diminished transverse plane forces transmitted to the knee joint. LLDs of approximately 4 cm or greater that are associated with microtrauma injuries may benefit from a heel lift.[77] The initial heel lift should attempt to correct no more than one half of the measured LLD.[78]

6. The patient was fitted with a patellofemoral knee sleeve on the right. The knee sleeve provides compression to control edema, and helps to reduce mobility of the patella tendon during activity.

V. EVALUATING EFFECTIVENESS OF THE METHOD OF RESOLUTION

Reassessment

Four weeks after the initial assessment, the patient reported a 50 percent reduction in symptoms in the right knee and complete resolution of symptoms in the left knee. She still experienced pain after volleyball practice, but no longer at the outset of practice. Therefore, her case could be reclassified as a phase 1 patella tendinitis (see Table 6–3). Tenderness remained over the inferior pole of the right patella. Repeated isokinetic strength testing at 90 degrees per second showed improvement to 55 percent of peak-torque-to-body-weight ratio of the quadriceps femoris muscle on the left. This ratio is considered acceptable for the patient's sex and age.[101] Peak torque deficit of the quadriceps muscle in 20 degrees of flexion had diminished to 25 percent. Ankle dorsiflexion had improved, with the right now equal to the left.

VI. MODIFYING MANAGEMENT

1. The patient was started on gradual plyometric exercises using a sled in the supine position (Fig. 6–14). She began with minimal resistance and 3 time bouts of 30 seconds each, with 90-second rest periods between bouts. Time bouts were gradually increased to 10. At that point, resistance was increased with addition of more surgical tubing, and time bouts were reduced to 3. The

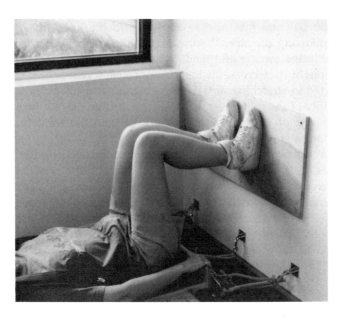

FIGURE 6–14. Plyometric sled. Controlled, gravity-eliminated jumping exercises can be used to train for sports activities.

cycle was repeated. The plyometric program adapts the quadriceps femoris muscles and patella tendon by simulating a jumping manuver in a gravity-eliminated position. Jumping requires a quick, powerful, eccentric contraction, followed by a concentric contraction of the quadriceps femoris muscles.[108]

2. Permanent orthoses will probably not be needed. When symptoms resolve and quadriceps muscle strength is improved on the right, adequate ankle joint dorsiflexion range of motion and the use of a heel lift on the left side will likely limit the amount of compensatory pronation occurring on the right side.

CASE STUDY 3

I. IDENTIFYING THE PATIENT'S PROBLEM

The patient is a 16-year-old high school drill team member with an insidious onset of left knee pain, beginning 3 months ago during drill team practice. The pain has gradually worsened. She also reported aching in her left knee with prolonged sitting at school or when driving, which she could relieve by extending the knee.

II. IDENTIFYING CHARACTERISTICS OF THE PROBLEM

1. The pain increases with weight bearing activities that produce greater knee joint reaction forces than does ambulation.
2. The pain increases during prolonged rest with a flexed knee joint.
3. The pain increases during stair climbing.

III. IDENTIFYING FACTORS AFFECTING THE PROBLEM

Evaluation

There was tenderness to palpation over the left lateral retinaculum, lateral patellar facet, and inferior pole of the patella. Range of motion of the knee joint was full. Hamstring muscle flexibility was decreased. Multiple intrinsic predisposing factors were identified as noted below. In the standing position, excessive calcaneal valgus, "squinting patellae," and tibial torsion were noted. Apprehension sign was positive (Fig. 6–15).

Extrinsic Factor

Sudden onset of weight bearing activity.

Intrinsic Factors

1. Q angle of 25 degrees bilaterally.
2. Standing calcaneal valgus angle of 10 degrees on the left and 8 degrees on the right.

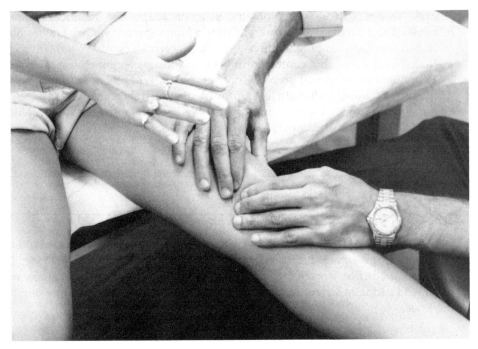

FIGURE 6–15. Apprehension sign. The examiner attempts to displace the patella laterally. A positive test is indicated by the patients subjective report of pain and a feeling of instability.

3. Forefoot varus deformities of 14 degrees on the left and 10 degrees on the right.
4. Excessive pronation, worse on the left, noted during gait assessment on the treadmill.
5. Quadriceps femoris muscles demonstrated 50 percent peak-torque-to-body-weight ratios bilaterally.
6. Palpable atrophy of the vastus medialis obliquus muscle bilaterally.
7. Possible femoral anteversion, suggested by 60 degrees of hip internal rotation (in the prone position) on the left, and 50 degrees on the right (Fig. 6–16).
8. Passive SLR limited to 70 degrees bilaterally due to hamstring musculotendinous tightness.
9. Tightness of the lateral retinaculum, suggested by decreased medial patellar gliding.

IV. DETERMINING A METHOD TO RESOLVE THE PROBLEM

Assessment

"Miserable malalignment" with femoral anteversion, external tibial torsion, and excessive foot pronation (see Fig. 6–7). Onset of new activity with higher demands than ambulation brought the condition to a symptomatic level.

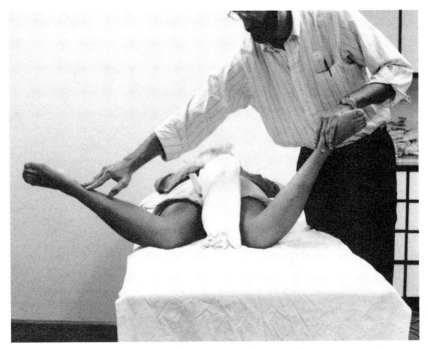

FIGURE 6-16. Hip joint rotation range of motion, tested prone. Excessive internal rotation of the left hip suggests femoral anteversion.

Program of Treatment

1. Application of moist heat before activity and ice after activity. Heat before activity increases circulation within the muscle, improving efficiency of subsequent muscle contractions.[35] Ice reduces a potential inflammatory response to activity.[99]

2. Fabrication of foot orthoses with 5-mm forefoot varus posting on the left and 4 mm on the right. Rearfoot varus posting of 4 mm bilaterally. Compensatory abnormal tibial and femoral internal rotation that result from abnormal STJ pronation may result in lateral tracking of the patella along the femoral trochlear groove, increasing the lateral patellofemoral joint compression forces.[39]

3. PRE program of quadriceps femoris muscle strengthening to emphasize the vastus medialis muscle, using terminal knee extension, and SLR in slight external rotation of the hip joint (Figs. 6-17 and 6-18). Increased vastus medialis muscle strength corrects the muscle imbalance at the patellofemoral joint and also reduces the lateral tracking of the patella and the subsequent joint compression forces along the lateral patellar facet.[17,40,72]

4. Stretching of lateral retinaculum (Fig. 6-19). An extensible lateral retinaculum is a prerequisite for normal tracking of the patella.[72] The objective is to reduce the muscle imbalance at the patellofemoral joint by decreasing passive resistance to the contraction of the vastus medialis obliquus muscle.

5. Contract-relax hamstring muscle stretching. Contract-relax muscle stretching is

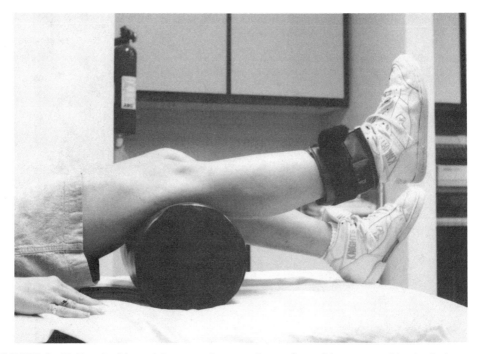

FIGURE 6–17. Terminal knee joint extension exercise performed in an open kinetic chain.

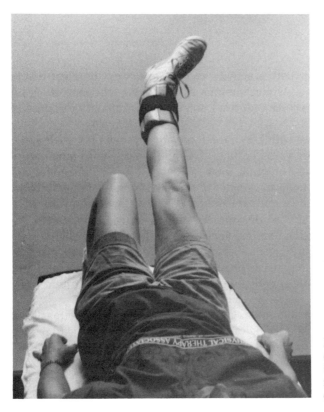

FIGURE 6–18. Straight-leg raise exercise with the leg externally rotated 30 to 40 degrees to facilitate recruitment of the vastus medialis obliquus muscle.

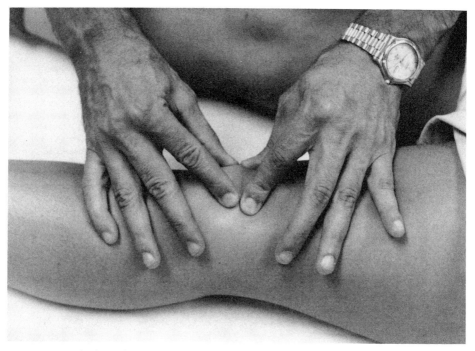

FIGURE 6-19. The lateral retinaculum can be stretched by passive medial glide while everting the patella.

superior to ballistic stretching, prolonged stretching, or passive mobilization in increasing hamstring muscle flexibility.[109,110]

V. EVALUATING EFFECTIVENESS OF THE METHOD OF RESOLUTION

Reassessment

After 2 weeks, the patient reported 40 percent improvement in symptoms, based on a subjective improvement scale of 0 to 10. Passive SLR had increased to 80 degrees on the left. Medial gliding of the patella on the left had improved, but remained restricted compared with the right. Vastus medialis obliquus muscle tone had improved. An isokinetic strength retest demonstrated that peak-torque-to-body-weight ratios of the quadriceps femoris muscle had increased to 60 percent on the right and 55 percent on the left.

VI. MODIFYING MANAGEMENT

1. Forefoot varus post on the left was increased to 7 mm. The patient was tolerating the orthoses well, and posting on the left side was increased to further support the forefoot varus deformity and reduce compensatory STJ pronation.
2. Closed kinetic chain exercises were begun, including leg press, stairclimber, and step-ups (Figs. 6–20, 6–21, and 6–22A,B). Quadriceps femoris muscle exer-

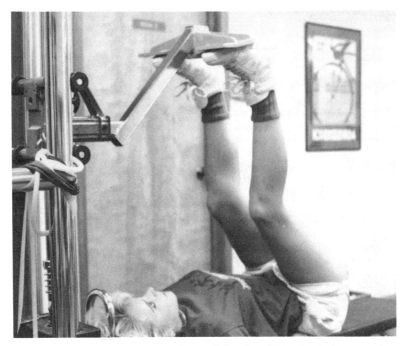

FIGURE 6–20. The leg press exercise may be used for closed kinetic chain strengthening of the quadriceps, gluteal, and gastrocnemius-soleus muscles.

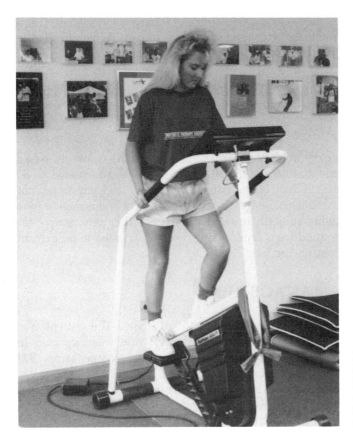

FIGURE 6–21. A stairclimbing machine provides closed kinetic chain endurance exercise for the quadriceps, gluteal, and gastrocnemius-soleus muscles.

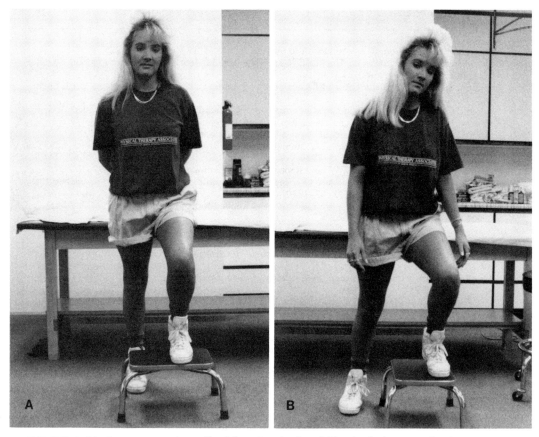

FIGURE 6–22. Step-up exercises afford functional, closed kinetic chain strengthening exercises for the knee and hip joint musculature. *A*) Forward step-up exercise. *B*) Side-step exercise.

cises performed from full extension to 30 degrees of flexion during weight bearing results in lesser patellofemoral joint reaction forces than when the limb is non–weight bearing.[111]

SUMMARY

A review of microtrauma or overuse injuries to the knee included a discussion of the incidence of overuse injuries; their etiology and evaluation; treatment strategies and principles for common overuse injuries; and cases that incorporated problem solving and the principles of treatment. The importance of identifying the underlying factors of microtrauma injury was emphasized. Factors intrinsic to the individual include muscle imbalances and lower extremity malalignment. Extrinsic factors include training errors and equipment problems. The premise of this chapter is that failure to identify both the extrinsic and intrinsic factors in the clarifying evaluation, and to modify and/or correct these factors in treatment, will result in ineffective and incomplete treatment results. To assist the reader in identifying and correcting both extrinsic and intrinsic factors, specific strategies and related information were presented. This included discussion of proper running shoes and surfaces, orthotic therapy, and evaluation and treatment of muscle imbalances and malalignment syndromes in the lower extremities.

REFERENCES

1. Herring, SA and Nilson, KL: Introduction to overuse injuries. Clin Sports Med 6:225, 1987.
2. Engles, M: Tissue response. In Donatelli, R and Wooden, MJ (eds): Orthopaedic Physical Therapy. Churchill Livingstone, New York, 1989.
3. Cummings, GS, Crutchfield, CA, and Barnes, MR: Soft Tissue Changes in Contractures, Vol 1. Stokesville Publishing, Atlanta, 1983.
4. Kloth, LC and Miller, KH: The inflammatory response to wounding. In Kloth, LC, McCulloch, JM, and Feedar, JA (eds): Wound Healing: Alternatives in Management. FA Davis, Philadelphia, 1990.
5. Arem, AJ and Madden, JW: Effects of stress on healing wounds. J Surg Res 20:93, 1976.
6. Akeson, WH, Amiel, D, and Woo, SL-Y: Immobility effects on synovial joints: The pathomechanics of joint contracture. Biorheology 17:95, 1980.
7. Peacock, EP and VanWinkle, W: Wound Repair, ed 2. WB Saunders, Philadelphia, 1976.
8. Madden, JW and Smith, HC: The rate of collagen synthesis and deposition in dehisced and resutured wounds. Surg Gynecol Obstet 130:487, 1970.
9. Madden, JW: Current concepts in wound healing as applied to hand surgery. Orthop Clin North Am 1:325, 1970.
10. Cain, SD and Janos, SC: Clinical pharmacology for the physical therapist. In Boissonnault, WG (ed): Examination in Physical Therapy Practice. Churchill Livingstone, New York, 1991, pp 279–312.
11. Abramson, SB: Nonsteroidal anti-inflammatory drugs: Mechanisms of action and therapeutic considerations. In Leadbetter, WB, Buckwalter, JA, and Gordon, SL (eds): Sports-Induced Inflammation: Clinical and Basic Science Concepts. American Academy of Orthopaedic Surgeons, Park Ridge, IL, 1990, pp 421–441.
12. Leadbetter, WB: An introduction to sports-induced soft-tissue inflammation. In Leadbetter, WB, Buckwalter, JA, and Gordon, SL (eds): Sports-Induced Inflammation: Clinical and Basic Science Concepts. American Academy of Orthopaedic Surgeons, Park Ridge, IL, 1990, pp 3–23.
13. Clancy, WG: Tendinitis and plantar fasciitis in runners. In D'Ambrosia, R and Drez, D (eds): Prevention and Treatment of Running Injuries. Slack, Thorofare, NJ, 1982, pp 77–87.
14. Cavanagh, P: The biomechanics of lower extremity action in distance running. Foot Ankle 7:197, 1987.
15. Murphy, P: Ultrasports are in—in spite of injuries. The Physician and Sportsmedicine 14:180, 1986.
16. Renstrom, P and Johnson, RJ: Overuse injuries in sports: A review. Sports Med 2:316, 1985.
17. Taunton, JE, et al: Non-surgical management of overuse knee injuries in runners. Can J Sports Sci 12:11, 1987.
18. Marti, B, et al: On the epidemiology of running injuries: The 1984 Bern grand-prix study. Am J Sports Med 16:285, 1988.
19. Lutter, LL: Injuries in the runner and jogger. Minn Med 63:45, 1980.
20. James, SL, Bates, BT, and Osternig, LR: Injuries to runners. Am J Sports Med 6:40, 1978.
21. Weiss, BD: Nontraumatic injuries in amateur long distance bicyclists. Am J Sports Med 13:187, 1985.
22. Clancey, WG: Runner's injuries. Am J Sports Med 8:137, 1980.
23. Andrews, JR: Overuse injuries of the lower extremity. Clin Sports Med 2:139, 1983.
24. Solomonow, M and D'Ambrosia, RD: Biomechanics of muscle overuse injuries: A theoretical approach. Clin Sports Med 6:241, 1987.
25. Mann, RA: Biomechanics of walking, running, and sprinting. Am J Sports Med 8:345, 1980.
26. Mann, RA: Biomechanics of running. In Mack, R (ed): Symposium the Foot and Leg in Running Sports. CV Mosby, St Louis, 1982, pp 1–29.
27. Smith, WB: Environmental factors in running. In Clancy, WG: Runner's injuries. Am J Sports Med 8:138, 1980.
28. Renne, JW: The iliotibial band friction syndrome. J Bone Joint Surg[Am] 57:1110, 1975.
29. Noble, CA: Iliotibial band friction syndrome in runners. Am J Sports Med 8:232, 1980.
30. Lindenberg, G, Pinshaw, R, and Noakes, TD: Iliotibial band friction syndrome in runners. The Physician and Sportsmedicine 12:118, 1984.
31. Messier, SP and Pittala, KA: Etiologic factors associated with selected running injuries. Med Sci Sports Exerc 20:501, 1988.
32. Drez, D: Running footwear. In Clancy, WG: Runner's injuries. Am J Sports Med 8:140, 1980.
33. Ellis: The match game. Runner's World. October 1985.
34. Roy, S and Irwin, R: Sports Medicine: Prevention, Education, Management, and Rehabilitation. Prentice Hall, Englewood Cliffs, NJ, 1983.
35. Kulund, DW: The Injured Athlete, ed 2. JB Lippincott, Philadelphia, 1988.
36. Ciullo, JA and Jackson, DW: Track and field. In Schneider, RC, Kennedy, JC, and Plant, MC (eds): Sports Injuries: Mechanism, Prevention, and Treatment. Williams & Wilkins, Baltimore, 1985.
37. Ramig, D, et al: The foot and sports medicine: Biomechanical foot faults as related to chondromalacia patellae. Journal of Orthopaedic and Sports Physical Therapy 2:48, 1980.
38. Antich, TJ, et al: Evaluation of knee extensor mechanism disorders: Clinical presentation of 112 patients. Journal of Orthopaedic and Sports Physical Therapy 8:248, 1986.
39. Tiberio, D: The effect of excessive subtalar joint pronation on patellofemoral mechanics: A theoretical model. Journal of Orthopaedic and Sports Physical Therapy 9:160, 1987.

40. James, SL: Chondromalacia of the patellae in the adolescent. In Kennedy, JC (ed): The Injured Adolescent Knee. Williams & Wilkins, Baltimore, 1979.

41. Insall, J, Falvo, KA, and Wise, DW: Chondromalacia patellae. J Bone Joint Surg[Am] 58:1, 1976.

42. Lutter, LD: Foot-related knee problems in the long distance runner. Foot Ankle 1:112, 1980.

43. Buchbinder, MR, Napora, NJ, and Biggs, EW: The relationship of abnormal pronation to chondromalacia of the patella in distance runners. J Am Podiatr Med Assoc 69:159, 1979.

44. Grana, WA and Coniglione, TC: Knee disorders in runners. The Physician and Sportsmedicine 13:127, 1985.

45. Donatelli, R: Abnormal biomechanics. In Donatelli, R (ed): The Biomechanics of the Foot and Ankle. FA Davis, Philadelphia, 1990, pp 32–65.

46. Tachdjian, MO: The Child's Foot. WB Saunders, Philadelphia, 1985.

47. McCrea, JD: Pediatric Orthopaedics of the Lower Extremity. Futura Publishing, Mount Kisco, NY, 1989.

48. Root, ML, Orien, WP, and Weed, JN: Clinical Biomechanics, Vol 2, Normal and Abnormal Function of the Foot. Clinical Biomechanics, Los Angeles, 1977.

49. Hlavac, HF: Compensated forefoot varus. J Am Podiatr Med Assoc 60:229, 1970.

50. Taunton, JE, et al: A triplanar electrogoniometer investigation of running mechanics in runners with compensatory overpronation. Can J Sports Sci 10:104, 1985.

51. Garbalosa, J and McClure, M: Normal angular relationship of the forefoot to the rearfoot in the frontal plane. Graduate Thesis. Division of Physical Therapy, Department of Rehabilitative Medicine, Emory University. Atlanta, 1987.

52. Schoenhaus, HD, et al: Computerized analysis of gait. J Am Podiatr Med Assoc 69:11, 1979.

53. Blake, RL and Denton, JA: Functional foot orthoses for athletic injuries. J Am Podiatr Med Assoc 75:359, 1985.

54. D'Ambrosia, RD: Orthotic devices in running injuries. Clin Sports Med 4:611, 1985.

55. Eggold, JF: Orthotics in the prevention of runner's overuse injuries. The Physician and Sportsmedicine 9:125, 1981.

56. Subotnick, SI: Foot orthotics: An update. The Physician and Sportsmedicine 11:103, 1983.

57. Subotnick, SI: Biomechanics of the subtalar and midtarsal joints. J Am Podiatr Med Assoc 65:756, 1975.

58. Bates, BT, et al: Functional variability of the lower extremity during the support phase of running. Med Sci Sports Exerc 11:328, 1979.

59. Wright, DG, Desai, SM, and Henderson, WH: Action of the subtalar and ankle-joint complex during the stance phase of walking. J Bone Joint Surg[Am] 46:361, 1964.

60. Lilievre, J: Current concepts and correction in the valgus foot. Clin Orthop 70:43, 1970.

61. Bates, BT, et al: Lower extremity function during the support phase of running. In Asmussen, E and Jorgensen, K (eds): Biomechanics VI-B. University Park Press, Baltimore, MD, 1978.

62. Bates, BT, et al: Foot orthotic devices to modify selected aspects of lower extremity mechanics. Am J Sports Med 7:338, 1979.

63. Perry, J: Anatomy and biomechanics of the hindfoot. Clin Orthop 177:9, 1983.

64. Soutes-Little, RW, et al: Analysis of foot motion during running using a joint co-ordinate system. Med Sci Sports Exerc 19:285, 1987.

65. Inman, VT: The Joints of the Ankle. Williams & Wilkins, Baltimore, 1976.

66. Inman, VT, Rolston, HJ, and Todd, F: Human Walking. Williams & Wilkins, Baltimore, 1981.

67. Scranton, PE, Pedegana, LR, and Whitesel, JP: Gait analysis: Alterations in support phase forces using supportive devices. Am J Sports Med 10:6, 1982.

68. Rose, GK: Correction of the pronated foot. J Bone Joint Surg[Br] 44:642, 1962.

69. Lundberg, A, et al: Kinematics of the ankle/foot complex. III. Influence of leg rotation. Foot Ankle 9:304, 1989.

70. Jones, DC and James, SL: Overuse injuries of the lower extremity: Shin splints, iliotibial band friction syndrome, and exertional compartment syndromes. Clin Sports Med 6:273, 1987.

71. Taunton, JE and Clement, DB: Iliotibial tract friction syndrome in athletes. Can J Sports Sci 6:76, 1981.

72. Kramer, PG: Patella malalignment syndrome: Rationale to reduce excessive lateral pressure. Journal of Orthopaedic and Sports Physical Therapy 8:301, 1986.

73. Micheli, LJ, et al: Patella alta and the adolescent growth spurt. Clin Orthop 213:159, 1986.

74. Fulkerson, JP: The etiology of patellofemoral pain in young, active patients. Clin Orthop 179:129, 1983.

75. Lutter, LD: Cavus foot in runners. Foot Ankle 1:225, 1981.

76. Friberg, O: Clinical symptoms and biomechanics of lumbar spine and hip joint in leg length inequality. Spine 8:643, 1983.

77. Subotnick, SI: Limb length discrepancies of the lower extremity (the short leg syndrome). Journal of Orthopaedic and Sports Physical Therapy 3:11, 1981.

78. Blustein, SM and D'Amico, JC: Leg length discrepancy. J Am Podiatr Med Assoc 75:200, 1985.

79. Powls, B: Leg length discrepancy. Orthopaedic Division Newsletter. Canadian Physical Therapy Association, March–April, 1985.

80. Janda, V and Schmid, HJ: Muscles as a pathogenic factor in back pain. Paper presented at the 4th Conference of the International Federation of Manipulative Therapy, Christchurch, New Zealand, 1988.

81. Jull, GA and Janda, V: Muscles and motor control in low back pain: Assessment and management. In Grant, R (ed): Physical Therapy of the Cervical and Thoracic Spine. Churchill Livingstone, New York, 1989, pp 253–278.

82. Bennett, JG and Stauber, WT: Evaluation and treatment of anterior knee pain using eccentric exercise. Med Sci Sports Exerc 18:526, 1986.
83. Hunter, SC and Poole, RM: The chronically inflamed tendon. Clin Sports Med 6:371, 1987.
84. Burns, LT, Burns, MJ, and Burns, GA: A clinical application of biomechanics. I. J Am Podiatr Med Assoc 63:394, 1973.
85. Reilly, JP and Nicholas, JA: The chronically inflamed bursa. Clin Sports Med 6:345, 1987.
86. Kessler, RM and Hertling, D: Management of Common Musculoskeletal Disorders. JB Lippincott, Philadelphia, 1983, p 401.
87. Hoppenfeld, S: Examination of the Spine and Extremities. Appleton-Century-Crofts, New York, 1976, p 180.
88. Pick, TP and Howden, R (eds): Gray's Anatomy. Bounty Books, New York, 1977.
89. Barfred, T: Experimental rupture of Achilles tendon: Comparison of various types of experimental ruptures in rats. Acta Orthop Scand 42:528, 1971.
90. D'Ambrosia, RD: Musculoskeletal Disorders. JB Lippincott, Philadelphia, 1977, p 469.
91. Blazina, ME, et al: Jumper's knee. Orthop Clin North Am 4:665, 1973.
92. Roels, J, et al: Patellar tendinitis (jumper's knee). Am J Sports Med 6:362, 1978.
93. Albert, M: Eccentrics: Clinical program design and delayed onset muscle soreness. In Albert, M (ed): Eccentric Muscle Training in Sports and Orthopaedics. Churchill Livingstone, New York, 1991.
94. Curwin, S and Stanish, WD: Tendinitis: Its etiology and treatment. DC Heath, Lexington, MA, 1984.
95. Turek, SL (ed): Orthopaedics: Principles and their application, ed 3. JB Lippincott, Philadelphia, 1977.
96. Glass, JM, Stephen, RL, and Jacobson, SC: The quantity and distribution of radiolabeled dexamethasone delivered to tissue by iontophoresis. Int J Dermatol 19:519, 1980.
97. Harris, PR: Iontophoresis: Clinical research in musculoskeletal inflammatory conditions. Journal of Orthopaedic and Sports Physical Therapy 4:109, 1982.
98. Bertolucci, LE: Introduction of antiinflammatory drugs by iontophoresis: Double blind study. Journal of Orthopaedic and Sports Physical Therapy 4:103, 1982.
99. Gieck, JH and Saliba, EN: Application of modalities in overuse syndromes. Clin Sports Med 6:427, 1987.
100. Noble, HB, Hajek, MR, and Porter, M: Diagnosis and treatment of iliotibial band tightness in runners. The Physician and Sportsmedicine 10:67, 1982.
101. Davies, GJ: A Compendium of Isokinetics in Clinical Usage. S & S Publishers, Onalaska, WI, 1987, p 167.
102. Griffin, JE, et al: Patients treated with ultrasonic driven cortisone and with ultrasound alone. Phys Ther 47:594, 1967.
103. Kleinkort, JA and Wood, F: Phonophoresis with 1 percent versus 10 percent hydrocortisone. Phys Ther 55:1320, 1975.
104. Albert, M: Physiologic and clinical principles of eccentrics. In Albert, M (ed): Eccentric Muscle Training in Sports and Orthopaedics. Churchill Livingstone, New York, 1991, pp 11–23.
105. Novick, A and Kelley, DL: Position and movement changes of the foot with orthotic intervention during the loading response of gait. Journal of Orthopaedic and Sports Physical Therapy 11:301, 1990.
106. Bates, BT, et al: Foot orthotic devices to modify selected aspects of lower extremity mechanics. Am J Sports Med 7:338, 1979.
107. Smith, LS, et al: The effects of soft and semi-rigid orthoses upon rearfoot movement in running. J Am Podiatr Med Assoc 76:227, 1986.
108. Voight, ML and Draovitch, P: Plyometrics. In Albert, M (ed): Eccentric Muscle Training in Sports and Orthopaedics. Churchill Livingstone, New York, 1991.
109. Holt, LE, Travis, TM, and Okita, T: Comparative study of three stretching techniques. Percept Mot Skills 31:611, 1970.
110. Tanigawa, MC: Comparison of the hold-relax procedure and passive mobilization on increasing muscle length. Phys Ther 52:725, 1972.
111. Hungerford, DS and Barry, M: Biomechanics of the patellofemoral joint. Clin Orthop 144:9, 1979.

CHAPTER 7

Rehabilitation of Patellofemoral Joint Dysfunction

J. Gregory Bennett, MS, PT

Maladies of the patellofemoral joint are among the most common knee complaints experienced by athletes.[1,2,3] However, difficulties at the patellofemoral joint are not peculiar to athletes. Children, particularly adolescent females, frequently suffer from pain and instability at the patellofemoral joint.[4] Late adolescents and young adults are often afflicted with tendinitis, stress syndromes, and instability.[5,6] Older individuals are not immune either, due to the consequences of osteoarthritis of this heavily used joint.[2,7]

Numerous diagnostic categories fall under the general heading of patellofemoral joint dysfunction (Table 7–1). Most common is nondifferentiated anterior knee pain, which is frequently diagnosed as patellalgia or patellofemoral joint syndrome (PFJS) but is known by a variety of other names as well. The clinician must distinguish between these nondifferentiated pathologies and other diagnoses of the patellofemoral joint. Conditions such as subluxation or dislocation require increased attention to prevent further incidence of the malady and a potentially more significant injury, such as a fractured patella. Degenerative diseases, such as osteoarthritis and chondromalacia, will also be discussed, with emphasis on conservative management of patellofemoral maladies. However, the treatment principles covered can be applied to both surgically and conservatively managed cases. Care must be taken to allow for the additional soft-tissue healing constraints encountered in postoperative cases.

The intent of this chapter is to discuss the numerous anatomic and mechanical variances at the patellofemoral joint and the consequences of those variances. A number of successful treatment approaches will also be explored along with the rationale for those treatments. Ideally, the clinician will be able to form an eclectic approach to the wide variety of problems associated with the patellofemoral joint. Case studies reviewing the problem-solving approach for rehabilitation of selected patellofemoral injuries are presented at the end of the chapter.

TABLE 7–1 Pathologies of the Patellofemoral Joint

Diagnosis	Symptoms/Characteristics	Intervention
Patellalgia Patellofemoral joint syndrome Anterior knee pain syndrome Patellofemoral arthralgia	Nondifferentiated pain below and around the patella, often characterized by increased lateral patella tracking. Pain is increased by activity, especially by running and by climbing or descending stairs.	Conservative treatment consisting of rest, modalities, and emphasizing progressive exercise is the treatment of choice. Orthotics for the knee and foot are helpful. Surgery is usually not necessary.
Patella subluxation Patella dislocation	Symptoms and characteristics of patella subluxation and dislocation are the same as above. The difference is that instability is present and must be addressed.	Rehabilitation is similar to the above. Care must be taken to protect the patient from further incidence of the instability. Surgery is more frequent.
Chondromalacia Degenerative joint disease	The above symptoms are present. In addition, these patients often experience significant crepitation and pain at rest.	Rehabilitation remains as above. Exercise is tolerated less well, and frequent modification of intensity and range of motion may be necessary.

Emphasis is also placed on the clinical management of patellofemoral joint problems. Certainly, home exercise and management are an integral and necessary part of any treatment program for the patellofemoral joint. In some cases, home management is all that is necessary to successfully relieve patellofemoral pain syndromes. The principles for strengthening and stretching exercises are the same whether the exercises are done clinically or at home.

ANATOMIC CONSIDERATIONS

A comprehensive study of knee anatomy is presented in Chapter 1. This chapter will briefly review the static and dynamic structures of the knee that have primary or secondary effects on patellofemoral joint function. Emphasis is placed on understanding the anatomy of the patellofemoral joint and its effect on biomechanics and function.

Static Stabilizers

Osseous structures have a major role in patellofemoral joint function and stability. Particular importance is ascribed to the patellar facets and their relationships to the articular surface of the trochlear groove of the femur.

The patella is a multifaceted sesamoid bone integral with the quadriceps femoris musculature and the capsule of the knee. The posterior surface is divided longitudinally by a smooth ridge.[8] The patella's articulating surface has five distinct areas: the lateral, medial, and odd facets, and the superior and inferior regions (Fig. 7–1).[9] The odd facet, which lies at the extreme medial border of the patella, comes into contact with the femur during the end range of knee flexion.[10] Wiberg[11] describes six variations in patellar

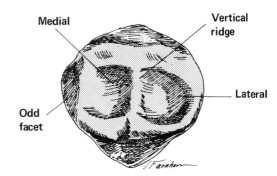

FIGURE 7-1. The posterior surface of the patella. (From Norkin and Levangie,[9] p 321.)

shape (see Chapter 1) and notes that the depth of the femoral trochlear groove and the pattern of patellar facets are important to patellofemoral joint stability.

The patellar (trochlear) surface of the femur is grooved to accommodate the ridge of the posterior surface of the patella. The patellar surface extends over both the medial and lateral condyles, with the much larger articular surface being lateral. The femoral condylar surface extends higher on the lateral side, which adds some margin of stability to the patella and reduces lateral subluxation.[8] The importance of this anatomic variance is obvious given the nature of the patella to dislocate laterally, as will be discussed later in the chapter.

Additional static stability is provided by the capsule of the knee joint and the patellofemoral retinaculum. Henry[2] describes thickenings of the lateral retinaculum called the lateral patellofemoral ligaments, which can contribute to lateral tilt and possible lateral subluxation of the patella in cases of hypomobility (Fig. 7-2). Medial stability is enhanced by the medial patellar retinaculum, which extends from the margin of the patella to the collateral ligament and patella.[8] Similarly, hypermobility of the medial structures from trauma or congenital maldevelopment can increase the likelihood of lateral patella tracking or instability.

The fibrous capsule of the knee joint is extensive and complex (see Chapter 1). Although the capsule itself is composed of noncontractile tissue, several muscles are

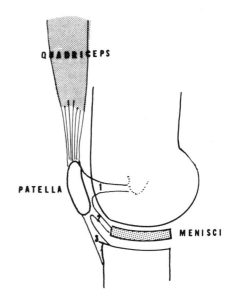

FIGURE 7-2. The quadriceps mechanism with three ligamentous extensions: 1) the lateral patellofemoral ligament attaches to the epicondyle eminence of the femur; 2) the meniscopatellar ligament attaches to and pulls the meniscus forward during knee extension; 3) the infrapatellar tendon. (From Cailliet, R: Knee Pain and Disability, ed 3. FA Davis, Philadelphia, 1992, p 31.)

contiguous with the capsule and play an important role in patellar dynamics.[8] (That role is discussed in the next section of this chapter.) An important point is that capsular pathologies such as fibrosis and synovitis can affect the patellofemoral joint by interrupting or disturbing the continuity of the capsule with the patella; therefore, it is important to evaluate the knee joint capsule when investigating anterior knee pain.

Dynamic Influences on the Patellofemoral Joint

Several muscles play a direct role in patellofemoral joint function and dysfunction. Muscular strength and tightness and neuromotor control are important factors in rehabilitating patients with patellar pain syndromes.

The quadriceps femoris musculature exerts the most direct effect on the relationship of the patella to the trochlear groove. The rectus femoris and vastus intermedius muscles exert an essentially cephalad pull, with angles of insertion, respectively, of 10 and 0 degrees medial from the vertical.[2] The vastus lateralis muscle inserts at 15 degrees laterally, and the vastus medialis muscle inserts at 20 degrees medially, with the oblique head more sharply angled at 55 to 60 degrees medially (Fig. 7–3). The vastus medialis

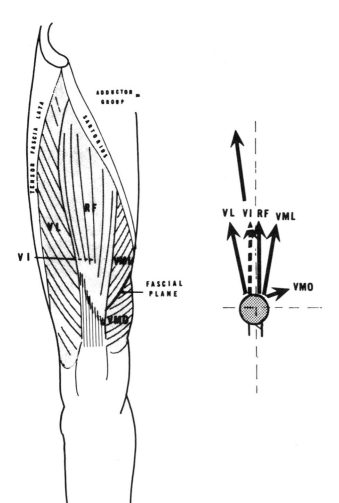

FIGURE 7–3. The quadriceps femoris musculature and its line of pull relative to the femur: RF, rectus femoris; VL, vastus lateralis; VI, vastus intermedius; VM, vastus medialis; VMO, vastus medialis obliquus. (From Calliet, R: Knee Pain and Disability, ed 3. FA Davis, Philadelphia, 1992, p 28.)

and vastus medialis obliquus muscles, by virtue of their insertions, play a major role in rehabilitating dislocations, subluxations, and conditions caused by excessive lateral tracking.

Other muscles affect patellofemoral dynamics because of their integral relationship with the capsule of the knee. Posteriorly, the gastrocnemius and semimembranosus muscles blend with the capsule (Fig. 7–4). Laterally, a slip of the iliotibial tract (the iliopatellar band) extends to the capsule (Fig. 7–5). Medially, expansions from the semitendinosus and sartorius muscles blend with the capsule.[8] The congruous relationship of these muscles with the patella and capsule necessitates their evaluation in cases of anterior knee pain syndromes. Conditions involving abnormal patellofemoral joint compression forces and lateral tracking are particularly aggravated by tightness of these muscles. Such tightness would restrict capsular mobility and therefore potentially in-

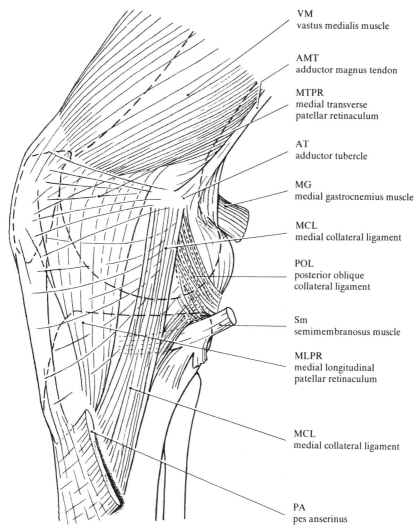

VM
vastus medialis muscle

AMT
adductor magnus tendon

MTPR
medial transverse
patellar retinaculum

AT
adductor tubercle

MG
medial gastrocnemius muscle

MCL
medial collateral ligament

POL
posterior oblique
collateral ligament

Sm
semimembranosus muscle

MLPR
medial longitudinal
patellar retinaculum

MCL
medial collateral ligament

PA
pes anserinus

FIGURE 7–4. The knee joint with its main anatomic structures viewed from the medial and posteromedial aspect. Note the integration of the contractile tissues, i.e., semimembranosus, medial gastrocnemius, adductor magnus, and vastus medialis muscles, to the capsule. (From Müller, W: The Knee: Form, Function, and Ligament Reconstruction. Springer-Verlag, Berlin, 1982, p 4, with permission.)

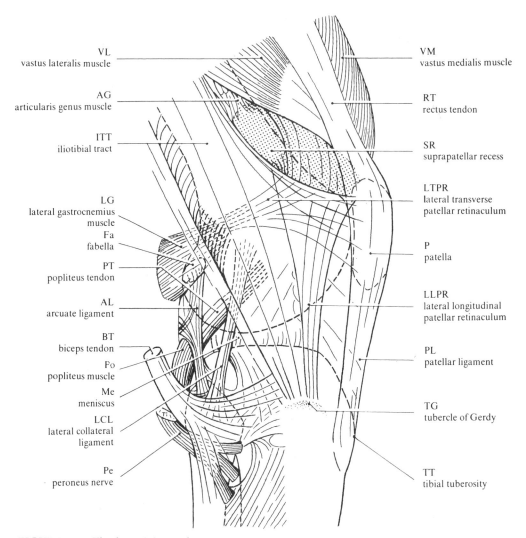

FIGURE 7–5. The knee joint with its main anatomic structures viewed from the lateral aspect. Note the iliotibial tract with its expansion (iliopatellar band) into the lateral transverse patellar retinaculum. (From Müller, W: The Knee: Form, Function, and Ligament Reconstruction. Springer-Verlag, Berlin, 1982, p 5, with permission.)

crease patellofemoral compression forces. Tightness of the iliopatellar band or the iliotibial band may increase lateral tracking of the patella contributing to lateral subluxation, dislocation, and increased lateral facet pressure.

PATELLOFEMORAL JOINT MECHANICS

Of the numerous mechanical variances that affect the patellofemoral joint, most occur in patellar placement or orientation. As stated earlier, the patella is a sesamoid bone integral with quadriceps femoris muscle function but also greatly affected by other musculature. The primary role of the patella is to enhance the function of the quadriceps femoris musculature via increased leverage. Quadriceps femoris muscle force output would diminish by as much as 30 percent without a patella, because the mechanical torque produced is greatly enhanced by the increased moment arm created by the presence of the patella.[9]

The vertical orientation of the patella also is important to normal mechanics. The patella is occasionally abnormally high (patella alta) or low (patella baja or infera). The patella's anatomic position is usually determined by roentgenogram comparing patellar length with patellar tendon length. This relationship is normally 1 to 1. Higher or lower ratios would indicate patella alta or baja, respectively.[3,12] Both conditions have potentially adverse consequences. Patella alta, or high-riding patella, may be unstable and more prone to subluxation and dislocation.[13] Patients with patella alta often exhibit structural abnormalities, such as "grasshopper-eye" or "frog-eye" patella as described by Hughston and colleagues.[3] In the presence of grasshopper-eye patellae, when viewed from the front, the patellae face outward. The opposite abnormality is "squinting" patellae, in which the patellae face inward. Patella baja or infera can cause anterior knee pain syndromes due to increased patellofemoral contact forces, because the patella sits lower in the trochlear groove and therefore contact occurs earlier as the knee is flexed.[1,3,12]

"Miserable malalignment" syndrome, frequently associated with patellofemoral dysfunction (Fig. 7–6), is described as excessive internal rotation of the femurs, with a secondary external rotation of the tibias with pronated feet.[1,14,15] The net effect is genu valgus with increased lateral tracking of the patella and syndromes ranging from pain to the potential for dislocation (see Chapter 6).

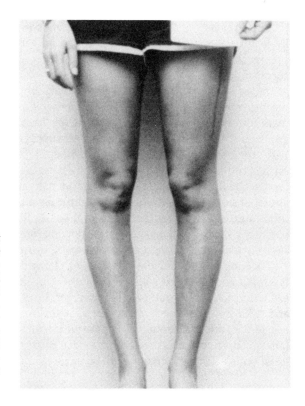

FIGURE 7–6. Miserable malalignment is a series of compensatory transverse and frontal plane changes characterized by femoral anteversion, proximal tibial external torsion, distal tibial varum, and subtalar joint pronation. Note the "squinting patellae" which indicate femoral anteversion with excessive femoral internal rotation. Proximal external tibial torsion results in an increased Q angle of the extensor mechanism.

Patellofemoral joint compression forces and retropatellar crepitation are significant and controversial in assessing anterior knee pain syndromes. Patellofemoral contact forces have been demonstrated to increase as knee flexion increases. Morrison[16] reports compression forces during normal walking as being one half of the individual's body weight. However, during more stressful activities such as ascending or descending stairs, compression forces reach more than three times the body weight.[17,18,19] Varying levels of crepitance often correlate with the amount of retropatellar contact force. However, crepitance is not necessarily indicative of joint pathology and is frequently found in normal knees.[20] It should be noted that whereas retropatellar crepitation may not be indicative of pathology, its presence is never desirable and should be included as an objective finding.

Analyzing compression forces of the knee as a diagnostic tool requires careful consideration. MacDonald and colleagues[21] demonstrated significantly lower patellofemoral joint contact forces in patients with chondromalacia when tested isometrically except at 30 degrees of knee flexion. Patients with anterior knee pain but no chondromalacia had normal contact forces. Bennett and Stauber[22] Dvir[23] found diminished eccentric but not concentric forces in a patient sample with anterior knee pain tested isokinetically. These studies point out that if contact forces were the cause of pain, then the concentric force production would also have been inhibited. The importance of this observation becomes more apparent during discussion of rehabilitation techniques later in the chapter, but in at least these instances, patellofemoral contact forces may not be considered as the primary cause of symptomatology.

EXAMINATION

Several tests and signs help to evaluate patellofemoral joint dysfunction. Necessarily included in the examination is a careful scrutiny of the anatomic variances noted previously. Patellar orientation and muscular condition assessment are paramount to successful treatment of patellofemoral joint disorders.

Assessment of patellar stability is very important. The consequences of misdiagnosis or mismanagement of an unstable patella are much more severe than for that of mere anterior knee pain. Assessment of the stability of the patella in the trochlear groove is frequently accomplished via the apprehension sign.[12,24] The patient lies supine with the leg muscles relaxed and the knee flexed to 30 degrees. The examiner slowly pushes the patella laterally. The test is positive when the patient activates the quadriceps to stabilize the patella or experiences pain and/or apprehension about the test. The apprehension test should be done at multiple angles of knee flexion, because the patella drops into the femoral trochlear groove at 30 degrees of knee flexion and thereby enhances stability. A positive sign beyond 30 degrees of knee flexion may indicate severe instability and be very problematic during rehabilitation.

A common test for the presence of chondromalacia or a compression syndrome is the *grind test* or *Clarke's sign.*[12,24] The patient lies relaxed in the supine position. The examiner places the web of his or her hand just above the proximal pole of the patella and asks the patient to contract the quadriceps muscle. The patella is forced down, causing a grinding, catching, or painful response. Unfortunately, this test elicits many false-positive results due to the pressure of the examiner's hand, and its usefulness is questionable.[12] The *Perkins* sign or *synovial pinch test* gives far fewer false-positive results. The patient lies supine with the musculature relaxed and the knee extended. The examiner pushes the patella medially and laterally and then pinches the soft tissues against the exposed underside of the patella. The test result is positive in the presence of pain and is indicative of synovial or articular irritation.

Another useful indication is cinema sign, or *moviegoer's knee*, a frequent complaint of pain induced from long periods of sitting immobile with the knee flexed, such as occurs when sitting in a theater.[3,25] Hughston and associates[3] described the cinema sign as an aching pain resulting from static pressure and ischemia around the patella. Numerous authors point to the need for motion to prevent the negative effects of immobilization (including pain, as in the cinema sign) and to promote healing of injured tissues regardless of pathology.[26-28]

A final concern is examining the entire lower kinetic chain when anterior knee pain syndromes are present. As discussed earlier in the chapter, in case of "miserable malalignment" syndrome, compensatory abnormalities occur throughout the lower extremity. Abnormalities in foot mechanics, especially excessive pronation, are commonly associated with anterior knee pain.[5,29,30] Chapter 6 reviews common pathomechanical conditions in the lower extremities, including the foot and ankle, that can result in patellofemoral joint dysfunction. In addition, referred pain from pathologies at the hip or low back must be ruled out as part of a comprehensive evaluation.

REHABILITATION

Four separate areas must be addressed when discussing patellofemoral joint rehabilitation. Individual attention is given to *orthotics* (including taping), *modalities, conservative* management, and *postoperative* management. Although dealt with individually, a combination of orthotics, modalities, and exercise is usually prescribed and effective.

Modalities as an adjunct to patellofemoral rehabilitation are used as in other orthopedic diagnosis and will not be discussed in detail. The use of ice, heat, and various electrical modalities for management of pain, inflammation, and edema are effective and desirable for comprehensive management. Additionally, functional electrical stimulation (FES), or neuromuscular electrical stimulation (NMES), has been effectively used for muscle re-education, particularly of the vastus medialis complex.[31,32] NMES can also be used to overcome problems of muscular inhibition due to pain and effusion. However, the use of electrical versus volitionally induced muscle contraction is not without controversy[33,34] and concerns as to whether NMES increases muscle strength apart from, or in conjunction with, volitional exercises (e.g., isometric contractions). An in-depth discussion of this controversy is beyond the scope of this chapter. An excellent review of the efficacy and clinical use of NMES is available by Snyder-Macklen and Robinson.[35] The reader is referred to this source for general guidelines for clinical applications of NMES. A compilation of clinical and research literature performed by Snyder-Macklen and Robinson indicates that whereas NMES demonstrates no advantage for muscle strengthening over volitional exercises in healthy subjects, NMES does increase strength when used either alone or in conjunction with volitional exercises in patients with muscle weakness. Numerous differences exist between electrically and volitionally induced muscle contractions (Table 7–2). The effect of the electrically induced contraction on both the muscle and joint should be considered prior to application.

TABLE 7-2 Electric versus Volitional (Voluntary) Muscle Contraction

Contraction Type	Characteristics	Purpose
Electrical	Numerous protocols exist using selected frequency, intensity, waveform, current type, and other variables to create involuntary or electrically enhanced muscle contraction.	Electrically induced contractions are primarily used when patients have difficulty achieving voluntary contraction. Increasingly, stimulation is being used to enhance voluntary effort and compliance. In patellofemoral pathologies, emphasis is placed on activation of the vastus medialis obliquus muscle.
Volitional	Voluntary contraction of the muscle initiated and controlled by the patient. Intensity and range of motion are the primary variables.	Volitional contractions appear to create greater long-term strengthening, but research is ongoing. Here, too, emphasis is placed on activation of the vastus medialis obliquus muscle in cases of patellofemoral pathology.
Biofeedback	Muscular contraction (or relaxation) accompanied by visual or auditory feedback via surface electrodes or dynamometry.	To enhance (vastus medialis) or diminish (vastus lateralis) muscular activity in order to achieve the goals of the applied exercise.

Orthotics

Various external means of support are often used to treat patellofemoral joint dysfunction. Prescription biomechanical foot orthotics balance and control the subtalar joint, improve lower extremity alignment, and improve patellofemoral joint mechanics. The reader is encouraged to seek appropriate references for foot mechanics and its effect on the kinetic chain and for the use of prescription orthotics.[36,37] For additional description of the use of biomechanical foot orthotics in patients with abnormal mechanics, see the case studies in Chapter 6.

Patellar stabilizing braces are frequently used as an adjunct to patellar rehabilitation (Table 7-3). Palumbo,[38] Levine,[39] and Henry and Crosland[40] have all advocated using a variety of braces for patellar support. All of the braces use various straps as buttresses to stabilize the patella and reduce maltracking; all have been used with considerable success. Numerous types of patellar stabilizing braces exist, giving the clinician a wide variety of materials and sizes to choose from. As pointed out by Henry,[2] while neither should be used alone, exercise is more important than bracing.

Recently, patellar taping has been advocated as part of a comprehensive plan for managing patients with patellar pain syndromes. McConnell[41] supports a complete understanding of the mechanics of the patellofemoral joint, with appropriate exercise prescription and patellar taping used for rehabilitation. Strips of tape are applied to correct various deviations from normal patellar mechanics including glide, tilt, and rotation of the patella (Fig. 7-7). At the same time, patients are given careful instruction in appropriate exercises and extensive feedback via visualization and touch. Positive results are reported in up to 90 percent of the patients treated with this method.[34,42]

TABLE 7-3 Orthotics for Patellofemoral Pathologies

Type	Purpose
Taping	Strong adhesive tape may be applied to correct abnormalities in patella location and tracking. The primary areas of correction are patellar glide (medial to lateral), tilt (medial versus lateral), and rotation (superior to inferior).
Bracing	Elastic or neoprene support for the patellofemoral joint. Desirable features include a medial buttress, open patella, and superior or inferior patella support as indicated.
Foot orthotics	Correction of abnormal foot and lower limb mechanics that contribute to patellofemoral dysfunction. Examples of abnormalities contributing to patellofemoral pain would be "miserable malalignment" syndrome and pes planus.

In an effort to lend objective data to the empirical success of patellar taping, further study has been conducted. Bennett and Thal (unpublished data) have conducted magnetic resonance imaging (MRI) of the patellofemoral joint with and without taping of the patella (Fig. 7-7, C and D). These results clearly demonstrate medialization, medial tilt, and increased compression of the patella under static conditions. In addition, cine MRI is being used in dynamic studies to evaluate the position of the patella with and without tape during exercise. Although not as dramatic as static MRI, cine MRI does reveal alterations of the patellofemoral mechanics during exercise (Thal and Bennett, unpublished observations). Together, these data give strong objective reasons for the use of patella taping in selected cases (documented patellofemoral incongruency), although considerably more research is needed.

Conservative Management

Research literature overwhelmingly supports the use of exercise in managing patellofemoral pain syndromes.[5,15,22,25,30] Emphasis is placed on strengthening the quadriceps femoris musculature and especially the vastus medialis and the vastus medialis oblique muscles. These muscles are emphasized because of their ability to stabilize the patella superiorly and, more importantly, medially. The superior medial pull of the vastus medialis muscle complex directly counteracts lateral tracking syndromes and most subluxations and dislocations of the patella. Hughston[43] describes medial patellar dislocation, but its occurrence is rare and usually results from poor surgical management of lateral instability.

Methods for recruiting and strengthening the quadriceps femoris musculature vary significantly in form and function. Open and closed kinetic chain exercises, isometrics, isokinetics, and free weights have all been incorporated in successful rehabilitation programs. General principles concerning the implementation and progression of these exercises are described in Chapter 5. The clinician should choose an eclectic approach when prescribing and performing rehabilitative exercises. Some studies have indicated that certain exercise programs can help considerably in achieving appropriate response of the quadriceps femoris muscles in general and the vastus medialis muscle complex in particular. Several investigators have used electromyography (EMG) to try to distinguish exercises that promote activity in the vastus medialis and vastus medialis obliquus muscles from those that promote activity in the other quadriceps femoris muscles.

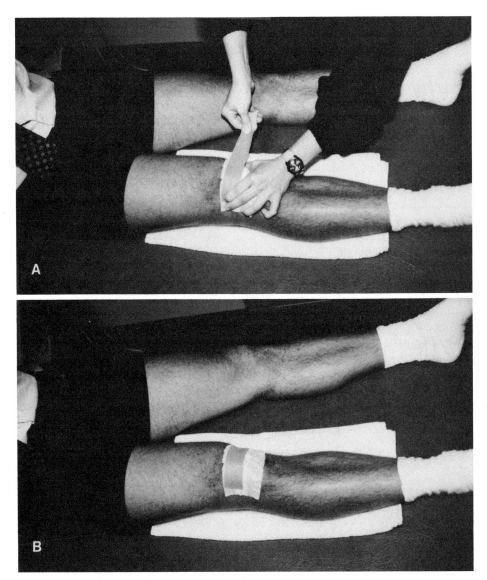

FIGURE 7-7. Patella taping is used to correct abnormalities in patella position and tracking. *A)* Tape is applied to the lateral border of the patella and pulled across toward the medial femoral condyle to correct a lateral patella glide in the right patellofemoral joint. *B)* The final disposition of the taping technique to correct a lateral patella glide. The tape may be worn continuously during the day to improve patella tracking, stretch the lateral retinaculum and iliopatellar band, and enhance VMO muscle contraction.

Clinicians frequently prescribe terminal extension exercises (static quads, straight leg raises, short-arc quads) to promote vastus medialis muscle strength and to avoid pain.[13,25,44,45] Although such exercises may help in limiting pain, EMG studies have shown no discrete increase in vastus medialis muscle activity during terminal knee joint extension during these exercises.[46,47]

Lieb and Perry[47] found that the vastus medialis muscles, along with the entire quadriceps femoris muscle complex, were active throughout the range of knee extension. The vastus medialis obliquus muscle has the same fascial origin as the hip adductor musculature. Hanten and Schulthies[46] advocate isometric contraction of the hip adduc-

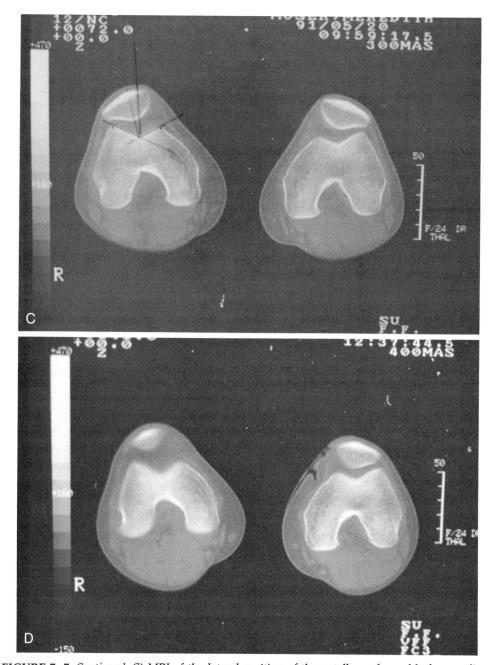

FIGURE 7–7. *Continued.* C) MRI of the lateral position of the patella performed before application of McConnell taping (bilateral knees). Note both lateral translation and lateral tilt of both patellae. D) MRI performed after tape application demonstrates medialization and medial tilt of the left patella (Bennett and Thal, unpublished observations). Note the diminished joint space and skin folds located medially. The right patella remains untaped.

tor musculature and have demonstrated excellent recruitment of the vastus medialis muscle during this exercise. Clinicians at our facility have incorporated hip adduction in knee extension exercises by instructing patients to squeeze a pillow between their knees while doing the knee extension exercises. In principle, this maneuver facilitates vastus medialis muscle contraction.

Rehabilitation programs often focus on reducing patellofemoral joint contact forces and crepitation. This is frequently accomplished by limiting the arc of motion of the knee during knee extension exercises. Numerous authors advocate exercises emphasizing the last 30 degrees of knee extension.[3,13,39,40,44,45] Previously it was thought that the vastus medialis muscle was most active in terminal extension. This arc of motion was also used to limit patellofemoral joint contact and reduce the possibility of traumatic subluxation or dislocation of the patella.[1,3]

Malek and Mangine[25] and Sczepanski and colleagues[31] have investigated terminal flexion exercises from 60 to 120 degrees of flexion. In this position the patella is very stable and contact forces are low because of the larger area of distribution of force via the patellar facets. Also, as terminal flexion is approached, the patella sits over the femoral condylar notch and not over bone. Sczepanski and colleagues also demonstrated a more favorable EMG ratio of the vastus medialis obliquus muscle compared with the vastus lateralis muscle when exercising in the range of 60 to 85 degrees of knee joint flexion. Clinicians are reminded, however, that carryover from strengthening exercises to angles outside the arc of motion in which the exercise was performed are minimal, and that at some point exercising throughout the range of motion (ROM) is often desirable.

Diagnoses of patella subluxation and dislocation require special consideration whether they are conservatively or surgically managed. Subluxation can lead to dislocations, and dislocations can recur if managed inappropriately. Hughston and colleagues[3] described most dislocations as occurring laterally and during deceleration activities (eccentric quadriceps femoris muscle action), especially when changing directions. They also described the quadriceps femoris muscle as the "decelerator mechanism of the body" and alluded to errors in this mechanism as a cause of pain and dysfunction at the patellofemoral joint. Since the original investigations by Houston and colleagues, other authors have noted variances in eccentric force production in a population with anterior knee pain, lending further support to this theory.[22,23]

The occurrence of subluxations and dislocations primarily during eccentric contractions, coupled with documented deficits in eccentric muscle action, requires that clinicians address motor control and eccentric muscle action in rehabilitation. First, caution must be used to protect the patient from recurrence, especially during loaded or weighted exercises and, in particular, the eccentric component of quadriceps femoris muscle action. Second, sequential progression must be used to adequately prepare the patient for resumption of function. Merely avoiding the activity in rehabilitation is not feasible, because at some point athletic function or simply walking down stairs will be a goal of rehabilitation.

Motor control plays an important role in rehabilitation in general and patellofemoral joint problems in particular. Teaching the patient to better use the muscular stabilizers of the patella is a primary goal of many rehabilitation programs. McConnell,[41] Bennett and Stauber,[22] and Knight[48] have all demonstrated the body's ability to adapt rapidly and via motor learning to enhance both strength and function. Biofeedback methods, including visualization, EMG, and exercise, have all been effective in muscular re-education as well as in the more common application for strength gain[49,50] (Fig. 7–8).

Stretching exercises, particularly as part of a comprehensive home exercise program, are integral to long-term success. Tightness of the hamstring and gastrocnemius musculature can contribute to abnormal patellofemoral joint contact and compression, as mentioned earlier (Fig. 7–9). Because tightness of the iliopatellar band contributes to lateral tracking, it too must be stretched. Integration of stretching with appropriate

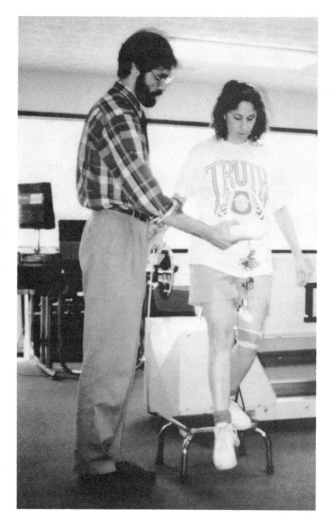

FIGURE 7-8. Biofeedback is used to enhance VMO muscle activity. A dual-channel biofeedback unit (Cyborg Dual Channel J53, Cyborg Corp., Boston, MA) is used with an electrode placed over the VMO muscle. The patient is instructed to perform an 8-inch step-down and step-up while maintaining a VMO muscle contraction. (The patient is receiving both visual and auditory feedback from the Cyborg unit to maintain her VMO muscle contraction to a preset threshold level of excitation. The additional channel provides the clinician with an option to inhibit VL muscle activity, while facilitating VMO muscle activity. This particular patient has been taped to correct both a lateral patellar glide and tilt. Additionally, the VMO electrode in this patient was placed slightly above the central portion of the muscle belly, and was subsequently lowered to an optimum position.)

strengthening exercises provides a multifaceted program that patients can and should carry over to a home program for better long-term success.

Mobilization of the patella is also desirable in enhancing patellar mobility[41,52] (Fig. 7-10). Patellar gliding techniques can be especially helpful in cases of lateral tracking and patella infera. In particular, medial glides of the patella to stretch the lateral knee structures are almost always indicated. Superior and inferior patellar mobilization techniques must be applied with more discretion and careful consideration given to existing joint mechanics.

Appropriate rates of progression are a concern of many clinicians when prescribing and advancing exercise programs. The clinician having ensured adequate stability of the patellofemoral joint and adequate tissue healing time in cases of trauma, the course of exercise can then follow a logical progression. Excluding isometric contractions, most exercise programs vary in range of motion, load (resistance), and speed of exercise, whether isokinetic or isotonic.

Additional factors that can be adjusted within the above parameters are open kinetic chain versus closed kinetic chain exercise and concentric and/or eccentric mus-

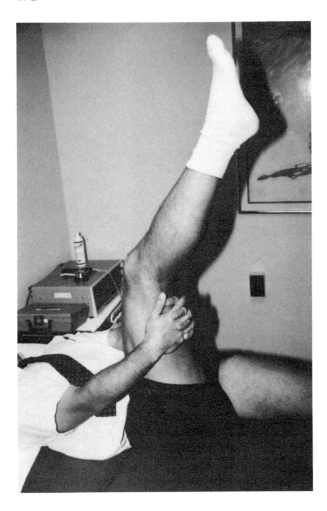

FIGURE 7-9. Tight hamstring muscles contribute to syndromes of the patellofemoral joint. With the hip flexed to 90 degrees, the patient should be able to extend the right knee joint.

cular action. Isokinetically, patients exercise through a pain-free range of motion at varying velocities. As the patient progresses, the arc of motion is increased until full range or function is achieved. Resistance to isokinetics is accommodative, and empirically patients increase effort as pain subsides. Multiple speeds are used to allow the patient to experience, and accommodate to, a variety of contractile velocities.

Isotonic exercise can include the same parameters for progression. The range of motion should be pain-free and progressive. Loads are progressive as tolerated, and the patients should exercise at a variety of speeds. In general, isotonic exercise in rehabilitation settings involves high-repetition, low-weight exercise with gradual transition to high-load, maximal-strength activities as indicated and tolerated by the involved tissues.

Chapter 5 provides a more complete analysis of isotonic and isokinetic exercises and appropriate rates of progression.

Postoperative Management

General guidelines only will be presented for postoperative patellofemoral joint rehabilitation. Pain, inflammation control, and adequate tissue healing time follow the

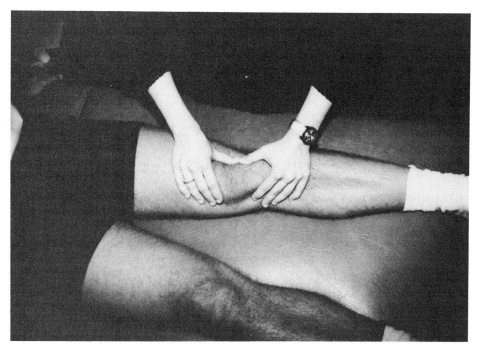

FIGURE 7-10. Mobilization, particularly medial glides of the patella, can be used to stretch tight lateral structures, such as the lateral retinaculum and iliopatellar band. Improved lateral soft-tissue flexibility can result in enhanced VMO muscle contraction and improved patellar tracking.

guidelines discussed earlier and as determined by the physician. Tissue healing is variable for the type of surgery, and exercises should be coordinated with, and approved by, the attending surgeon. Several types of surgery may be encountered and will be classed as either conservative or radical interventions.

CONSERVATIVE SURGERIES

Lateral Capsular Release

Lateral capsular release involves either an open or arthroscopic release of the lateral patellar retinaculum, sometimes combined with medial capsular reefing. Some surgeons also release the distal fibers of the vastus lateralis muscle.[52,53]

The rehabilitation approach is similar to that for nonoperative cases, because there is minimal tissue compromise. Attention must be given to regaining full ROM, especially flexion, which can be compromised. Adequate incision healing must be allowed, usually 7 to 10 days before moderate to vigorous stress is allowed. General guidelines for rehabilitation are as follows:

Week 1

- Active ROM, passive ROM and mobilization as needed
- Isometrics (multi-angular)
- Bike, primarily for ROM
- Submaximal quadriceps and hamstring muscle exercise

Weeks 2 to 4

- Progressive strength and endurance exercises
- Mobilize as needed, emphasize full ROM

Weeks 4 to 6

- Assumes normal postoperative response (full ROM without joint effusion)
- Normalize strength
- Resume functional activities via functional progression

Complications from a simple lateral release are relatively uncommon. As with any operative procedure, infection and reflex sympathetic dystrophy can occur. Also, medial instability can result if the surgery is too aggressive. Probably the most common complication of simple lateral release surgery is failure to achieve symptomatic relief.

The criteria for discharge following a simple lateral release are full ROM without effusion, symmetrical strength, and adequate stability. Ideally, the patient will be asymptomatic as well.

Chondroplasty and Abrasion Arthroplasty

Chrondroplastic or abrasion arthroplastic surgery involves shaving and/or drilling holes through the femoral or patellar articular surface or both to promote new bony ingrowth and perfusion.[54] This approach is used in instances of moderate to severe degenerative changes of the articular surfaces, as in osteoarthritis and chondromalacia patella. Weight bearing inhibits cartilage regeneration, and therefore these patients remain non-weight bearing for 4 to 6 weeks with progressive weight bearing to 8 weeks postoperatively. In addition, only open kinetic chain exercises are performed during this time so as to minimize weight bearing of the joint. General rehabilitation guidelines are as follows:

Weeks 1 to 3

- Postoperative inflammation control
- Active ROM to tolerance
- Patellar mobilization as needed
- Bike without tension
- Open chain quadriceps and hamstring muscle exercise, 25 to 50 percent effort

Weeks 4 to 6

- Continue as above
- Promote full ROM
- Increase exercise intensity
- Introduce weight bearing (physician discretion)

Weeks 6 to 12

- Progress to full weight bearing
- Normalize strength, add closed chain exercise
- Functional integration

RADICAL SURGERIES

Distal Realignment

In instances of severe patellofemoral joint dysfunction, comprehensive surgical intervention may be necessary. A variety of surgical techniques are used to change patellofemoral joint mechanics, including, but not limited to, the Hauser, Elmslie-Trillat, Fulkerson, and Maquet procedures. Distal realignment surgeries usually involve some combination of elevation, distalization, and medialization of the patella with respect to the femoral groove.[7,55] This realignment of the patella is usually accomplished by moving the tibial tubercle and utilizing screw fixation.

Rehabilitation guidelines follow those of the patellectomized knee, outlined later in this chapter. Occasionally, a more aggressive approach to rehabilitation may be undertaken (at the surgeon's discretion), as compared with the patellectomized knee.

Patellectomy

Occasionally, in cases of severe degeneration or trauma, a patellectomy may be performed. Ideally, the patella is "shelled," and continuity of the patellar tendon is not compromised. If continuity of the patellar tendon is lost, a considerably more conservative approach to rehabilitation is necessary. The following protocol is offered as a guideline only and must be adapted according to circumstances and at the discretion of the surgeon.

Rehabilitation Guidelines for Distal Realignment/Patellectomy*
Weeks 1 and 2

1. Cast or immobilizer for 10 days, non- or touch weight bearing for 4 to 6 weeks
2. Continuous passive motion
3. ROM as established in the operating room
4. Hamstring muscle isometrics and active range of motion to 100 degrees or limit
5. Multiposition straight or bent leg raises without weight (in brace)
6. Neuromuscular electrical stimulation of the quadriceps muscle (vaster medialis oblique in particular)
7. Cocontractions
8. Inflammation control
9. Distal patellar mobilization (realignment surgeries)

Weeks 3 to 6

1. Continue as above, touch to partial weight bearing 4 to 6 weeks
2. Active quadriceps muscle exercise, begin side-lying (Fig. 7–11)
3. Range of motion to 100–120 degrees flexion
4. Emphasize ROM
5. Hamstring muscle strengthening from 0 to between 100 and 120 degrees of flexion

Post Week 6

1. Continue as above

---

*Assumes screw fixation, noncompromised patellar tendon.

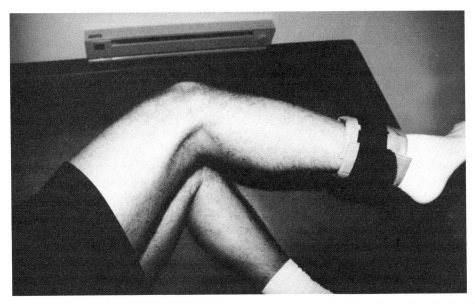

FIGURE 7-11. Side-lying quadriceps femoris muscle exercise can be tolerated early in the rehabilitation program and is less stressful than are supine exercises.

2. Establish full ROM as tolerated
3. Progressive strengthening of the lower quarter
4. Functional progression

Normal (symmetrical) strength is not expected, particuarly in the patellectomized knee. Deficits of 30 to 40 percent are common in the quadriceps muscles but strength still sufficient for most activities of daily living. Restriction of ROM is generally not a problem, but knee flexion of 125 degrees is usually acceptable.

CASE STUDIES

CASE STUDY 1

HISTORY

A 16-year-old male active in several high school varsity sports was referred to physical therapy because of right anterior knee pain and dysfunction. The patient reported that traumatic onset of symptoms occurred while running around second base during a game. The patient reported a sensation of his knee giving way but was able to continue in the game.

The patient awoke the next day with pain, stiffness, and swelling in the knee and was referred to an orthopedic surgeon by the school's athletic trainer. The physician placed the patient's affected leg in a neoprene sleeve with a patella cut-out and referred him to physical therapy with a diagnosis of sub-luxation of the right patella. Quadriceps-to-tibia angle (Q angle) was normal on the roentgenogram.

The physical therapy prescription was for evaluation and treatment of an acute subluxation of the right patella. Emphasis was to be placed on pain control with progressive exercise to tolerance. Physician follow-up was scheduled for 3 weeks after physical therapy was initiated.

EVALUATION

The patient presented in physical therapy with a normal gait and the affected leg was fully weight bearing with the neoprene sleeve. The right knee was moderately effused and warm to palpation. The patient demonstrated full active ROM, with moderate pain in full flexion. The ligaments were stable and symmetrical. The patient had a positive ballottement sign and a positive apprehension test. In addition, there was a positive synovial pinch test with universal peripatellar tenderness. There was no measurable quadriceps muscle atrophy. Manual muscle testing caused pain and apprehension and was abandoned for the quadriceps muscles. Other musculature was unremarkable except for generalized tightness of the hamstring muscles bilaterally.

Initial treatments focused on controlling the inflammatory response and preserving range of motion and strength. Pain-free exercises were emphasized and included stationary biking, straight and bent leg raises, and active ROM. Additionally, one-quarter squats with bilateral weight bearing and leg press activities with light weight were prescribed and tolerated well (Fig. 7–12). The patient

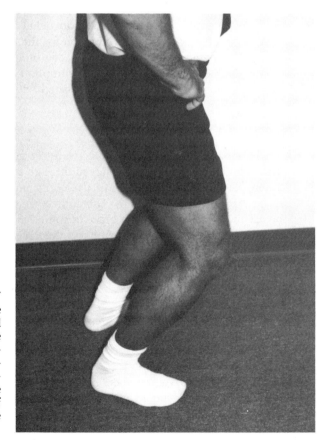

FIGURE 7–12. "Quarter squats" using the initial 45 degrees of knee flexion are usually tolerated well and are an effective exercise for the gluteal, quadriceps, and gastrocnemius-soleus muscles. Slight external rotation of the hips while performing this exercise places the VMO muscle an optimum "line of pull" to enhance the muscle contraction.

received electrical stimulation, ice, compression, and elevation postexercise and was seen 3 times a week.

At 10 days postinjury, the patient was progressing extremely well. ROM and girth remained normal and pain was resolved. Minimal effusion without warmth persisted.

TREATMENT

Exercise intensity was increased to tolerance. The patient was able to tolerate a full arc of motion without pain, and therefore concentric isokinetic exercise was introduced (quadriceps/hamstrings) at 60, 120, and 180 degrees per second. Weights were added to the leg raises and short-arc quadriceps femoris muscle exercises.

At 21 days postinjury, the patient continued to do well. Eccentric isokinetic quadriceps muscle exercise (submaximal) was instituted in a pain-free range of motion (0 to 45 degrees). Care was taken to monitor instability; however, the patient progressed without incident. Isokinetic speeds were reduced to 30, 60, and 90 degrees per second to incorporate the force velocity principle of increased force with increased speed in eccentric contractions.

Functional activities were introduced at 4 weeks postinjury. Light running was encouraged along with clinic activities of tilt board, mini-tramp, and proprioception band exercises. In addition, exercise intensity was increased and tolerated without incident (Fig. 7–13).

Maximal concentric and eccentric isokinetic testing of the quadriceps femoris and hamstring muscle groups was conducted at 5 weeks postinjury. A right-to-left comparison of average force production for the entire range of motion yielded no deficit. The patient was instructed to continue the home exercises for at least another six weeks and discharged. Resumption of sports activities while wearing the neoprene sleeve and was accomplished without incident.

CASE STUDY SUMMARY

This patient presented with a relatively classic case of anterior knee pain. Successful management was achieved through a multifaceted approach to rehabilitation. The treatment program focused on symptom management while improving strength and biomechanics. These goals were accomplished primarily through the use of a patella-stabilizing brace in conjunction with exercise to strengthen the quadriceps musculature in general and the vastus medialis complex in particular. As with most cases of anterior knee pain, symptomatic relief was achieved conservatively, and the patient returned to normal activity, including sports.

CASE STUDY 2

HISTORY

A 29-year-old woman was referred to physical therapy for preoperative and postoperative management of long-standing left anterior knee pain. The patient presented with a diagnosis of chondromalacia patella and significant osteoarthritis

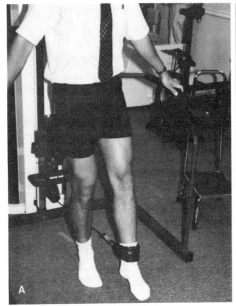

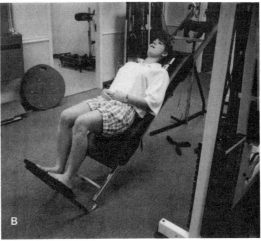

FIGURE 7-13. Proprioceptive and closed-chain exercises are important in patellofemoral rehabilitation. *A*) Standing hip flexion is performed by the uninvolved lower extremity to enhance balance, joint proprioception, and muscle cocontractions in the involved lower extremity. *B*) Partial (¼) squats performed along an incline bench is an excellent closed kinetic-chain exercise that can be used for concentric and eccentric VMO muscle contractions. This is an alternative method for standing ¼ squats shown in Figure 7-12 to enhance dynamic stability to joints in the lower extremities and therefore may be used in patients with reduced lower extremity strength and proprioception.

secondary to multiple minor traumas incurred during and since adolescence. These injuries included multiple episodes of falling on both knees, and pain during and after running, especially downhill. None of the injuries required medical intervention. The patient reported a lifetime battle with morbid obesity, with weight loss of greater than 100 pounds over the 2 years prior to referral.

Debilitating pain was the primary reason for referral. Pain was episodic and severe, with diminished activities of daily living and diminished function. Pain increased with activity and prolonged sitting. Walking, especially stairs and hills, was painful. Running and sports activities could not be tolerated.

The prescribed treatment was for intervention as indicated for pain, motion, and muscle strength and function for 1 to 3 months as needed. Patient and physician anticipated the need for surgical distal realignment (Maquet procedure) at approximately 3 months from referral.

EVALUATION

The patient presented with an antalgic gait evidenced by decreased stance on the involved leg. She was mildly to moderately obese with generally fair to good muscle tone and condition except for the involved extremity.

Inspection revealed a classic "miserable malalignment" syndrome with femoral anteversion, genu valgum, and pes planus. Genu recurvatum of 10 degrees was also noted bilaterally. General quadriceps muscle tone was fair, but the vastus medialis portion was poorly defined. Atrophy of 0.5 inch as compared with the right was noted for the thigh musculature at three points of comparison. Inspection also showed moderate peripatellar effusion with no appreciable change in joint temperature.

Physical examination revealed full active ROM with significant (3+/3) patellofemoral crepitance and pain throughout the range of 20 to 120 degrees of flexion. The ligaments were stable symmetrically, and special ligament testing was unremarkable except for pain. The patient had a positive synovial pinch test and a positive grind test. Pain was noted with the patellar apprehension test but not associated with instability. Vertical patellar alignment was essentially normal; however, there was increased lateral tilt and "frog-eye" patellae with the knees flexed to 90 degrees. Tenderness to palpation was universal and moderately severe. Hamstring, hip, and lower leg muscle strength was manually assessed as normal. The quadriceps musculature tested manually at 3 + /5 with pain at all angles. Isokinetic testing was not tolerated.

TREATMENT

Surgery for this patient was a foregone conclusion on the part of both the patient and physician. However, preoperative physical therapy was indicated for several reasons. The following preoperative goals were established.

First, to control pain and inflammation. The active-joint inflammatory response, as indicated by pain and effusion, would potentially complicate surgery. As with most conditions, pain control must be achieved for the patient to progress to other forms of therapy, especially exercise.

Second, to preserve ROM and strength. Because of the acute pain present, there was concern that the patient would progressively lose flexibility and strength due to disuse.

Third, to improve strength as tolerated. This patient suffered significantly diminished quadriceps strength, whether physiologic or secondary to pain. In general, the quadriceps muscle should be as strong as possible prior to surgery, because of the natural consequence of weakness postoperatively.

Initial intervention centered on physical therapy modalities for control of pain and inflammation. Specifically, ice packs combined with galvanic stimulation were used extensively, especially postexercise. Pulsed ultrasound was also used to promote circulation and symptomatic relief.

For the patient, compliance with exercise prescription was tedious at best because of the presence of pain universally. Active ROM (without resistance) exercise was encouraged even though it was painful. Additionally, range-promoting exercises such as walking in water and stationary biking without resistance were encouraged.

Multiple-angle isometric quadriceps muscle contractions were taught at 25-to-30-degree intervals and tolerated well. Similarly, multiangular bent-to-straight leg raises (static knee, dynamic hip) were taught and tolerated well (Fig. 7–14).

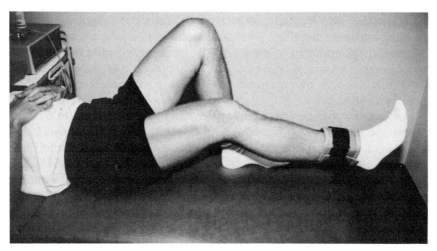

FIGURE 7-14. Bent and straight leg lifts at multiple angles of knee flexion isometrically exercise the quadriceps femoris muscles and avoid patellofemoral joint irritation.

Attempts to integrate dynamic quadriceps muscle exercise met with little success. Open and closed chain, isotonic, and isokinetic exercises all exacerbated pain. Little effect was achieved thereby, even as ROM, speed, and resistance were manipulated.

Prescription biomechanical foot orthotics had been tried previously with no success. Patellar taping and bracing were used to decrease lateral tracking of the patella and increase comfort during exercise, but with minimal benefit. A neoprene knee sleeve with a lateral patella buttress did increase the patient's comfort during activities of daily living.

After 4 weeks of treatment (two to three times weekly), the patient's condition remained essentially the same. She did report an increased tolerance for activities of daily living, but objectively her findings were unchanged. The patient was subsequently discharged to a home program for active ROM, exercise to tolerance, and copious use of ice packs pending surgical intervention.

POSTOPERATIVE TREATMENT

The patient subsequently underwent a modified Maquet procedure whereby the left tibial tubercle was excised, medialized, and elevated with an iliac bone graft. Screw fixation of the tubercle to the tibia through the graft was achieved, and the patient was casted for 3 weeks.

The patient returned to physical therapy 3 weeks postoperatively. She was ambulatory, touch weight bearing, and was wearing a long-leg knee immobilizer. Her physical therapy prescription was for unloaded active ROM only, with modalities for pain and inflammation.

The patient's active ROM was measured goniometrically at 10 to 30 degrees of flexion. There was marked increase in joint temperature and marked effusion. The incision was healed. One inch of thigh atrophy was noted at 5, 7, and 9 inches above the medial joint line.

The patient was instructed in active ROM exercises including heel slides and side-lying knee bending (Fig. 7–15). Additionally, she was encouraged to sit with the lower leg unsupported to encourage knee flexion. A continuous passive motion machine was used in the home for 2 to 10 hours per day. Passive distal patellar mobilization by both therapist and patient was permissible because it would not stress the fixation site.

At 5 weeks postoperatively the patient had progressed to 5 to 60 degrees of active ROM. Partial weight bearing was allowed up to approximately 25 percent of body weight. Pain and effusion were resolving and subjectively diminished by 50 percent.

Active assistive ROM was initiated along with gentle to moderate mobilization techniques to both the patellofemoral and tibiofemoral joints. Weights (1 to 5 lbs) were added to the exercise program of hamstring curls, multiposition straight leg raises, and short-arc quads.

At 8 weeks post-operatively, the patient was progressing in all areas except active ROM, which had plateaued at 0 to 85 degrees of flexion. Pain and effusion continued to abate, and thigh atrophy was reduced by one quarter inch.

Vigorous mobilization was instituted, and the patient was encouraged to progress to full weight bearing. Progressive exercise was encouraged, and low-speed concentric and eccentric submaximal isokinetic exercises were used in a pain-free arc of motion.

At 10 weeks, manipulation under anesthesia was performed due to failure to surpass 90 degrees of active or passive knee flexion. Physical therapy resumed the day after manipulation, emphasizing ROM, which was 0 to 120 degrees. Vigorous mobilization, stationary biking, active ROM, and modalities were used to preserve and progress the ROM.

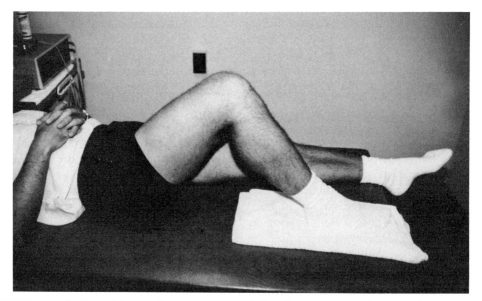

FIGURE 7–15. Heel slide exercises are incorporated early in postoperative cases to encourage knee joint mobility and circulation.

The patient continued uneventfully after manipulation. At 12 weeks after the Maquet procedure, the active ROM was 0 to 125 degrees and de-emphasized but closely monitored.

Exercise including open and closed chain, isotonic, and isokinetic activities were continued and tolerated well, although pain was transient. Normal activities of daily living were encouraged, but not high-stress activities, because of residual degenerative changes.

The patient was discharged to a home exercise program 15 weeks postoperatively. Active ROM was 0 to 125 degrees with thigh atrophy of one half inch. Isokinetic testing was not conducted. Pain was subjectively decreased by 80 percent as compared with preoperative levels. Effusion was minimal but transient. The patient was scheduled for physician follow-up at 6 months and 1 year and progressed uneventfully, although further intervention is anticipated due to the severe nature of the degenerative disease.

CASE STUDY SUMMARY

This patient presented with a worst-case scenario relative to anterior knee pain syndromes. Conservative management using numerous treatment approaches was not effective. Radical surgical intervention was necessary to provide symptomatic relief of pain. Unfortunately, further surgery may be required as the degenerative changes continue. Efforts must be made to preserve existing strength, range of motion, and function. A lifetime effort by this patient is needed to maintain normal activities of daily living. Participation in stressful activities such as sports will not be possible.

SUMMARY

This chapter reviewed the evaluation and treatment of patellofemoral dysfunction and pathology from a problem-solving standpoint. A major premise of this chapter is that variations from the normal anatomy and mechanics of the patellofemoral joint and lower extremities are major predisposing factors in patellofemoral problems. An understanding of normal and abnormal anatomy and mechanics of the patellofemoral joint and lower extremity is therefore an essential prerequisite for successful treatment. Specific anatomic variations and aberrations that are factors in patellofemoral dysfunction include imbalances of the static and dynamic soft tissues attached to the patellofemoral joint; patellofemoral malalignment, including an increased Q angle, patella alta, and patella baja; and lower extremity malalignment. Theories concerning precipitation of patellofemoral dysfunction include a neuromuscular eccentric control problem of the quadriceps femoris muscle, altered recruitment pattern between the vastus lateralis and vastus medialis obliquus muscle, and excessive and repetitive retropatellar contact stresses. An eclectic approach to treatment was reviewed based on the individual case and included a combination of exercises, orthotics, and modalities. Surgical alternatives were briefly reviewed, with emphasis on specific considerations and differences in rehabilitation for each type of surgery. Finally, case studies were presented to illustrate the implementation of treatment principles for individual pathologies.

REFERENCES

1. Ficat, RP and Hungerford, DS: Disorders of the patellofemoral joint. Williams & Wilkins, Baltimore, 1977.
2. Henry, JH: The patellofemoral joint. In Nicholas, JA and Hershman, EB (eds): The Lower Extremity and Spine in Sports Medicine. CV Mosby, St Louis, MO, 1986, pp 1013–1054.
3. Hughston, JC, Walsh, WM, and Puddu, G: Patellar Subluxation and Dislocation, WB Saunders, Philadelphia, 1984.
4. Micheli, LJ: Special considerations in children's rehabilitation programs. In Hunter, LY and Funk, FJ, Jr (eds): Rehabilitation of the Injured Knee, CV Mosby, St Louis, MO, 1984, pp 406–413.
5. Cox, JS: Patellofemoral problems in runners. Clin Sports Med 4:699, 1985.
6. Devas, MB: Stress fractures of the patella. J Bone Joint Surg [Br] 42:71, 1960.
7. Cox, JS: Evaluation of the Roux-Elmslie-Trillat procedure for knee extensor realignment. Am J Sports Med 10:303, 1982.
8. Gross, M: Gray's Anatomy, ed 29. Lea & Febiger, Philadelphia, 1973.
9. Norkin, C and Levangie, P: Joint Structure and Function: A Comprehensive Analysis. FA Davis, Philadelphia, 1983.
10. Warwick, R and Williams, PL (eds): Gray's Anatomy, ed 35. Churchill Livingstone, New York, 1973.
11. Wiberg, G: Roetgenographs and anatomic studies on the femoropatellar joint with special references to chondromalacia patella. Acta Orthop Scand 12:319, 1941.
12. Magee, DJ: Orthopedic Physical Assessment. WB Saunders, Philadelphia, 1987.
13. Smillie, IS: Injuries of the Knee Joint, Churchill Livingstone, London, 1978.
14. Hunter, LY: Aspects of injuries to the lower extremity unique to the female athlete. In Nicholas, JA and Hershman, EB (eds): The Lower Extremity and Spine in Sports Medicine. CV Mosby, St. Louis, MO, 1986.
15. Paulos, L, et al: Patellar malalignment. Phys Ther 60:1624, 1980.
16. Morrison, JB: The mechanics of the knee joint in relation to normal walking. J Biomech 3:51, 1970.
17. Perry, J, Antonellis, D, and Ford, W: Analysis of knee-joint forces during flexed knee stance. J Bone Joint Surg [Am] 57:961, 1975.
18. Reilly, DT and Martens, M: Experimental analysis of the quadriceps muscle force and patellofemoral joint reaction force for various activities. Acta Orthop Scand 43:126, 1972.
19. Smidt, GL: Biomechanical analysis of knee flexion and extension. J Biomech 6:79, 1973.
20. Abernathy, PJ, et al: Is chrondro-malacia patellae a separate clinical entity? J Bone Joint Surg [Br] 60:205, 1978.
21. MacDonald, DA, Hulton, JF, and Kelly, IG: Maximal isometric patellorfemoral contact force in patients with anterior knee pain. J Bone Joint Surg [Br] 71:296, 1989.
22. Bennett, JG and Stauber, WT: Evaluation and treatment of anterior knee pain using eccentric exercise. Med Sci Sports Exerc 18:528, 1986.
23. Dvir, A, et al: Concentric and eccentric torque variations of the quadriceps femoris in patellofemoral pain syndrome. Clinical Biomechanics 5:68, 1990.
24. Hoppenfield, S: Physical Examination of the Spine and Extremities. Appleton-Century-Crofts, New York, 1976.
25. Malek, MM and Mangine, RE: Patellofemoral pain syndromes: A comprehensive and conservative approach. The Journal of Orthopedic and Sports Physical Therapy 2:3, 1981.
26. Amiel, D, et al: The effect of immobilization on collagen turnover in connective tissue: A biochemical-biomechanical correlation. Acta Orthop Scand 53:325, 1982.
27. Enneking, F and Horowitz, M: The intra-articular effects of immobilization on the human knee. J Bone Joint Surg [Am] 54:5, 973, 1972.
28. Gamble, JG, Edwards, CC, and Max, SR: Enzymatic adaptation in ligaments during immobilization. Am J Sports Med 12(3):221, 1984.
29. Eggold, JF: Orthotics in the prevention of runners' overuse injuries. The Physician and Sportsmedicine 9(3):125, 1981.
30. Steadman, JR: Nonoperative measures for patellofemoral problems. Am J Sports Med 7:374, 1979.
31. Sczepanski, TL, et al: Effect of contraction type, angular velocity, and arc of motion on VMO:VL EMG ratio. The Journal of Orthopedic and Sports Physical Therapy 14:256, 1991.
32. Johnson, D, Thurston, P, and Ashcroft, P: The Russian technique of faradism in the treatment of chondromalacia patellae. Physiotherapy Canada 29:2, 1977.
33. Bohannon, RW: Effect of electrical stimulation to the vastus medialis muscle in a patient with chronically dislocating patellae. Phys Ther 63:1445, 1983.
34. Currier, DP, Lehman, J, and Lightfoot, P: Electrical stimulation in exercise of the quadriceps femoris muscle. Phys Ther 59:1508, 1979.
35. Snyder-Macklen, L, Robinson, A (eds): Clinical Electrophysiology: Electrotherapy and Electrophysiologic Testing. William & Wilkins, Baltimore, 1989, p 98.
36. Wooden, MJ: Biomechanical evaluation for functional orthotics. In Donatelli, R (ed): The Biomechanics of the Foot and Ankle. FA Davis, Philadelphia, 1990.
37. Fisher, RL: Conservative treatment of patellofemoral pain. Orthop Clin North Am 17:269, 1986.

38. Palumbo, PM, Jr: Dynamic patellar brace: A new orthosis in the management of patellofemoral disorders. Am J Sports Med 9:45, 1981.
39. Levine, J: A new brace for chondromalacia patella and kindred conditions. Am J Sports Med 6:137, 1978.
40. Henry, JH, and Crosland, JW: Conservative treatment of patellofemoral subluxation. Am J Sports Med 7:12, 1979.
41. McConnell, J: The management of chondromalacia patellae: A long term solution. Australian Journal of Physical Therapy 32:4, 1986.
42. Gerrard, B: The patellofemoral pain syndrome: A clinical trial of the McConnell Programme. Australian Journal of Physical Therapy 35:2, 1989.
43. Hughston, JC and Deese, M: Medial subluxation of the patella as a complication of lateral retinacular release. Am J Sports Med 16:4, 1988.
44. Larson, E and Lauridsen, F: Conservative treatment of patellar dislocation. Clin Orthop 171:131, 1982.
45. Lyssholm, J, et al: The affect of a patellar brace on performance in a knee extension strength test in patients with patellar pain. Am J Sports Med 12:110, 1984.
46. Hanten, WP and Schulthies, SS: Exercise effect on electromyographic activity of the vastus medialis oblique and vastus lateralis muscles. Phys Ther 70:9, 1990.
47. Lieb, FJ and Perry, J: Quadriceps function and electromyographic study under isometric conditions. J Bone Joint Surg [Am] 53:749, 1971.
48. Knight, KL: Quadriceps strengthening with the DAPRE technique: Case studies with neurological implications. Med Sci Sports Exerc 17:646, 1985.
49. Delitto, A and Lehman, RC: Rehabilitation of the athlete with a knee injury. Clin Sports Med 8:805, 1989.
50. LeVeau, BF and Rogers, C: Selective training of the vastus medialis muscle using EMG biofeedback. Phys Ther 60:1410, 1980.
51. Kramer, PG: Patellar malalignment syndrome: Rationale to reduce excessive lateral pressure. The Journal of Orthopedic and Sports Physical Therapy 8:301, 1986.
52. Merchant, AC and Mercer, RL: Lateral release of the patella: A preliminary report. Clin Orthop 103:40, 1974.
53. Metcalf, RW: An arthroscopic method for lateral release of the subluxating or dislocating patella. Clin Orthop 167:9, 1982.
54. Johnson, LL: Arthroscopic abrasion arthroplasty historical and pathologic perspective: Present status. Arthroscopy 2(1):54, 1986.
55. Maquet, P: Advancement of the tibial tuberosity. Clin Orthop 115:225, 1976.

CHAPTER 8

Rehabilitation of the Knee with Arthritis

Deborah E. Lechner, MS, PT

The knee joint is frequently affected in both osteoarthritis (OA) and rheumatoid arthritis (RA). Arthritic changes in the knee can create difficulties in a number of functional activities, such as squatting, climbing stairs, getting in and out of the bathtub, and rising from a chair. Individuals with arthritis affecting the knee walk more slowly and with reduced rates and ranges of knee flexion and extension compared with healthy subjects.[1] Due to the functional impairment and pain, physical therapy is often indicated in patients with arthritis involving the knee.

Physical therapy management of the arthritic knee is influenced by the type of arthritis, the severity of joint disease, and the patient's life-style and personal goals. This chapter reviews the clinical features of both RA and OA, highlighting their similarities and differences. The pathology and stage of reactivity of the disease are related to clinical signs and symptoms. Components of a sequential evaluation are delineated to determine the clinical signs and symptoms to be treated. The advantages and disadvantages of various treatment techniques for the arthritic knee are discussed. The chapter concludes with case presentations of an OA and an RA patient. The objective of this chapter is to provide guidelines for decision making in the physical therapy management of patients with arthritis involving the knee.

CLINICAL FEATURES OF OSTEOARTHRITIS

OA involves gradual degeneration and loss of the articular cartilage, with secondary changes in the subchondral bone. Two types of OA, primary and secondary, have been described.[2] OA is classified as *secondary* when the causative factor is known to be trauma or systemic illness, and *primary* in the absence of a causative factor. The cartilage in both types of OA develops fissures and begins to erode in small local areas. These small cartilage lesions then progress to denude larger areas until, in some instances, there is complete loss of articular cartilage.[2] In addition, osteophytes and bony enlargement occur at the joint margins, and the subchondral bone begins to sclerose. The exact pathogenesis of OA is unknown.[2,4] Obesity and repetitive stress may be influencing factors. One study indicated that obesity cannot be correlated with OA,[5] whereas other studies indicated that there is a positive correlation,[6,7] especially in weight bearing joints. Excess body weight produces an increase in mechanical stress to the weight bearing joint.[7] Repetitive stress has been postulated to produce microscopic stress fractures in the subchondral bone. The healing of these stress fractures results in sclerosis of the subchondral bone.[8] Sclerotic subchondral bone is unable to attenuate the compressive forces, which results in an increase in compressive force within the hyaline cartilage matrix.

The American Rheumatism Association (ARA) has proposed a classification criteria for primary OA of the knee that is designed to help researchers classify the disease on the basis of clinical and radiologic findings. The presence of knee pain along with at least two of the following six criteria—age over 50 years, morning joint stiffness of less than 30 minutes, crepitus, bony tenderness, bony enlargement, and no palpable warmth—provides a fairly sensitive and specific classification scheme for research.[2]

The osteoarthritic knee is often tender to palpation along the articular structures and painful during both active and passive movement. Audible and palpable crepitus is usually present, along with quadriceps femoris muscle weakness and atrophy[2] secondary to knee joint effusion[9-12] and/or pain.[13-15] Articular cartilage loss is often asymmetrical within the knee joint, with either the medial or lateral compartment being more involved. A disproportionate loss of hyaline cartilage in one of the compartments may create either a varus or valgus deformity. In the advanced stages, synovitis (or an inflammation and thickening of the synovial lining)[2] and intra-articular effusions (or increases in the volume of intra-articular fluid)[2] are common.[3]

CLINICAL FEATURES OF RHEUMATOID ARTHRITIS

Rheumatoid arthritis is defined as "a chronic, systemic inflammatory disorder of unknown etiology" involving the joints.[2] The inflammatory process begins in the synovial lining: the synovium thickens and protrudes into the joint cavity and is referred to as a *pannus*. Collagenase, a proteolytic enzyme, is released from the pannus and damages the joint capsule and supporting ligaments. Leukocytes migrate into the synovium and release lysosomes, which eventually destroy the articular cartilage and erode the periarticular bone.[2]

The ARA has defined criteria to assist with diagnosis of RA.[2] These include morning stiffness, pain on motion or tenderness in at least one joint, swelling (not bony overgrowth) present in at least one joint, symmetrical involvement, subcutaneous nodules, roentgenographic changes typical of RA (bony decalcification adjacent to the involved joints), and a positive rheumatoid factor.

Knee joint involvement in RA is common and usually begins with effusion and synovitis. As the disease progresses, quadriceps femoris muscle atrophy develops secondary to muscle inhibition[2] caused by pain, joint effusion, and disuse.[9-15] A synovial cyst, also called a *Baker's Cyst*, may develop in the semimembranosus or popliteus bursa as a result of their communication with the synovial joint cavity.[16] The cyst may enlarge into the popliteal fossa. Occasionally a Baker's cyst will rupture, giving rise to symptoms similar to acute thrombophlebitis.

Because of the quadriceps femoris muscle atrophy, and concomitant reflex muscle spasm in the hamstring muscle,[17] the common position of deformity in the RA knee is one of knee joint flexion. Approximately 30 degrees of knee joint flexion is the loose-pack position of the knee joint[18] and allows more space for an intra-articular effusion. Therefore, a joint effusion further encourages the development of a knee joint flexion deformity. A deformity that progresses to the severe stage may result in a posterior subluxation of the tibia. Destruction of the soft tissues supporting the knee can lead to joint hypermobility and instability. In other cases, adhesions between the two joint surfaces can develop and result in hypomobility and joint stiffness. Either hypermobility or hypomobility can alter the mechanics of normal knee joint function.

COMPARISON OF OSTEOARTHRITIS AND RHEUMATOID ARTHRITIS

The following sections discuss the similarities and differences in OA and RA involvement of the knee. A recognition of these similarities and differences will assist the clinician in developing appropriate treatment goals, time frames for achieving those goals, and a prognosis for treatment.

Similarities

Both the RA and OA knee may present with pain, tenderness, and swelling. In either case the swelling is either intra-articular or secondary to thickened synovium and does not respond to intermittent compression treatments, which are effective in decreasing lymphedema. In both diseases, reflex inhibition of the quadriceps femoris muscle occurs when pain or joint effusion is present.[9-15,17] The vastus medialis portion of the quadriceps muscle has been shown to be particularly affected by reflex muscle inhibition.[9-11] Patients with painful, swollen joints often limit their activity level,[19] which can result in further muscle atrophy and strength declines of up to 3 percent per week.[20] If the knee is painful or unstable, or if significant muscle atrophy has developed, the patient will demonstrate a decreased single-limb stance time on the painful lower extremity, decreased rate and range of motion of the knee joint during ambulation, and decreased plantarflexion of the ankle joint at the end of stance.[1]

Physical therapy is more effective if applied in the early stages of either OA or RA, before the surrounding connective tissue has become fibrotic and contracted or weakened. Correction or reversal of a severe knee joint flexion, valgus, or varus deformity is difficult if not impossible to achieve without surgical intervention. Once these changes in soft tissues have occurred, strengthening and stretching exercises are less likely to produce the desired functional changes.

Differences

The initial pathologic process in OA is cartilage destruction; joint effusion and synovitis occur less frequently and later in the disease process than in patients with RA. The initial pathologic process in RA is inflammation of the synovium resulting in joint effusion, with cartilage and subchondral bone destruction occurring later in the disease. Although flexion, varus, and valgus deformities can occur in either diagnosis, joint flexion deformities are often more severe in the RA knee. Varus or valgus deformities are present more frequently in the OA knee joint due to the asymmetrical compartment involvement. Obesity is more often a problem in the OA knee, whereas the RA patient often experiences a loss of appetite and weight. The OA knee is more likely to be stiff and hypomobile, whereas the RA knee is hypermobile as often as hypomobile.

The subchondral bone in OA is sclerotic. Radin[8] suggests that this sclerosis is secondary to healing of microfractures in the subchondral bone. The increased density of the sclerotic subchondral bone reduces the shock-absorbing ability of the bone and results in accelerating the degeneration of the overlying cartilage. In contrast, the subchondral bone in RA is usually osteopenic, or soft, and does not accelerate the degeneration of overlying cartiliage.

EVALUATION

Components of the evaluation for clinical problem solving include the disease severity, reactivity, functional status, and physical characteristics of the patient. Determining severity enables the therapist to make a prognosis as to functional rehabilitation (Fig. 8–1). The state of disease reactivity indicates the desired level of aggressiveness in treatment (Fig. 8–2). Figure 8–3 shows the information to be obtained from each evaluation procedure and the use to which the therapist puts that information. Table 8–1 summarizes the purpose of each procedure in the decision-making process.

Observation

Examination of the knee joint begins with visual observation of the patient rising from the chair in the waiting room and walking to the treatment area. The patient has just performed two functions that are affected when arthritis involves the knee: rising from a chair and walking. The speed and ease with which the patient rises are noted by the clinician. The amount of pain in the knee joint is reflected by the time spent on the involved leg during the single-limb stance phase of the gait cycle. The degree of stiffness will be reflected in the patient's cadence. Once the patient reaches the treatment area and exposes the knee for closer inspection, the amount of swelling and presence of deformity will be evident. At this point, the clinician can make some initial judgments about the severity and stage of reactivity of the diseased knee joint. The patient with severe joint destruction will rise slowly from the chair using his or her arms to assist by pushing to standing. If the knee is painful, patient will spend less time in stance on the involved leg and may also exhibit decreased knee flexion during swing. The knee joint will be significantly swollen, and deformity is likely to be obvious. These initial observations are useful in guiding the remainder of the evaluation and classifying the severity of the disease, which in turn, when combined with other information, assists in making a physical therapy prognosis (see Figs. 8–1 and 8–3).

Pain

Questioning the patient regarding pain early in the evaluation develops empathy and trust between clinician and patient. The intensity of pain will assist the clinician in judging the acuteness of the disease and will guide the selection of other clinical evaluation procedures (see Figs. 8–2 and 8–3). Pain will also guide the aggressiveness

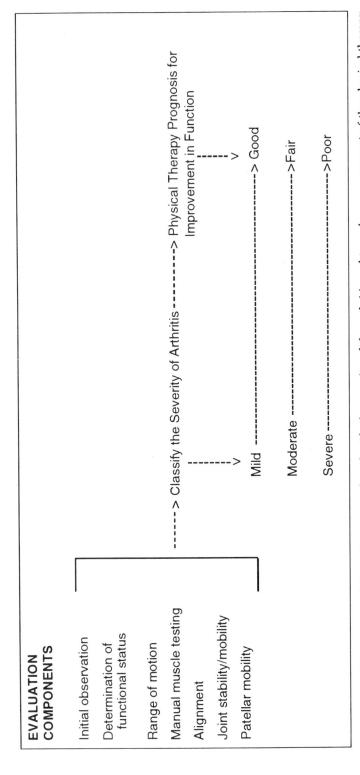

FIGURE 8–1. Components of the evaluation used to classify the severity of the arthritis and to make an assessment of the physical therapy prognosis.

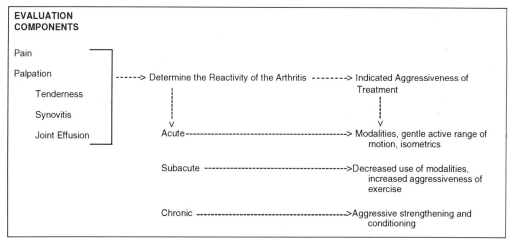

FIGURE 8-2. Components of the evaluation used to determine the reactivity of the disease and to guide the aggressiveness of treatment.

of the treatment approach, and is an important indication of the effectiveness of treatment. The intensity of pain is measured objectively and reliably using the visual-analog scale or a numerical 1-to-10 scoring system. The location of pain is outlined on a figure drawing. The clinician should ask whether the pain is present at rest. Rest pain is an indication that the patient is in an acute phase of the disease process. The clinician should ask specific questions concerning activities that increase pain. Asking the patient to list three activities that increase knee pain will serve as a basis for further quantification of the intensity of knee pain. A numerical or visual-analog pain score can then be determined for each of the activities that the patient identifies as causing or increasing knee pain. These pain scores provide objective measures that can be repeated after treatment to document improvement. Other questions regarding how long various functional activities can be performed before the onset of pain, or how great a distance can be walked before onset of pain, can provide further objective measures. Objective measures of pain allow the clinician to accurately monitor changes secondary to treatment.

Functional Status

Functional status should be addressed early in the evaluation. Loss of function or painful function is usually a major complaint of patients with arthritis. The extent of the functional impairment provides a prognosis for functional improvement, and assists the clinician in ordering the sequence of the evaluation (see Figs. 8-1 and 8-3).

Measures of functional performance are extremely useful for assessing the efficacy of treatment. The velocity of walking or stair climbing, and the time required to squat or rise from sitting are examples of objective functional measures. These measures can be obtained easily in the clinic using a stopwatch and are good indicators of progress. Asking the patient to rate the degree of difficulty of functional tasks on a visual-analog or 1-to-10 scale will provide an objective measurement for later comparison.

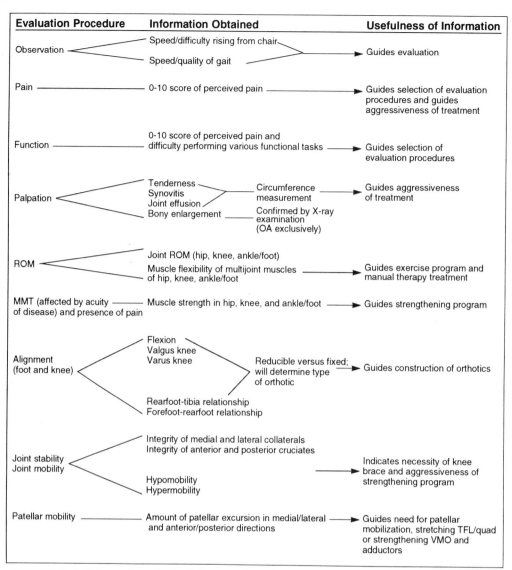

Evaluation Procedure	Information Obtained	Usefulness of Information

Observation — Speed/difficulty rising from chair / Speed/quality of gait → Guides evaluation

Pain — 0-10 score of perceived pain → Guides selection of evaluation procedures and guides aggressiveness of treatment

Function — 0-10 score of perceived pain and difficulty performing various functional tasks → Guides selection of evaluation procedures

Palpation — Tenderness / Synovitis / Joint effusion → Circumference measurement; Bony enlargement → Confirmed by X-ray examination (OA exclusively) → Guides aggressiveness of treatment

ROM — Joint ROM (hip, knee, ankle/foot) / Muscle flexibility of multijoint muscles of hip, knee, ankle/foot → Guides exercise program and manual therapy treatment

MMT (affected by acuity of disease) and presence of pain — Muscle strength in hip, knee, and ankle/foot → Guides strengthening program

Alignment (foot and knee) — Flexion / Valgus knee / Varus knee → Reducible versus fixed; will determine type of orthotic → Guides construction of orthotics; Rearfoot-tibia relationship / Forefoot-rearfoot relationship

Joint stability / Joint mobility — Integrity of medial and lateral collaterals / Integrity of anterior and posterior cruciates / Hypomobility / Hypermobility → Indicates necessity of knee brace and aggressiveness of strengthening program

Patellar mobility — Amount of patellar excursion in medial/lateral and anterior/posterior directions → Guides need for patellar mobilization, stretching TFL/quad or strengthening VMO and adductors

FIGURE 8–3. Information obtained from each evaluation procedure that is used to formulate treatment strategies.

TABLE 8–1 Summary of the Evaluation Information

Evaluation Procedure	Classify Severity	Stage/ Acuteness	Rehabilitation Prognosis	Guides Evaluation	Guides Treatment	Document Change
Initial observation	X	X	X	X		
Pain		X		X	X	X
Functional status	X		X	X		X
Palpation		X			X	
ROM	X		X		X	X
MMT*	X		X		X	X
Alignment	X		X		X	X
Joint stability/ mobility	X		X		X	
Patellar mobility	X		X		X	

*MMT = manual muscle test.

212

Palpation

Palpation of the joint enables the therapist to locate tenderness and establish the presence of joint effusion, synovitis, or bony enlargement. Palpation provides information about the acuteness of the arthritis that assists in guiding treatment (see Figs. 8–2 and 8–3). For example, in the presence of a major knee joint effusion, treatment is directed toward reducing the effusion and using gentle active or active-assisted range of motion (ROM) exercises. Extremes of ROM, which would further stretch the joint capsule or produce pain, are avoided. Conversely, the resolution of effusion accompanied by only minimal tenderness indicates that a more aggressive program of active and resistive quadriceps femoris muscle-strengthening exercises through a pain-free ROM can be initiated.

Both OA and RA knee joints are likely to be tender to palpation. In the early stages of either disease, the tenderness is more localized. In later stages of the disease, tenderness is likely to be quite diffuse. Joint effusions and synovial thickening are more common in RA but occur also in advanced stages of OA. Bony enlargement of the periarticular bone is present only in OA.

In the presence of synovial thickening or knee joint effusion, documentation of knee joint circumference is useful to monitor the changes in these conditions with treatment. Circumferential measurements are made by palpating the joint line medially and laterally and placing the tape measure at this level. Distinguishing between an effusion, synovial thickening, and bony enlargement can be difficult but is nonetheless quite important. All can make the knee joint appear larger. A bony enlargement feels firmer on palpation than either synovitis or joint effusion and is also visualized on a roentgenogram. Synovitis can be recognized by palpating the medial and lateral joint lines. Healthy joint capsule can be palpated as a narrow band about 2 to 3 mm in diameter running parallel to the joint line. Joint capsules with thickened synovial linings due to chronic synovitis will feel much thicker and wider in diameter.

A knee joint effusion can be recognized by performing one of two tests.[21] If there appears to be a large amount of excess synovial fluid in the joint, the knee joint should be placed in extension with the quadriceps femoris muscle relaxed. When the patella is pushed into the trochlear groove and then released, joint fluid will be forced to the sides of the joint and then rebound to the center, forcing the patella to return to its original position.[21] Hoppenfeld[21] refers to this test as the *ballotable patella*. A minimal effusion may be detected by maintaining the patient's knee relaxed in extension and applying pressure from above and lateral to the patella in an effort to force the synovial fluid into the anteromedial knee compartment. A slight bulge medial to the patella can be observed or palpated if a minimal effusion is present. When pressure is applied to this medial bulge, the joint fluid then traverses to the lateral compartment, and lateral bulge can be observed or palpated. Unfortunately, many patients with OA are overweight and have an excess of adipose tissue around the knee, making a joint effusion more difficult to detect.

Range of Motion, Muscle Flexibility, and Muscle Strength

The lower extremity is an interdependent system of joints and muscles which function primarily in a closed kinetic chain. Dysfunction in any joint can lead to altered mechanics throughout the entire lower extremity. Therefore, ROM, muscle flexibility, and muscle strength should be assessed throughout the entire extremity. Procedures for

ROM and strength testing are covered adequately by others and will not be elaborated in this chapter.[22-24] Flexibility of the muscles that cross more than one joint, such as the hamstrings, iliopsoas, gastrocnemius, tensor fascia lata (TFL) and rectus femoris muscles, are evaluated. Manual muscle testing (MMT) or isokinetic strength testing can be confounded by the presence of pain. If the patient states that pain limited his ability to perform, documentation of the degree of pain is important for comparison with follow-up strength testing. Occasionally patients will be in too much pain to attempt strength testing. The benefits of the added information must be weighed against the cost to the patient. In the presence of a severe joint effusion, placing a joint in its closed-pack position and then requesting a maximal quadriceps femoris muscle contraction is contraindicated. The joint effusion stretches the joint capsule and supporting ligaments. Joint compression due to maximal muscle tension at the end of knee joint range is likely to further stretch soft tissue structures and may eventually result in knee joint instability. Overstretching secondary to effusion is more common and of more concern in the RA knee.

Evaluation of ROM and muscle strength can provide information that will indicate the level of disease severity (see Fig. 8–1). Knowing disease severity will aid in making a physical therapy prognosis and will guide and monitor treatment. For example, a patient in the advanced stage of arthritis with severely limited ROM and Fair (3/5) quadriceps femoris muscle strength is less likely to tolerate aggressive treatment. The more severely involved patient is also unlikely to show as much improvement from treatment as is a patient with less severe disease.

Lower Extremity Alignment

Assessment of lower extremity and foot/ankle alignment is used to guide the fabrication of biomechanical orthoses (see Fig. 8–3) and to classify the severity of joint involvement. Joints with severe malalignment will have a poor prognosis for improvement in function. Capsular end feel will determine the need for joint mobilization, which may in turn change alignment.

Evaluation of lower extremity alignment should include an assessment of the relationship of the tibia to the floor and of the tibia to the calcaneus in standing.[25] The position of the forefoot relative to the rearfoot should be measured in prone.[25] The amount of knee flexion/extension/hyperextension in standing should also be measured. Abnormal subtalar joint pronation or supination can result in pathomechanical changes in the knee and patellofemoral joints. For example, prolonged subtalar joint pronation during stance may result in an obligatory internal rotation of the tibia, which can produce a functional genu valgus. The result is increased stress along the medial capsule of the knee joint, as well as an increased Q angle affecting the patellofemoral joint. A rearfoot varus restricts the normal subtalar joint pronation that should occur at heelstrike to allow normal dissipation of ground reaction forces. The result is increased joint reaction forces imparted up the lower extremity, especially through the knee joint.

Lower extremity alignment should be measured by a goniometer, documented in degrees, and classified as either fixed or reducible. A fixed deformity indicates that no further correction with passive movement is possible. The end feel in a fixed deformity is hard and usually means that the restriction is secondary to a bony block. Improvement of the deformity is unlikely in this case. A reducible deformity is one in which either complete or partial correction can be achieved with passive movement. In some cases the deformity can be completely corrected and normal alignment attained. These deformities are most often seen in rheumatoid arthritis and are an indication of muscle imbalances or capsular hypermobility. Other reducible deformities cannot be corrected fully but have a capsular end feel. The capsular end feel indicates that the joint restriction can be improved with mobilization. The degree of foot and ankle joint malalignment, the reducibility of the deformity, and the end feel all influence the type of orthotic used. For example, in the presence of a fixed rearfoot varus deformity with a bony end feel in the subtalar joint, a flexible, cushioned orthotic will help dissipate ground reaction forces at heelstrike. In the presence of forefoot varus and a reducible, mobile subtalar joint, an orthotic may be used with a rigid or firm forefoot wedge to control subtalar joint pronation in late stance.

Joint and Patellar Mobility

In both RA and OA the knee joint can be either hypomobile or hypermobile. Both hypermobility and hypomobility can exist concomitantly in different planes of rotation in the same knee. A single knee joint can be unstable in a varus/valgus or medial/lateral direction in the frontal plane while full extension and flexion are lacking in the sagittal plane. Varus/valgus, anterior/posterior, and rotary joint accessory movement should be assessed.[21] Joint effusion and pain with muscle guarding may produce hypomobility in a joint that is actually hypermobile. In such cases, joint mobility/stability testing should be deferred until the effusion and muscle guarding are at least partially resolved.

For the knee joint to fully flex and extend, the patella must glide in both a superior and inferior direction along the femoral trochlear groove (see Chapter 1). Often, patella mobility is limited in patients with arthritis. Patellar hypermobility or dislocating/sub-luxating patella is rarely a problem in either OA or RA. Manual displacement of the patella to determine mobility in superior/inferior and medial/lateral directions is an important assessment. Observation of patellar tracking is also important if the patient describes patellofemoral joint pain. Selective strengthening of the vastus mediales obliquus muscle or stretching of the vastus lateralis muscle and lateral retinaculum may be indicated in patellar tracking problems. Evaluation of knee joint and patellar mobility provides information that determines the need for knee joint or patella mobilization or stabilization and aids in classifying the severity of the disease (see Fig. 8–1).

INCORPORATING THE PROBLEM-SOLVING APPROACH

The problem-solving approach was discussed in detail in Chapter 3. A brief discussion using the problem-solving approach within the framework of evaluation and treatment of the arthritic knee, however, merits discussion. During the evaluation, the clinician will be making decisions about which of the procedures are important to perform and the sequence in which they should be completed. At the culmination of the evaluation the therapist should have a clear idea of the patient's major problems. Recent studies have shown that most therapists agree upon the need for systematic, methodical data collection methods, reserving judgment until all data have been collected (i.e., inductive reasoning process).[26] Other research in clinical decision making indicates that a working hypothesis is often developed early in the evaluation session, and the remainder of the evaluation is spent confirming or rejecting the working hypothesis (i.e., deductive reasoning process).[27] In reality, the point at which the working hypothesis is developed varies between therapists and patients. What is important in problem solving is to listen carefully to the patient's responses to questioning and to allow the responses to guide the sequence of the evaluation procedure.[28]

In treating OA or RA involving the knee joint, most often the patient presents to the physical therapist with a medical diagnosis. In either case, however, a host of biomechanical and musculoskeletal problems can be associated with the diagnosis. Typical dysfunctional patterns may arise frequently, but no two OA or RA patients are ever exactly alike. The physical therapist must identify the accompanying biomechanical and musculoskeletal problems and their possible causes. After factors influencing the problems are identified in the initial evaluation, the clinician determines treatment for addressing these problems. Continued re-evaluation of selected signs and symptoms over the course of the treatment determines the efficacy of the program.

Each piece of data that is collected should have a clear use. Some information will be used to classify the severity of the patient's disease and formulate a prognosis for change (see Fig. 8–1). Other information is used to determine disease acuity and to guide the selection of treatments (see Fig. 8–2). Most components of the evaluation will have more than one purpose, and each component should be used to assist with clinical decisions (see Fig. 8–3 and Table 8–1).

TREATMENT

The following sections discuss the various treatments available for use with patients with OA or RA involving the knee joint. The indications and contraindications for each modality are presented.

Modalities

Use of modalities such as heat, cold, transcutaneous electrical neuromuscular stimulation (TENS), and hydrotherapy to minimize swelling and/or decrease pain are important components of the treatment for patients with arthritis.[29-31] Both heat and cold have been shown to relieve pain secondary to arthritis, with neither having a clear advantage over the other in decreasing pain and improving ROM and function.[32-34] Cold may be more effective in the acute stages, whereas heat may be more effective in the subacute or chronic stages and in noninflammatory arthritis such as OA.[34,35] The use of heat or cold in conjunction with stretching techniques depends on the tissue being treated. Heat may be more effective in increasing the extensibility of connective tissue.[31,36] The choice of a specific modality should be based on the problem-solving approach and patient preference, because there is a paucity of well-controlled comparative research regarding the efficacy of most modalities.[30,37] A more in-depth discussion on the physiologic basis for heat, cold, and electrical modalities in the treatment of arthritis is beyond the scope of this chapter and can be gathered from other sources.[30,31,37] A summary of the important physiologic responses to heat and cold, however, is presented in the following paragraphs.

Heat therapy can be used to decrease pain, joint stiffness, and muscle spasm and increase the extensibility of contracted connective tissues.[30] Heat delivery can be either superficial or deep, depending on the mode of application. Superficial heat, such as hot packs, penetrates only a few millimeters into the subcutaneous tissue, whereas deep heat, such as diathermy and ultrasound, can penetrate to the level of the joint.[38,39] (The application of deep heat to superficial joint structures, such as those in the hand, is an exception to this guideline.) Manardi and associates[40] have shown that superficial heat applied to the hand of a healthy individual raised the intra-articular temperature of the metatarsophalangeal and interphalangeal joints 8.0°C. Diathermy has been shown to raise the intra-articular temperature 4.8°C,[39] whereas ultrasound may increase it as much as 11.5°C.[41] Some studies indicate that raising the intra-articular temperature as little as 3°C may increase disease activity and encourage the destruction of cartilage.[42-44] Other researchers have shown that heat treatments elevating joint temperature 8°C daily for 2 years did not result in a progression of joint erosion on roentgenogram.[40] Until further research clarifies the effects of joint warming, continuous ultrasound over arthritic joints should be applied with caution. One possible therapeutic approach is to decrease ultrasound intensity if joint warming is of concern. Perhaps ultrasound should be reserved for connective tissue that does not lie directly over the arthritic joint. Regardless of the heat modality chosen, the main purpose of the modality is to increase the patient's tolerance to and benefit from exercise and should seldom be used as the sole rehabilitation treatment.[30]

The use of cryotherapy has been advocated for the management of pain and swelling in acute musculoskeletal trauma and after surgical procedures.[45-47] Cryotherapy decreases pain and muscle spasm and increases range of motion.[32,48,49] However, in some instances cold application may also decrease connective tissue extensibility[50] and increase joint stiffness.[36,51,52] Nevertheless, if pain reduction in the acute phase is the primary goal, cold may produce rapid pain reduction.[53]

Some clinicians advocate using cryotherapy for up to, but not exceeding, 15 minutes to avoid a rebound vasodilation of the blood vessels within the cooled tissues. *Rebound vasodilation*, also known as the "hunting response," is defined as vasodilation of the blood vessels after an initial period of vasoconstriction.[31] Results from studies have indicated that this rebound vasodilation occurs in tissues cooled for more than 15 minutes or to a temperature of less than 10°C.[54-56] However, vasodilation responses were found primarily in skin and muscle, and there is no clear evidence to link vasodilation to increased intra-articular swelling. Whether rebound vasodilation occurs in the knee joint may depend upon the depth of penetration of the cooling response, which is a function of the length of application. Subcutaneous tissue at a depth of 4 cm can be cooled to 2°C in 30 minutes.[57] Ten minutes of ice packs to dog's knees decreases blood flow to the joint by 56 percent with a return to precooled temperatures in 25 minutes.[58] A study by Kern and associates[59] demonstrated that applying cold to animals for 30 minutes resulted in a mean intra-articular temperature of 6.6°C. The joints in this study returned to their original temperature in 3.5 hours. The effect of this treatment on vasodilation and intra-articular swelling was not reported. Because the perimeter of the human knee is fairly superficial, cryotherapy should probably be limited to 15 minutes if rebound vasodilation is of concern. The most practical clinical approach is to apply the modality for a given time, monitor the swelling, and modify the treatment based on the results.

Methods of application of cold appropriate for the knee include ice/cold packs, and ice massage. Neither of these forms of cold is more effective than the other in relieving pain and muscle spasm.[30] Ice or cold packs wrapped in some form of insulation can be applied for 5 to 20 minutes.[30,31,49] Ice massage is usually administered for 5 to 10 minutes[30] and lowers the skin temperature to 15°C only. Therefore, the concerns of rebound vasodilation do not apply to ice massage.

Transcutaneous electrical neuromuscular stimulation (TENS) is another useful adjunct for temporarily decreasing pain in both RA and OA.[60-64] Specific optimal electrode placement and settings for stimulus parameters have not been systematically evaluated.[30] Mannheimer and Carlson[65] studied various pulse patterns in patients with rheumatoid arthritis and found better pain relief using high-intensity stimulation. The suggested electrode placement for reduction of joint pain is to place the electrodes directly over the area of pain.[61] Clinicians should rely upon the patient's response to determine optimal electrode placement, stimulus parameters, and efficacy of TENS as a treatment modality.[30]

Both patient and therapist should realize that the use of modalities will bring temporary relief and should be used in conjunction with an oral anti-inflammatory or remittive drug therapy. A combination of medication and physical modalities is an important component of overall patient management and reduction of joint inflammation. Regular compliance with patient medication may help the patient to be more compliant with an exercise program. An in-depth discussion of drug therapy in arthritis is beyond the scope of this work and can be found elsewhere.[2]

Exercise

Exercise is an important component of an overall rehabilitation program for patients with arthritis.[19,35,66-69,70] Exercise for arthritic patients is used to increase joint ROM, muscle flexibility, strength, and endurance. These goals can be achieved with either exercise or recreational activity.[19,71] Research demonstrating that exercise prevents deformity in arthritis does not exist.[72] However, ROM and strengthening exercises can increase strength, joint mobility, and function.[73,74] Special considerations, however, must be made in the presence of the painful swollen knee. In general, increased pain lasting for more than 2 hours after exercise or activity is an indication that exercise intensity should be decreased.[72]

MUSCLE STRENGTHENING

In the presence of a symptomatic knee, strengthening exercises are chosen that best achieve the desired goal of increased strength and yet will not create increased inflammation in the joint.[75] Strengthening exercises are performed at the hip, knee, and ankle musculature. In the knee joint, swelling can produce quadriceps femoris muscle inhibition, resulting in weakness and muscle atrophy.[9-15,17,76] Hip musculature, especially in the gluteus maximus muscle can become significantly weak with inactivity. A shortening of single-limb stance time of the affected limb may create disuse weakness in both the gastrocnemius-soleus and gluteus medius muscles.

Researchers have attempted to determine the optimal type, frequency, intensity, and duration of exercise to increase muscle strength.[77-95] However, no controlled studies have compared the effectiveness of various forms of exercise in the presence of arthritis. Therefore, the clinician should use problem-solving with each patient to determine the type, frequency, intensity, and duration of each exercise. A training regimen should incorporate several types of exercise modes—for example, isometric, isotonic, and isokinetic exercises (see Chapter 5, Multimodal Training). Figure 8–4 shows the exercise variables to be considered in treatment planning for patients with osteoarthritis or rheumatoid arthritis, and their relationship to the stage of reactivity. As reactivity

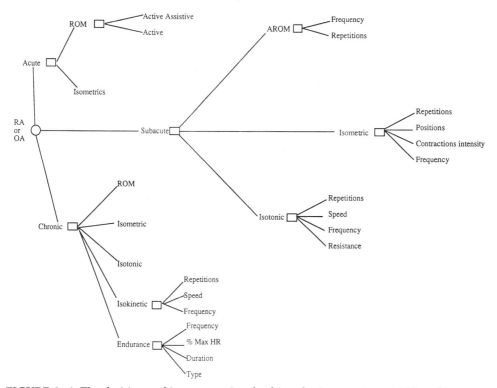

FIGURE 8–4. The decision-making process involved in selecting exercise variables of intensity, duration of exercises, frequency, and mode or type of exercise. Note that there is an inverse relationship between the reactivity of the disease and the number of exercise variables. For example, as the reactivity of the disease increases, the number of exercise variables that are used in a specific case decreases. Conversely, as the reactivity of the disease decreases, the number of exercise variables increases. Based on the relationship between reactivity and exercise variables, the clinician must continually reevaluate the patient's status to assure the proper implementation of the exercise program.

improves (e.g., from acute to chronic), the number of exercise variables and the complexity of exercise increase. In the acute stage, exercises are usually limited to active range of motion (ROM) or active-assisted ROM exercises and isometric muscle contractions. In the subacute stage, multiple-angle isometrics and partial- to full-range isotonic exercises can be added. Finally, in the chronic phase, several additional modes of exercise can be added, including isokinetic training that can encompass the use of mutiple speeds and high repetitions.

In the acute phase, the clinician should choose the type of exercise mode that creates the least amount of joint stress and yet is adequate to maintain or minimize the loss of strength. Isometric exercise produces a greater amount of tension in the muscle than do concentric contractions[96], and is therefore effective in increasing muscle strength.[72,79–83,85–87] Isometric exercise minimizes stress to the knee joint by eliminating the rolling and sliding forces present during concentric or eccentric isotonic or isokinetic exercises. In addition, isometric exercise does not cause inflammation or juxta-articular bone destruction, when used to increase knee strength in patients with RA.[87] However, the increased tension developed in the muscle during isometric contraction may result in joint compression that is painful to patients with an effused knee. Therefore, in the presence of knee joint effusion, isometric contractions of the quadriceps femoris muscle should be performed in ranges that avoid terminal extension and flexion.

Three maximal isometric contractions with 20-second rest periods between contractions increase strength in RA patients when performed three times per week for a month.[87] A two-thirds maximal contraction maintained for 6 seconds and performed daily increases strength in healthy males.[77] Increased strength gains of 7 to 20 percent were correlated with the use of maximal isometric contractions.[77] However, maximal isometric contractions probably should be reserved for patients who are in the chronic stage of their disease. Increasing the frequency of exercise to daily sessions and the length of contraction time to 15 seconds resulted in greater strength gains.[77] As a general guideline, strengthening should be initiated at a submaximal level and slowly increased to maximal effort as joint effusion and inflammation resolve.

Another consideration for isometric exercise is the appropriate position for strengthening while maintaining minimal stress on the joint. In the presence of a significant intra-articular effusion, isometric contractions of the quadriceps femoris muscle should not be performed in the closed-pack position (i.e., full extension). Full knee joint extension combined with quadriceps femoris isometric muscle contraction will increase intra-articular pressure[98] and overstretch the joint capsule and supporting soft tissues. Increasing the intra-articular pressure will also inhibit quadriceps femoris muscle contraction. Isometric muscle strengthening in the presence of a major joint effusion should be performed with the patient's knee joint flexed at least 30 degrees.[75,99] As the effusion resolves, quadriceps femoris muscle isometric contractions should be performed in full knee joint extension to reduce quadriceps lag (the inability to fully and actively extend the knee joint), which is often present after prolonged knee swelling and pain. Several studies have shown that isometric strengthening is specific to the training position, with little carryover to other angles.[79,85,86] Functional strength gains with isometric exercises therefore require that contractions be performed at various angles throughout the ROM.

Breathing exercises should be taught in conjunction with isometric exercises to minimize the Valsalva maneuver and attenuate the body's pressor response to isometric exercise.[84] The pressor response also can be minimized by decreasing the isometric contraction time from 20 seconds to 3 to 6 seconds and providing a 20-second rest between contractions.[66,19]

Muscle strengthening should be progressed to include isotonic contractions as soon as possible to incorporate functional movement into the exercise program.[89] Concentric and eccentric exercises, in both open and closed kinetic chain positions, should be performed. Much of functional lower extremity muscle activity is eccentric and occurs in the range of 0 to 45 degrees of knee flexion.[75] Incorporating eccentric strengthening in this range, therefore, is an important technique. Closed kinetic chain exercises are appropriate functionally, because the lower extremity functions primarily during weight bearing. However, full weight bearing creates forces in the knee joint that are equal to approximately three times body weight.[18,100] Full weight bearing strengthening exercises, therefore, should be used judiciously in the subacute or chronic phases and avoided in the acute phase of arthritis. Exercises such as leg presses (with the weight kept below body weight) or weight bearing in water, however, are methods of initiating closed kinetic chain exercises in the more acute phase of disease. Antich and Brewster[101] have outlined a strengthening method for open kinetic chain strengthening exercises for the quadriceps femoris muscle.

When used in the chronic stages, isokinetic exercise may be very helpful for the patient with arthritis affecting the knee. Isokinetic exercise allows for the development of maximal tension throughout the full ROM at speeds that more closely resemble that of function.[94] Isokinetic exercise is an accommodating resistive exercise in which the speed of movement remains constant throughout the ROM. The amount of force exerted by the device can never exceed the amount of effort the patient imparts to the dynamometer. The patient with arthritis can reduce the amount of force at particularly painful angles in the ROM by simply reducing speed of movement. Force-velocity curves indicate that with increased velocity of movement, the torque produced by the muscle decreases. This force-velocity relationship indicates that the patient with arthritis should be exercised isokinetically at an angular velocity of at least 180 degrees per second.[19,102] Isokinetic strenghtening is an effective exercise mode to be used with either isotonic or isometric strengthening[90,94,95,102] in rehabilitation of the OA or RA knee.

The use of biofeedback and electromyostimulation of muscles during exercise may enhance strength gains.[83,103,104,105] An in-depth discussion of these two adjuncts to exercise is beyond the scope of this chapter. For a more thorough discussion of biofeedback or electromyostimulation, please consult the work of Krebs[103] and Morrisey.[104]

RANGE OF MOTION

Basic ROM exercises are particularly important in the acute phase to minimize permanent loss of range. In the presence of a major joint effusion, care should be taken not to force the knee into end range, thus overstretching the joint capsule.[99] For the same reason, aggressive passive range of motion (PROM) should never be used when a major effusion is present.

MUSCLE FLEXIBILITY

Flexibility of two-joint and multiple-joint muscles such as the hip flexors, hamstrings, and gastrocnemius muscles, is often lacking in patients with arthritis affecting the knee joint. Due to secondary reflex muscle spasm/tone of the hamstring muscles when the knee joint capsule is distended by a joint effusion,[17] the hamstring muscles often become inflexible or tight (i.e., less than 60 degrees of straight leg raising is available). Additionally, the hamstring and hip flexor muscles can become tight as a result of patient inactivity. When patients spend much of their time sitting, the hip flexor and hamstring muscles are placed in an adaptively shortened position. Muscle tightness in these muscle groups will facilitate a lack of hip and knee extension and a lack of ankle plantar flexion at the end of single-limb stance, thereby increasing the force generated within these joints during walking.[106,107] Early initiation of lower extremity flexibility exercises is important in maintaining a normal gait pattern and minimizing knee joint stress.

ENDURANCE

Poor cardiovascular status and deconditioning are significant problems in patients with arthritis due to decreased activity levels.[4,108-110] A cardiovascular exercise program should be initiated once the knee joint is less acute. Much has been written recently regarding endurance exercise in arthritis.[109,111-116] These studies have shown that in general, even fairly aggressive cardiovascular fitness programs do not harm, or create an increased reactivity in, joints with arthritis and may in fact improve function and decrease pain.[109,111-116]

Because running and jogging cause repetitive stress in the knee joint,[4] walking, stationary biking, and swimming are three forms of fitness training often recommended because of the low-impact nature of these activities.[19,117] Bicycling at 120 W at 60 rpm helps to develop a mean peak tibiofemoral joint compression of just 1.2 times body weight.[118] Both raising the seat height and decreasing the workload will decrease the amount of compression force across the knee.[119-121] Knee loading during bicycling is independent of the individual's body weight because body weight is supported by the seat.[120,121] Walking creates forces across the knee joint that are about three times the body weight.[100] Water walking further reduces the weight bearing forces across the knee joint and is an excellent way to increase heart rate while allowing the buoyancy of the water to decrease the force of gravity affecting the weight bearing joints.[122] The amount of weight experienced in water can be adjusted by changing the depth of the water (neck height = 10 percent body weight; chest height = 25 percent body weight; and waist height = 50 percent body weight).[122-124]

A 30-minute session of any of these types of cardiovascular exercise for three times per week, during which the patient's heart rate is at least 60 to 80 percent of maximum, is generally adequate for conditioning.[19]

Incorporating pool therapy into a theraputic exercise program for arthritis can be very helpful in all stages of the disease.[31] In the acute stage, when maintenance of ROM and of muscle flexibility is the major focus, the buoyancy of the water can assist ROM and muscle flexibility exercises.[29,66] When the patient is ready to begin resistive exercise, water can provide resistance if the speed of the movement is increased. As previously mentioned, water walking is an excellent form of cardiovascular endurance exercise that does not place a great deal of force on the joints. A water temperature of 86°F is usually recommended.[66]

Orthotics

Most patients with knee joint arthritis have lower extremity alignment problems in the knee joint and foot, which may create additional joint stress. Use of a foot orthosis can minimize these stresses and decrease pain at the knee. The goal of a biomechanical foot orthosis is to control and support the subtalar and midtarsal joints. Because the feet of patients with OA or RA are often rigid and inflexible, effective foot orthoses in these patients should be flexible and shock absorbing and assist in accommodating the weight bearing surface to the foot.[125,126]

Younger patients with RA, who have excessive movement in the foot that needs to be blocked or modified with a more rigid orthosis, are the exception to this rule.[125] Foot orthoses are commercially available in a variety of materials with varying degrees of stiffness. Finding the correct combination for a patient often involves some experimentation. Depending on the status of the ankle, subtalar, and midtarsal joints, a trial of joint mobilization in effort to increase ankle and foot mobility may be indicated (see discussion below on joint mobilization). As the mobility of the foot changes, the orthotic may require alteration as well.

Theoretically the use of a knee joint splint or bracing could minimize pain and the progression of deformity. However, clinical experience indicates that knee splints are usually not effective in controlling knee deformity in adults with RA or OA and are quite uncomfortable and poorly tolerated by most patients. The primary use of a knee splint is for correction of knee joint flexion deformities greater than 5 to 10 degrees. In such cases a serial splint or cast is used to gradually increase knee joint extension. Correction of knee joint flexion contractures of greater then 30 degrees without the undesired complication of posterior tibial subluxation is difficult. Once the flexion deformity has progressed to 30 degrees or greater, the use of skeletal traction may be required to prevent tibial subluxation while the knee joint is pulled into extension.[127]

Joint Mobilization

Advocates of the use of joint mobilization have cautioned against use of the techniques for patients with RA. The rationale is that joints affected by RA can be hypermobile with weakened joint capsules and therefore should not be passively stretched.[128] Hypermobility and weakened joint capsules in RA are certainly common and should not be further stretched with mobilization. However, hypomobility, joint capsule tightness, and fibrous adhesions can also be problems in RA, and patients may benefit from careful joint mobilization.

If a major joint effusion is present, the joint can appear hypomobile. The hypomobility is created by the effusion, which puts stretching force on the joint capsule. Further joint stretching through mobilization is contraindicated at this time.

The critical first step in determining the appropriateness of joint mobilization is to determine whether a joint effusion is present. If no effusion is present, the joint mobility testing is more likely to be valid. If the results of joint mobility testing indicate that the knee or patella is hypomobile, then joint mobilization is indicated.

Patient Education

An important component of management of either OA or RA of the knee is patient understanding of the disease process and self-efficacy skills in managing pain and protection of the joint.[129] A problem-solving approach seems warranted, in that each patient has a different level of understanding and different life-styles and goals. Incorporating questions into the evaluation and/or treatment sessions can provide insight into the patient's understanding of his or her problems. Questions such as "What has your doctor told you about the problem with your knee?" "What aggravates your knee?" and "How do you relieve the pain in your knee?" will provide information regarding the patient's understanding of his or her diagnosis and management. Once the patient's knowledge level has been determined, teaching can begin. If the patient can be an active participant in this process, rather than a passive recipient of information, he or she is more likely to apply the new knowledge to everyday activities. The Arthritis Foundation is a valuable resource for teaching and patient education materials.

CASE STUDIES

CASE STUDY 1: OSTEOARTHRITIS

HISTORY

The patient was a 64-year-old woman with a diagnosis of primary OA affecting both knees, with the right knee joint more involved than the left. Her arthritis began 3 years previously with insidious onset of knee pain. She could not recall a traumatic incident that initiated the onset of pain. Pain was present daily at a level of 5 on the 0 to 10 scale when walking or standing, descending stairs, and with movement. At the time the patient entered therapy, she was not participating in a regular exercise program and was employed in sedentary work. Roentgenograms of the knee joints revealed osteophytes at the joint margins, subchondral sclerosis, and narrowing of the joint spaces, with the medial compartment being more narrowed than the lateral.

EVALUATION

Mild tenderness to palpation was present at the medial knee joint line and inferomedial to the patella. Bilaterally, mild knee joint crepitus on active motion was also present. Synovitis was present only on the right knee joint, with no evidence of a joint effusion. Circumference at the joint line measured about 44 cm bilaterally.

The patient's pelvis was level and there was no leg length discrepancy. Genu varus was present in standing bilaterally, with the left measuring 5 degrees and the right measuring 8 to 10 degrees. Her calcaneus, in standing, was in 5 degrees of varus on the right and 1 to 2 degrees of valgus on the left (Fig. 8–5). Subtalar neutral was in 5 degrees of inversion bilaterally (Fig. 8–6). When compared with

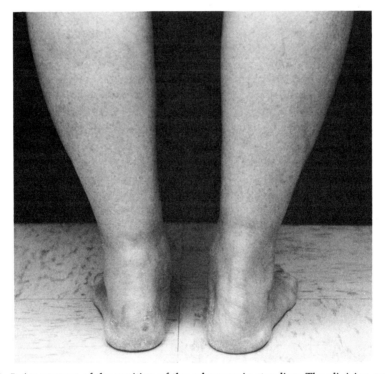

FIGURE 8–5. Assessment of the position of the calcaneus in standing. The clinician assesses the relationship between the midline of the patient's distal tibia and the midline of the calcaneus. Relative to the midline of the tibia, the calcaneus is in varus (inversion) in the right subtalar joint, and in valgus (eversion) in the left. OA patient.

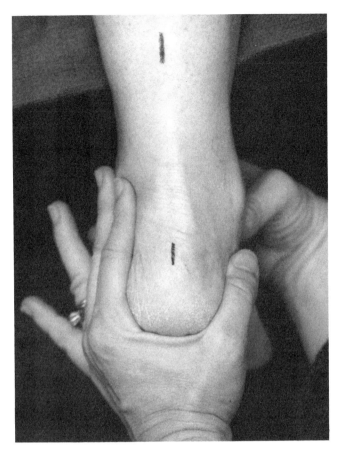

FIGURE 8-6. Subtalar joint neutral position is assessed with the patient non–weight bearing. The rearfoot is positioned in neutral by palpating the head of the talus with the thumb and the forefingers while the patient is prone. The foot is maximally pronated (everted), then maximally supinated (inverted). The subtalar joint neutral is thought to be at the point in the range at which the head of the talus is felt equally on the lateral and medial sides. Although this test is a quick clinical method, the validity and reliability of the method has not been conclusively established. Subtalar neutral was approximately 5 degrees of inversion in the right. Right foot of an OA patient.

the rearfoot, the forefoot was in slight varus bilaterally, with the right forefoot being in more varus than the left (Fig. 8–7).

In general, ROM at the hips was within normal limits. She had 125 degrees of knee joint flexion but lacked 5 degrees from full knee joint extension bilaterally. Ankle dorsiflexion with the knee joint flexed was within normal limits, but plantarflexion was limited to about 30 degrees. The subtalar joint could be passively inverted to 16 degrees on the right and 10 degrees on the left. Passively the subtalar joint could be everted to 10 degrees from the 5-degree inverted neutral position. On the left there was 8 degrees of eversion from the 5-degree inverted neutral position. The lack of eversion was considered to be a reducible deformity because a capsular end-feel was present. Therefore, the potential to improve subtalar eversion with mobilization and stretching was good.

The patient demonstrated moderate tightness in all major two-joint muscle groups except for the rectus femoris muscle. Hip extension with the knee in extension and the pelvis stabilized lacked 25 degrees from neutral on the right and 20 degrees from neutral on the left. Passive straight leg raise (SLR) was 55 degrees bilaterally. With the knee extended, the ankle lacked about 5 degrees from neutral dorsiflexion. The TFL muscle was mildly tight, as demonstrated by thigh abduction during the test for hip flexor tightness (Thomas test).

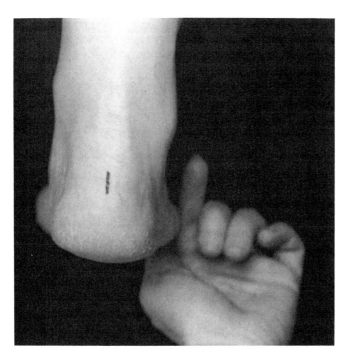

FIGURE 8-7. The forefoot is in varus (inversion) relative to the rearfoot. The forefoot/rearfoot relationship is determined with the rearfoot positioned in neutral. Right foot of an OA patient.

Strength in the iliopsoas, anterior tibialis, and gastrocnemius-soleus muscles was normal on manual muscle testing. Gluteus maximus and medius, and hamstring muscles appeared to have only $3 + /5$ strength, whereas the quadriceps femoris muscle was rated as $4 - /5$. Manual muscle testing did not produce pain.

Knee joint mobility (tested with the patient in supine position with the knee joint flexed to approximately 60 degrees) was moderately restricted in anterior gliding of the tibia on the femur. Posterior gliding of the tibia (tested in the same position as anterior gliding) on the femur was within normal limits. External rotation of the tibia on the femur was also slightly decreased. Patellar mobility was within normal limits, and no joint or patellar instability was noted.

The patient reported difficulty and pain with prolonged weight bearing in both standing and walking, climbing stairs, and squatting to pick up objects from the floor. She rated these activities on a 0-to-10 scale of pain and a 0-to-10 scale of difficulty as being at a level 5 for both scales.

ASSESSMENT

The patient appeared to have moderate OA of the knee joint, with evidence of early varus and flexion deformities. Her arthritis appeared to be in the chronic phase, with little evidence of acute inflammation. The patient's major problems were (1) decreased lower extremity muscle flexibility and strength; (2) tibial varum, weight bearing subtalar joint varus on the right and valgus on the left, and forefoot varus bilaterally; (3) joint hypomobility at the knee, ankle, and subtalar joints; (4) impaired function of the lower extremities; and (5) pain in both knees. The judgment was made that the patient could likely benefit from strengthening, muscle stretching, joint mobilization, and use of a foot orthosis.

FACTORS AFFECTING THE PROBLEMS

Factors that affect all patients' problems include the severity of disease, age, premorbid activity level, motivation to improve the problem, general health, financial resources, and family support system. At the time of this evaluation she was considered to have a moderate disease severity level with mild to moderate malalignment present, which would indicate a good prognosis for improvement. Although beyond middle age, she was young enough to expect considerable improvement with a rehabilitation program. Unfortunately, she had never been particularly oriented toward physical activities or exercise. However, she was active in community projects that required a considerable amount of functional mobility. She was highly motivated to maintain this level of community involvement and was willing to comply with an exercise program, because she was convinced such a program would help to maintain her functional status and decrease her pain. Other than OA, her general health was good, and her family encouraged her to begin a program to minimize the deleterious effects of OA.

GOALS

Goals were projected to be achieved in 8 weeks, a period selected based on anecdotal experience of the clinician, who felt that at least 8 weeks is usually needed to make significant changes in a 64-year-old patient with a diagnosis of OA. Goals were as follows:

1. Pain level 1 to 2/10
2. Neutral calcaneal alignment in standing
3. Improved forefoot and midfoot flexibility
4. Difficulty in functional activities at 1 to 2/10
5. Normal strength in all lower extremity muscle groups
6. Improve flexibility of the lower extremity two-joint muscles (SLR = 65 to 70 degrees, ankle joint dorsiflexion with the knee joint extended = 5 degrees, hip joint extension to neutral)
7. Improve comfort and minimize stresses at the foot, ankle, and knee joints in weight bearing
8. Weight loss of 10 lb

TREATMENT

The patient attended physical therapy twice a week for 8 weeks, receiving 1 hour of therapy at each visit.

Treatments 1 to 3

During treatments 1 to 3, grade III and IV mobilizations of the knee joint, gliding the tibia anteriorly and into external rotation, were carried out. The rationale for joint mobilization at the knee was to increase knee extension. Anterior gliding of the tibia on the femur is thought to improve knee joint extension, because the concave tibial plateaus move anteriorly during the joint extension.[18] The subtalar joint was mobilized to increase eversion by tilting the calcaneus laterally. The navicular, cuneiforms, and first three metatarsal bones were mobilized in a plantar direction to increase forefoot valgus. The overall purpose of subtalar and forefoot mobilization was to improve foot alignment and mobility and thereby decrease mechanical stresses at the knee joint. Contract-relax stretching for the hamstrings, iliopsoas, TFL, and gastrocnemius-soleus muscles were also performed with the therapist. Improvement in lower extremity muscle flexibility would correct muscle imbalances and result in improved lower extremity alignment. Improved muscle flexibility would also improve the shock absorption property of the muscle, aiding in muscular protection of the knee joint. The patient also began strengthening for the hamstrings, quadriceps femoris, gluteus medius and maximus, and hip adductor muscles. The rationale for muscle strengthening was that stronger muscles could protect and support the joints. The quadriceps femoris and hamstring muscles were exercised by performing leg lifts with the knee in extension in the supine and prone positions, respectively. The rationale for choosing leg lifts with the knee joint maintained in extension was to avoid repetitive stress to the knee joint. Exercises initially were performed with the resistance provided by the weight of the limb for 10 repetitions and gradually increased to 30 repetitions. By the third treatment a 1-lb cuff weight was added. Low resistance was used and progressed slowly so as to minimize the likelihood of trauma to the joint. At the second visit the patient was instructed in a home program to be performed daily and advised to purchase cuff weights in increments of 1 to 5 lb. By doing a home program, the patient was able to maintain gains made in the therapy session and to progress more rapidly in gaining muscle strength and flexibility.

First Reassessment

On the fourth treatment, re-evaluation revealed a pain level of 4/10 while weight bearing. Palpation elicited decreased tenderness along the joint line. Alignment of the calcaneal-floor angle in standing and the rearfoot-forefoot relationship were unchanged. Knee joint extension was measured at -3 degrees from full extension. Pain and difficulty in climbing stairs was 4 on a 10-point scale. Difficulty in squatting was still rated at 5 on a 10-point scale. Manual muscle testing showed no change from the initial evaluation. Overall assessment at this time was that the patient was making improvement in pain level, function, and ROM but could benefit from further treatment with the short-term goals of a 2/10 level of pain and full knee extension, with functional difficulty in stair climbing rated at 3/10 and squatting at 4/10.

Treatments 4 to 6

The previously described program of joint mobilization and stretching and strengthening of lower extremity muscles was continued. By the fifth treatment, the cuff weight was increased to 2 lbs. The decision was made to increase the cuff weight because the patient found the 1-lb weight was no longer a challenge and she was having no pain with the exercises. On the fifth treatment, a program of stationary cycling was added. The cycling program was initiated to help the patient expend calories and, hopefully, to lose weight, improving her overall conditioning as well as the tone and strength in her lower extremities. The repetitive nature of cycling was also felt to help nourish the articular cartilage of the patellofemoral and tibiofemoral joints. She started at a low intensity of cycling, 10 minutes with minimal resistance so as to not irritate her knee or patellofemoral joints. The seat was elevated so that during the downstroke of the pedal, the knee was in full extension. This seat height was chosen to minimize the amount of knee flexion and patellofemoral joint compression. On the sixth treatment, the patient was advised to begin a water-walking program at her local YMCA on the days she did not come to therapy. The purpose of this suggestion was the same as for the stationary bicycle. Both activities were performed with monitoring of the heart rate. The patient was encouraged to achieve an exercise intensity level that created a heart rate of 60 percent of her maximum heart rate (calculated using the formula of 220 − age). Performing walking in the water provides buoyancy to decrease the knee joint compression in weight bearing while the water provides resistance to the forward progression of walking.

Second Reassessment

On the seventh treatment, the second re-evaluation revealed a pain level of 3/10, with no tenderness to palpation at the joint line. Her calcaneal-floor alignment in standing was improved on the right. The calcaneus was in only 2 degrees of inversion (as compared with 5 degrees in the initial evaluation). Bilaterally, both forefeet appeared to be in less varus (i.e., the forefeet/rearfeet alignment was closer to parallel with the calcaneus positioned in neutral.) Both midtarsal joints and forefeet also seemed slightly more flexible, based on assessment of end feel. The patient had gained full active and passive knee joint extension. Pain and difficulty on climbing stairs was rated 3/10 and squatting was rated 4/10. Manual muscle testing elicited 4/5 strength in the hamstring, gluteus maximus, and gluteus medius muscles. The overall assessment was that the patient's pain level was decreasing. Lower extremity alignment, function, and strength were improving. Full ROM was achieved. The revised short-term goals for the next three treatment sessions were (1) pain level of 2/10; (2) neutral calcaneal position in standing (vertical calcaneus relative to the midline of the tibia); (3) improvement in midfoot and forefoot mobility; (4) maintainance of full knee extension; (5) functional difficulty at a level of 2/10 for climbing stairs, and 3/10 for squatting; (6) 4 + /5 strength in hamstrings, gluteus maximus, and gluteus medius muscles; and (7) Increase SLR to 65 degrees, hip extension to 10 degrees from neutral, and ankle dorsiflexion with the knee extended to 5 degrees.

Treatments 7 to 11

On the seventh treatment, knee joint mobilization was discontinued because full active and passive knee joint extension had been achieved. Ankle joint and subtalar joint mobilization were continued. Contract-relax stretching for hip flexors, hamstrings, gastrocnemius, and TFL muscles was continued. Cuff weights on the strengthening program were increased to 3 lbs because 2 lb weights were no longer a challenge. On the seventh treatment, a program of isokinetic strengthening for the quadriceps femoris and hamstring muscles was added. The patient began with three sets of 5 repetitions each and quickly worked up to three sets of 10 repetitions. Initially, peak torque production was 30 lb at 180 degrees per second. The rationale for using isokinetic strengthening was to provide a safe method of giving dynamic resistance that accommodates to the patient's strength and pain throughout the ROM. Another reason for using isokinetics was that the visual feedback provided from the isokinetic computer screen would help maintain the patient's interest and motivation for the treatment program. Time on the stationary bike was increased to 20 minutes by the seventh treatment, 25 minutes by the eighth treatment, and 30 minutes by the ninth treatment. On the ninth treatment, the resistance was slightly increased to provide a little more challenge to the patient. The patient continued the water-walking program on her own.

Third Reassessment

On the 12th treatment, the third re-evaluation was performed. The patient's overall pain score was 2/10. The right calcaneal-floor angle in standing was now in neutral. Flexibility and alignment of the forefeet were essentially unchanged from the second re-evaluation but were improved from the initial evaluation. The patient had maintained full knee joint extension. Pain and difficulty climbing stairs was now rated at 2/10, and squatting was rated at 3/10. Manual muscle testing of the hamstrings, gluteus maximus, and gluteus medius muscles revealed 4 + /5 strength in those muscle groups. SLR was 65 degrees bilaterally. The hips extended to 10 degrees from neutral extension, bilaterally, and ankle dorsiflexion with the knee extended was 5 degrees, bilaterally.

The overall assessment was that the patient's pain level was continuing to decline. Correction in calcaneal-floor alignment had plateaued. Full mobility of the subtalar, midtarsal, and talocrural joints had been achieved. Full knee extension had been maintained without weekly mobilization. Function, hip and knee muscle strength, and muscle flexibility of the hamstring, gastrocnemius, and hip flexor muscle groups were continuing to improve. Short-term goals for the final four sessions were (1) pain level 1/10; (2) maintain neutral calcaneal position in standing; (3) maintain forefoot and midfoot mobility; (4) maintain full knee extension; (5) functional difficulty at a level of 1/10 for climbing stairs and 2/10 for squatting; (6) 5/5 strength in hamstrings and gluteus medius and maximus muscles; and (7) maintain SLR at 65 degrees, dorsiflexion with knee extension at 5 degrees, and further improve hip extension to −5 degrees from neutral, bilaterally.

Treatments 12 to 15

On the 12th treatment, the patient was fitted with a custom-made flexible foot orthosis for both feet, with a medial wedge at the forefoot to accommodate for the forefoot varus and a medial wedge for the rearfoot to accommodate for the tibial varus and lack of rearfoot eversion. Special care was taken to provide only the amount of medial rearfoot posting to accommodate the rearfoot varus. Too much medial posting would overcorrect the deformity and predispose the patient to lateral ankle sprains. Mobilization of the foot and ankle joint was discontinued because maximum subtalar, forefoot, and midfoot flexibility had been achieved. Contract-relax stretching of the hamstrings and gastrocnemius muscles was discontinued because flexibility was thought to be within normal limits. However, the patient continued to stretch these muscles in her home program. Contract-relax stretching of the hip flexors was continued to further elongate this muscle group. By the 12th treatment, cuff weights had been increased to 5 lb. The isokinetic strengthening of quadriceps and hamstring muscles was continued at 180 degrees per second for three sets of 10. The stationary bike was maintained at 30 minutes with moderate resistance, and the patient was advised to purchase a stationary bike at home. The patient continued the 30-minute water-walking program three times per week on her own.

Treatment 16/Final Evaluation

The final evaluation revealed the patient's pain level had improved to 1/10. The right calcaneus was maintained in neutral alignment in standing. Forefoot and midfoot flexibility and full knee extension were maintained. Pain and difficulty climbing stairs was now 1/10, squatting was rated 2/10. Manual muscle testing revealed normal or 5/5 strength in all lower extremity muscle groups. SLR was maintained at 65 degrees, dorsiflexion with the knee extended was maintained at +5 degrees, and the hip now extended to neutral. The patient reported that the foot orthoses were very comfortable and helped to decrease her knee joint pain during ambulation. She had lost 10 lb since the initiation of treatment.

The patient was felt to have achieved all goals set out for her and was generally pleased with her progress. Figure 8–8 summarizes the patient's overall progress in the areas of pain, knee ROM, function, strength, and alignment. She stated that she planned to continue her exercise program daily and to alternate stationary biking with water walking. Follow-up phone calls at 1 and 6 months revealed that the patient was continuing her program as planned and that she had maintained her functional gains and low pain level.

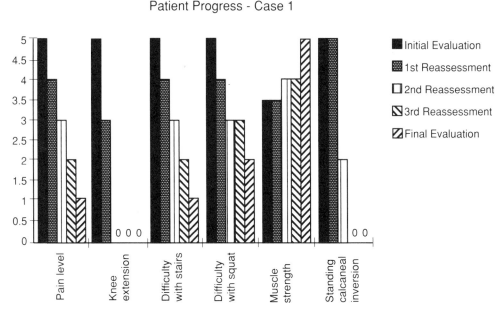

FIGURE 8–8. Summary of OA patient's progress in six areas: pain, knee extension, range of motion, squatting, stair climbing, strength, and calcaneal alignment in standing. 0 = full knee extension and neutral calcaneal alignment. Y axis indicates the following initial findings: pain level 5/10; knee extension 5 degrees from full extension; difficulty with stairs 5/10; difficulty with squat 5/5; muscle strength 3.5/5; and 5 degrees calcaneal varus in standing. See text in Case Study 1 for additional descriptions of these scales.

CASE STUDY 2: RHEUMATOID ARTHRITIS

HISTORY

The patient was a 57-year-old woman whose RA began approximately 17 years ago. Her initial symptoms included knee pain and swelling. Several months after onset, the knee pain and swelling resolved while symptoms in the upper extremities continued. Knee symptoms did not return until approximately 3 months ago, when she noted swelling and pain. The patient was admitted for a 7-day inpatient stay to control the current increase in acuity of her arthritis. The patient reported that her left knee joint was quite swollen and painful on admission. However, 2 days ago her knee joint was aspirated and injected with a corticosteroid. She reported a dramatic decrease in both swelling and pain after the aspiration and injection. On the day of the physical therapy initial evaluation, she reported a pain level of 4/10 at rest, which increased to 6/10 on weight bearing. At the time of admission the patient was doing minimal light housework and performing no regular exercise. Her roentgenograms of the knee joints revealed some erosions along the joint margins and juxta-articular osteoporosis.

EVALUATION

The patient arose very slowly from her chair, ambulating slowly with an antalgic gait, with a significant decrease in limb stance time on the left. Stride length and cadence were both decreased. The amount of ankle joint plantarflexion in the late stance phase of gait was decreased, resulting in a "shuffling" gait pattern.

Palpation of the left knee revealed minimal tenderness over the lateral joint line. There was no knee joint effusion but there was a pocket of swelling posteriorly, which appeared to be in the semimembranosus bursa.

The patient's pelvis was level, and no leg length discrepancy was noted. The right tibia was in neutral alignment relative to the floor. The left tibia was in 4 degrees of varus relative to the floor (Fig. 8–9). On the right, the vertical line through the calcaneus was perpendicular to the floor (forming the calcaneal-floor angle); on the left, the vertical line through the calcaneus was in 5 degrees of varus relative to the floor (Fig. 8–9). Subtalar neutral was at 10 degrees of inversion on the right and 5 degrees of inversion on the left. With the subtalar joint in neutral, the forefoot had a rigid plantarflexed first ray bilaterally. Figure 8–10 illustrates both subtalar neutral and the forefoot-to-rearfoot relationship on the right. Figure 8–11 illustrates subtalar neutral and the forefoot-to-rearfoot relationship on the left.

Hip ROM was grossly within normal limits bilaterally. Right knee and ankle ROM were also within normal limits bilaterally. The left knee had full flexion but lacked 5 degrees from full extension. Left ankle dorsiflexion was 5 degrees with the knee flexed. Plantarflexion on the left was within normal limits. Subtalar inversion on the right was 25 degrees and on the left 15 degrees. Subtalar eversion was 5 degrees on the right and lacked 5 degrees on the left. The subtalar deformity/alignment problem was reducible, with a capsular or soft tissue end feel. Therefore, improvement of subtalar eversion with joint mobilization was thought to be possible. Muscle flexibility of the iliopsoas and TFL muscles was within

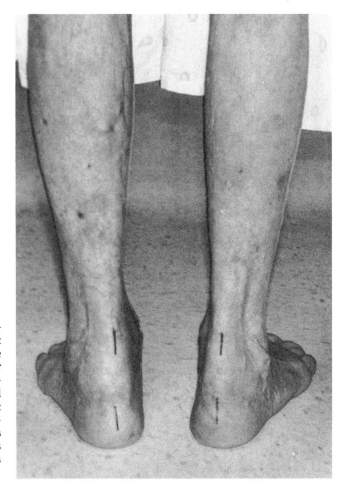

FIGURE 8-9. Position of calcaneus in standing. The right calcaneus is in line with the vertical line along the tibia, or perpendicular to the floor. Although there is pronounced swelling surrounding the left medial malleolus, the relationship between the vertical lines on the tibia and the calcaneus indicates that the left calcaneus is in varus. RA patient.

normal limits. Tightness was recorded in the hamstring muscles, with SLR measuring 60 degrees bilaterally. The rectus femoris muscle tightness was demonstrated with the Ely test, being positive bilaterally at 45 degrees. (In the Ely test, the patient is placed in prone position with the hip and knee extended. The knee is passively flexed. If rectus femoris muscle tightness is present, the hip will begin to flex as the knee is being passively flexed. The knee joint angle is recorded when hip flexion is first observed.) Gastrocnemius muscle tightness was demonstrated by a lack of dorsiflexion 5 degrees from neutral with the knee extended.

Muscle strength was decreased throughout the lower extremities, with proximal hip girdle musculature being weaker than the more distal muscle groups. Hip extensor and abductor muscles had 3/5 strength, hamstrings were 4 − /5, and the remainder of the lower extremity muscles (including the quadriceps femoris muscles) were 4 + /5.

Joint mobility and stability of the right knee was within normal limits. Joint mobility in medial, lateral, anterior, and posterior gliding and tibial rotation were slightly increased on the left. Patellar mobility was within normal limits on the right but decreased in superior, inferior, and lateral gliding on the left.

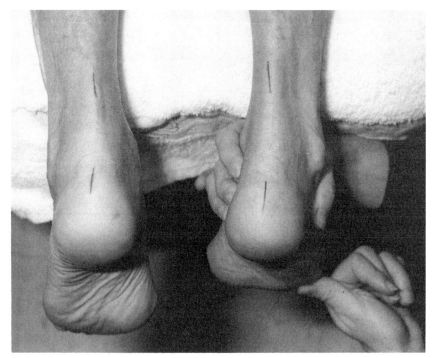

FIGURE 8–10. Right forefoot/rearfoot relationship indicates a plantar-flexed first ray. A plantar-flexed first ray is present when the first metatarsal is in valgus (eversion) relative to the neutral position of the rearfoot. The mobility of the plantar-flexed first ray is assessed by the examiner as either fixed or reducible. A fixed or rigid plantar-flexed first ray usually requires a lateral forefoot post to control the subtalar joint during standing and walking. Right foot of an RA patient.

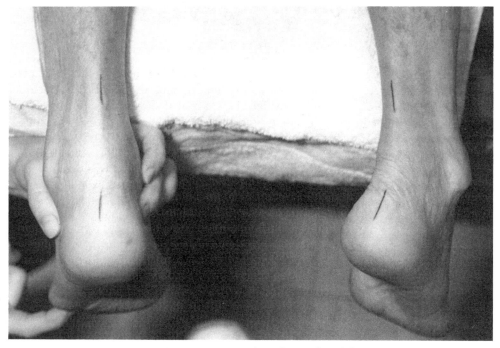

FIGURE 8–11. Subtalar neutral in inversion with a plantar-flexed first ray. RA patient.

The patient related difficulty getting in and out of a car at a level of 5 on a scale of 0 to 10. Getting out of the bathtub and going upstairs were rated at a level of 4/10.

ASSESSMENT

The patient had a long history of RA with previous involvement being in the upper extremities and with the knee joints fairly well preserved. She was now resolving a generalized increase in the acuity of her RA that had involved the left knee. Evidence of residual inflammation was present, and the patient appeared to be in a subacute stage of her disease. Minimal deformity and loss of motion, and moderate loss of function indicated that her prognosis for rehabilitation was good. The major problems at this time were: (1) slight evidence of swelling; (2) slight loss of knee extension, ankle dorsiflexion, and subtalar inversion and eversion in the left lower extremity; (3) decreased muscle flexibility of hamstrings, rectus femoris, and gastrocnemius muscles; (4) alignment problems of rearfoot and forefoot in the left lower extremity; (5) tibiofemoral joint hypermobility with patellar hypomobility on the left; (6) impaired function; and (7) pain in the left knee.

TREATMENT

The patient was treated for 6 consecutive days as an inpatient, then discharged to outpatient physical therapy twice a week for 4 weeks. The patient spent 1 hour in physical therapy at each visit. Part of the treatment addressed upper extremity problems; these aspects of the treatment will not be discussed here.

Treatments 1 to 6

Treatments 1 to 6 were initiated with an ice pack applied to the patient's left knee for 20 minutes to minimize the swelling in her left posterior knee. The ice packs were followed by gentle AROM, and patella and subtalar mobilization of grades III and IV. Gentle AROM was chosen as a way of "loosening" and warming up the joint prior to stretching. Patellar mobilization was performed primarily in a superior direction to facilitate knee extension but also in an inferior direction to promote extensibility of the rectus femoris muscle. The subtalar joint was mobilized into eversion to improve alignment of the calcaneus in standing. An improved alignment was intended to minimize stress on the knee and to provide the needed calcaneal eversion, which is required just after heelstrike and through the early stance phase of gait.

Contract-relax stretching of all tight muscle groups was carried out for the same reasons noted in case 1. A strengthening program similar to that used in case 1 was implemented for a similar reason. One difference in the program was that cuff weights were not used and the patient began with only five repetitions and advised to add one repetition each day. The rationale for beginning the strengthening at a lower intensity for this patient was twofold. First, she was weaker and in generally poorer condition than the patient in case 1. Second, she was in a more acute stage of her arthritis than was the first case. The patient was also seen in the pool daily for a water-walking program and for strengthening and flexibility exercises. The rationale for adding a pool program at this time was to use the mild warmth of the water to minimize joint stiffness and the buoyancy of the water to decrease compressive forces on the joint. The water also provides resistance that can be controlled by the patient's speeding up or slowing down the movement of her exercise.

Reassessment

Upon discharge from the hospital, the patient had no evidence of knee swelling and had regained full knee extension. Dorsiflexion with the knee flexed was 10 degrees. Subtalar joint inversion was 20 degrees, and subtalar joint eversion was 0 degrees on the left. SLR was 70 degrees bilaterally, the Ely test was positive bilaterally at 65 degrees, and left ankle dorsiflexion with the knee straight was 0 degrees (neutral). Hip extensor and abductor muscles were 3 + /5, hamstrings were 4/5, and the quadriceps femoris muscle had increased to 5/5. Alignment in standing had not changed from the initial evaluation. Patellar mobility was slightly increased. Pain and difficulty getting in and out of a car was now rated as 3/10. Getting in and out of the bathtub and going upstairs were both unchanged from the initial evaluation. Based on these measurements, the patient seemed to have improved in all areas except standing alignment. Range, strength, muscle flexibility, patellar mobility, and function had all shown significant improvement clinically.

Treatments 7 to 13

Because pain and swelling were minimal at this time, the ice was discontinued at the time of the first outpatient treatment (treatment 7). Patella and subtalar joint mobilization were continued along with contract-relax stretching. A 1 lb weight was added to the strengthening exercises. Isometric quadriceps femoris and hamstring muscle strengthening exercises were continued so as not to aggravate the joint. Muscles surrounding the hip joint were strengthened isotonically. After discharge the patient continued the pool program at her local YMCA.

On the 13th treatment, flexible orthoses were added to the patient's shoes, since gains in subtalar motion had plateaued. A medial wedge was added to both rearfeet since the subtalar neutral was in inversion bilaterally. Again, care was taken to provide only enough medial posting to accommodate the deformity. A lateral forefoot wedge was added to compensate for the rigid plantarflexed first ray on the left foot.

Final Evaluation

At the time of discharge from the 4-week outpatient program, the patient had no evidence of swelling and had full range of motion at the knee and talocrural joints. Subtalar inversion on the left was now 25 degrees with subtalar eversion lacking 5 degrees from neutral. SLR tests were 75 degrees bilaterally. The Ely test was negative at this time. Dorsiflexion with the knee extended was 5 degrees. Hip extensor and abductor muscles had increased to 4/5 (Good). Hamstrings had increased to 4 + /5 and quadriceps femoris muscle had maintained the 5/5 strength achieved as an inpatient. Patellar mobility on the left now seemed essentially the same as on the right. The left tibiofemoral joint continued to be slightly hypermobile but not grossly unstable. The increase in muscle strength will hope-

Patient Progress - Case 2

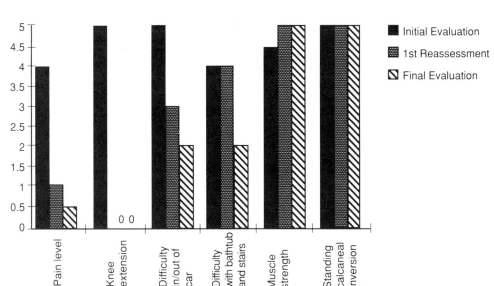

FIGURE 8-12. Summary of RA patient's progress in six areas: pain, knee extension, range of motion, getting in and out of the car and bathtub, going up and down stairs, muscle strength, and the position of the calcaneus in standing. 0 = full knee extension. Y axis indicates the following initial findings: pain level 4/10; knee extension 5 degrees from full extension; difficulty in/out of car 5/10; difficulty with bathtub and stairs 4/10; muscle strength 4.5/5; and 5 degrees of calcaneal varus in standing. See text in Case Study 2 for additional descriptions of these scales.

fully minimize this mild instability. The difficulty of all functional activities were rated at 2 on the 0-to-10 scale. The patient's gait pattern had significantly improved. She no longer exhibited an antalgic limp. Stride length, cadence, and gait velocity had increased. The patient was tolerating the wedges and flexible shock-absorbing orthoses very well and felt that she had less knee pain when she used them. She was encouraged to continued a strengthening and stretching home program 3 to 4 days per week and to continue her water exercise 2 to 3 days per week.

The patient had achieved most of our goals and was committed to continuing her home program. Figure 8-12 summarizes the patient's overall progress in pain reduction, knee extension, function, strength, and alignment. Follow-up phone calls at 1 and 6 months indicated that she was following through with the program except during an occasional small flare-up. Functional difficulty scores were slightly higher (indicating a minimal loss of function) at 6 months, and pain level had risen only slightly. Overall the patient had significantly benefited from the combination inpatient-outpatient program.

SUMMARY

This chapter reviewed the clinical features and problem-solving approach to management of patients with OA and RA involving the knee joint. Emphasis was placed on a thorough musculoskeletal evaluation, a clear delineation of the patient's problems and goals, and development of a treatment plan based on a physical therapy problem list. The problem list and goals modified in a timely manner based on regular reassessment. The importance of stage or acuity of disease and early intervention was emphasized. A systematic approach to evaluation and treatment improves the functional states in arthritic patients who otherwise present with a limited prognosis for recovery.

REFERENCES

1. Brinkman, JR and Perry, J: Rate and range of knee motion during ambulation in healthy and arthritic subjects. Phys Ther 65:7, 1985.
2. Schumacher, HR (ed): Primer on the Rheumatic Diseases, ed 9. Arthritis Foundation, Atlanta, 1988.
3. Goldenberg, DL, Egan, MS, and Cohen, AS: Inflammatory synovitis in degenerative joint disease. J Rheumatol 9:204, 1982.
4. Panush, RS and Brown, DG: Exercise in arthritis. Sports Med 4:54, 1987.
5. Goldin, RH, et al: Clinical and radiological survey of the incidence of osteoarthritis among obese patients. Ann Rheum Dis 35:349, 1976.
6. Leach, RE, Baumgard, S, and Broom, J: Obesity: Its relationship to OA of the knee. Clin Orthop 93:271, 1973.
7. Hartz, AS, et al: The association of obesity with joint pain and osteoarthritis in the HANES data. Journal of Chronic Disease 39:311, 1986.
8. Radin, EL and Rose, RM: Role of subchondral bone in initiation and progress of cartilage damage. Clin Orthop 213:34, 1986.
9. Kennedy, JC, Alexander, IJ, and Hayes, KC: Nerve supply of the human knee and its functional importance. Sports Med 10:329, 1982.
10. Stratford, P: Electromyography of the quads in subjects with normal knees and acutely effused knees. Phys Ther 62:279, 1981.
11. Spencer, JD, Hayes, KC, and Alexander, IJ: Knee joint effusion and quadriceps reflex inhibition in man. Arch Phys Med Rehabil 65:171, 1984.
12. Fahrer, H, et al: Knee effusion and reflex inhibition of the quadriceps. J Bone Joint Surg [Br] 70:635, 1988.
13. Doxey, GE: The influence of patellofemoral pain on electromyographic activity during submaximal isometric contractions. Master's thesis. University of Utah, Salt Lake City, 1986.
14. Mariani, PP and Caruso, I: An electromyographic investigation of subluxation of the patella. J Bone Joint Surg [Br] 61:169, 1979.
15. Morrissey, MC: Reflex inhibition of thigh muscles in knee injury causes and treatment. Sports Med 7:263, 1989.
16. Moore, KL: Clinically Oriented Anatomy, ed 2. Williams & Wilkins, Baltimore, 1985, p 529.
17. deAndrae, JR, et al: Joint distention and reflex muscle inhibition in the knee. J Bone Joint Surg [Am] 47:313, 1965.
18. Norkin, CC and Levangie, PK: Joint Structure and Function: A Comprehensive Analysis. FA Davis, Philadelphia, 1983.
19. Hicks, JE: Exercise in patients with inflammatory arthritis and connective tissue disease. Rheum Dis Clin North Am (16):4, November 1990.
20. Muller, EA: Influence of training and of inactivity on muscle strength. Arch Phys Med Rehabil 51:449, 1970.
21. Hoppenfeld, S: Physical Examination of the Spine and Extremities. Appleton-Century-Crofts, New York, 1976.
22. Kendall, FP and Kendall, EK: Muscles Testing and Function. Williams & Wilkins, Baltimore, 1983.
23. Daniels, L and Worthingham, C: Muscle Testing. WB Saunders, Philadelphia, 1972.
24. Moore, ML: The measurement of joint motion. II. The technique of goniometry. Physical Therapy Review 29:256, 1949.
25. Root, M, et al: Normal and Abnormal Function of the Foot, Vol 2. Clinical Biomechanics Corporation, Los Angeles, 1976.
26. May, BJ and Dennis, JK: Expert decision making in physical therapy: A survey of practitioners. Phys Ther 71:190, 1991.
27. Payton, OD: Clinical reasoning process in physical therapy. Phys Ther 65:924, 1985.
28. Jensen, GM, et al: The novice versus the experienced clinician: Insights into the work of the physical therapist. Phys Ther 70:314, 1990.
29. Banwell, BF: Exercise for arthritis. In Banwell, BF and Gall, V, (eds): Physical Therapy Management of Arthritis. Churchill Livingstone, New York, 1987.
30. Haralson, K: Physical modalities. In Banwell, BF and Gall, V, (eds): Physical Therapy Management of Arthritis. Churchill Livingstone, New York, 1987.

31. Michlovitz, SL: The use of heat and cold in the management of rheumatic diseases. In Michlovitz, SL (ed): Thermal Agents in Rehabilitation. FA Davis, Philadelphia, 1990.
32. Kirk, JA and Kersley, GD: Heat and cold in the physical treatment of rheumatoid arthritis of the knee: A controlled clinical trial. Annals of Physical Medicine 9:270, 1968.
33. Williams, J, Harvey, J, and Tannebaum, H: Use of superficial heat versus ice for the rheumatoid arthritic shoulder: A pilot study. Physiotherapy Canada 38:8, 1986.
34. Utsinger, PD, Bonner, F, and Hogan, N: Efficacy of cryotherapy and thermotherapy in the management of rheumatoid arthritis pain: Evidence for endorphin effect (abstr). Arthritis Rheum (Suppl) 25:113, 1982.
35. Swezey, RL: Essentials of physical management and rehabilitation in arthritis. Semin Arthritis Rheum 3:349, 1974.
36. Warren, CG, Lehmann, JD, and Koblanski, JN: Heat and stretch procedures: An evaluation using rat tail tendon. Arch Phys Med Rehabil 52:465, 1971.
37. Banwell, BF: Therapeutic heat and cold. In Riggs, GK and Gall, EP (eds): Rheumatic Diseases: Rehabilitation and Management. Butterworth & Co, Boston, 1984.
38. Downey, JA: Physiological effects of heat and cold. Phys Ther 44:713, 1964.
39. Hollander, JL and Horvath, SM: Influence of physical therapy procedures on intra-articular temperatures of normal and arthritic subjects. Am J Med Sci 218:543, 1949.
40. Mainardi, C, et al: Rheumatoid arthritis: Failure of daily heat therapy to affect its progression. Arch Phys Med Rehabil 60:390, 1979.
41. Lehmann, JR and DeLateur, B: Therapeutic heat and cold in arthritis. In Licht, S (ed): Arthritis and Physical Medicine, Vol 2. Physical Medicine Library. Elizabeth Licht Publisher, New Haven, 1969.
42. Horvath, SM and Hollander, JL: Intra-articular temperature as a measure of joint reaction. J Clin Invest 28:469, 1949.
43. Harris, ED, Jr and McCroskey, JA: Influence of temperature and fibril stability on degradation of cartilage collagen by rheumatoid synovial collagenase. N Engl J Med 290:1, 1974.
44. Freibal, A and Fast, A: Deep heating of joints: A reconsideration. Arch Phys Med Rehabil 57:513, 1976.
45. Grant, AE: Massage with ice (cryokinetics) in the treatment of painful conditions of the musculoskeletal system. Arch Phys Med Rehabil 45:233, 1964.
46. Rembe, EC: Use of cryotherapy on the postsurgical rheumatoid hand. Phys Ther 50:19, 1970.
47. Lane, LE: Localized hypothermia for the relief of pain in musculoskeletal injuries. Phys Ther 51:182, 1871.
48. Kangilaski, J: Baggie therapy: Simple relief for arthritic knees. JAMA 247:317, 1981.
49. Pegg, SMH, Littler, TR, and Littler, EN: A trial of ice therapy and exercise in chronic arthritis. Physiotherapy 55:51, 1969.
50. Tepperman, PS and Devlin, M: Therapeutic heat and cold: A practitioner's guide. Postgrad Med 73:69, 1983.
51. Wright, V and Johns, RJ: Physical factors concerned with the stiffness of normal and diseased joints. Bulletin of the Johns Hopkins Hospital 106:215, 1960.
52. Backlund, L and Tiselius, P: Objective measurement of joint stiffness in rheumatoid arthritis. Acta Rheumatologica Scandinavica 12:275, 1967.
53. Clarke, GR, et al: Evaluation of physiotheraphy in the treatment of osteoarthrosis of the knee. Rheumatology and Rehabilitation 13:190, 1974.
54. Lewis, T: Observations upon the reactions of the vessels of the human skin to cold. Heart 15:177, 1930.
55. Fox, RH and Wyatt, HT: Cold-induced vasodilation in various areas of the body surface in man. J Physiol (Lond) 162:289, 1962.
56. Major, TC, Schwinghamer, JM, and Winston, S: Cutaneous and skeletal muscle vascular responses to hypothermia. Am J Physiol 240:868, 1981.
57. Bierman, W and Friedlander, M: The penetration effect of cold. Archives of Physical Therapy 21:585, 1940.
58. Cobbold, AF and Lewis, OJ: Blood flow to the knee joint of the dog: Effect of heating, cooling and adrenaline. J Physiol (Lond) 132:379, 1956.
59. Kern, H, et al: Kryotherapie. Das verhalten der gelenkstemperatur unter eisapplikation: Grundlage für die praktische anwendung. Wren-Klin-Wochenschr 96:832, 1984.
60. Kumar, N and Redford, SB: Transcutaneous nerve stimulation in rheumatoid arthritis. Arch Phys Med Rehabil 63:595, 1982.
61. Mannheimer, C, Lund, S, and Carlsson, CA: The effect of transcutaneous electrical nerve stimulation on joint pain in patients with rheumatoid arthritis. Scand J Rheumatol 7:13, 1978.
62. Abelson, K, et al: Transcutaneous electrical nerve stimulation in rheumatoid arthritis. N Z Med J 96:156, 1983.
63. Lewis, D, Lewis, B, and Sturrock, RD: Transcutaneous electrical nerve stimulation in osteoarthrosis: A therapeutic alternative? Ann Rheum Dis 43:47, 1984.
64. Taylor, P, Hallett, M, and Flaherty, L: Treatment of osteoarthritis of the knee with TENS. Pain 11:233, 1981.
65. Mannheimer, C and Carlson, CA: The analgesic effect of transcutaneous electrical nerve stimulation in patients with rheumatoid arthritis: A comparative study of different pulse patterns. Pain 6:329, 1979.

66. Gerber, LH and Hicks, JE: Exercise in the rheumatic diseases. In Basmajian, JV and Wolf, SL (eds): Therapeutic Exercise. Williams & Wilkins, Baltimore, 1990.
67. Gerber, L and Hicks, J: Rehabilitative management of rheumatic diseases. In Hicks, JE, Nicholas, JJ, and Swezey, R (eds): Handbook of Rehabilitative Rheumatology. Contact Associates, Bayport, NY, 1988, p. 82.
68. Hicks, JE and Nicholas, JJ: Treatment utilized in rehabilitative rheumatology. In Hicks, JE, Nicholas, JJ, and Swezey, R (eds): Handbook of Rehabilitative Rheumatology. Contact Associates, Bayport, NY, 1988, p 31.
69. Fred, DM: Rest versus activity in arthritis and physical medicine. In Licht, S (ed): Arthritis and Physical Medicine. Waverly Press, Baltimore, 1969.
70. Calabro, JJ and Wykert, J: The Truth About Arthritis Care. David McKay, New York, 1977.
71. Banwell BF: Exercise and mobility in arthritis. Nurs Clin North Am 19:6054, 1984.
72. Wickersham, BA: The exercise program. In Riggs, GK and Gall, EP (eds): Rheumatic Diseases: Rehabilitation and Management. Butterworth & Co, Boston, 1984.
73. Gerber, LH: Principles and their application in rehabilitation of patients with rheumatic diseases. In Kelley, WN, et al (eds): Textbook of Rheumatology. WB Saunders, Philadelphia, 1981.
74. Swezey, RL: Rehabilitation aspects in arthritis. In McCarty, DJ (ed): Arthritis and Related Disorders, ed 9. Lea & Febiger, Philadelphia, 1979.
75. Morrissey, MC: Reflex inhibition of thigh muscles in knee injury causes and treatment. Sports Med 7:263, 1989.
76. Moynes, DR: Patellar malalignment. Unpublished material. Centinela Hospital Medical Center Biomechanics Laboratory. Inglewood, CA, 1985.
77. Hislop, HJ: Quantitative changes in human muscular strength during isometric exercise. Phys Ther 43:21, 1963.
78. Bos, RR and Blosser, TG: An electromyographic study of vastus medialis and vastus lateralis during selected isometric exercises. Medicine and Science in Sports 2:218, 1970.
79. Lindh, M: Increase of muscle strength from isometric quadriceps exercises at different knee angles. Scand J Rehabil Med 11:33, 1979.
80. Graves, JE, et al: Effect of training frequency and specificity on isometric lumbar extension strength. Spine 15:504, 1990.
81. Pelletier, JR, Findley, TW, and Gemma, SA: Isometric exercise for an individual with hemophilic arthropathy. Phys Ther 67:1359, 1987.
82. Currier, OP, Lehman, J, and Lightfoot, P: Electrical stimulation in exercise of the quadriceps femoris muscle. Phys Ther 59:1508, 1979.
83. Lucca, JA and Recchiuti, SJ: Effect of electromyographic biofeedback on an isometric strengthening program. Phys Ther 63:200, 1983.
84. O'Connor, P: Effect of breathing instruction on blood pressure responses during isometric exercise. Phys Ther 69:757, 1989.
85. Bender, JA and Kaplan, HM: The multiple angle testing method for the evaluation of muscle strength. J Bone Joint Surg [Am] 45:135, 1963.
86. Gardner, GW: Specificity of strength changes of the exercised and nonexercised limb following isometric training. Research Quarterly 34:98, 1963.
87. Machover, S and Sapecky, AJ: Effect of isometric exercise on the quadriceps muscle in patients with RA. Arch Phys Med Rehabil 69:928, 1988.
88. DeLateur, BJ and Lehmann, JF: A test of the DeLorme axiom. Arch Phys Med Rehabil 49:245, 1968.
89. Delateur, BJ, Lehmann, J, and Stonebridge, J: Isotonic versus isometric exercise: A double shift transfer of training study. Arch Phys Med Rehabil 53:212, 1972.
90. Delateur, BJ, et al: Comparison of effectiveness of isokinetic and isotonic exercise in quadriceps strengthening. Arch Phys Med Rehabil 53:60, 1982.
91. DeLorme, TL and Watkins, AL: Techniques of progressive resistance exercises. Arch Phys Med Rehabil 47:737, 1966.
92. Noble, L: Relative effects of isometric and isotonic exercise programs on selected circumferential measures. American Corrective Therapy Journal. September–October, 1972.
93. Souza, DR and Gross, MT: Comparison of vastus medialis obliquus: Vastus lateralis muscle integrated electrographic ratios between healthy subjects and patients with patellofemoral pain. Phys Ther 7:310, 1991.
94. Pipes, TV and Wilmore, JH: Isokinetic vs isotonic strength training in adult men. Sports Med 7:463, 1975.
95. Timm, KE: Postsurgical knee rehabilitation: A five year study of four methods and 5,381 patients. Am J Sports Med 16:463, 1988.
96. Van Eijden, TMGJ, de Borr, W, and Verburg, J: A dynamometer for the measurement of the extension torque of the lower leg during static and dynamic contractions of the quadriceps femoris muscle. J Biomech 16:1019, 1983.
97. Soderberg, GL: Kinesiology: Application to Pathological Movement. Williams & Wilkins, Baltimore, 1986, p 208.

98. Smidt, GL: Biomechanical analysis of knee flexion and extension. J Biomech 79, 1973.

99. Jayson, MIVB and Dixon, SJ: Intra-articular pressure in rheumatoid arthritis of the knee. III. Pressure changes during joint use. Ann Rheum Dis 29:401, 1970.

100. Morrison, JB: The mechanics of the knee joint in relation to normal walking. J Biomech 3:51, 1970.

101. Antich, TJ and Brewster, CE: Modification of quadriceps femoris muscle exercises during knee rehabilitation. Phys Ther 66:1246, 1986.

102. Wessel, J and Quinney, HA: Pain experienced by persons with rheumatoid arthritis during isometric exercise and isokinetic exercise. Physiotherapy Canada 36:131, 1984.

103. Krebs, DE: Biofeedback in therapeutic exercise. In Basmajian, JV and Wolf, SL (eds): Therapeutic Exercise. Williams & Wilkins, Baltimore, 1990.

104. Morrissey, MC: Electromyostimulation from a clinical perspective: A review. Sports Med 6:29, 1988.

105. Eriksson, E and Haggmark, T: Comparison of isometric muscle training and electrical stimulation supplementing isometric muscle training in the recovery after major knee ligament surgery: A preliminary report. Am J Sports Med 7:3, 1979.

106. Morrison, JB: Bioengineering analysis of force actions transmitted by the knee joint. Biomedical Engineering 3:164, 1960.

107. Paul, JP: The biomechanics of the hip joint and its clinical relevance. Proc R Soc Lond [Biol] 59:943, 1966.

108. Burckhardt, CS, et al: Assessing physical fitness of women with rheumatic disease. Arthritis Care and Research 1:38, 1988.

109. Nordemar, R: Physical training in rheumatoid arthritis: A controlled long-term study. II. Functional capacity and general attitudes. Scand J Rheumatol 10:25, 1981.

110. Harkcom, TM, et al: Therapeutic value of graded aerobic exercise training in rheumatoid arthritis. Arthritis Rheum 28:32, 1985.

111. Minor, MA, et al: Efficacy of physical conditioning exercise in patients with rheumatoid arthritis and osteoarthritis. Arthritis Rheum 32:1396, 1989.

112. Ekblom, B, et al: Physical performance in patients with rheumatoid arthritis. Scand J Rheumatol 3:121, 1974.

113. Ekblom, B, et al: Effect of short-term physical training on patients with rheumatoid arthritis: A 6-month follow-up study. Scand J Rheumatol 4:87, 1975.

114. Ekblom, B, et al: Effect of short-term physical training on patients with rheumatoid arthritis. Scand J Rheumatol 4:80, 1985.

115. Beals, C, et al: Oxygen cost of work in rheumatoid arthritis patients. Clin Res 28:752A, 1980.

116. Minor, MA, et al: Efficacy of physical conditioning exercise in patients with rheumatoid arthritis and osteoarthritis. Arthritis Rheum, 32:11, 1989.

117. Cavanagh, PR and Lafortune, MA: Ground reaction forces in distance running. J Biomech 13:397, 1980.

118. Allen, ME: Arthritis and adaptive walking and running. Rheum Dis Clin North Am 16:4, 1990.

119. O'Toole, ML, et al: Overuse injuries in ultraendurance triathletes. Am J Sports Med 17:514, 1989.

120. Ericson, MO and Nisell, R: Tibiofemoral forces during ergometer cycling. Am J Sports Med 14:285, 1986.

121. Namey, TC: Adaptive bicycling. Rheum Dis Clin North Am 16:4, 1990.

122. Golland, A: Basic hydrotherapy. Physiotherapy 67:258, 1981.

123. Huss, D and Rud, A: Unpublished material. Memorial Hospital, Boulder, CO, 1986.

124. Whalen, S, et al: An Introduction to Aquatic Therapy. Bryn Mawr Rehabilitation Hospital, Malvern, PA, 1985.

125. Levin, R: Gait and mobility. In Banwell, BF and Gall, V (eds): Physical Therapy Management of Arthritis. Churchill Livingstone, New York, 1988.

126. Moncur, C and Shields, ML: Gait and ambulation. In Riggs, GK and Gall, EP (eds): Rheumatic Diseases: Rehabilitation and Management, Butterworth & Co, Boston, 1984.

127. Brasher, HR and Raney, RB: Shand's Handbook of Orthopedic Surgery, ed 9. CV Mosby, St Louis, 1978, p 283.

128. Paris, SV: Spinal Dysfunction: Course Notes. Institute of Graduate Health Sciences, Atlanta, 1979, p 452.

129. Lorig, KL and Fries, JF: The Arthritis Helpbook. Addison-Wesley, Reading, MA, 1990.

Protective Injuries to the Knee

CHAPTER 9

Rehabilitation of Intra-articular Reconstructions

Andrew R. Einhorn, PT, ATC
Michael Sawyer, PT
Brian Tovin, MMSc, PT, ATC

More, perhaps, than that of any other orthopedic injury, the surgical management and rehabilitation of patients with anterior cruciate ligament (ACL) injuries have evolved a great deal in the last few decades. Surgical management, for instance, has progressed from procedures that violated knee joint integrity without addressing normal ACL anatomy and mechanics to less invasive techniques that result in minimal tissue trauma and restore knee mechanics. Rehabilitation has changed from the use of cautious protocols that took as long as 12 months to accelerated programs incorporating a wide variety of exercise variables. A corollary to these changes is that the rehabilitation specialist now must thoroughly understand knee anatomy and mechanics, the sequalae of ACL injury, and the surgical variables affecting the rehabilitation period.

The medical/surgical management of patients with ACL injury has included conservative treatment without repair,[1-4] extra-articular reconstruction,[5] primary repair of the torn ligament without augmentation,[6,7] intra-articular reconstruction using a graft,[8] and combined extra-articular and intra-articular reconstructions.[9] The use of long-term prospective studies has provided some conclusive information concerning the efficacy of each procedure to restore knee function.

Nonsurgical management is used in the presence of both partial- and full-thickness tears of the ACL, but this approach has led to functional disability in patients who desire to return to their preinjury levels of activity.[1-3] Therefore, management of patients with ACL injuries who are active in sports or exercise usually involves surgery.[4]

Different surgical procedures for ACL injury are reported in the literature. Isolated extra-articular procedures are advocated by Andrews and Carson[5] for mild to moderate, chronic anterolateral rotatory instability of the knee and in those patients having meniscal repairs without intra-articular stabilization. Extra-articular procedures reduce the healing and rehabilitation time compared with that for patients who undergo intra-articular ACL reconstruction. Extra-articular grafts are sometimes used to augment intra-articular reconstructions, although most surgeons have discarded this procedure as ineffective in re-establishing the biomechanical integrity of the knee joint.[9]

Direct repairs without augmentation of the injured ACL yields poor clinical results.[6,7] The healing capability of a torn ACL is poor and will be discussed later in this chapter. Most surgeons prefer isolated intra-articular reconstructions because these procedures directly restore the anatomic and biomechanical deficits of the injured ACL.[8] The controversy, therefore, has shifted focus from the surgical management of ACL injuries to rehabilitation.[10]

This chapter reviews the principles of rehabilitation for patients with intra-articular ACL reconstructions. The initial sections review the basic surgical considerations associated with ACL reconstruction that are necessary to understand and incorporate in the development of a rehabilitation program. The middle portion reviews the general biomechanical guidelines for rehabilitation of the ACL-reconstructed knee. The final portion presents case studies of rehabilitation of patients who underwent intra-articular ACL reconstructions. These studies illustrate the problem-solving approach in rehabilitation. This chapter is not intended as a review of surgical techniques that are associated with intra-articular ACL reconstruction. That information has been described elsewhere.[11] Rather, this chapter provides information on the surgical and biomechanical factors relevant to the rehabilitation program and their influence on the problem-solving process in patients with intra-articular ACL reconstructions.

SURGICAL FACTORS IN REHABILITATION

Rehabilitation is integral to restore normal function in the ACL-reconstructed knee.[12] Because the type and length of rehabilitation is influenced by the surgical procedure, the therapist must understand the variables associated with ACL reconstruction.[12–14] Some of these variables include the type of surgical approach (arthrotomy and arthroscopy), the type of graft, the method of graft placement, the method of graft fixation, and the timing of surgical intervention relative to the initial injury.

Arthrotomy versus Arthroscopically Assisted Procedures

Two types of surgical approaches commonly used for ACL reconstruction are arthrotomy and arthroscopically-assisted techniques.[15] The type of approach may influence the rate of exercise progression, as well as the patient's rate of improvement during the early phases of rehabilitation. The more traditional of the two approaches is *arthrotomy*, which is sometimes referred to as an *open technique*. This approach involves exposing the knee joint through a parapatellar incision. The advantage of this approach is that the surgeon is provided with an extensive exposure into the knee joint and has a thorough visualization of the injured tissues. The subsequent techniques of careful surgical preparation and placement of the osseous tunnels through the tibia and femur, along with careful preparation and placement of the graft, can result in good long-term results with an open technique. To facilitate early motion of the knee joint, some surgeons perform lateral parapatellar incisions rather than the traditional medial parapatellar incisions.[16] By placing the incisions along the lateral aspect of the knee joint, the surgeon can avoid disrupting the vastus medialis muscle, thereby enhancing postoperative muscle reeducation progress.

The disadvantages of arthrotomy result directly from the surgical disruption of the knee joint capsule. In addition, when using a parapatellar incision, the surgeon must sublux or dislocate the patella to see the intra-articular structures. The disturbance of the knee joint capsule and patellofemoral joint usually causes increased pain and decreased range of motion (ROM). Early postoperative rehabilitation is further delayed by pain inhibition of the quadriceps femoris muscles. The patient will usually have difficulty performing a satisfactory contraction of the quadriceps femoris muscle and specific difficulty in attempting to selectively recruit and contract the vastus medialis muscle. The delay in quadriceps femoris muscle re-education results in a longer period of ambulation using assistive devices, because the patient will be unable to safely stabilize and control the knee joint. The large parapatellar incision can result in a painful and indurated scar and delay restoration of full ROM of the knee joint.

Current advances in technology have resulted in the use of *arthroscopically-assisted* intra-articular ACL reconstructions. The advantages of arthroscopy result directly from preserving the integrity of the knee joint capsule. In addition, the posterior horns of the meniscus and the intercondylar notch of the femur are better visualized through the arthroscope because the structures are magnified and the joint distention enhances the field of vision in a tight knee. This approach results in the avoidance of a large parapatellar incision, a lower risk of infection, less postoperative pain, enhanced quadriceps femoris muscle contraction, and fewer adhesions in both the patellofemoral and tibiofemoral joints. Postoperative rehabilitation is usually aggressive, focusing on restoring early passive ROM to the knee joint, strength to both the quadriceps femoris and hamstring muscles, and independent ambulation within the first 4 postoperative weeks.

Graft Selection

The type of graft selected for intra-articular ACL reconstruction can influence the activities performed during the early phases of rehabilitation.[13,14] According to Noyes and associates,[13] an ideal graft should possess the following characteristics: mechanical properties similar to the replaced ligament; availability for use as a graft without compromising the harvest site; and bone fragments at each end to ensure rigid fixation within the osseous tunnels of the tibia and femur.

The three types of graft materials that are used for intra-articular ACL reconstruction are artificial ligaments, allografts, and autografts. *Artificial ligaments* are synthetic materials that are developed in laboratories. *Allografts* are biologic tissues taken from another human body. *Autografts* are biologic tissues taken from the body of the individual having ACL reconstruction. The biomechanical characteristics and strength of each graft material, as well as the advantages and disadvantages of using each graft material for ACL reconstruction, are presented in Tables 9–1 and 9–2, respectively. *Tensile strength* (breaking point) is the level of force at which all components in the graft material fail; *stiffness* is defined as an object's resistance to deformation as a result of a change in force.[17]

TABLE 9–1 Mechanical Properties of ACL Replacements

Graft Material	Tensile Strength (N)	Stiffness (N/mm)
Normal ACL	1730	175
Synthetics*		
Gore-Tex	4830	219
Leeds-Keio	2100	X
Meadox	3045	420
Polyethylene Richards	420	X
Proplast	1500	1900
Xenotech	3000	527
Carbon fiber	1600	230×10^9
Dexon	910	3100
LAD	1700	360
Autografts†		
Patellar tendon	2900	208
Semitendinosus	1216	X
Gracilis	838	X
Iliotibial tract	769	44

*Based on the data of Bonnarens and Drez[17], pp 24–249.
†Based on the data of Noyes et al.,[27] p 347.
X = Data not available.

ARTIFICIAL LIGAMENTS

The use of artificial ligaments has gained popularity over the past few years as the research in this area has increased.[17-23] The advantage of using artificial ligaments for ACL reconstruction is to avoid tissue dissection around the knee joint. Artificial ligaments are used in the reconstruction of previously failed ACL surgeries or when no biologic alternative exists.

The three general classifications of artificial ligaments include prosthetic devices, scaffold devices, and augmentation devices (see Tables 9–1 and 9–2). Each group is designed to serve a specific purpose.

Prosthetic devices are designed to take the place of the injured ligament. The greatest advantage of using a prosthetic ligament is that these grafts are at maximum strength directly after implantation, allowing a rapid and aggressive rehabilitation program. In addition, artificial ligaments have no chance of disease transmission, and the surgeon does not need to dissect or harvest tissue from the injured knee. Experimental evidence indicates that the Gore-Tex (W. L. Gore & Co., Flagstaff, AZ) polytetrafluoroethylene device possesses the strongest mechanical properties[17] and yields encouraging clinical results comparable with other prosthetic devices.[18-20] However, follow-up studies indicate that mechanical properties of this graft deteriorate with time.[21,22] A possible reason for this deterioration process is that artificial materials are not capable of adapting to the stress-strain loads like biologic materials. A partially damaged graft will not heal and will eventually wear out.

The concept of a *scaffold device* is to use the biologic tissues of the body to "develop" a new ligament. The carbon fiber scaffold device is designed to facilitate collagen ingrowth.[17] The rapid ingrowth of collagen enhances the mechanical properties of the ligament. However, carbon fiber debris has been found to accumulate in the joint and the stiffness property of this device has resulted in failure.

TABLE 9–2 Graft Materials in Intra-articular
ACL Reconstruction

Graft Material	Advantages	Disadvantages
Artificial ligaments		

Prosthetic devices	No harvest site damage
	Strong mechanical properties
	Allows accelerated
	  rehabilitation
	No risk of disease
	  transmission
		Lack of biologic fixation
		Possible tissue rejection
		Weakens over time
		May not be strong enough
		  for use as a substitute

Scaffold devices	Allows accelerated
	  rehabilitation
	Rapid collagen ingrowth
	No harvest site damage
	No risk of disease
	  transmission
		Carbon fiber debris
		  accumulates within the
		  joint
		Possible tissue rejection
		Lack of biologic fixation

Augmentation devices	Helps support biologic
	  tissues during healing
	No risk of disease
	  transmission
		May share too much of the
		  load to facilitate proper
		  soft tissue healing and
		  collagen alignment
		Possible tissue rejection

Allografts	No harvest site damage Strong mechanical properties Biologic fixation	Risk of infection and tissue rejection
Autografts		

Patellar tendon	Strongest autograft
	Bone-to-bone fixation
	Low risk of tissue rejection
		Harvest site problems:
		  patellofemoral joint
		  dysfunction, quadriceps
		  muscle weakness, risk of
		  patellar tendon or
		  quadriceps tendon rupture

Semitendinosus tendon	Expendable autograft
	Second strongest autograft
	  (when doubled)
	Low risk of tissue rejection
		Not as strong as patellar
		  tendon autograft
		Bone-to-bone fixation only at
		  one end

Others (Gracilis tendon,
  fascia lata, quadriceps
  muscle tendon)
	Readily available
	Low risk of tissue rejection
		Not as strong as above
		  autografts
		Must rely on mechanical
		  fixation

A *ligament augmentation device* (LAD) is designed to be used with another biologic material to reduce the stress on the graft during the period of remodeling.[23] This concept is known as *load sharing*. The advantage of load sharing is that the LAD can support up to 45 percent of the force, thus reducing the risk of injury during the period of remodeling. Therefore, the main advantage of this graft material is that it provides the biologic graft with increased tensile strength, allowing aggressive rehabilitation during the early phases. The disadvantage of a LAD is that the autograft or allograft requires a certain level of stress to facilitate collagen regeneration and alignment, and the LAD may inhibit this process. The use of a biodegradable LAD would theoretically support the ligament during the early remodeling stages and disintegrate when the ligament is no longer at risk, but more research is needed in this area.

ALLOGRAFTS

Allografts offer several potential advantages over the use of autografts. First, the knee joint is preserved because there is no harvesting of surrounding tissues. (The harvest site is the area that is affected by removal of the autograft material.) This minimizes potential morbidity in the already injured knee by avoiding steps necessary to harvest the autograft. Second, extensor mechanism problems may be reduced by the use of allografts. Harvesting of the patient's bone–patellar tendon–bone tissue is spared, avoiding further damage of the previously damaged periarticular knee tissues. Third, the results of animal studies indicate that patellar tendon allografts possess biologic and biomechanical properties similar to patellar tendon autografts and may be an ideal material for ACL reconstruction.[24]

Finally, surgical time is decreased and cosmesis is improved with allografts by avoiding the incisions and surgical procedures necessary to harvest autogenous tissues.

Allotransplantation still has several inherent risks. The possible transmission of disease and the immunogenicity of the graft present two serious problems with this type of surgery. Another potential problem with allografts is the sterilization procedure that is used to reduce the risk of disease transmission. Because complete screening of allografts is not always possible, most allografts undergo secondary sterilization.

The most common methods of secondary sterilization include the use of ethylene oxide, and gamma irradiation. The use of ethylene oxide as a means of secondary sterilization has encountered complications. Jackson and associates[25] reviewed 109 patients who underwent ACL reconstruction with freeze-dried, ethylene oxide–sterilized bone–patellar tendon–bone allografts. Seven (6.4 percent) patients developed an intra-articular reaction characterized by persistent synovial effusion and cellular inflammatory response. Most tissue banks no longer use ethylene oxide as a means of secondary sterilization because the intra-articular environment of the knee joint appears to participate in reactions to tendon allografts.

Allograft storage is accomplished by deep-freezing or freeze-drying techniques. These techniques were once considered to be appropriate methods for graft immunogenicity. However, bacteria and viruses have recently been reported to survive these methods of sterilization. Therefore, deep freezing and freeze drying are now considered acceptable only for allograft preservation, but not sterilization.[26]

AUTOGENOUS GRAFTS

Autogenous grafts are the most common structures used for ACL reconstruction. Many autogenous tissues have been used for intra-articular ACL reconstruction (see Tables 9–1 and 9–2). The research that has analyzed the different biomechanical properties of these autografts indicates that only the patellar tendon and semitendinosus tendon have mechanical strength properties similar to the ACL.[27]

The *patellar tendon graft* is the most common autograft used for intra-articular ACL reconstruction. The advantages of using a patellar tendon autograft include the mechanical strength of the tissue and the bone plugs at both ends of the graft to maintain the strongest possible fixation. The main disadvantage of using the patellar tendon is the damage that results at the harvest site.[13] Removal of one third of the patellar tendon may cause patellofemoral pain and significantly weaken the quadriceps femoris muscle. Follow-up studies of ACL reconstructions using the patellar tendon autograft have found problems with quadriceps femoris muscle weakness, anterior knee joint pain, knee joint flexion contractures, radiographic changes within the tibiofemoral and patellofemoral joints, rupture of the patellar tendon, and rupture of the quadriceps tendon.[28-30] However, interpretation of these results is difficult because the complications may be due to either inadequate or inappropriate rehabilitation, or to poor surgical procedures.

The semitendinosus tendon possesses similar biomechanical properties to the patellar tendon, but only when the graft is doubled in thickness (see related graft strengths listed in Table 9–1). Doubling the semitendinosus tendon is a common surgical procedure that is used to increase graft strength.[31,32] The semitendinosus tendon is more accessible and easier to harvest, due to less dissection, than the patellar tendon.[33] A follow-up study of reconstructions using the semitendinosus tendon indicated that removal of the graft only minimally affected knee flexion strength.[33] Another study indicated a significant loss of knee flexion strength when the semitendinosus tendon was used in conjunction with the gracilis tendon.[32] The semitendinosus tendon autograft does not possess the mechanical strength properties of the patellar tendon autograft and does not provide bone-to-bone fixation at each end of the graft. Therefore, accelerated rehabilitation may not be recommended for a patient having ACL reconstruction with a semitendinosus autograft.[10]

Intra-articular ACL reconstructions using the gracilis tendon, the iliotibial band, or the quadriceps tendon without additional support are rarely performed. The lack of strength in these grafts results from weak tissue composition or an inadequate method of fixation, making these autogenous grafts unpopular for intra-articular ACL reconstruction.

Graft Fixation

The postoperative strength of an autograft or allograft during the early phases of rehabilitation depends on the type of graft fixation as well as the graft material. The type of graft fixation has a vital impact on preserving integrity of the reconstruction. A graft is more likely to fail at the fixation site than at the bone-tendon junction or midportion of the graft.[34]

The three most common *types of fixation* include *sutures*, a *staple*, or an *interference screw*.[35] The *sutures* that are passed through the graft material are anchored to a screw. Suture fixation has been shown to be the weakest method of graft fixation because until the osseous tunnels close, the graft is essentially only as strong as the suture.[35] In addition, any sharp bony ridges can fray the sutures, contributing to early failure.

Different types of *staple fixation* have been used to anchor the graft material. Care must be taken when using a staple because when the legs of the staple do not pass through the graft material, there is a high risk of failure.[35] The use of a barbed staple and a "double-back" staple fixation procedure appears to provide the strongest staple fixation.[35]

The use of an *interference screw* is another option of graft fixation.[35] An interference screw is a large, headless screw that is placed parallel to the bone plug to compress it tightly in the osseous tunnel. The option of using bone-to-bone interference fixation depends on graft selection. The patellar tendon is the only graft that allows bone-to-bone fixation at both ends. This type of fixation offers the strongest means of fixation[34] and enhancement of bone-to-bone healing.

Recently, an "endoscopic" approach for intra-articular ACL reconstruction has been popularized for the patellar tendon autograft.[36,37] This approach eliminates the incision over the lateral thigh needed for the femoral drill hole. The femoral tunnel is drilled from within the joint by retrograding the drill through the tibial tunnel. Intra-articular fixation is achieved with a cannulated interference screw placed in the femoral tunnel. The advantage of this technique is that it eliminates the lateral thigh incision and thus the potential morbidity of the vastus lateralis muscle. Additionally, this technique provides better cosmesis and a faster surgery time.

Graft Placement

The method of graft placement has a significant impact on the clinical results.[38] *Isometry* is a currently used graft placement technique that permits early passive motion during rehabilitation.[39] Isometry is a conceptual term that is used to describe the placement of a graft in a similar position to the original ACL. Theoretically, an isometric graft will not move as the knee joint is flexed and extended.[39] However, Sapega and associates[39] have demonstrated that true isometry does not exist in the intact ACL. Instead of two exact isometric points on the femur and tibia, a small range of isometric points exists along the lateral femoral condyle and medial tibial plateau. The ability of the surgeon to position the graft within these points will ensure that the graft undergoes length-tension changes that are similar to the original ACL. Prior to isometry, immediate passive motion was contraindicated because any movement may have adversely over-stretched the graft, resulting in a lax knee. Improper graft placement can lead to poor clinical results, whereas an isometrically placed graft allows safe and early passive motion during the period of rehabilitation.[13]

Timing of Surgery and Related Surgical Procedures

Recently the importance of the timing of the surgical procedure has been shown to affect clinical results. Shelbourne and colleagues[40] concluded that acute ACL reconstructions should be delayed for at least 3 weeks following the initial injury to reduce the risk of arthrofibrosis. Given 3 weeks, the injured tissues will have time to heal and intra-articular scarring will have less of an effect on the healing of the reconstructed graft. Although surgery is deferred for the first 3 weeks, the patient should start physical therapy during this time to initiate knee ROM and quadriceps femoris strengthening.

Related surgical procedures can also influence the rehabilitation program. A *femoral notchplasty* is a procedure that is advocated to reduce the risk of arthrofibrosis.[41] A notchplasty removes bone from the lateral wall of the intercondylar notch so that possible impingement of the graft is reduced. The use of a notchplasty, in conjunction with proper timing of the surgery, can decrease postoperative complications.

Secondary Injuries

Secondary injuries to the surrounding structures of the knee joint will also affect the rehabilitation process. Repairs of the menisci or collateral ligaments are commonly performed during ACL reconstruction. Increased tension on the collateral ligaments of the knee and increased translation of the femur on the meniscus occur in terminal knee joint extension. Therefore, patients with collateral-ligament or meniscus repairs must avoid active and passive ROM in the end range of knee joint extension during the early phases of rehabilitation. Clinicians are encouraged to communicate with the surgeon to discuss these extenuating circumstances, given that each procedure may vary, even when performed by the same surgeon.

GRAFT REMODELING AND HEALING POTENTIAL DURING REHABILITATION

This section provides the clinician with an overview of ACL vascularity, graft revascularization, and healing potential. A thorough understanding of these areas is needed to provide appropriate ACL rehabilitation.

ACL Vascularity

The ACL is endowed with blood vessels that originate from branches of the genicular artery. Although the ACL has a rich blood supply, its vascular supply is considered fragile compared with other extra-articular tissues.[42,43]

Arnoczky[42] has noted that the synovial membrane forms an envelope over the ACL. This synovial fold originates at the posterior inlet of the intercondylar notch and extends to the anterior tibial insertion of the ligament, blending with the synovial tissue of the joint capsule distal to the infrapatellar fat pad. This unique arrangement places the ligament intracapsularly, but extrasynovial throughout its course within the knee.

The ACL has been recognized as a ligament with poor healing potential since the early 1900s.[44] Amiel, Kuiper, and Akeson[43] studied the cellular response following ACL injury and have referred to the ACL as a ligament living in a "hostile" environment. This study indicated that once the synovial sheath enveloping the ACL is torn, the frayed ligament ends are exposed to a host of potentially destructive enzymes contained in the hemarthrosis fluid of the injured joint. This fluid has a deleterious effect on the collagenous matrix and appears to inhibit the healing capabilities of the fibroblast cells contained within the ACL. Thus, once ruptured and exposed to the intra-articular knee joint environment, cellular and histologic changes in the ACL occur, which may be the reason for the high failure rates reported in primary ACL repairs.[8,9]

Revascularization and Remodeling of the Autograft

The success of the autograft transplant is dependent upon the ability of the selected graft to survive and function in the intra-articular environment of the reconstructed knee. Many studies have attempted to determine the optimum time frame for soft-tissue revascularization in animals.[45-47] Chapter 4 in this text reviews the soft-tissue healing process of various biologic tissues. Although animal studies should not be used to predict precise timing of soft-tissue healing in the human knee joint, the phases of revascularization are probably similar. The graft goes through a period of avascular necrosis in the first 6 to 8 weeks that is followed by a period of revascularization. Complete revascularization of the patellar tendon graft can take up to 20 weeks, and even more time is required for the graft to remodel and take on the structural and mechanical characteristics of a ligament.[42,48]

Biomechanical strength curves have been reported in the literature in an effort to correlate rehabilitation with graft remodeling.[14] A proposed strength curve indicates that at 3 months following implantation, graft strength is less than 50 percent of its maximum.[14] The time that a graft takes to reach full strength and maturity is controversial. Some authorities suggest that the graft takes at least a year to reach full maturity and may never regain its original strength.[12]

GENERAL GUIDELINES FOR REHABILITATION

The following section offers guidelines for rehabilitation of patients with intra-articular ACL reconstructions. These guidelines are based on empirical evidence of the authors, which is supported by basic science, applied science, and clinical research. A summary of these guidelines is presented in Table 9–3. The biomechanical constraints relative to anterior tibial shear force and ACL strain are discussed throughout this section.

The Rehabilitation Specialist's Role in Identifying Problems

The rehabilitation team consists of three important components: the *patient*, the *physician*, and the *rehabilitation specialist*. Each member plays a specific role during the rehabilitation process. Initially, the physician will evaluate and discuss treatment options—that is, surgical or nonsurgical approaches. The rehabilitation program is reviewed and a reasonable time frame for return to activity or work is established. When outpatient physical therapy is initiated, rehabilitation goals, time frames for adequate healing, and patient/therapist roles are established. Treatment is usually conducted three times per week following nonsurgical/postsurgical treatment.

The first line of recognition and assessment of potential problems lies with the therapist or athletic trainer. Early recognition and triage of problems such as deep vein thrombosis (DVT), sepsis, effusion, reflex sympathetic dystrophy, changes in laxity/instability, and early signs of arthrofibrosis need to be carefully monitored during the

TABLE 9–3 Exercise Guidelines for Rehabilitation after
ACL Reconstruction

Immobilization	
Knee brace locked at zero	10 d
Brace motion 0–60 degrees (daytime)	10 d–2 wk
Brace locked at 0 degrees (while sleeping)	6 wk

Ambulation	
Two-crutch ambulation in brace	
Partial weight bearing as tolerated	10 d–2 wk
Full weight bearing with two crutches	2–4 wk
D/C crutch when quad control is able to protect knee and extension is < 10 degrees	4 wk

(Continued)

TABLE 9–3 Exercise Guidelines for Rehabilitation after ACL Reconstruction (*Continued*)

*Range of Motion (Without Brace)**

Early ROM is encouraged. Passive flexion to full extension with uninvolved leg assisting.	2 d–4 wk
Passive extension with weighted assistance	2–6 wk
Patellar mobilization	1–8 wk

Strength Return†

Quadriceps

Quad set—Cocontraction with hamstrings	
Leg raises—Bent knee raise with cocontraction	10 d–6 wk
Knee dips with adduction squeeze	1–6 wk
Stationary bike	2 wk
Step ups/Step downs	4–8 wk
Wall sits	7 wk
Lunges	8–12 wk
Closed chain quadriceps exercises, including Stairmaster, squat machines, leg press, and ski machines	3 wk–6 mo
Open chain leg extensions and isokinetic exercises are not routinely conducted	

Hamstrings

Hamstring sets, slides	1–8 wk
Resisted ham curls	3 wk–6 mo
Resisted hip extension	2–8 wk
Hip and back machine.	
Universal total hip machine	8 wk–6 mo

Lower Extremity Conditioning

Isometric abduction and adduction	1–8 wk
Isometric calf exercises	1–3 wk
Hip abduction and adduction using machines	4 wk–6 mo
Soleus/calf raises	4 wk–6 mo
Hip flexion/extension	4 wk–6 mo
Road bicycle	4 mo

Functional Exercises

Weight shift	1 wk
Weight shift on trampoline	3 wk
One-leg bounce (supported)	4 wk
Form walking—gait evaluation	6 wk
Balance board	2 wk
Slide board†	12 wk
Return to activity:	
Running, straight line†	6 mo
Directional-change sports, e.g., tennis, racquetball, skiing‡	9–12 mo
Return to sports and progression of activity requires timely return of extension–flexion motion, good stability, and VMO control	

*Aggressive measures may be taken to regain extension. The use of a Dynasplint, lysis of adhesion, or manipulation is encouraged.

†VMO must be functioning to accelerate quadriceps femoris exercises.

‡Hop test must be 90% of uninvolved limb.

rehabilitation program. If problems arise, the physician should be notified at once to determine the proper course of action.

Guidelines for Progression

Many rehabilitation programs were based on the work of Paulos, Noyes, and co-workers,[14] who advocated a five-phase protocol based on biomechanical models that correlated healing properties of the graft with the strain imposed on the ACL during various activities. Patients progressed from knee joint immobilization and partial weight bearing activity to a gradual increase in ROM exercises and full weight bearing. The return to functional activity did not occur until approximately 1 year after surgery.

The estimated maturation of the graft was based on models extrapolated from animal research and dictated the time and progression of these programs. These models assume that the healing and maturation of collagen varies little from patient to patient. In clinical practice, each patient reacts differently to the surgical intervention. Loss of strength, swelling, and ROM are unpredictable. Patient personality, attitude, and pain tolerance vary greatly with each individual case. Specific cases that involve litigation or work-related injuries may present additional factors that can alter levels of motivation. Because of these factors, we do not advocate a time-based protocol with phases that correlate to the healing process of the graft.

Patients progress through phases of rehabilitation as they attain preset goals and criteria. For example, prior to advancing a patient to independent ambulation or high-load quadriceps femoris muscle exercise, a patient must have adequate control of knee joint extension (as evidenced by a straight leg raise without an extensor lag) and a visible contraction of the vastus medialis obliquus (VMO) muscle. Muscular control ensures stability around the tibiofemoral[49] and patellofemoral joints,[50] as well as compensating for the loss of knee proprioception that occurs following ACL reconstruction.[51] By observing quadriceps femoris muscle recruitment patterns for adequate control and ensuring that the patient obtains full ROM, careless progression of activities will be avoided.

Immobilization

The purpose of immobilization is to protect the newly damaged ligament or surgical reconstruction and allow healing of the graft. The time of immobilization prescribed by many physicians has decreased over the years as the detrimental effects of immobilization were documented and graft placement and fixation improved.[52,53] In an effort to facilitate knee joint extension ROM in our practice, a hinged knee brace (Fig. 9–1) is locked at 0 degrees and is worn for the first 10 postoperative days, except when performing home exercises. As the patient demonstrates adequate muscular control (between day 10 and 2 weeks), the daytime brace motion is increased from 0 to 60 degrees. The brace remains locked at 0 degrees at night, for a period of 6 to 8 weeks, to maintain full knee joint extension. If the patient has full knee joint extension and ROM is maintained throughout the day, the use of a brace at night can be discontinued. The brace is discontinued during the daytime about the fourth postoperative week. Removal of the daytime brace is based on the following criteria: no increase in knee joint laxity, sufficient proprioception, quadriceps femoris muscle control, and skill with crutches. A

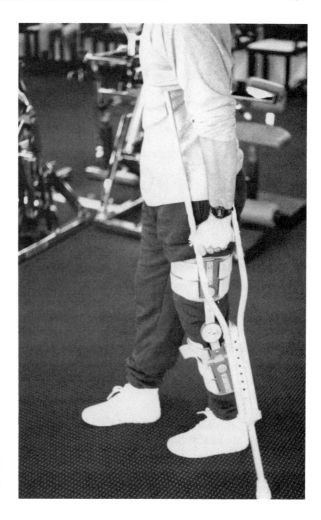

FIGURE 9-1. A hinged-knee brace, locked at 0 degrees, ensures immobilization during the first 10 days after surgery.

goal of our program is to expedite the period of immobilization by limiting the use of the brace and encouraging normal gait patterns and safe functional use.

Continuous Passive Motion (CPM) Devices

Postoperative immobilization of the knee has been associated with an increased incidence of arthrofibrosis, cartilage degeneration, muscle atrophy, and changes in ligament strength.[52-54] Early restoration of ROM following ACL reconstruction is obtained through early controlled active motion and the use of continuous passive motion (CPM) devices. Noyes and colleagues[55] demonstrated that the use of a CPM device did not increase knee joint laxity. However, a recent study cautioned against using the calf support with CPM units, because the support can increase anterior tibial translation and potentially stress the graft.[56] These authors recommended using only a thigh and heel support when a CPM device for patients with intra-articular ACL reconstructions is applied (Fig. 9-2). Although some studies indicated no significant difference in ROM at a 6-month follow-up between a group that used a CPM device and a group that did

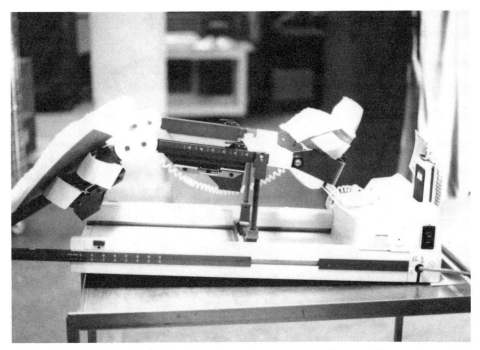

FIGURE 9-2. This continuous passive motion (CPM) unit can be used during the period of hospitalization.

not,[57] other studies indicated that CPM devices were beneficial in postoperative care for increasing the absorption rate of synovial joint hemarthrosis.[58] According to Paulos and co-workers,[12] "the judicious use of CPM devices will aid in preventing knee joint contracture and articular surface changes." Following these reports, many ACL rehabilitation protocols have incorporated the use of CPM units.[10,12,36,59,60]

The rehabilitation program presented in this chapter recommends CPM use during the period of hospitalization when the patient is recovering from surgery. The CPM unit is used during the daytime hours; the patient maintains knee joint extension at night by using the brace locked at full extension. Typically, the CPM is effective in gaining knee joint flexion ROM but is ineffective for gaining knee joint extension.

Outpatient rehabilitation begins during the first postoperative week, with an emphasis on early controlled active motion in conjunction with passive ROM (PROM) exercises. A CPM device is not typically used at home, due to the added expense to the patient and the limited value a CPM unit has over self-administered PROM exercises.[57] However, the CPM will be used in select patients who refuse to participate in the rehabilitation program, or require additional surgery secondary to arthrofibrosis. These cases are discussed in the section titled Complications Following ACL Surgery.

The Goals of Range of Motion (ROM) Exercises

Passive knee joint extension is a primary concern early in the rehabilitation process and is encouraged on the first postoperative day. Knee joint flexion contractures alter gait patterns, which changes lower extremity kinetics. ROM exercises are conducted out of the knee immobilizer with the nonoperative limb providing the knee flexion and extension forces while the patient is seated at a table (Fig. 9–3). The goal is to have the patient obtain a passive knee joint ROM of 0 to 120 degrees within the first 4 weeks. If self-administered ROM fails to yield the desired results, aggressive therapist intervention must be employed. These techniques include muscle and joint stretching, as well as friction massage along the surgical incision. Obtaining full ROM as early as possible is critical because as time passes, scar tissue will mature and thus make knee joint flexion and extension gains increasingly difficult.

Patellofemoral joint mobilization is initiated immediately following surgery and is continued as necessary (Fig. 9–4). *Patellar tracking* refers to the gliding of the patella along the femoral trochlear groove during knee motion in the sagittal plane. Research indicates that the patella should glide parallel, or slightly lateral, to the midline of the femoral trochlear groove.[61] The patella must glide inferiorly and superiorly to achieve normal flexion and extension at the knee joint, respectively.[61] Poor patellar mobility makes knee joint flexion-extension difficult to achieve and may result in patellofemoral joint dysfunction. Normal knee joint ROM (full extension to approximately 135 to 140 degrees) is expected by 3 months.

Factors that may slow the progression of motion include prolonged knee joint effusion; excessive pain causing inhibition of the quadriceps femoris muscles; and severe scar formation. Effusion must be controlled, and any increased effusion following a therapy session or home program must be addressed prior to progressing treatment. Anti-inflammatory modalities including cryotherapy, heat, and compression are used. Beyond these methods, anti-inflammatory medication or joint aspiration may be used by the physician, and the intensity and the frequency of rehabilitation may need to be reduced.

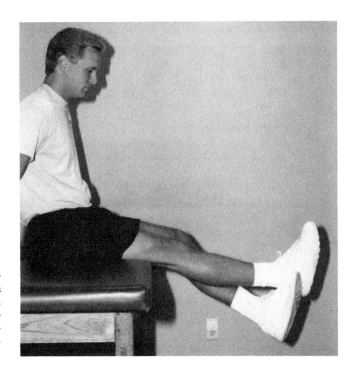

FIGURE 9–3. Self-administered passive range of motion exercise. During this exercise, the patient is out of the immobilizer and uses the uninvolved leg to support the involved leg.

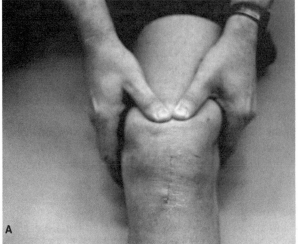
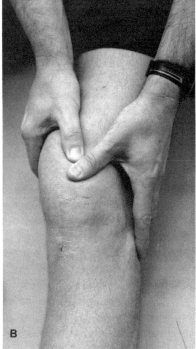

FIGURE 9-4. Mobilization of the patellofemoral joint can be accomplished by self-administered patellar tracking. The patient glides the patella along the femoral trochlear groove during knee motion in the sagittal plane. The patient should be able to accomplish *A*) inferior glide, and *B*) medial glide.

Patient compliance with exercise is essential, particularly when knee joint ROM does not return freely. The nature of aggressive therapy and self-administered mobilization will usually result in discomfort during the treatment, and the patient must know to expect this reaction. The patient must monitor the symptoms and be aware that any discomfort due to exercise should decrease after a few hours. If the patient's discomfort does not decrease, the therapist must explore the possibility of other complications and adjust the frequency and intensity of rehabilitation. By ruling out other problems and adjusting the frequency and intensity of the therapy, the clinician can ensure that patient comfort and compliance will increase, which will ultimately lead to positive results.

Specific exercises such as stationary cycling, wall slides (Fig. 9-5), and weighted knee extension in prone (Fig. 9-6) play a role in gaining knee joint ROM. The employment of these specific exercises is left to the discretion of the therapist. The use of aggressive measures to gain knee ROM is discussed later in this chapter.

Ambulation

Normal gait patterns are practiced early in the rehabilitation process. Early weight bearing reduces the effects of postoperative immobilization and proprioception impairment. Patients are discouraged from using a flexed knee during the midstance phase of gait. Knee joint extension is emphasized at heelstrike. Ambulation is started as soon as possible, and the patient is instructed to bear weight as tolerated with the assistance of crutches. The patient will increase weight bearing as lower extremity strength and ambulatory skills increase, while pain and knee joint effusion decrease. Full weight

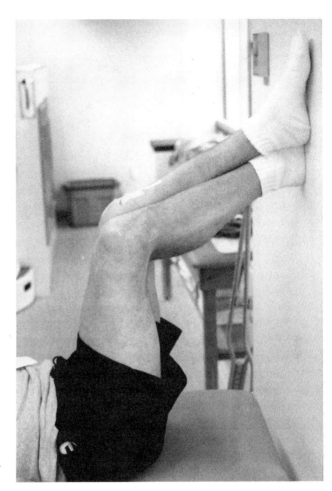

FIGURE 9-5. Wall slide performed with the patient supine.

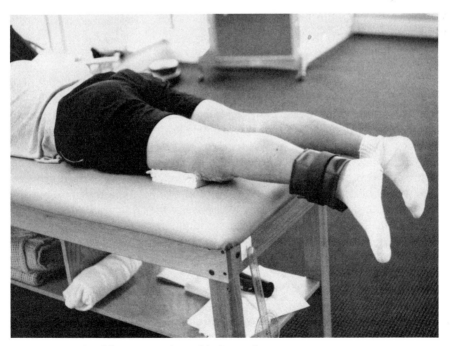

FIGURE 9-6. Weighted-knee extension with the patient prone.

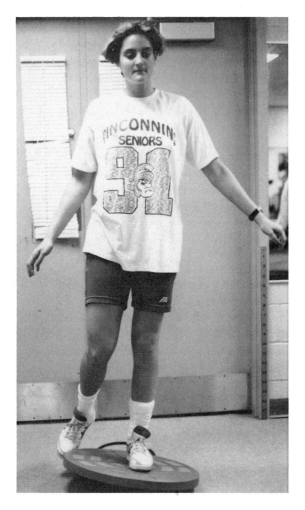

FIGURE 9-7. Before attempting full weight bearing after postoperative immobilization, the patient should demonstrate adequate proprioception by standing on a BAPS (Biomedical Ankle Platform System; Camp Medical Products, Jackson, MI) board with eyes closed.

bearing is encouraged by 2 to 4 weeks, and use of the crutches is discontinued at 4 weeks. The patient must have sufficient muscular control of the quadriceps femoris muscles (as evidenced by performing a straight leg raise without an extensor lag), adequate proprioception (as evidenced by balance testing; Fig. 9-7), minimal or absent knee effusion, and lack no more than 10 degrees of passive knee joint extension to begin independent ambulation. The use of one crutch may be recommended for ambulating long distances to prevent synovial irritation that is commonly seen during early or excessive weight bearing. The patient is not permitted to walk in the immobilizer alone; the use of the brace is discontinued prior to the use of the crutches. Walking in the brace alone can result in gait patterns that place undue stress on the graft, as well as the patellofemoral joint, the hip joints, and the lumbar spine.

Strengthening Exercises

The goal in strength training is to restore muscle function in order to return the patient to preinjury activity level without jeopardizing the implanted graft or causing further damage to periarticular structures. Patient and therapist expectations may need to be adjusted at times, depending on the preinjury level of conditioning or special limitations imposed by surgical complications. The return of muscle strength appears to correlate with the return of function. As the muscles around the knee joint are strengthened, joint protection and lower extremity function can be improved. However, exercises that place excessive anterior shear forces across the knee must be avoided.

Many biomechanical studies have been performed to determine the effects of active exercise in an open kinetic chain (see Chapters 1 and 5 for description of open kinetic chain exercises) on ACL strain.[49,62-65] Results from studies analyzing active hamstring contractions indicated that these exercises can be incorporated into the rehabilitation program without strain to the graft.[64,65] The results of studies analyzing active quadriceps femoris contractions in an open kinetic chain were less definitive.[62,63,65] These studies indicated that active knee joint extension in the final 30 to 44 degrees can be detrimental to the graft because of the increase in anterior tibial shear forces and increased strain in the ACL. The following sections on exercise progression and quadriceps femoris muscle strengthening reviews strategies for reducing anterior tibial shear forces across the knee joint.

The strengthening program described below is initiated on the first post-operative day and is continued for 12 to 18 months.

HAMSTRING MUSCLE

The hamstring muscles are believed to play a crucial role in the rehabilitation of patients with ACL injuries.[49,65] The hamstring muscles act as an ACL agonist, pulling the tibia posteriorly. As stated earlier, strengthening of this muscle group can be progressed rapidly without risk of damaging the graft.[64] Exercise progression is based on the severity of knee joint effusion, the degree of pain, and the ability to master the previous level of exercise without complications. The hamstring muscles can be exercised as hip extensors and hip stabilizers as well as knee joint flexors during functional exercise such as squats and step-ups. During closed kinetic chain exercise, the hamstring muscles are able to provide a posterior stabilizing force against the contracting quadriceps femoris muscle group.

Hamstring muscle setting (Fig. 9–8A), heel slides (Fig. 9–8B), and isotonic resistance provided by the healthy leg (Fig. 9–8C) are initiated in the first postoperative week. As strength and confidence improve, the patient can initiate hamstring curls in a standing position using cuff weights (Fig. 9–8D) and then advance to prone resistive exercises (Fig. 9–8E). Resisted hip joint extension is usually started 1 to 2 weeks postoperatively, and the patient is progressed from cuff weights to hip extension machines.

The progression of hamstring muscle strengthening exercises can be limited by patellofemoral joint problems such as pain, joint restriction, or tracking malalignment. A decrease in inferior glide of the patella may limit the amount of knee joint flexion.[61] A tight patellar retinaculum may also hinder patellar glide.[66] The patient can potentially develop retropatellar or parapatellar symptoms during resisted knee joint flexion if the patient has poor patellofemoral mobility or inadequate quadriceps femoris muscle control.

Hamstring muscle exercises are progressed more rapidly than quadriceps femoris muscle exercise because these exercises pose no threat to graft safety.[64] Additionally, knee flexion exercises can be less irritating to the knee joint.

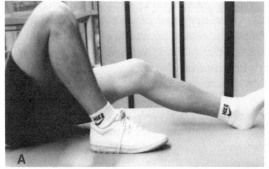
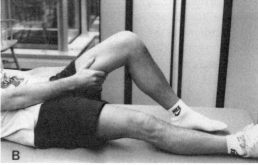
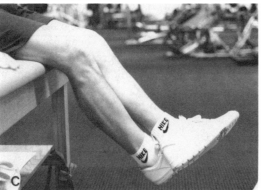

FIGURE 9–8. Exercises for strengthening hamstring muscles. *A*) "Heel dig" or hamstring muscle set with patient in long sitting position. *B*) Heel slide in supine position. *C*) Knee flexion in sitting position with resistance from the uninvolved leg.

QUADRICEPS FEMORIS MUSCLE

Quadriceps femoris muscle strengthening begins on the first postoperative day. However, caution must be taken to protect the newly reconstructed ligament. In addition to placing high shear forces across the knee joint, resistance of the knee joint extensors in an open kinetic chain does not duplicate functional activities. Therefore, these exercises are only used on a limited basis in this program to provide a foundation that allows progression to closed kinetic chain exercise.

If resistance to the knee extensors in an open kinetic chain is used, the patient must be prohibited from performing this exercise in the final 40 degrees of knee extension ROM because of the high tensile forces on the ACL. The application of resistance to the lower leg must be considered. Altering the site of resistance application along the tibia is one mechanism that is used to reduce anterior shear forces during open kinetic knee joint extension. Studies have demonstrated that during isometric and isokinetic (180 degrees per second) knee extensor exercises, placing the site of resistance proximally on the tibia significantly decreased the anterior tibial translation.[67,68] These studies also concluded that isometric contraction of the knee joint extensors performed at an angle greater than 90 degrees results in posterior tibial translation regardless of load placement.

Cocontraction exercises and closed kinetic chain exercises are the preferred methods used in this program for early quadriceps femoris muscle strengthening. Cocontracting the hamstring muscles simultaneously with the quadriceps femoris muscles reduces the anterior tibial shear forces and tension on the ACL graft.[65,69] A cocontraction requires the patient to perform a simultaneous contraction of the hamstring muscles during contraction of the quadriceps musculature, so as to counteract the anterior pull of the quadriceps muscles on the tibia.[49,65,69,70] This method was studied on

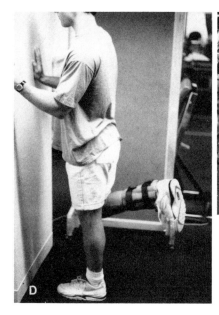

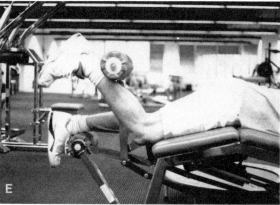

FIGURE 9-8 Continued. *D*) Standing knee flexion with cuff weights. *E*) Knee flexion in prone position on leg curl machine.

cadaveric extremities, using simulated cocontractions.[65] The results of this study suggest that cocontraction of the hamstring muscles during knee joint extension can reduce the strain on the ACL, but only in the range of 90 to 30 degrees of knee joint flexion. Voluntary cocontraction exercises were compared to electrically stimulated cocontractions, in patients who have had ACL reconstruction.[69,70] The results of these studies indicated that electrically stimulated cocontractions were more effective than voluntary cocontractions for improving isometric knee joint extension strength, isokinetic knee joint extension strength, and ambulation skills. Electrical muscle stimulation is also an effective method for muscle re-education of the quadriceps femoris muscles.

Cocontraction exercises are taught early using the following two methods: cocontraction muscle setting of the quadriceps femoris and hamstring muscles in a sitting position with the involved foot on the floor; and bent leg raises in the brace, with the patient contracting the hamstrings against the brace during the leg raise. A cocontraction is not easily taught to the patient, so the use of EMG biofeedback or electrical stimulation may need to be employed in the early phases of rehabilitation. As the quality of quadriceps femoris muscle contraction improves, the patient is progressed to closed kinetic chain exercises.

Closed kinetic chain exercises also control the amount of strain in the ACL. Weight bearing exercise, such as the squat, increases knee joint compression, which can enhance knee joint stabilization and increase graft protection.[71] In addition to knee joint compression, research findings indicate that cocontraction of the thigh musculature occurs during the half squat exercise.[72,73] Pope and associates[73] studied the effect of a squatting motion on the anterior tibial translation and ACL strain. The results of this study indicated that there is a reduction in ACL tension at angles greater than 17 degrees of knee joint flexion during squatting. Increasing the resistance by using an elastic rubber tube resulted in a decrease in ACL strain because of the increased joint compression. The calculated anterior tibial shear forces remained constant from full knee joint extension to 20 degrees of knee joint flexion, but the authors found that the strain in the ACL decreased sharply. The authors concluded that three possible mechanisms may be responsible for the decrease in ACL strain in the presence of anterior tibial

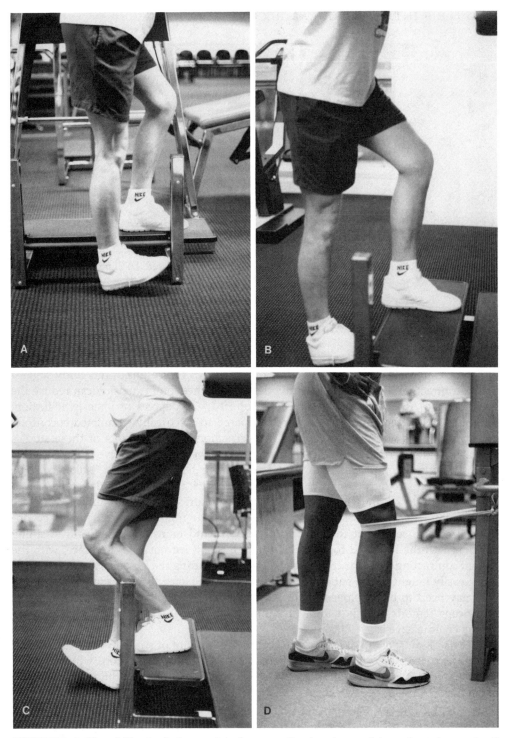

FIGURE 9-9. Closed kinetic chain exercises for strengthening the quadriceps femoris muscle. *A*) Knee dip off a step with the involved leg remaining on the step. *B*) Step-up with involved leg remaining on the step. (*B* from Greenfield, BH and Tovin, BJ: The application of open and closed kinematic chain exercises in rehabilitation of the lower extremity. Journal of Back and Musculoskeletal Rehabilitation 2[4]:38–51, 1992, with permission.) *C*) Step-down with the involved leg remaining on the step. *D*) Standing terminal knee extension with resistance from an elastic band positioned behind the popliteal fossa.

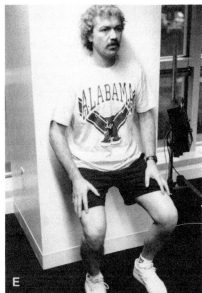

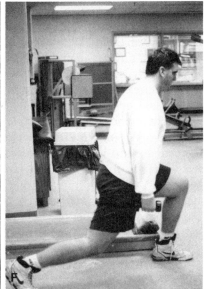

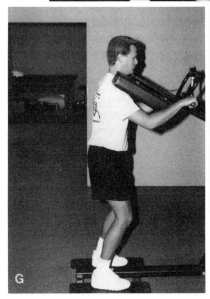

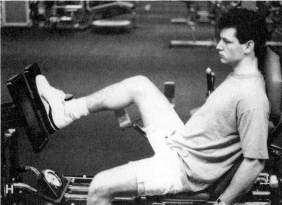

FIGURE 9-9 Continued. *E*) Wall sitting at 60 degrees of knee flexion. *F*) Lunges with light hand weights. *G*) Standing leg press machine. *H*) Sitting leg press machine. (*E, G,* and *H* from Greenfield, BH and Tovin, BJ: The application of open and closed kinematic chain exercises in rehabilitation of the lower extremity. Journal of Back and Musculoskeletal Rehabilitation 2[4]:38–51, 1992, with permission.)

shear forces. These mechanisms include difference in arthrokinematics during squatting compared with isolated knee extension (femur rolls on the fixed tibia rather than the tibia translating on the femur); cocontraction of the hamstring muscles to hold the tibia posteriorly; and an increase in joint compression between the articular surfaces. Other studies have reached similar conclusions.[72,74,75] The use of closed kinetic chain activities is advocated in current rehabilitation programs.[10,36]

Closed kinetic chain exercises such as knee dips with hip abduction (Fig. 9–9A), step-ups (Fig. 9–9B), step-downs (Fig. 9–9C), and stationary cycling are introduced between the second and fourth week. Standing resisted knee extension (Fig. 9–9D) and standing quadriceps femoris muscle setting are used to strengthen the quadriceps in a functional position. Wall-sitting exercises (Fig. 9–9E) and lunges (Fig. 9–9F) are started

6 to 8 weeks following surgery. Progressive quadriceps femoris muscle exercises including the Stairmaster (Randall Corp., Seattle, WA), squat machine, leg presses, and ski machines are implemented at 8 weeks following surgery. The criteria for progression includes minimal or no knee joint swelling, satisfactory completion of the previous level of exercise without increased symptoms, and a straight leg raise without an extensor lag.

The VMO muscle is monitored throughout the rehabilitation process with manual palpation and biofeedback. Progression of the quadriceps femoris muscle exercise regimen is contingent on the strength and control of the VMO muscle as well as tracking of the patella.[66] Normally the VMO muscle fires prior to the vastus lateralis muscle to hold the patella medially and within the femoral trochlear groove. Some studies have indicated that a reversal in the normal firing order of the vastus medialis and vastus lateralis muscles exists in patients with extensor mechanism dysfunction.[49,66] If an abnormal firing pattern exists, the therapist must train the patient to restore normal function by having the patient palpate the muscles and attempt to control the firing pattern.

Lower Extremity Conditioning

Intra-articular ACL reconstruction can affect the musculature of the entire lower extremity. A rehabilitation program that focuses only on strengthening exercises for the thigh musculature treats only a partial aspect of the clinical picture. Therefore, other muscles of the lower extremity and pelvis must be strengthened to ensure a desirable outcome. Most hip and ankle musculature exercises can be performed without placing the knee joint in jeopardy.

Isometric exercises for hip abduction and adduction, as well as isometric calf exercises to the gastrocnemius-soleus muscles, can be started in the first postoperative week. These exercises can be quickly progressed to isotonic exercises as strength gain dictates. Progressive resistive exercises in all planes of movement for the hip and ankle joint are implemented at 4 weeks following surgery.

Swimming and water resistance exercises are started after the surgical wounds heal. The water provides an ideal medium for exercise and gait training, in that the stresses imposed on the joints are reduced significantly. Additionally, water can be used to either resist or assist movement in functional planes of motion, depending on the speed of movement.[76] Ambulating forward and backward in shallow water can create resistance to movement and help restore normal gait patterns. Functional exercises such as step-ups, step-downs, and squatting can be initiated in the water with only minimal stress placed on the lower extremity. The patient can maintain cardiovascular status by advancing to deep-water jogging with flotation vests. Swimming is discouraged for the first 3 months, unless the patient is willing to use a pull buoy (Fig. 9–10A and B). The pull buoy will greatly reduce the use of the lower extremities and consequent stress on the knee joint. At approximately 8 weeks following surgery, the patient can begin some gentle kicking from the hip with the knee flexed. This pattern of kicking will ensure a cocontraction of the quadriceps femoris and hamstrings, thus minimizing anterior shear forces and graft deformation. Straight leg kicking or "flutter" kicking is allowed after the third month, provided the patient is a fairly good swimmer. Patients who are not efficient swimmers often do not kick properly and thus create a thrashing-type kick through the water in order to prevent sinking, putting increased stress on the graft. A breaststroke whipkick or "frog" kick is avoided during rehabilitation due to the increased valgus and rotatory stresses placed on the knee with this movement. A breaststroke-type kick involves the following movements occurring simultaneously: hip flex-

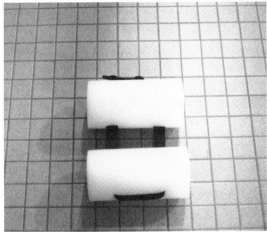

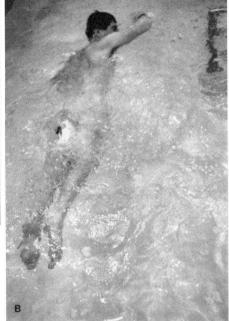

FIGURE 9-10. *A*) For the first 3 months after surgery, swimming should be done only with the pull-buoy. *B*) Held between the thighs, the device enables the swimmer to maintain the correct body position without kicking.

ion with abduction and internal rotation, knee flexion, tibial external rotation, and subtalar eversion. This initial position is followed by the propulsion phase, which consists of a forceful extension of the hips and knees with the lower extremities adducting and derotating (Fig. 9-11). This action creates a whipping motion through the water and can be detrimental to the healing graft. Hydrodynamic rehabilitation can create a positive setting for patients because the aqueous environment will allow them to perform activities they are unable to perform on dry land.

Stationary cycling may be used as a device to increase ROM, especially knee joint flexion, beginning the first postoperative week. As the mechanics of cycling become easier for the patient, the stationary bicycle serves as a lower extremity strengthening and conditioning tool. The patient is prohibited from using a road bicycle until 4 months

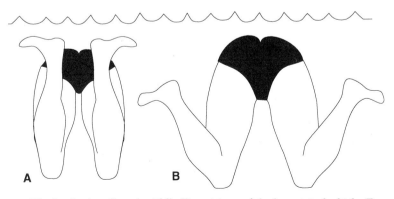

FIGURE 9-11. The beginning *A*) and middle *B*) positions of the breaststroke kick. (From Vizsolwi, P, Taunton, J, and Gordon, R, et al: Breaststroker's knee: An analysis of epidemiological and biomechanical factors. Am J Sports Med 15[1]:71, 1987, with permission.)

following surgery. This delay allows time for healing, coordination, and the return of strength to decrease the chances of injury on rough terrain.

Functional Exercise

Most injuries that require a period of immobilization usually result in some loss of proprioception. The rehabilitation of kinesthetic awareness must be addressed early in the rehabilitation program to prevent additional problems in the later phases.

Early weight shifting exercises allow the patient to gain confidence in the extremity and prepare for ambulation. Gradual weight bearing and weight shifting are initiated on a flat, immovable surface and progressed to weight shifting on dynamic surfaces such as a trampoline. As skill level permits, controlled one-leg bounces can begin at 4 weeks (Fig. 9–12).

Gait evaluation and correction of aberrant gait patterns continues throughout the rehabilitation program. As weight bearing increases, specific gait deviations may become apparent that need to be addressed in the treatment program. At 8 weeks, controlled dynamic exercises are initiated to facilitate directional change during ambu-

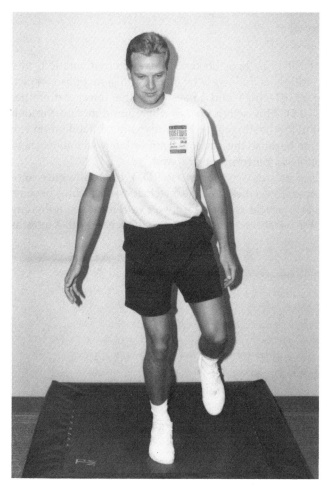

FIGURE 9–12. After gradual resumption of weight bearing and weight shifting on flat stable surfaces, controlled one-leg trampoline bounces can begin at 4 weeks. (From Greenfield, BH and Tovin, BJ: The application of open and closed kinematic chain exercises in rehabilitation of the lower extremity. Journal of Back and Musculoskeletal Rehabilitation 2[4]:38–51, 1992, with permission.)

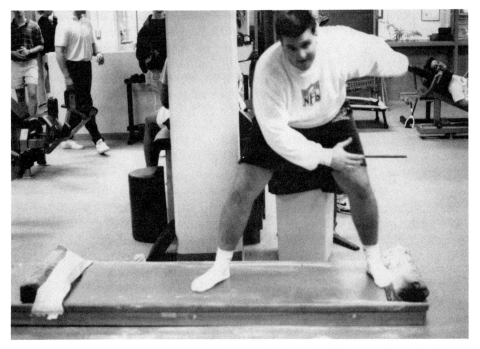

FIGURE 9-13. Slide board exercises can help restore timing and ability to make quick changes in direction.

lation. The patient's skill level is evaluated and progressed as indicated. Caution must be taken to control the amount of rotational torque on the knee during these exercises.

At 3 to 4 months following surgery, a slide board may be used to emphasize timing and directional change (Fig. 9-13). Determination of when to initiate this exercise will vary from patient to patient and is contingent on the skill level attained during the early phases of rehabilitation. Later in the rehabilitation program, progressive exercises such as skating or "roller blading" may be useful in gaining functional lower extremity strength while limiting repetitive compression on the joint. However, extreme caution and close monitoring are essential when using these exercises. Other functional exercises for this patient population have been documented in the literature.[36,77]

Return to Activity

The minimum time required before a patient can return to activity is based on the biomechanical factors previously mentioned. The limiting factors beyond the maturity of the graft are the return of quadriceps femoris muscle strength; lower extremity coordination; cardiovascular conditioning; and the absence of continuing symptoms such as knee joint effusion, instability, and pain.

Straight-line running can begin at 4 to 6 months following surgery if the potential problems listed above are not present. Progression in the duration and intensity of running must be performed slowly to avoid knee joint and patellofemoral joint inflammation and excessive articular cartilage loading.

High-risk sports that involve contact or sudden changes in direction can be resumed 9 to 12 months following surgery. Return to sports and progression of functional activity requires full knee joint ROM, return of quadriceps femoris muscle strength with an active VMO muscle, and sport-specific agility. Functional ability is assessed using the Noyes "Functional Hop" test (see Appendix I).[78] Isokinetic dynamometer scores can be used to test muscle force and endurance levels of the quadriceps femoris and hamstrings. However, dynamometer results do not test functional capacities of the rehabilitated knee.

Derotation Braces

The use of derotation braces during rehabilitation and during individual exercise and sports participation has been a common practice. Timing of implementation and ROM settings remain controversial. The American Academy of Orthopaedic Surgeons reviewed a wide variety of derotation braces in 1984.[79] As published in the Academy's 1985 knee seminar report, the use of braces on the market at that time did not prevent anterior tibial translation or rotation under the stresses of normal sports activity. A similar conclusion was noted in a recent review of the current literature on functional knee bracing.[80] For this reason, the effectiveness of derotation braces must be weighed against the patient's desire to wear a brace after surgery. Braces can be used but should not provide the patient with a false sense of security during activity.

COMPLICATIONS FOLLOWING SURGERY

Complications following ACL reconstruction have been discussed in the literature.[28-30,40,41,81-87] This section of the chapter addresses the complications associated with the surgical procedure, as well as complications associated with the rehabilitation process.

Some surgical complications that can be attributed to error in the operative technique include nonisometric graft positioning,[38,39] inappropriate graft tensioning, inadequate graft fixation, or inadequate notchplasty.[41] These problems usually become apparent in the postoperative period when decreased knee joint motion or increased knee joint laxity becomes evident. Complications such as ischemia, paresis, or even paralysis have been attributed to prolonged tourniquet application at high pressures during surgery.[41]

Other complications become evident during the period following surgery. Infection and deep vein thrombosis (DVT) are both serious complications that may occur after any surgical procedure. In a review of 103 ACL reconstructions, Graf and co-workers[41] reported a 1 percent incidence of both superficial infection and DVT. The use of preoperative and postoperative antibiotics, along with support stockings and early mobilization, can minimize these potentially disastrous complications.

Arthrofibrosis,[40,41,84] infrapatellar contracture syndrome,[85] and pain/irritation over the metallic fixation devices[41] are additional complications that can occur following ACL reconstruction. Soft tissue reaction to surgery can vary from case to case. The patient can develop excessive intercondylar adhesions or posterior compartment adhesions. All of these complications usually result in a loss of knee joint ROM, particularly extension. One reason for these complications, as stated earlier, may be the timing of the reconstruction following the initial injury.[40] To avoid these complications, Shelbourne[40] recommended waiting a minimum of 3 weeks following the initial injury before performing ACL reconstruction. Schaefer and Jackson[81] reported the loss of extension following intra-articular ACL reconstruction in certain patients. These authors noted that the loss of knee joint extension may occur due to a dense fibrous tissue mass anterior to the graft, which they have termed *cyclops syndrome*. In addition to loss of knee joint extension, an audible and palpable clunk is noted in terminal knee joint extension. Following manipulation and arthroscopic debridement of the "cyclops," all 13 patients in this study demonstrated significant improvement in knee joint extension. The precise etiology of the cyclops syndrome is not fully understood, but the authors believe this phenomenon may be partially stimulated by the drilling and preparation of the tibial bone tunnel.

Prolonged immobilization, poor patient compliance, and improper or inadequate rehabilitation techniques are additional reasons why a patient may not achieve full knee joint range of motion. Rehabilitation programs must emphasize immediate PROM exercises, patellar mobilization, and controlled quadriceps femoris muscle exercise to prevent the loss of knee joint extension. The patient must also be instructed in a home exercise program in the early postoperative stages that focuses on achieving full passive knee joint extension.

The long-term effects of knee joint extension loss can lead to permanent knee disability secondary to abnormalities in the lower kinetic chain.[82] Altered gait patterns due to loss of knee joint extension can lead to extensor mechanism dysfunction, patellar tendonitis, and chondrosis around the patellofemoral joint. Hip and lumbar spine dysfunction have also been reported in patients who lack knee joint extension ROM.

Reflex sympathetic dystrophy (RSD) is the term often used to describe the clinical syndrome of excessive or prolonged pain following surgery or accidental trauma.[86] The classic symptom of RSD is pain disproportionate to the physical findings of swelling, cyanosis, and stiffness. An abnormal amount of burning pain, hyperesthesia, and hyperhydrosis may also be present. Initial goals in the management of this condition should be the reduction of pain and swelling. Various modalities, such as transcutaneous electrical nerve stimulation (TENS) or the use of hot-cold contrast baths, may be therapeutic in the acute stages of this disorder. High-dose corticosteroids used in tapering dosages, followed by nonsteroidal anti-inflammatory medication, may also be beneficial in the treatment of RSD. Paravertebral sympathetic blockades are another method of treatment.

Ladd and DeHaven[87] have described a similar condition (reflex sympathetic imbalance [RSI]) in a patient who underwent surgical reconstruction of the ACL and tibial collateral ligament (TCL). The clinical presentation suggested an abnormal sympathetic response but lacked the cardinal signs and symptoms of RSD. The patient received a presumptive diagnosis of incomplete RSD, or RSI. The response of the patient was slow; at 3 months following surgery, the patient continued to experience knee joint stiffness, swelling, and sensation changes in the foot. The patient declined treatment with epidural blockade and continued with supervised physical therapy and anti-inflammatory medication. Most of the sympathetic signs decreased, but persistent signs of arthrofibrosis continued. An arthroscopic lysis of adhesions was performed about 21 months postoperatively, and a complete epidural blockade was used. The sympathetic component of the block was continued via an indwelling catheter for a period of 4 days because of the past history of RSI. Four months after the lysis procedure, the mechanical and sympathetic symptoms had resolved and the patient returned to sports with only minor discomfort.

The same patient sustained a hyperextension-rotational–type injury to the previously uninvolved knee joint, approximately 27 months following the initial injury. The patient experienced mild posteromedial knee joint pain for several months. At 17 months after the initial injury, an arthroscopy that was performed under complete epidural blockade revealed anteromedial synovial scar tissue. As a prophylactic measure prompted by the patient's history of RSI in the contralateral knee, a sympathetic block was continued through an indwelling catheter for several days following surgery. The patient received only transient relief following this procedure. Pain continued and appeared disproportionate to the injury and the operative procedure performed, suggesting a reflex sympathetic disorder. The patient was referred to a pain center at 24 months following the initial injury to this knee, for a possible second epidural. The patient also received a Minnesota Multiphasic Personality Inventory (MMPI) test, and overall scores revealed no abnormalities characteristic of individuals who may be prone to chronic pain problems. An outpatient epidural sympathetic block was repeated with complete resolution of pain. Outpatient physical therapy was resumed, with an emphasis on strength and ROM. The patient was seen at 68 months following the second injury and was actively participating in recreational sports.

CASE STUDIES

The following cases illustrate the problem-solving approach for treatment of patients with selected ACL injuries. The format of the case studies follows the elements of problem solving outlined in Chapter 3. These elements include a sequential evaluation that identifies characteristics and factors that affect the patient's problem, an assessment delineating a problem list, goals of treatment, and plan of treatment.

CASE STUDY 1: AN ACCELERATED REHABILITATION PROGRAM

HISTORY

An active, well-conditioned 32-year-old male sustained an injury to his left knee joint while rounding second base during a softball game. As he was accelerating, he heard a loud "pop" and had immediate knee joint pain and effusion. At the time, he was unable to bear weight on the injured extremity. He sought medical attention and was treated with ice, immobilization, and rest. The knee pain and effusion subsided after two weeks and he was able to continue activities of daily living.

At 6 weeks following the initial injury, he attempted to return to an exercise program consisting of jogging, weight lifting, and bicycling. These activities caused further pain and resulted in knee joint effusion after exercise. He was unable to return to his preinjury active lifestyle and sought an orthopedic consultation approximately 9 months after the initial injury.

EVALUATION

Upon examination by an orthopedist, the patient did not complain of locking, popping, or giving way of the knee. His chief complaint was an inability to return to his preinjury level of activity without knee pain or effusion. Physical evaluation revealed a normal gait pattern without symptoms or the need for an assistive device. Functional testing revealed that the patient was able to completely squat, hop on one leg, and run in place without knee joint symptoms. Knee ROM was 0 to 135 degrees bilaterally. Examination of muscle function in the lower extremities revealed no atrophy of the thigh musculature, and manual muscle testing failed to demonstrate a deficit between the right and left quadriceps femoris muscles. No intra-articular knee joint effusion or prepatellar swelling was present. Tracking of the patellofemoral joint was normal without retropatellar grating or popping, and no tenderness was present in the quadriceps tendon or the patellar tendon. A positive McMurray test was noted, with pain noted over the medial joint line of the knee. The patient had a positive (+3) anterior drawer, Lachman, and pivot shift test. Knee joint arthrometry, as measured using a KT-1000 (Med-Metric Company, San Diego, CA), revealed a 12-mm anterior tibial translation with a 15-lb force, and 16 mm of anterior tibial translation with a 20-lb force. In both tests, the uninvolved knee joint had 0 to 4 mm of anterior tibial translation. The remainder of the ligamentous examination was within normal limits.

The objective examination revealed a well-documented anterior cruciate deficient knee and a possible tear of the medial meniscus. This patient had a strong desire to return to his preinjury level of activity. Therefore, the decision was made to proceed with an ACL reconstruction, using a patellar tendon autograft.

SURGICAL TREATMENT

The patient was examined under anesthesia prior to ACL reconstruction. Arthrometric measurements were reproduced as previously noted. Arthroscopic inspection revealed a buckethandle tear of the medial meniscus and a complete tear of the ACL. The patient also had severe articular cartilage damage. Grade III articular cartilage changes (fibrillation larger than 0.5 inch in diameter) were found on both medial and lateral patellar facets and the medial femoral condyle. Grade II articular cartilage changes (fibrillation of less than 0.5 inch in diameter) were noted on the medial tibial plateau. All other joint surfaces were normal. No synovitis or loose bodies were found.

The buckethandle tear of the medial meniscus was trimmed, maintaining a well-balanced meniscal rim. Isometric placement of the carefully prepared patellar tendon graft was performed via arthroscopy and was fixated with an interference screw. The concept of graft isometry, as stated previously, is achieved when the length of the graft remains relatively unchanged as the knee joint is passively flexed or extended, in the absence of external load or muscle activity. Postsurgical arthrometric measurements confirmed adequate knee joint stability. Postoperative measurements were reduced from 12 mm on a 15-lb force, 16 mm on a 20-lb force, and 19 mm on a maximal force to 3 mm, 4 mm, and 5 mm, respectively.

POSTOPERATIVE CARE

The patient remained in the hospital for 3 days. The patient was placed in a hinged brace locked in full extension for the first 10 postoperative days. The brace was removed to perform exercises, including isometric contractions of the quadriceps femoris and hamstring muscles (see Fig. 9-8A) and PROM exercises (see Fig. 9-3). Additionally, the patient performed bent leg raises with the involved leg in the hinged brace, locked at 40 degrees. Emphasis was on achieving full passive knee joint extension (see Fig. 9–6).

When the patient was able to perform a leg raise independently, toe-touch ambulation was initiated with the use of crutches and a hinged knee brace. Gait training continued until the patient left the hospital.

Outpatient rehabilitation was initiated 1 week following surgery. The initial physical therapy visit included evaluation and treatment, which consisted of strengthening and ROM exercises. Knee joint PROM was −2 degrees of knee joint extension to 73 degrees of knee flexion. The Lachman test revealed a solid end-point. Moderate to severe knee joint effusion and mild soft tissue edema in the lower extremity were noted. Sensation was intact, and the wound showed no signs of infection. Homans' testing for DVT was negative, and palpation of the calf did not elicit any tenderness. The patient was unable to voluntarily perform an isolated contraction of the quadriceps femoris muscle and had a 15-degree knee joint extension lag when actively raising his leg without assistance. VMO muscle contraction was poor. Passive gliding of the patella revealed mild restriction in the superior direction.

PROBLEM LIST

1. Decreased knee joint PROM
2. Knee joint effusion
3. Quadriceps femoris muscle inhibition, characterized by an extensor lag
4. Atrophy and poor motor control of the VMO muscle, resulting in altered patellofemoral mechanics
5. Decreased patellofemoral passive mobility, particularly in a superior direction
6. Lower extremity anterior compartment edema
7. Lack of independent ambulation
8. Decreased cardiovascular conditioning

FACTORS AFFECTING THE PROBLEMS

1. Surgical procedure
   a. *Surgical approach:*   Arthroscopically assisted technique
   b. *Graft selection:*   Autogenous patella tendon
   c. *Graft fixation:*   Interference screws
   d. *Graft placement:*   Isometric
2. Other factors
   a. *Timing of surgery:*   Nine months after initial injury.
   b. *Secondary injuries:*   Buckethandle tear of medial meniscus was trimmed and balanced; chondromalacia of the medial and lateral patellar facets and medial femoral condyle was not debrided.
   c. *Immobilization:*   Locked in full extension for first 10 days only.
   d. *Continuous passive motion unit:*   Not used.
   e. Patient was young, active, healthy, and well-motivated.

TREATMENT GOALS AND PLAN

This patient presented with considerable quadriceps femoris muscle inhibition (as evidenced by the inability to fully contract his quadriceps femoris muscle), active knee extension lag, and decreased patellofemoral joint mobility. All of these findings may have been related to the moderate amount of knee joint effusion.

Based on the problem list and the characteristics of the problem (i.e., arthroscopically assisted patella tendon autograft, isometrically placed; and the fact that the patient was young and well motivated), an accelerated rehabilitation protocol was implemented. The following immediate goals and summary of the treatment plan are based on the problem list:

1. *Achieve full passive knee joint extension and flexion:* Weighted knee extension ("prone hangs") to achieve knee extension. Wall slides, active-assistive knee ROM (using the contralateral extremity), and stationary cycling to achieve knee flexion.
2. *Resolution of knee joint effusion:* Modalities.
3. *Increase strength of the quadriceps femoris and hamstring muscles:* Quadriceps femoris/hamstring muscle setting, closed kinetic chain exercises, progressive-resistive exercises.
4. *Increased motor recruitment of the VMO muscle:* Patient taught manual palpation for selective recruitment of the VMO muscle.
5. *Increase patellofemoral joint mobility:* Patient educated in patellofemoral self-mobilization for medial and superior-inferior glides.
6. *Decrease lower extremity compartment edema:* Soft-tissue massage, elevation of the lower extremity, and ROM exercises to help decrease lower extremity edema. The patient lies supine with the involved lower extremity elevated above the heart. In this position, soft-tissue massage is performed distally to proximally along the lower extremity, followed by the patient's actively performing "ankle pumps" (i.e., repetitive active dorsiflexion and plantar flexion movements).
7. *Promote early independent ambulation:* Full weight bearing is permitted immediately, with the patient using a knee brace and crutches. The use of the brace is discontinued by week 4 and the crutches are discontinued by week 6. Weight shifting and one-legged bouncing are used to facilitate ambulation skills.
8. *Improve conditioning:* Stationary cycling and swimming.

Outpatient physical therapy was initiated with an emphasis on decreasing the knee joint effusion, gaining quadriceps femoris muscle control, improving knee proprioception, and maximizing PROM.

The initial exercises included quadriceps femoris and hamstring muscle co-contraction, hip muscle strengthening, and PROM to the knee joint. All of the exercises were done without the brace. Weighted knee extension in prone (see Fig. 9–6), wall slides (see Fig. 9–5), patellar mobilization (see Fig. 9–4), and active-assistive ROM (see Fig. 9–3) were used at home to help gain knee joint ROM. Ice was applied immediately following exercise and intermittently throughout the day to control postoperative knee joint effusion, and soft-tissue massage was used to reduce lower extremity edema. A stationary bicycle was used on the second outpatient visit to gain knee joint ROM.

ROM of the knee had increased to 0 to 115 degrees within 2 weeks. Continued knee joint effusion appeared to interfere with the patient's ability to regain muscular control. In an effort to reduce knee joint effusion, the patient was asked to reduce ambulation time and the use of ice was continued. Knee joint effusion was reduced by the following week, and the full therapy program was resumed. Closed kinetic chain knee dips in the range of 0 to 60 degrees were added to help increase the strength of the quadriceps and hamstring muscles. The patient was also taught manual palpation of the VMO muscle to enhance recruitment, as well as self-mobilization of the patellofemoral joint (see Fig. 9–4). These exercises were advanced as noted in the Appendix.

The exercise program was increased at 4 weeks to include hip muscle strengthening on exercise equipment. Functional activities such as weight shifting, one-legged bouncing (see Fig. 9–12), and gait exercises were also added at this time, and the hinged knee brace was discontinued.

The patient demonstrated rapid improvement with the strengthening program over the next 4 to 8 weeks. VMO muscle strengthening had improved and was providing adequate tracking of the patella in the femoral trochlear groove. The quadriceps femoris muscle was graded as 3/5, as determined by manual muscle testing. Tibiofemoral joint ROM at 8 weeks had increased to 0 to 135 degrees of flexion. The knee joint remained stable during this phase of rehabilitation. Less than 4 mm of anterior tibial translation was noted during an instrumented Lachman test. The patient experienced mild synovial pain on the medial aspect of the knee joint, but only after prolonged ambulation. This complaint continued for several weeks, but decreased as his VMO muscle strength and control improved.

The patient was able to ambulate without a flexed knee gait pattern by the eighth postoperative week. The patient's attitude, motivation, and dedication to the rehabilitation program were excellent, and he was off the crutches by week 6.

During the second and third postoperative months, emphasis was placed on functional strengthening of the lower extremity. Activities included continued gait training, progressive-resistive exercises for the hip, and squatting with resistance. Leg press machines (see Fig. 9–9G) and lunges (see Fig. 9–9F) were initiated during this time. The home program consisted of cycling, swimming, and closed kinetic chain strengthening exercises.

The third to fourth postoperative month focused on advanced quadriceps femoris muscle strengthening with increased resistance. The patient performed the exercises listed previously, and added the use of the slide board (see Fig. 9–13). The slide board was added earlier than usual because the patient demonstrated good ligamentous stability, excellent VMO muscle control, and high-level proprioception.

Formal physical therapy was discontinued at the end of the fourth postoperative month. The patient was instructed to continue with cycling, swimming, and strengthening exercises independently.

The patient was seen during the fifth postoperative month for a follow-up visit to review the home exercise program. Upon re-evaluation, the patient had full knee joint extension and 135 degrees of knee joint evaluation. Quadriceps femoris and hamstring muscle strength were graded 4+/5 by a manual muscle test, and a visible VMO muscle contraction was evident. Knee joint stability remained intact, with no evidence of increased laxity. The patient had a normal gait and was able to hop on one leg, run in place, and perform a full squat. Resistance was increased for all his hip, quadriceps femoris, and hamstring muscle exercises. A running program was initiated and was progressed as symptoms dictated. After 4 weeks on a running program, the patient was able to complete 2 miles, three times per week, without knee joint pain or effusion.

COMMENTS

This patient represents an ideal case, where rehabilitation following intra-articular ACL reconstruction progressed without difficulty. The only complication encountered was postoperative knee joint effusion. This patient was highly motivated and was compliant with the full rehabilitation program. He did not have severe quadriceps femoris muscle atrophy, which is often seen in patients having a similar surgical procedure. These factors made an accelerated rehabilitation program possible.

Therapists often see patients who have a slower progression of exercise than was presented in this case study. The protocol must consider the entire knee joint and related structures. Patients who have undergone additional procedures such as meniscal repairs or collateral ligament injuries often require a less aggressive postoperative program to allow adequate healing to take place.

CASE STUDY 2: THE PROBLEM KNEE

HISTORY

A 25-year-old athlete sustained a tear of his left ACL and medial meniscus in a local recreational basketball game. He underwent ACL reconstruction using a patellar tendon autograft. The patient was placed in a hinged knee brace locked at 30 degrees of knee joint flexion and began physical therapy 5 weeks following surgery. The patient failed to regain functional motion and underwent arthroscopic lysis and manipulation 6 months following the initial surgery. Physical therapy was resumed and a Dynasplint (Dynasplint Systems, Inc., Baltimore, MD) was used to help decrease his loss of knee joint extension. The subjective comments included the inability to completely straighten or completely flex the involved knee joint. The patient continued to ambulate with a limp and was unable to walk more than $\frac{1}{2}$ mile. Knee pain was aggravated by standing and hindered stair climbing. The patient continued to have problems with knee joint effusion and also complained of grating and grinding within the patellofemoral joint during ambulation.

This patient presented a difficult problem for the rehabilitation team. The case history revealed a severe case of arthrofibrosis in the knee joint. The patient was a dedicated recreational athlete who lost the ability to ambulate normally. In reviewing the case, past medical care appeared to be appropriate, but extenuating circumstances prevented the patient from initiating physical therapy until 5 weeks following surgery. This delay, in conjunction with the patient's highly reactive soft-tissue response to the initial surgery, appears to have been the reason for the complications. Scar tissue developed rapidly, and by the time ROM was initiated, early signs of arthrofibrosis had already developed. Early controlled ROM has reduced the cases of arthrofibrosis, but certain patients are still susceptible to this problem.

EVALUATION

The patient was evaluated in our office 8 months following the initial ACL reconstruction and 2 months following arthroscopic lysis and manipulation. Active knee joint ROM was −20 degrees of extension to 80 degrees of flexion. Passive knee joint flexion-extension movements revealed a firm end feel in both directions, indicating mature scar formation. Quadriceps femoris muscle inhibition was evidenced by the patient's inability to perform a quad set. Patellofemoral joint mobility was significantly restricted in all directions. A mild knee joint effusion was present, and the patient complained of a dull ache around the knee. Tenderness was noted around the graft fixation device on the tibia. The patient also complained of mild retropatellar pain during knee joint flexion-extension movements. Radiographs showed good position of the fixation devices, and no evidence of foreign bodies blocking knee joint ROM was detected. These findings suggested that the patient had arthrofibrosis with extensive patellar entrapment.

SURGICAL TREATMENT

Following the evaluation by the new treatment team, the initial lysis was considered a failure and another attempt at lysis and manipulation was recommended. The second lysis and manipulation was performed 9 months following the initial ACL reconstruction and 3 months after the patient's previous lysis.

The patient underwent an arthroscopic evaluation of the knee joint, which revealed such extensive scarring in the femoral intercondylar notch that an open arthrotomy approach was required. A lateral retinacular and parapatellar incision was made, and scar tissues in these areas were released. Adhesions were lysed in both the lateral gutter and suprapatellar pouch. A cyclops lesion was removed, along with extensive scar tissue under the patellar tendon. Manipulation was performed several times during the procedure as adhesions were cut. After several manipulations were performed, knee joint ROM on the operating table was −4 degrees of extension to 130 degrees of flexion. The tourniquet was released, and the areas of bleeding were ligated. A medium Hemovac drain was inserted, the incisions were stapled, and Ted hose were applied. The patient remained in the hospital overnight, and the involved knee was placed in a CPM device.

PROBLEM LIST

1. Decreased knee ROM
2. Knee joint effusion
3. Quadriceps femoris muscle inhibition
4. Decreased patellofemoral mobility
5. Pain
6. Decreased ambulation skills

FACTORS AFFECTING THE PROBLEMS

1. Surgical factors
   a. Initial ACL reconstruction secure at this time.
   b. Knee joint arthrotomy performed; disruption of patellofemoral and tibio-femoral joints, disruption of quadriceps femoris muscle, and adhesions torn.
2. Other factors
   a. Rehabilitation initiated very late.
   b. Patient has highly reactive scar formation, increasing risk of arthrofibrosis.
   c. Patient has had ROM problems for 9 months.

TREATMENT GOALS AND PLAN

This patient presented with considerable ROM problems, decreased patellofemoral mobility, increased quadriceps femoris muscle inhibition, and postoperative pain. All of these findings may be due to the arthrofibrosis and excessive scar formation leading to surgery. These problems may have been prevented if the original medical team had initiated physical therapy immediately.

Based on the problem list and the related factors affecting the problem (history of arthrofibrosis and recent knee arthrotomy), a rehabilitation program addressing the following goals and treatment techniques was implemented:

1. *Increase knee ROM and decrease risk of arthrofibrosis:* Use of CPM, Dynasplint, self-administered PROM techniques, and eventually a stationary bicycle.
2. *Decrease knee effusion:* Use of a Hemovac, CPM, and self-administered ROM exercises.
3. *Reduce quadriceps femoris muscle inhibition:* Use of muscle stimulation, isometric quad sets, and eventually progressive-resistive exercises as the knee effusion decreases.
4. *Increase patellofemoral mobility:* Teach the patient self-mobilization techniques to restore superior, inferior, and medial glides. Implement stationary cycling to maintain patellofemoral mobility.
5. *Decrease postoperative pain:* Cryotherapy.
6. *Improve ambulation skills:* Gait training as ROM and strength increase.

EARLY REHABILITATION FOLLOWING LYSIS

Physical therapy was initiated on the first postoperative day. Active knee joint ROM prior to treatment was −22 degrees of extension to 63 degrees of flexion. The incisions were healing nicely and no signs of infection were noted. The patient used a CPM device during the day to help gain knee joint flexion ROM. The Dynasplint was used at night to help maintain knee joint extension. The patient was educated in self-administered ROM techniques to restore patellofemoral mobility (see Fig. 9–4). The focus of the rehabilitation during this time was to regain knee joint ROM. Heat was used during passive extension to increase tissue extensibility, and ice was applied following heat to theoretically help stabilize the collagenous microstructure in the newly stretched length.[88,89]

Examination of the knee on the second postoperative day revealed severe joint effusion. The staples were intact and the incision was clean and dry. A large, palpable hematoma was noted around the knee. Further limitation of ROM was noted secondary to the knee joint effusion and pain. Neurovascular status around the knee and throughout the lower extremity was normal. The patient was then seen by his physician, and evacuation of the hematoma was performed the same day. A large hematoma with thick, clotted blood was evacuated from the knee joint during this procedure. Irrigation of the knee was performed after the bleeding was controlled. The incisions were closed and a large Hemovac drain was applied. The patient was discharged on the following day; the CPM unit was used at home during the waking hours, and the Dynasplint was used at night. The patient returned 3 days after the procedure, and physical therapy was resumed. Active ROM prior to treatment was −10 degrees of extension to 75 degrees of knee joint flexion. The incisions were healing well with no signs of infection. Patellofemoral joint mobility was improved, and quadriceps femoris muscle strength was considered 3/5, as noted by a manual muscle test. The patient was advised to continue using both crutches, weight bearing as tolerated. The focus of rehabilitation continued to be decreasing knee joint effusion and increasing knee joint ROM.

A superficial stitch abscess developed over the portal entry of the inflow cannula 10 days following the evacuation of the hematoma. The patient presented no signs of knee joint infection and was afebrile. The infection was treated locally and no antibiotics were administered. Six days later, the incision was completely closed and a decrease in redness was noted.

The patient's gait pattern continued to improve as knee joint ROM returned. The use of quad sets was the primary means of strengthening exercises. Quadriceps femoris muscle control improved as knee joint effusion decreased.

INTERMEDIATE REHABILITATION

Physical therapy continued with an emphasis on restoring knee joint ROM. Joint mobilization procedures were administered to the tibiofemoral joint to gain knee joint flexion and extension. Patellofemoral mobilization continued, emphasizing superior and inferior gliding. The CPM was continued during the daytime for 3 weeks, while the Dynasplint continued to be used at night to gain knee joint extension. A customized seated bike that allows change in crankshaft length was used to accommodate the lack of knee joint motion (Fig. 9–14). Neuromuscular electrical stimulation was used to help maintain quadriceps femoris muscle tone during this period of rehabilitation. Various quadriceps-hamstring muscle isometrics and hip muscle strengthening exercises were performed as knee joint effusion decreased. Active knee joint ROM at this time measured 0 degrees extension to 80 degrees of flexion. The patient had 8 degrees of knee joint hypertension to 130 degrees of flexion on the uninvolved side.

LATE REHABILITATION

The patient was evaluated 11 months after his initial ACL reconstruction and 9 months after his second lysis of adhesions, manipulation, lateral release, removal of hardware, and evacuation of his hematoma. Clearly the patient's postoperative

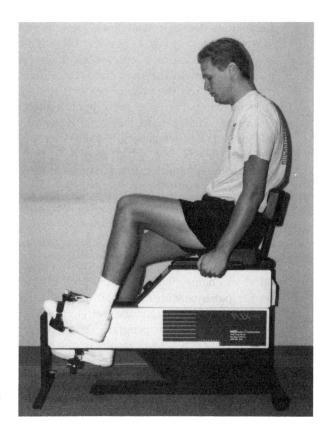

FIGURE 9–14. Customized bicycle with adjustable crank shaft arms.

course had been difficult. The patient was ambulating well and without pain. Active ROM of the knee joint was 4 degrees of knee hyperextension to 100 degrees flexion. Knee joint stability was good, with a firm end feel to the Lachman test and no pivot shift. The patellofemoral joint presented mild crepitus without pain, and a trace of knee joint effusion was present when the patient walked for a long distance. Control of the quadriceps femoris and hamstring muscles continued to improve. The patient discontinued the use of the Dynasplint, and formal physical therapy and a home exercise program was initiated.

COMMENTS

This patient underwent four surgeries and represents a case of the "problem knee." The focus of the early and intermediate phases of rehabilitation was ROM.

The use of short-duration cryotherapy was helpful during the early postoperative phases of this difficult case. Once knee joint effusion was controlled, the use of hot-cold contrast treatments helped to reduce the remaining effusion.

Protection of the patellofemoral joint was another consideration during the early and intermediate rehabilitation phases. Both passive flexion and extension movements of the knee joint were emphasized. The therapist must be concerned about increased patellofemoral forces during passive knee joint flexion. Passive knee joint flexion is an important part of the rehabilitation program, but the overzealous use of forced knee joint flexion was avoided in the intermediate phases of this program to prevent excessive trauma to the patellofemoral joint

This particular case represents a unique history. On reviewing the entire case history, one might question the factors that contributed to the development of arthrofibrosis and the precautions that could have been taken to prevent this case scenario. This patient may represent the select population that has a high reactivity to surgery. Each patient will react differently to surgery and produce different levels of soft-tissue reaction. Physical therapy was initiated on the fifth postoperative week in this case, which may have been the primary problem. By the time physical therapy had begun, a major soft tissue reaction had already occurred and early signs of joint fibrosis were already present.

SUMMARY

The rehabilitation programs presented in this chapter emphasize consideration of the surgical and biomechanical factors necessary for providing safe and effective rehabilitation for patients who have had intra-articular ACL reconstructions. The timely implementation of functional muscle strengthening and joint ROM exercises is the main focus of this rehabilitation program. The use of these exercises, based on scientific evidence and clinical research, results in a safe and effective return of muscle strength and joint ROM. By rehabilitating patients in this manner, the therapist can ensure graft safety and avoid the detrimental effects of immobility and disuse.

REFERENCES

1. Fetto, JF and Marshall, JL: The natural history and diagnosis of anterior cruciate ligament insufficiency. Clin Orthop 147:29, 1980.
2. Noyes, FR, et al: The symptomatic anterior cruciate-deficient knee. I. The long-term functional disability in athletically active individuals. J Bone Joint Surg [Am] 65:154, 1983.
3. Noyes, FR and McGinniss, GH: Controversy about treatment of the knee with anterior cruciate laxity. Clin Orthop 198:61, 1985.
4. Noyes, FR, et al: The symptomatic anterior cruciate-deficient knee. II. The results of rehabilitation, activity modification, and counseling on functional disability. J Bone Joint Surg [Am] 65:163, 1983.
5. Andrews, JR and Carson, WG: The role of extra-articular anterior cruciate ligament stabilization. In Jackson, DW and Drez, D, Jr (eds): The Anterior Cruciate Deficient Knee: New Concepts in Ligament Repair. CV Mosby, St Louis, MO, 1987, p 168.
6. Kaplan, N, Wickiewicz, TL, and Warren, RF: Primary surgical treatment of anterior cruciate ligament ruptures: A long-term follow-up study. Am J Sports Med 18:354, 1990.
7. Weaver, JK, et al: Primary knee ligament repair—revisited. Clin Orthop 199:185, 1985.
8. Hefzy, MS, Grood, ES, and Noyes, FR: Factors affecting the region of most isometric femoral attachments: II. The anterior cruciate ligament. Am J Sports Med 17:208, 1989.
9. O'Brien, SJ, et al: The iliotibial band sling procedure and its effect on the results of anterior cruciate ligament reconstruction. Am J Sports Med 19:21, 1991.
10. Shelbourne, KD and Nitz, P: Accelerated rehabilitation after anterior cruciate ligament reconstruction. Am J Sports Med 18:292, 1990.
11. Ihle, CL and Jackson, DW: Intra-articular surgical considerations. In Jackson, DW and Drez, D, Jr (eds): The Anterior Cruciate Deficient Knee: New Concepts in Ligament Repair. CV Mosby, St Louis, MO, 1987, p 142.
12. Paulos, LE, Payne, FC, and Rosenberg, TD: Rehabilitation after anterior cruciate ligament surgery. In Jackson, DW and Drez, D, Jr (eds): The Anterior Cruciate Deficient Knee: New Concepts in Ligament Repair. CV Mosby. St Louis, MO, 1987, p 291.
13. Noyes, FR, et al: Intra-articular cruciate reconstruction. I. Perspectives on graft strength, vascularization, and immediate motion after replacement. Clin Orthop 172:71, 1983.
14. Paulos, LE, et al: Knee rehabilitation after anterior cruciate ligament reconstruction and repair. Am J Sports Med 9:140, 1981.

15. Jackson, DW and Reiman, PR: Principles of arthroscopic anterior cruciate reconstruction. In Jackson, DW and Drez, D, Jr (eds): The Anterior Cruciate Deficient Knee: New Concepts in Ligament Repair. CV Mosby, St Louis, MO, 1987, p 273.

16. Wilcox, PG and Jackson, DW: Factors affecting choices of anterior cruciate ligament surgery. In Jackson, DW and Drez, D, Jr (eds): The Anterior Cruciate Deficient Knee: New Concepts in Ligament Repair. CV Mosby, St Louis, MO, 1987, p 127.

17. Bonnarens, FO and Drez, D, Jr: Biomechanics of artificial ligaments and associated problems. In Jackson, DW and Drez, D, Jr (eds): The Anterior Cruciate Deficient Knee: New Concepts in Ligament Repair. CV Mosby, St Louis, MO, 1987, p 239.

18. Ahlfeld, SK, Larson, RL, and Collins HR: Anterior cruciate reconstruction in the chronically unstable knee using an expanded polytetrafluoroethylene (PTFE) prosthetic ligament. Am J Sports Med 15:326, 1987.

19. Arnoczky, SP, et al: Biologic fixations of ligament prostheses and augmentations: An evaluation of bone ingrowth in the dog. Am J Sports Med 16:106, 1988.

20. Macnicol, MF, Penny, ID, and Sheppard, L: Early results with the Leeds-Keio anterior cruciate ligament replacement. J Bone Joint Surg [Br] 73:377, 1991.

21. Glousman, R, et al: Gore-Tex prosthetic ligament in anterior cruciate deficient knees. Am J Sports Med 16:321, 1988.

22. Woods, GA, Indelicato, PA, and Prevot, TJ: The Gore-Tex anterior cruciate ligament prosthesis: Two versus three year results. Am J Sports Med 19:48, 1991.

23. Hanley, P, et al: Load sharing and graft forces in anterior cruciate ligament reconstructions with the Ligament Augmentation Device. Am J Sports Med 17:414, 1989.

24. Drez, D, Jr, et al: Anterior cruciate ligament reconstruction using bone-patellar tendon-bone allografts: A biological and biochemical evaluation in goats. Am J Sports Med 19:256, 1991.

25. Jackson, DW, Windler, GE, and Simon, TM: Intra-articular reaction with the use of freeze-dried, ethylene oxide-sterilized bone-patellar tendon-bone allografts in the reconstruction of the anterior cruciate ligament. Am J Sports Med 18:1, 1990.

26. Jackson, DW and Kurzweil, PK: Allografts in knee ligament surgery. In Scott, WN (ed): Ligament and Extensor Mechanism Injuries of the Knee: Diagnosis and Treatment. Mosby–Yearbook, St. Louis, 1991, pp 349–360.

27. Noyes, FR, et al: Biomechanical analysis of human ligaments used in knee-ligament repairs and reconstructions. J Bone Joint Surg [Am] 66:344, 1984.

28. DeLee, JC and Craviotto, DF: Rupture of the quadriceps tendon after a central third patellar tendon anterior cruciate ligament reconstruction. Am J Sports Med 19:415, 1991.

29. Sachs, RA, et al: Patellofemoral problems after anterior cruciate ligament reconstruction. Am J Sports Med 17:760, 1989.

30. Tibone, JE and Antich, TJ: A biomechanical analysis of anterior cruciate ligament reconstruction with the patellar tendon: A two year followup. Am J Sports Med 16:332, 1988.

31. Gomes, JLE and Marczyk, LRS: Anterior cruciate ligament reconstruction with a loop or double thickness of the semitendinosus tendon. Am J Sports Med 3:199, 1984.

32. Marder, RA, Raskind, JR, and Carroll, M: Prospective evaluation of arthroscopically assisted anterior cruciate ligament reconstruction: Patellar tendon versus semitendinosus and gracillis tendons. Am J Sports Med 19:478, 1991.

33. Sgaglione, NA, et al: Primary repair with semitendinosus tendon augmentation of anterior cruciate ligament injuries. Am J Sports Med 18:64, 1990.

34. Kurosaka, M, Yoshiya, S, and Andrish, JT: A biomechanical comparison of different surgical techniques of graft fixation in anterior cruciate ligament reconstruction. Am J Sports Med 15:225, 1987.

35. Daniel, DM, et al: Fixation of soft tissue. In Jackson, DW and Drez, D, Jr (eds): The Anterior Cruciate Deficient Knee: New Concepts in Ligament Repair. CV Mosby, St Louis, MO, 1987, p 114.

36. Blair, DF and Wills, RP: Rapid rehabilitation following anterior cruciate ligament reconstruction. Athletic Training 26:32, 1991.

37. Indelicato, PA: Current concepts in ACL reconstruction and rehabilitation. Presented at Combined Sections Meeting of The American Physical Therapy Association, Orlando, FL, February 1991.

38. Penner, DA, et al: An in vitro study of anterior cruciate ligament graft placement and isometry. Am J Sports Med 16:238, 1988.

39. Sapega, AA, et al: Testing for isometry during reconstruction of the anterior cruciate ligament: Anatomical and biomechanical considerations. J Bone Joint Surg [Am] 72:259, 1990.

40. Shelbourne, KD, et al: Arthrofibrosis in acute anterior cruciate ligament reconstruction: The effect of timing of reconstruction and rehabilitation. Am J Sports Med 19:332, 1991.

41. Graf, B and Uhr, F: Complications of intra-articular anterior cruciate ligament reconstruction. In Indelicato, PA (ed): Treatment of the Anterior Cruciate Ligament-Deficient Knee. Clin Sports Med 7:4, 1988.

42. Arnoczky, SP: The vascularity of the anterior cruciate ligament and associated structures: Its role in repair and reconstruction. In Jackson, DW and Drez, D, Jr (eds): The Anterior Cruciate Deficient Knee: New Concepts in Ligament Repair. CV Mosby, St Louis, MO, 1987, pp 27–54.

43. Ameil, D, Kuiper, S, and Akeson, WH: Cruciate ligaments: Response to injury. In Daniel, D, Akeson, W, and O'Conner, J. (eds): Knee Ligaments: Structure, Function, Injury, and Repair. Raven Press, New York 1990, pp 365–377.

44. Palmer, I: On the injuries of the ligaments of the knee joint: A clinical study. Acta Chir Scand Suppl 53:1, 1938.
45. Butler, DL: Anterior cruciate ligament: Its normal response and replacement. J Orthop Res 7:910, 1989.
46. Clancy, WE, et al: Anterior and posterior cruciate ligament reconstruction in rhesus monkeys. J Bone Joint Surg [Am] 8:1270, 1981.
47. Noyes, FR, et al: Biomechanics of ligament failure. II. An analysis of immobilization, exercise, and reconditioning effects in primates. J Bone Joint Surg [Am] 56:1406, 1974.
48. Amiel, D, et al: The phenomenon of "ligamentization": Anterior cruciate ligament reconstruction with the autogenous patellar tendon. J Orthop Res 4:162, 1986.
49. Solomonow, M, et al: The synergistic action of the anterior cruciate ligament and thigh muscles in maintaining joint stability. Am J Sports Med 15:207, 1987.
50. Voight, MI and Weider, DL: Comparative reflex response times of the vastus medialis obliquus and vastus lateralis in normal subjects and subjects with extensor mechanism dysfunction. Am J Sports Med 19:2, 1991.
51. Barrack, RL, Skinner, HB, and Buckley, SL: Proprioception in the anterior cruciate ligament deficient knee. Am J Sports Med 17:1, 1989.
52. Noyes, FR: Functional properties of knee ligaments and alterations induced by immobilization. Clin Orthop 123:210, 1977.
53. Salter, RB, et al: The biological effect of continuous passive motion on the healing of full-thickness defects in articular cartilage: An experimental investigation in the rabbit. J Bone Joint Surg [Am] 62:1232, 1980.
54. Arvidsson, I and Eriksson, E: Counteracting muscle atrophy after ACL surgery: Scientific bases for a rehabilitation program. In Feagin, JA (ed): The Crucial Ligaments. Churchill Livingstone, New York, 1988 p 451.
55. Noyes, FR, Mangine, RE, and Barber, S: Early knee motion after open and arthroscopic anterior cruciate ligament reconstruction. Am J Sports Med 15:149, 1987.
56. Drez, D, Jr, et al: In vivo measurement of anterior tibial translation using continuous passive motion devices. Am J Sports Med 19:381, 1991.
57. Rosen, MA, Jackson, DW, and Atwell, EA: A comparison of immediate continuous passive and active motion in the rehabilitation of anterior cruciate ligament reconstructions. Am J Sports Med 15:2, 1987.
58. O'Driscoll, SW, Kumar, A, and Salter, RB: The effect of continuous passive motion on the clearance of a hemarthrosis from a synovial joint. Clin Orthop 176:305, 1983.
59. Anderson, AF and Lipscomb, AB: Analysis of rehabilitation techniques after anterior cruciate reconstruction. Am J Sports Med 17:154, 1989.
60. Seto, JL, et al: Rehabilitation of the knee after anterior cruciate ligament reconstruction. The Journal of Orthopaedic and Sports Physical Therapy 11:1, 1989.
61. Frankel, VH and Nordin, M: Biomechanics of the knee. In Hunter, CW and Funk, FJ (eds): Rehabilitation of the Injured Knee. CV Mosby, St Louis, MO, 1984, p 37.
62. Arms, SW, et al: The biomechanics of anterior cruciate ligament rehabilitation and reconstruction. Am J Sports Med 12:8, 1984.
63. Grood, ES, et al: Biomechanics of knee-extension exercise. J Bone Joint Surg [Am] 66:725, 1984.
64. Henning, CE, Lynch, MA, and Glick, KR: An in vivo strain gauge study of elongation of the anterior cruciate ligament. Am J Sports Med 13:22, 1985.
65. Renstrom, P, et al: Strain within the anterior cruciate ligament during hamstring and quadriceps activity. Am J Sports Med 14:83, 1986.
66. McConnell, J: Patella alignment an quadriceps strength. In Proceedings of the Fifth Biennial Conference of the Manipulative Therapists Association of Australia, Melbourne. 1987, p 399.
67. Jurist, KA and Otis, JC: Anteroposterior tibiofemoral displacements during isometric extension efforts: The roles of external load and knee flexion angle. Am J Sports Med 13:254, 1985.
68. Nisell, R, et al: Tibiofemoral joint forces during isokinetic knee extension. Am J Sports Med 17:49, 1989.
69. Delitto, A, et al: Electrical stimulation versus voluntary exercise in strengthening thigh musculature after anterior cruciate ligament surgery. Phys Ther 68:661, 1988.
70. Snyder-Mackler, L, et al: Electrical stimulation of the thigh muscles after reconstruction of the anterior cruciate ligament. J Bone Joint Surg [Am] 73:1205, 1991.
71. Engle, RP, et al: Immediate post-op anterior cruciate ligament rehabilitation: role of quadriceps facilitation techniques in full extension. Presented at the Annual Conference of the American Physical Therapy Association, Anaheim, CA, June 1990.
72. Ohkoshi, Y and Yasuda, K: Biomechanical analysis of shear force exerted on anterior cruciate ligament during half squat exercise. Presented at the 35th annual meeting of the Orthopedic Research Society, Las Vegas, NV, February 6–9, 1989.
73. Pope, MH, et al: Effect of knee musculature on anterior cruciate ligament strain in vivo. J Elect Kinesiol 1:191, 1991.
74. Chandler, TJ, Wilson, GD, and Store, MH: The effects of the squat exercise on knee stability. Med Sci Sports Exerc 21:299, 1989.
75. Whieldon, T, Yack, J, and Collins, C: Anterior tibial displacement during weight bearing and non-weight bearing rehabilitation exercises in the anterior cruciate deficient knee (abstr). Phys Ther 69:151, 1989.

76. Edlich, RF, et al: Bioengineering principles of hydrotherapy. J Burn Care Rehabil 8:580, 1987.
77. Lephart, SM, et al: Functional performance tests for the anterior cruciate ligament insufficient athlete. Athletic Training 26:44, 1991.
78. Noyes, FR, Barber SD, and Mangine, RE: Abnormal lower limb symmetry determined by function lap tests after anterior cruciate ligament rupture. Am J Sports Med 19(5):513, 1991.
79. Knee Braces Seminar Report. American Academy of Orthopaedic Surgeons, Park Ridge, IL, 1985.
80. Cawley, PW, France, EP, and Paulos, LE: The current state of functional knee bracing research: A review of the literature. Am J Sports Med 19:226, 1991.
81. Jackson, DW and Schaefer, RK: Cyclops syndrome: Loss of extension following intra-articular ACL reconstruction. Arthroscopy 6:171, 1990.
82. Einhorn, AE and Sawyer, M: The problem knee: Soft tissue considerations. In Engle, RP (ed): Knee Ligament Rehabilitation. Churchill Livingston, New York, 1991, pp 197–219.
83. Sprague, NF, O'Conner, RL, and Fox, JM: Arthroscopic treatment of postoperative knee fibroarthrosis. Clin Orthop 166:165, 1982.
84. Sprague, NF: Motion-limiting arthrofibrosis of the knee: The role of arthroscopic management. Clin Sports Med 6:537, 1987.
85. Paulos, LE, et al: Infrapatellar contracture syndrome: An unrecognized cause of knee stiffness with patella entrapment and patella infera. Am J Sports Med 15:4, 1987.
86. Pillemer, FG and Micheli, LJ: Psychological considerations in youth sports. In Micheli, LJ (ed): Injuries in the Young Athlete. Clinics in Sports Medicine 7:3, 1988.
87. Ladd, A and DeHaven, KE: The problem: Reflex sympathetic imbalance. In Ferguson, AB (ed): Orthopaedic Consultation, 11:4, HP Publishing Company, New York, 1990.
88. Sapega, AA, et al: Biophysical factors in range of motion exercise. The Physician and Sportsmedicine 9:57, 1981.
89. Sapega, AA: Advances in the nonsurgical treatment of joint contracture: A biophysical perspective. Presented at the Conference on Postgraduate Advances in Sports Medicine, Philadelphia, 1988.

CHAPTER 10

Rehabilitation of Extra-articular Reconstructions

Terry R. Malone, EdD, PT, ATC

The history of extra-articular (E-A) surgery is not as brief as many clinicians may believe. Surgical procedures and concepts popularized during the 1970s had their origins in much earlier times.[1-5] Those pioneering efforts provided the basis for the modern surgical era. During the 1970s, two patterns of surgical procedures developed to address anterior cruciate ligament (ACL) disruption. The first involved the replacement of the damaged cruciate with an intra-articular (I-A) graft (see Chapter 9); the second used an extra-articular tissue realignment to minimize the abnormal biomechanics that develop following ACL rupture. This chapter focuses on the E-A procedures and the rehabilitation techniques used following such surgeries. A case study will illustrate the problem solving for rehabilitation in a patient who has undergone E-A surgery. The intervening 20 years have allowed much scrutiny, additional development, and more appropriate selection and use of surgical procedures. Today, the E-A reconstruction is used much less frequently and according to very specific criteria, such as in adolescents with open epiphyses, and in minimally ligamentously 1ax/low-functional-demand patients. However, E-A surgery has played a major role in the evolution of ACL surgery and in the presently popular aggressive rehabilitation techniques now applied to intra-articular surgical procedures.

The modern development of E-A reconstruction can be traced to the work of Galway, Beaupre, and MacIntosh.[6] These authors described the role of the iliotibial band (ITB) in relationship to the "pivot shift" phenomenon. They demonstrated how the biomechanics of the pivot shift evolved and how altering the ITB could prevent this phenomenon. The *pivot shift* can best be described as the forceful internal rotation of the tibia or external rotation of the femur over a fixed tibia, allowing a subluxation of the lateral tibial plateau in relation to the femur with the knee near full extension. As

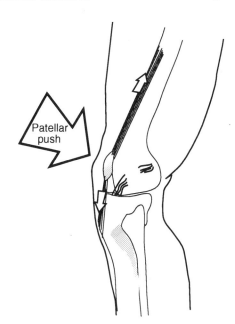

FIGURE 10-1. The slingshot effect of the quadriceps as described by Losee. The lateral femoral
complex is subluxated posteriorly because the anterior cruciate ligament is insufficient. The patellar
mechanism acts as a pushing agent. (Adapted from
Losee,[7] p 46.)

the subject flexes the knee, a forceful reduction of the subluxation occurs through the
tension of the ITB as it moves from anterior to posterior to the axis of rotation.[7] Losee
described these concepts in detail as well as the functional sequence of this maneuver
being related to the inherent interaction of the ITB and the quadriceps mechanism[7] (Figs.
10-1 and 10-2). The E-A reconstructive procedures were designed to function primarily as "check reins" to prevent the pivot shift from engaging during function. The
procedures could be based either distally or proximally, but all were dependent on
maintaining the ITB posterior to the axis of rotation. Rehabilitation associated with these
surgeries was specific to the structure and the healing/maturation constraints of the
tissues used. The rehabilitation sequence was based extensively on a functional progression of sequenced activities.[8]

SURGICAL PROCEDURES AND RELATED
REHABILITATION PROCEDURES

Four of the more popular surgical procedures used during the 1970s are presented
with their rehabilitation protocols. Each of these procedures has its inherent advantages
and disadvantages.

MacIntosh Procedure

The MacIntosh procedure was designed to use a strip of ITB approximately 1.5 cm
wide and 30 cm in length. The graft was anchored distally and detached proximally to
allow the development of a strip. This strip was then passed under the lateral collateral
ligament through an osteo-periosteal tunnel as the surgeon externally rotated the tibia
and then looped back upon itself through the intermuscular septum, and back to

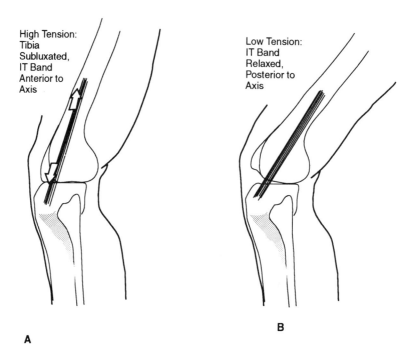

FIGURE 10–2. The iliotibial band functions to pull the tibia posteriorly from its anteriorly subluxated position during the pivot-shift phenomenon. A) When the knee is near extension, the IT band is anterior to the axis of rotation and under tension. B) As the knee is flexed, the reduction from this subluxated position occurs through the IT band, which causes it to become relaxed after 30 to 40 degrees of flexion. (Adapted from Losee,[7] p 49.)

Gerdy's tubercle (Fig. 10–3A–D). The physician closed the defect in the ITB, thus further tightening the lateral complex. Postoperative management included the maintenance of the externally rotated and posteriorly placed tibia for 6 to 8 weeks. Immobilization was performed with the patient placed in a postoperative cast for 7 days, followed by an additional 5 to 7 weeks using a hinge cast or hinge orthosis to allow a protected range of motion (ROM). The early ROM (weeks 2 to 4) was from 90 to 60 degrees, and later weeks (4 to 6) from 90 to 30 degrees. During hinge casting the patient was allowed to perform both isotonic and isometric exercises. Patients were encouraged to work very aggressively on their hamstring muscles and in the ROM of 90 to 40 degrees during isometric and isotonic quadriceps femoris exercises. The patient remained non–weight bearing until cast removal at 7 to 8 weeks.

EARLY REHABILITATION: CAST REMOVAL TO FULL WEIGHT BEARING

Patients were urged not to attempt to bear full weight until they had active control of knee extension. Most patients achieved full active knee extension within 5 to 8 days after removal of the hinge cast. Patients were allowed to work on active ROM and whirlpool activities to achieve greater knee range, but they were urged to achieve extension through muscular control. These patients achieved full extension at 10 days following hinge cast removal and were weight bearing to tolerance, progressing on to full weight bearing typically within 2 weeks of cast removal. We allowed full active knee extension because concomitant external rotation of the tibia during open kinetic chain

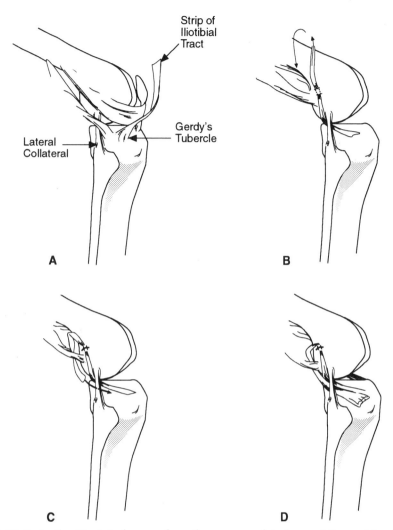

FIGURE 10-3. In the MacIntosh procedure the surgeon detaches a 1.5-cm strip of IT band proximally (*A*) and passes it under the fibular collateral ligament through an osteoperiosteal tunnel (*B*), then through the lateral intramuscular septum. After posteriorly positioning and externally rotating the tibia, the surgeon fixes the graft at the osteoperiosteal tunnel with a staple (*C*), then continues the graft back upon itself and stabilized it to Gerdy's tubercle (*D*). This makes a passive checkrein on anterior displacement of the lateral tibial plateau. (Adapted from Bassett, F.: Anterolateral rotatory instability of the knee. Phys Ther, 16:1635, 1980.)

knee extension protected this surgical procedure. Abductor and adductor muscle strengthening was emphasized to provide dynamic stability to the knee.

INTERMEDIATE REHABILITATION: 2 TO 5 WEEKS FROM CAST REMOVAL

The majority of patients had achieved full knee extension and essentially full ROM through the first 2 weeks of mobilization. They were fully weight bearing and were beginning what we termed a "protected strengthening environment." Patients worked on terminal extension but avoided heavy progressive resistive exercises (PREs) to terminal extension. Isokinetic exercises were performed at high angular velocities. We used lower speed isokinetics only on a submaximal level and advanced to moderate and higher speeds as quickly as possible. This approach allowed us to minimize compression and shear forces within the patellofemoral joint articular surfaces. Cycling and step-ups were two of the activities we used extensively during the intermediate phase.

ADVANCED REHABILITATION

At 3 to 4 months postoperatively, the advanced phase of rehabilitation began. Strength was approximately 80 percent and endurance was 80 percent, as assessed with isokinetic bilateral comparisons of involved versus uninvolved knees. The patients performed a functional progression as dictated by their chosen activities. Running was begun 3 to 4 months postoperatively, and a return to full competitive athletics was allowed somewhere between 6 and 8 months. Our experience indicated that 2 to 3 months of functional training in a particular activity were required before full competition would be advisable. This time frame was required for normalization of muscular responses through neural enhancement.[8]

We recently published a long-term follow-up of our patients treated with this procedure.[9] Our experience indicated that patients with a relatively low functional demand on their reconstructed knee returned to preinjury level of function, whereas patients who demanded high knee function, patients with varus knees, and individuals who had previous meniscectomies, active recurvatum, or generalized knee laxity were not performing at their preinjury level of function when evaluated after 5 or more years.

Unique in the rehabilitation of these patients was the ability to perform terminal knee extension activities safely, as external tibial rotation was a desired position. A second important factor was allowing early limited ROM through hinge casting, providing movement at 7 to 10 postoperative days. A third hallmark was promoting exercises with a hamstring muscle emphasis but also with active quadriceps femoris muscle work starting during the hinge cast immobilization phase. These patients were allowed to return to full activity at approximately 6 to 8 months and were involved in an advanced rehabilitation phase at 3 to 4 months. Finally, the rehabilitation was designed around functional progression as dictated by the demands of the individual patient.

Sling and Reef Procedure

Losee and associates described a diagnostic test and operative repair using a distally based ITB transfer, which they described as the sling and reef procedure.[10] This procedure was quite similar to the previously described MacIntosh procedure but varied in the placement and stabilization of the graft. The procedure used a 2.5-cm-wide and 16-cm-long strip of distally based ITB routed through an osseus tunnel in the lateral condyle of the femur, passed through the posterior capsule and lateral gastrocnemius, then brought distally under the lateral collateral ligament and returned to Gerdy's tubercle. The posterior lateral capsule and gastrocnemius muscle were tightened and sutured as the graft was brought posteriorly and begun on its return path toward the lateral collateral ligament. The tibia was held in external rotation with the knee flexed to approximately 45 degrees during this procedure and maintained in a flexed position postoperatively. The lateral defect in the fascia lata was approximated in those patients in whom it could be sutured without excessive tension, but otherwise it was frequently left open, allowing the development of a harmless asymptomatic hernia (Fig. 10–4). The knee was maintained postoperatively in a flexed position from 30 to 45 degrees for the first 6 to 8 weeks. Losee and associates recommended the use of an external rotation long leg brace for 3 months after discontinuing the cast. They allowed partial weight bearing until the patient had regained full extension, and allowed exercises while in the brace, concentrating on the biceps femoris muscle and low-ROM quadriceps femoris muscle strengthening (90 to 30 degrees). This approach requires a fairly lengthy period to provide some level of immobilization/protected mobilization. To maintain tibial external rotation during this 3-month sequence was difficult, and frequently patients were noncompliant with wearing the unit.

Losee and associates reported strong subjective satisfaction with this procedure and better than 80 percent objectively good or better results in short-term follow-up. As with the previously described MacIntosh procedure, this procedure attempted to prevent the pivot shift from occurring, as well as reefing, or plicating, the posterolateral structures that may have become stretched in patients who had experienced chronic ACL insufficiency. Losee and associates emphasized the importance of longer follow-up in their article and expressed concern that these procedures may not be sufficient in the relatively severe ligamentous instability or global instability seen with some ACL deficient patients. His early results demonstrated that patients achieved inconsistent ROM. The rehabilitation sequence recommended for these patients required a very slow progression, in that the effort to minimize internal tibial rotation stress and to protect the advanced/sutured posterolateral structures required a careful, gradual resumption of forceful extension activities. This approach contrasted somewhat to the early aggressive activities allowed with the MacIntosh procedure alone, inasmuch as that procedure did not require the healing of the advanced posterolateral structures.

Proximally Based Iliotibial Band (ITB) Procedure

Ellison[11] presented the distal ITB transfer for anterolateral rotatory instability in 1979. This procedure incorporated a 1.5-cm-wide strip of iliotibial tract routed beneath the fibular collateral ligament, allowing an advancement and distal fixation of this portion of the ITB. This technique is accomplished with the knee in approximately 90 degrees of flexion, and the knee is extended to determine the tension of this advanced tissue (Fig. 10–5). The author felt that if the knee could be extended beyond 30 degrees, the graft had not been advanced distally enough and thus the transfer was too loose. This procedure was designed to function as a check rein, which tightened to prevent the anterior displacement of the tibia. Ellison recommended complete closure of the iliotibial tract unless the proximal base was too wide to allow adequate closure. One of the problems with not getting closure of the lateral defect was the residual one-plane lateral instability that could develop. This procedure was designed as a dynamic functional transfer, and the author emphasized the importance of not having any suture or any other tissues that would interfere with the free movement of this graft.

Postoperative management began with a long leg cast and with the knee in 60 degrees of flexion and neutral or external rotation. The patients were immobilized for a minimum of 6 weeks, with many surgeons using 8 weeks of strict immobilization. Gentle ROM activities were initiated following cast immobilization, but full extension was not encouraged for a minimum of 12 weeks, and the authors emphasized the attempted avoidance of knee hyperextension.

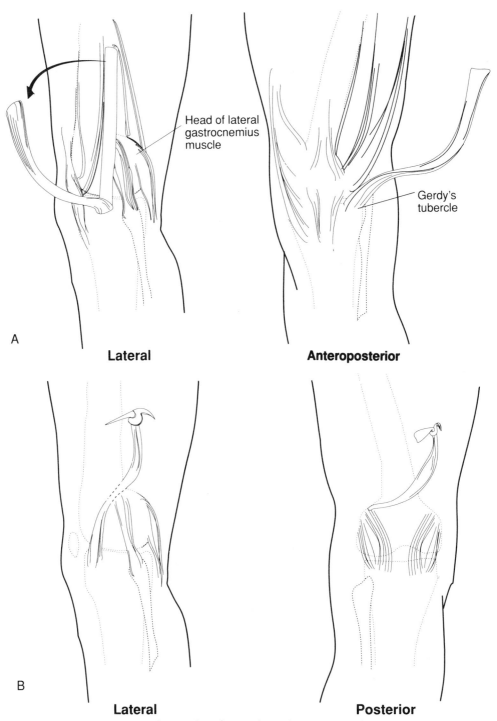

FIGURE 10-4. In the Losee sling and reef procedure, the surgeon splits the IT tract to create a strip about 16 cm long, still attached distally to Gerdy's tubercle (A). The surgeon routes the strip through a tunnel created in the lateral femoral condyle, then (with the knee flexed and held in external rotation) through the posterior capsule and the lateral gastrocnemius muscle (B), suturing the strip along this path and finally anchoring it back at Gerdy's tubercle (C). (Adapted from Losee,[10] pp 1019, 1023.)

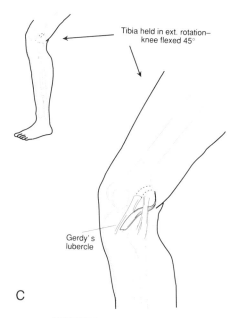

Tibia held in ext. rotation–
knee flexed 45°

Gerdy's
tubercle

C

FIGURE 10–4. *Continued.*

Early rehabilitation highlighted hamstring muscle strengthening, and the authors recommended the development of hamstring-to-quadriceps-femoris muscle parity prior to the development of additional quadriceps femoris muscle work.[11] The use of a derotation brace in the early months of convalescence was also recommended. The first 3 months of postoperative management were designed to minimize full extension and aggressive strengthening. Hamstring muscle-strengthening emphasis was similar to that of today, but we are now more aware of the importance of a balanced approach (multiple exercise patterns and functions) in our rehabilitation sequence and how difficult it is for the advanced material to be sufficient to control global instability. The dynamic function of the advanced ITB proposed by Ellison has not been documented by electromyography, and the positive early results were somewhat tempered by the experience of other authors.[12] One of the primary criticisms of the Ellison procedure involved the persistence of the pivot shift phenomenon during postoperative evaluation. Rehabilitation of these patients involved ROM within the protection or limitations of the procedure. The majority of surgeons recommend 6 to 8 weeks of protected immobilization followed by 4 to 8 weeks of protected mobilization. Weight bearing was advanced as the patient achieved active knee extension, but the patient had to demonstrate excellent control of knee extension prior to full weight bearing. As ROM was normalized, tibial rotation became a very important portion of this sequence. Because proximally based dynamic control is the active portion of the repair, 90-degree knee flexion combined with tibial rotation activities are quite useful. Thus, in our isokinetic programs we included tibial rotation exercises as well as knee flexion-extension. Adductor and abductor muscle strengthening exercises were emphasized because these muscle groups are dynamic stabilizers to the knee.[8] Submaximal isokinetic exercise is useful to recruit type I muscle fibers, and range limiting may be required to minimize terminal extension. Typically, the advanced phase of rehabilitation began at approximately 6 months postoperatively, and a functional progression of activities was then imple-

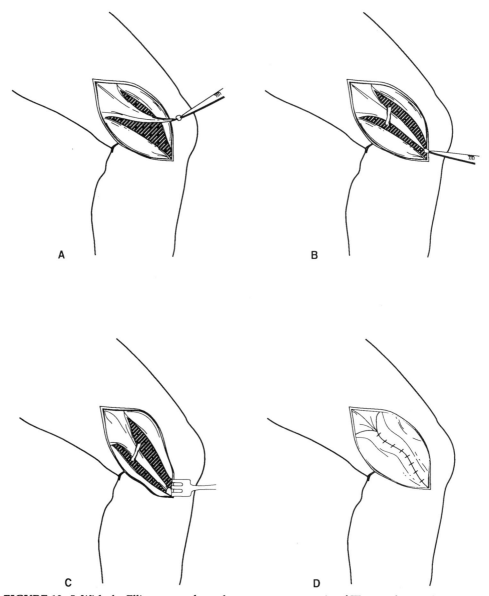

FIGURE 10-5. With the Ellison procedure, the surgeon cuts a strip of IT, complete with a terminal button of bone from Gerdy's tubercle (*A*), and passes it under the lateral collateral ligament. Then with the knee held in flexion (*B*), the surgeon fixes the strip into a trough on the tibia (*C*) and closes the IT tract over the graft (*D*). (Adapted from Ellison,[11] pp 331–333.)

mented. Dynamic control of the tibia is a required and important part of successful implementation of this sequence, in that the reconstruction is based proximally.

The majority of clinicians who rehabilitated patients with the Ellison procedure found difficulty in preventing a fairly rapid return of knee extension, and frequently a hyperextended state. The use of the Ellison procedure alone has become relatively uncommon, because the procedure fails to prevent the pivot shift phenomenon. Some surgeons continue to use this procedure as a backup during the performance of an intra-articular primary reconstructive procedure.[12] Although the surgical procedure was designed to function dynamically, no author has been able to document this action.

Minireconstruction

The Andrews procedure is a tenodesis of the iliotibial tract consisting of two parallel bundles or fiber strips that are attached to the lateral femoral condyle[13] (Fig. 10–6). This approach was basically designed to create two "ligaments" to duplicate the two bands of the ACL. The stabilization occurs through suture and by exposing the surface of the lateral femoral condyle to allow fibrous opposition and ingrowth. The tibia is slightly externally rotated during this procedure but not so greatly as to prevent normal tibial rotations required with function. Postoperatively, the lower extremity was placed in a 45-degree splint or cylinder cast. The majority of patients treated with this procedure were suffering chronic ACL insufficiency and were immobilized in the 45-degree position for approximately 6 weeks. After cast removal, progressive resistance quadriceps femoris muscle exercises were performed in a 45-to-90-degree restricted ROM, and hamstring muscle exercises were aggressively pursued. Early return of extension was not allowed, and the patients were typically kept partially weight bearing for approximately 3 months. Cycling was one of the activities used extensively with these patients. A functional progression of activity was permitted at 4 to 5 months, and approximately 7 months following surgery most patients were allowed to return to a competitive athletic environment.

These patients were sometimes very difficult to prevent from moving more aggressively into early weight bearing and full extension than the surgeon would prefer. The surgeon may have difficulty making sure that proper tension and orientation of this graft has been achieved. As Andrews noted, "In spite of its strength, however, reconstruction and repair relying on the iliotibial tract can have several disadvantages. With time, the tract can stretch and loosen. In addition, devascularization can occur, as well as division of the linear integrity of the fibers and disruption of its anatomic continuity with the lateral capsule."[13] The technique should probably not be used for chronic "global instability," and long-term results may not be as positive as the 2 year follow-up data on which the Andrews[13] article was based.

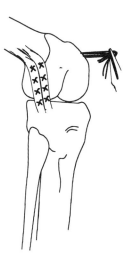

FIGURE 10–6. The Andrews minireconstruction uses two bundles of IT tract fibers to approximate the function of the ACL. The procedure involves creating two bundles of IT tract fibers and attaching them with sutures passed through holes drilled in the femoral condyle. To promote fibrous ingrowth from the IT bands, the surface of the condyle is roughened (fishscaled) before the bands are sutured. (Adapted from Andrews and Sanders,[13] p 94.)

CASE STUDY: REHABILITATION FOLLOWING EXTRA-ARTICULAR RECONSTRUCTION

The following case presents problem solving during the formulation and progression of a patient with an E-A surgery. The elements of problem solving include a clarifying evaluation, an assessment with a problem list, factors that affect the problem, short-term and long-term goals, and a treatment plan. Periodic reevaluation and modification of treatment is emphasized throughout rehabilitation.

HISTORY

The patient was a middle-aged healthy male attorney who sustained a varus-internal tibial rotation injury to his right knee while playing tennis. He was not a particularly avid tennis player, usually only playing once or twice each month. He felt a "pop" in his right knee, developed immediate swelling and pain, and was unable to walk. Subsequent clinical and magnetic resonance imaging evaluation confirmed an isolated ACL tear.

INITIAL COURSE OF ACTION

Because the patient was 55 years old and relatively sedentary, the surgeon and patient together decided not to reconstruct the ACL. The patient underwent 3 months of rehabilitation directed by a physical therapist and returned to his previous preinjury life-style without major difficulty.

Approximately 1 year after the patient was discharged from formal physical therapy, he began to experience a "slipping" sensation in his knee joint. He complained to his orthopedic surgeon that his knee felt unstable and he was having difficulty performing daily activities of living.

Subsequent evaluation indicated the following:

1. Mild effusion right knee
2. Full active/passive ROM
3. 2+ Lachman test
4. 1+ Jerk and Pivot Shift tests
5. Atrophy, most obvious in vastus medialis muscle
6. Meniscal tests (McMurray test and Appley's Grind test) were negative.

The diagnosis was made of an ACL deficient knee with anterolateral instability due to chronic stretching of the anterolateral knee capsule. Because of the age and activity level of the patient, the decision was made to perform an E-A reconstruction using a MacIntosh procedure and to avoid an I-A reconstruction of the ACL.

The MacIntosh procedure was performed (see Fig. 3A–D), and the patient was immobilized in a cast with the knee flexed to 45 degrees for 7 days. After 7 days the patient was fitted with a hinge brace set at 90 to 60 degrees of motion. The ROM of the hinge brace was increased at week 4 to 90 to 30 degrees. The brace remained on for 5 weeks. The patient was instructed to perform hourly active and passive knee ROM exercises, as well as multiple-angle isometric contractions to both his quadriceps femoris and hamstring muscles. The patient was non–weight bearing during this time and was referred for formal physical therapy after the brace was removed (6 weeks after surgery).

PHYSICAL THERAPY EVALUATION

Initial physical therapy evaluation indicated the following:

1. Severe atrophy of the vastus medialis obliquus muscle, right knee
2. Active range of motion (AROM) 90 degrees flexion to 20 degrees extension
3. Passive range of motion (PROM) 95 degrees flexion to 20 degrees extension — pain and soft-tissue resistance occurred simultaneously at end of ranges
4. Limited inferior, superior, and medial patellar glide
5. 1+ effusion as per fluctuation test (see Chapter 2)
6. Instrumented laxity testing (KT-2000 arthrometer) 6-mm anterior tibial translation, right knee; 2 mm greater than left knee
7. Well-healed, slightly indurated surgical scar along lateral aspect of the knee
8. Tight gastrocnemius-soleus muscle group
9. Non–weight bearing with crutches

Assessment

Formulation of a physical therapy problem list included:

1. Decreased AROM/PROM, right knee
2. Weakness of the quadriceps femoris muscle, especially the VMO muscle, with poor medial dynamic patellar stabilization
3. Restricted patellar mobility due to soft peripatellar tissue tightness, especially the lateral retinaculum
4. Nonfunctional and tender surgical scar
5. Mild knee joint effusion
6. Muscle imbalances of the right lower extremity, with weakness and reduced flexibility of gastrocnemius-soleus muscle groups
7. Weakness in most of the major muscles of the involved lower extremity
8. Reduced functional status and dependent ambulation with assistive device.

Factors Affecting the Problems

1. ACL deficient knee with multiplanar instability
2. Six weeks partial ROM immobilization of the right knee joint, with limited ROM
3. Older, relatively sedentary patient with probable generalized muscle weakness and deconditioning

Because this patient was slightly older than middle age, and his preinjury life-style was relatively sedentary, the goals of rehabilitation were limited to reestablishing adequate muscle strength in his involved knee through a functional ROM. Advanced rehabilitation requiring high-level functional training (e.g., high-speed isokinetics, agility drills, and plyometrics) was not considered an essential element in the long-term planning of this patient's rehabilitation program. Prior to surgery this patient had an ACL deficient knee with significant anterior tibial clinical laxity, which is an additional factor that limits the long-range goal to reestablish a highly functional knee.

EARLY REHABILITATION

Goals:

1. Attain full active knee extension and flexion
2. Facilitate motor recruitment of the VMO muscle
3. Maximize patellar mobility
4. Increase hamstring muscle strength
5. Eliminate knee joint effusion
6. Increase flexibility in the gastrocnemius and soleus muscles
7. Promote nontender, mobile surgical scar
8. Increase proximal strength in hip musculature and distal strength in the foot and ankle
9. Independent weight bearing

Treatment Plan

The patient was seen three times weekly for physical therapy. Initial treatments consisted of mobilization to the patella using manual gliding in medial, inferior, and superior directions. The patient was instructed to stretch his gastrocnemius-soleus muscle group. High-frequency stimulation (35 pps, 10 seconds on, 15 seconds off) was applied to the VMO muscle for 20 minutes each session, with the patient encouraged to voluntarily contract the muscle during electrical stimulation. The patient performed straight leg raises 4 ways: hip flexion, extension, abduction, and adduction. Initially no weight was used, and the patient was encouraged to work toward high repetitions (e.g., 60 for each movement). The goal was to facilitate total lower-extremity strengthening as well as to improve muscular endurance. The patient was also instructed to perform prone-lying hamstring curls, with the tibia maintained in external rotation to protect the healing repair. Once the patient was able to perform an adequate number of repetitions for each exercise, a 1-lb cuff weight was added to his ankle. The weights were added slowly to ensure that high repetitions were performed for each exercise. The patient was also instructed in toe raises, and closed kinetic chain knee extension (30 to 60 degrees), with surgical tubing placed behind the popliteal fossa for resistance. To regain full PROM he was instructed in wall slides and stationary cycling. He was instructed to massage his surgical scar 10 minutes daily, to facilitate collagen realignment. Ice was used for 20 minutes after each treatment session. The patient continued this program for 3 weeks.

Reevaluation

After 3 weeks, the patient had full PROM of his involved knee. He was able to actively perform straight leg raises without an extensor lag. The knee effusion had resolved, and his surgical scar was less tender and more mobile than initially. He attained excellent patellar mobility and was able to recruit his VMO muscle with what the therapist subjectively judged to be a fair contraction. The patient was fully weight bearing without crutches.

INTERMEDIATE REHABILITATION

Goals:

1. Increase muscular strength and endurance in the major muscle groups of the involved lower extremity
2. Increase lower-extremity proprioception/balance and flexibility
3. Improve cardiovascular conditioning

Treatment Plan

The patient continued his previous strengthening regimen, adding resistance in 1-lb increments while continuing to perform 60 repetitions for each exercise. His stationary cycling increased to 30 minutes each session, and he progressed to a stairclimber for continued cardiovascular training, as well as closed kinetic chain exercise (75 to 20 degrees). Additional closed kinetic chain exercises included continuing his standing terminal knee extension exercises, and performing 5-inch forward and lateral step-ups. He began intermediate-speed isokinetic training (120 degrees per second), which was considered slow enough so that the patient was able to consistently "catch" the lever arm and produce resistance, but fast enough to minimize retropatellar compressive forces. He was trained initially at 30 repetitions but increased to 60 repetitions during each session.

Reevaluation

At 4 months postsurgery, an isokinetic strength test of the involved knee was performed at an angular velocity of 120 degrees per second. The patient demonstrated bilateral differences of peak torque and power in the hamstring and quadriceps femoris muscles of slightly less than 20 percent. Over the last few weeks of therapy, mild (1+) effusion occurred in the involved knee. A KT-2000 arthrometry test indicated a 3.5 mm difference in anterior tibial translation compared with the uninvolved extremity. The clinical instability due to the ACL deficiency was believed by both the therapist and the orthopedist to be the cause of the low-grade knee effusion. The patient was fitted with a functional brace in an effort to control/minimize some of this instability and reduce stress to the tibiofemoral joint. He was instructed to begin a walk-jogging program while wearing the functional brace. He increased his total distance to approximately 2 miles, four times weekly. He was discharged from formal physical therapy 4 months after surgery and was instructed to continue a home program similar to the exercises instructed in the early phase of his rehabilitation and adding some functional progressions. He was able to return to tennis approximately 7 months after his surgery but played only on a limited basis.

COMMENTS

This patient represented an ideal candidate for an E-A procedure. The reasons include his relatively older age and the fact that his preinjury life-style placed minimal functional demands on his knee. Because of his ACL deficiency there remains a question of the long-term functional status of his knee. Because the normal biomechanics in his knee joint were not restored, one may expect attrition of secondary structures to occur. This attrition would be especially likely in a younger, active patient. Therefore the treatment of choice for patients with an ACL injury who require a high functional demand on their knee has become an intra-articular reconstruction.

SUMMARY

Each of the above described surgical procedures has been modified or performed with different fixation or slight reorientation by a variety of authors.[14-17] The common goal of each of these procedures is to maintain control of the tibia during function. The abnormal anterior subluxation of the tibial plateau (pivot shift), which manifests as functional instability, can be prevented if tissue restructuring is successfully provided on the lateral aspect of the knee. Although the pivot shift is thereby eliminated, normal biomechanics are not restored, and thus the majority of surgeons are attempting to use an intra-articular approach to duplicate the normal pivoting and guiding action of coupled rotation provided by the normal ACL. The long-term follow-up of E-A procedures has provided better recommendations for their use in a very select group of patients. These patients should not be hyperelastic, exhibit varus laxity, or have had previous meniscectomies. These procedures may be performed in conjunction with an I-A procedure to augment primary reconstructive action and to minimize previously developed varus laxity. Also, the early aggressive rehabilitation techniques pioneered in the E-A surgery patient have now been safely applied to the I-A surgery patient. The E-A procedure may in fact be one of the greatest contributions to the rehabilitation program of today, known as "accelerated rehabilitation after ACL reconstruction." The rehabilitation procedure is very much in line with those seen with the early MacIntosh procedures.[18] Clinicians must be mindful of the individual treatment plan required for patients undergoing any reconstructive procedure, particularly in the case of knee reconstructions that require soft-tissue healing and fixation. We often search for a fine line between aggressive and protected actions in both ROM and strength. Perhaps the best compromise is to use a functional progression, yet be mindful of healing constraints.

REFERENCES

1. Bosworth, DM and Bosworth, BM: Use of fascia lata to stabilize the knee in cases of ruptured crucial ligaments. J Bone Joint Surg [Am] 18:178, 1936.
2. Campbell, WC: Repair of the ligaments of the knee joint. Surg Gynecol Obstet 62:964, 1936.
3. Hey-Groves, EW: Operation for the repair of the crucial ligaments. Lancet 2:674, 1917.
4. Palmer, I: On the injuries to the ligaments of the knee joint. Acta Chir Scand Suppl 53:1, 1938.
5. Brantigan, OC and Voshell, AF: The mechanics of the ligaments and menisci of the knee joint. J Bone Joint Surg [Am] 23:44, 1941.
6. Galway, RD, Beaupre, A, and MacIntosh, DL: Pivot shift: A clinical sign of symptomatic anterior cruciate insufficiency. J Bone Joint Surg [Br] 54:763, 1972.
7. Losee, RE: Concepts of the pivot shift. Clin Orthop 172:45, 1983.
8. Malone, TR: Rotatory surgery and rehabilitation guidelines. In, Davies, G (ed): Rehabilitation of the Surgical Knee. Cypress, Ronkonkoma, NY, 1984, p. 29.
9. Vail, T, Malone, TR, and Bassett, FH: Long-term follow-up of patients with anterolateral rotary instability surgically corrected with a proximal IT-band transfer. Am J Sports Med 20(3):274, 1992.
10. Losee, RE, Johnson, TR, and Southwick, WO: Anterior subluxation of the lateral tibial plateau: A diagnostic test and operative repair. J Bone Joint Surg [Am] 60:1015, 1978.
11. Ellison, AE: Distal iliotibial-band transfer for anterolateral rotatory instability of the knee. J Bone Joint Surg [Am] 61:330, 1979.
12. Kennedy, JC, Stewart, R, and Walker, DM: Anterolateral rotary instability of the knee joint: An early analysis of the Ellison procedure. J Bone Joint Surg [Am] 60:1031, 1978.
13. Andrews, JR and Sanders, R: A "mini-reconstruction" technique in treating anterolateral rotary instability (ALRI). Clin Orthop 172:93, 1983.
14. Higgins, RW and Steadman, JR: Anterior cruciate ligament repairs in world-class skiers. Am J Sports Med 15:439, 1987.
15. Arnold, JA: A lateral extra-articular tenodesis for anterior cruciate ligament deficiency of the knee. Orthop Clin North Am 16:213, 1985.
16. Hughston, JC: Surgical repair of acute and chronic lesions of the lateral capsular ligamentous complex of the knee. In Feagin, JA (ed): The Crucial Ligaments. Churchill Livingstone, New York, 1988, p 425.
17. James, SL: Knee ligament reconstruction. In Evarts, CM (ed): Surgery of the Musculoskeletal System. Churchill Livingstone, New York, 1983, p 31.
18. Shelbourne, KD and Nitz, PA: Accelerated rehabilitation after anterior cruciate ligament reconstruction. Am J Sports Med 18:292, 1990.

SUGGESTED READINGS

Davies, G (ed): Rehabilitation of the Surgical Knee. Cypress, Ronkonkoma, NY, 1984.

Daniel, D, Akeson, W, O'Connor, J (eds): Knee Ligaments: Structure, Function, Injury, and Repair. Raven Press, New York, 1990.

Feagin, JA (ed): The Crucial Ligaments. Churchill Livingstone, New York, 1988.

Feagin, JA (ed): The Anterior Cruciate Ligament Deficient Knee. Clinical Orthop, vol 172, 1983.

Indelicato, PA (ed): Treatment of the Anterior Cruciate Ligament-Deficient Knee. Clin Sports Med 7(4), 1988.

Jackson, DW and Drez, D, (eds): The Anterior Cruciate Deficient Knee: New Concepts in Ligament Repair. CV Mosby, St Louis, MO, 1987.

Mangine, RE (ed): Physical Therapy of the Knee. Clinics in Physical Therapy 19, vol 19. Churchill Livingstone, New York, 1988.

CHAPTER 11

Rehabilitation of Posterior Cruciate Ligament Injuries

Robert P. Engle, PT, ATC
Thomas D. Meade, MD
Gary C. Canner, MD

Posterior cruciate ligament (PCL) injury presents a challenge to both the physician and the rehabilitation specialist. Although the PCL is an important stabilizing ligament, PCL injury is less likely than anterior cruciate ligament (ACL) injury to result in functional instability. Posterior cruciate ligament injury can, however, lead to significant long-term joint surface erosion and functional disability.[1,2] The incidence of ACL injury is higher than that of PCL injury, which means that there is less information about, and consensus on, the success of surgical management versus more conventional methods of rehabilitation for PCL deficient knees. To help clarify the issue, this chapter presents the rationale for, and case studies of, both surgical and nonsurgical treatment of selected patients with PCL injuries. In these cases, the process of examination and clinical diagnosis is based on the problem-solving model elaborated in Chapter 3.

The distal attachment of the PCL is the posterior aspect of the tibia; the proximal attachment is at the intercondylar notch of the medial femoral condyle. The ligament limits posterior translation of the tibia relative to the femur and is crucial, in concert with the ACL and the menisci, to normal kinematics of the knee (see Chapter 1).

SURGICAL MANAGEMENT VERSUS CONSERVATIVE MANAGEMENT

Controversy exists regarding whether to use surgery to repair or reconstruct a PCL deficient knee. Analysis of published literature reveals varying observations on the presence and degree of instabilities that occur with a torn PCL.[1-21] The direction and severity of a potential instability depend on the mechanism of injury and whether other structures are concomitantly injured in the knee. Hughston[22] found that acute PCL injuries may present with a negative posterior drawer test, the most common objective sign of a complete PCL tear. Hughston observed this finding may occur with isolated PCL injury as opposed to chronic cases and in cases with combined injury of the PCL and medial or lateral ligament complex structures. Hughston further reported that a significant number of patients with isolated PCL injuries can do well functionally without surgical repair or reconstruction.[1,2,4,5,9,15,19,22] However, Hughston[2] advocated surgery for combined instabilities that result in functional disability to the knee joint.

Although Clancy[1] has found that certain patients achieve acceptable results (i.e., return to their preinjury functional levels) with nonoperative treatment of isolated PCL injuries, many other patients with a similar injury progress to medial compartment or patellofemoral joint arthrosis. Clancy reports that early surgical intervention to reconstruct the PCL can negate future problems of knee degeneration, but stresses the need for effective postoperative graft function.[1] Clancy defines satisfactory postoperative graft function as posterior tibia translation of 5 mm or less than the uninvolved knee on follow-up examination.[1]

Therefore, according to Hughston and Clancy, some patients do well with PCL deficient knees, whereas others develop problems. One may deduce that additional factors influence the course of function of PCL-injured knees, and therefore should be used as determinants of whether surgery is a feasible option. These factors include the patient's age, preinjury activity level, vocation, motivation for rehabilitation, family support, and financial status. Generally, the younger, active, or athletic patient, whose knee requires a high level of functional stability, is appropriate for early surgical intervention. This profile is in contrast to the older, sedentary individual who makes fewer functional demands of his or her knee. The other consideration is the status of the other structures in the knee and whether secondary injuries occurred in conjunction with the injury to the PCL. Combined injuries (e.g., PCL and meniscal, or PCL and arcuate complex) result in a significantly unstable knee and increase the likelihood of operative repair/reconstruction of the PCL. However, the planning of every case should be done individually, and the final decision whether to operate is made with consultation of all significant parties — patient, family, surgeon, and rehabilitation specialist.

CLINICAL DIAGNOSIS AND EXAMINATION

The clinical evaluation of a patient with a suspected PCL injury should follow the sequential approach described in Chapter 2. A summary of the exam and special tests pertinent to evaluate the integrity of the PCL is presented in the following section.

Diagnosis of a PCL tear begins with a subjective history. Mechanisms of injury may include a direct blow to the anterior tibia driving the bone posteriorly. PCL injuries may occur with falls, motor vehicle accidents, or athletic trauma.[2] Hyperextension of the knee joint also has been associated with PCL ruptures.

The PCL is also torn with a posterolaterally directed force at the anterior tibia that first tears the arcuate complex and then the PCL.[2] Valgus and varus injuries with the knee in full extension have also been reported with PCL and associated tibial or lateral ligament tears.[3,23]

Following acute injury to the PCL, patients typically do not experience the tense hemarthrosis seen in ACL tears. Patients also will not necessarily experience giving way or severe pain with the initial injury, although weight bearing may be difficult. These facts make diagnosis of a major ligamentous injury to the PCL, based on the initial exam, sometimes difficult. However, if injuries to the tibial or lateral ligament complex or osteochondral lesions accompany the PCL tear, more pain and swelling may be present, and diagnosis may be more obvious.

Patients with chronic PCL deficiency commonly present with no prior knowledge of an acute episode of injury. Other patients recall the mechanism of injury but, because there is no significant instability in the knee joint after injury, do not seek treatment. Patellofemoral joint and/or medial compartment discomfort, instability with stairs and inclines, and recurrent swelling are the main complaints that ultimately bring these patients to the clinic. Increasing laxity of secondary restraints, primarily the posterolateral structures, makes functional laxity more perceptible to the patient.

Contusions to the subcutaneous peripheral nerves, including the saphenous nerve, must be evaluated with traumas that typically result in PCL disruption. Although they are difficult to diagnose and treat, nerve injuries or reflex sympathetic dystrophy (RSD) must be considered if the patient has suffered a blow to the anterior tibia.

Significant loss of motion in the knee joint is rare in the PCL deficient patient group. The end range of knee flexion may be painful. Limited active knee extension can be present secondary to quadriceps femoris muscle and extensor mechanism dysfunction or RSD.

Several clinical laxity tests have been used to determine PCL integrity. These include tibial sag or drop-off test, posterior drawer with tibia neutral, anterior drawer with tibia internally rotated, and valgus and varus stress tests in full extension.[2,3,22,24-27]

With the knee joint flexed 75 to 90 degrees in the drawer test position, posterior gravity-aided sagging of the tibia is present on bilateral comparison (Fig. 11–1). The examiner palpates the amount of posterior shift or dropback of tibial condyles relative to the femur. This dropback can also be demonstrated by holding the hips and knees in 90 degrees of flexion with the patient supine to increase gravity's effect on the tibial subluxation posteriorly (see Appendix, Fig. A–6).

From the 75-to-90-degree drawer position, a quadriceps femoris muscle active displacement test as described by Daniel and associates[28] is used. In this test, quadriceps

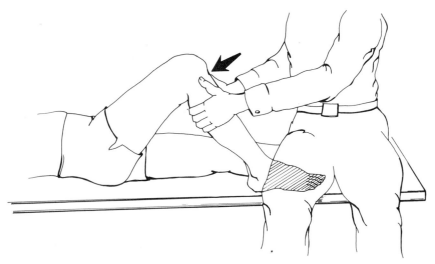

FIGURE 11–1. Tibial sag test. (From Engle, RP: Knee Ligament Rehabilitation. Churchill Livingstone, New York, 1991, p 30, with permission.)

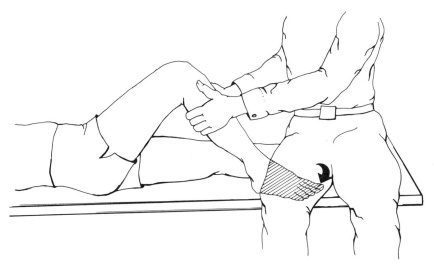

FIGURE 11-2. Posterolateral drawer test. (From Engle, RP: Knee Ligament Rehabilitation. Churchill Livingstone, New York, 1991, p 30, with permission.)

femoris muscle isometric contraction translates the tibia anteriorly from a posteriorly subluxed position, that is, a reduced position. Posterior drawer testing from this position passively translates the tibia. The magnitude of displacement can vary from 1 to 2 mm in acute, to greater than 15 mm in chronic, PCL deficiencies (relative to the uninvolved side).

External rotation with the posterior drawer test, or posterolateral drawer test, is positive with lesions of the arcuate complex and is markedly increased with PCL injury (Fig. 11-2). This combination of posterior and posterolateral instability is typically unappreciated in the diagnostic process but very important in both conservative and operative treatment.[3,22,24,25,29] Other important tests for accompanying posterolateral instability include the extension/recurvatum, dynamic posterior shift, reverse pivot shift, and rotation tests (Fig. 11-3). Hughston[26,27] reports positive valgus and varus stress test findings with PCL and accompanying tibial/lateral ligament tears at full extension (Fig. 11-4).

Patellofemoral joint assessment should include patella position (i.e., Q angle, patella alta or baja), dynamic stability, and functional tests. An accompanying functional and structural examination of the lower quarter is essential to evaluate patellofemoral and tibiofemoral joint alignment and function. (These tests are reviewed in Chapters 2, 6, and 7.)

Evaluation of the function of the quadriceps femoris muscle is performed in a number of ways. Methods of evaluation include isolated knee joint extension in an open kinetic chain with the tibia internally/externally rotated or in neutral; various closed kinetic chain techniques, such as squats on one or both lower extremities; and functional tests such as the single-leg hop or timed leg hop tests (see Appendix, Fig. A-12). The quadriceps femoris muscle should be tested both qualitatively and quantitatively; for example, isokinetic muscle strength parameters such as peak torque, power, or work. Qualitative assessment is largely subjective due to the paucity of valid and reliable tests. However, clinical experience indicates that useful information is available if several functional tests are performed. Examples of functional tests are partial knee squats and step-ups and step-downs. The clinician looks for the smoothness or control of the

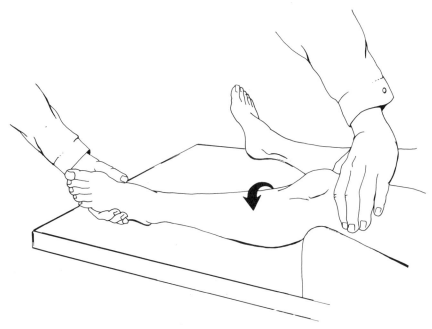

FIGURE 11-3. Rotation test. The clinician grasps the bottom of the patient's foot and applies an external rotation force through the tibia. Excessive external tibial rotation on the involved knee compared with the uninvolved knee may indicate posterolateral knee capsule laxity or instability. (From Engle, RP: Knee Ligament Rehabilitation. Churchill Livingstone, New York, 1991, p 28, with permission.)

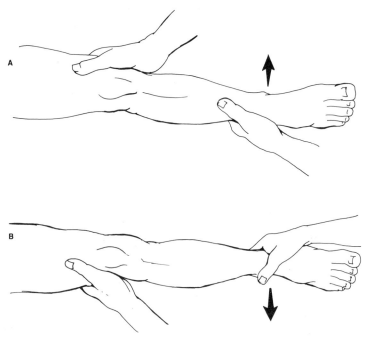

FIGURE 11-4. *A*). Varus stress test. *B*) Valgus stress test. (From Engle, RP: Knee Ligament Rehabilitation. Churchill Livingstone, New York, 1991, p 28, with permission.)

muscle contraction and the absence of muscle juddering that may indicate motor weakness. Sudden loss of knee flexion, substitution patterns using other muscle groups, or altered movement patterns may occur during these tests, especially with repetition. These changes may indicate either abnormal neuromuscular control, joint instability, joint proprioceptive deficits, or muscular endurance deficits. Neuromuscular examination and reexamination for proprioception, balance, coordination, flexibility, and strength of components other than the quadriceps femoris muscle are necessary. This evaluation includes assessment of the motor capabilities of the major muscle groups in the involved extremity.

PRINCIPLES OF POSTERIOR CRUCIATE LIGAMENT (PCL) REHABILITATION

Both conservative and surgical rehabilitation of the PCL-injured knee are directed at optimizing quadriceps femoris muscle control to reduce posterior tibial subluxation. Along with the quadriceps femoris muscle, the gastrocnemius and popliteus muscles are synergistic stabilizers to the PCL, and rehabilitation in the presence of PCL deficiency is directed at developing their functional strength.[19] An important principle is to delay hamstring muscle strengthening, particularly in the open kinetic chain position, until healing has occurred in the reconstructed knee. This delay is usually from 6 to 12 weeks after surgery to allow the graft to develop a functional scar (see Chapter 4). The hamstring muscles are antagonistic to the function of the PCL. Contraction of the hamstring muscles produces posterior translation of the tibia on the femur and places stress on the PCL. Closed kinetic chain exercises, including one-quarter squats and standing terminal knee extension as a way of strengthening the hamstring muscles, may be started earlier than 6 weeks. Closed kinetic chain exercises provide the advantages of producing cocontraction between the quadriceps femoris and hamstring muscles, increasing tibiofemoral joint stability through weight bearing compressive forces, and allowing the patient to perform slow, controlled movements (see Chapter 5). These factors assist in reducing posterior tibial translation and strain on the healing PCL graft.

Acute and chronic PCLl patients present differently. The acute patient with a saphenous nerve injury and/or RSD accompanying a combined PCL and posterior insufficiency will have significantly more pain and disability than in the case of an isolated PCL rupture with a barely perceptible posterior tibial sag. Chronic cases typically progress to stretching of the posterolateral secondary restraints and consequently to greatly increased overall instability as well as medial compartment and patellar arthrosis.[1] Minimizing these components of instability and joint surface problems throughout the rehabilitation program are essential to success.

Comprehensive PCL rehabilitation is achieved through a combination of manual therapeutic exercises and functional training techniques. Overall goals include restoration of full active/passive range of motion (ROM), redevelopment of full neuromuscular function of the affected lower extremity (strength, endurance, stability, proprioception, balance, coordination, muscle balance, and flexibility). The objective is to return the patient to full unrestricted activity without symptoms.[32] The clinician should be aware that these are the ideal goals desired for any patient with a knee injury, and that in reality they may not be fully attainable in all patients. The establishment of realistic treatment goals for each patient is based on problem solving in each individual case.

The selection of postoperative rehabilitation goals and treatment depends on the specific operative procedure. Most recently a bone–patellar tendon–bone autograft or allograft placed with arthroscopic assistance has been the preferred method of PCL substitution.[1,33,34] Noyes and associates[35] have shown the advantages of the patellar tendon as a substitute over several weaker but commonly used structures. Repair of the posterolateral structures, in addition, has been stressed by both Hughston and Clancy.[1,2,9] The use of a strong graft placed isometrically with repair of secondary structures restores a stable knee and allows the rehabilitation specialist to formulate an accelerated rehabilitation program that produces a highly functional knee.

RATIONALE FOR SELECTED TREATMENT AND/OR EXERCISE

Following surgery immediate motion is advocated to prevent motion loss, inhibit arthrofibrosis, promote articular cartilage nourishment, and stimulate the joint mechanoreceptors. ROM is controlled by a postoperative brace to reduce stresses on the healing PCL graft (Fig. 11–5). Accompanying repairs or injuries of the menisci and the collateral and capsular ligaments will further influence ROM guidelines. Weight bearing progression is generally more conservative with PCL than with ACL reconstruction. Full weight bearing is generally allowed between 4 and 6 weeks (sometimes longer) depend-

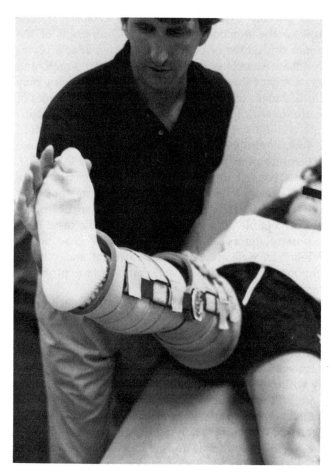

FIGURE 11–5. Postoperative passive flexion/abduction diagonal range of motion (ROM) exercise with knee maintained in full extension in a cast/brace system.

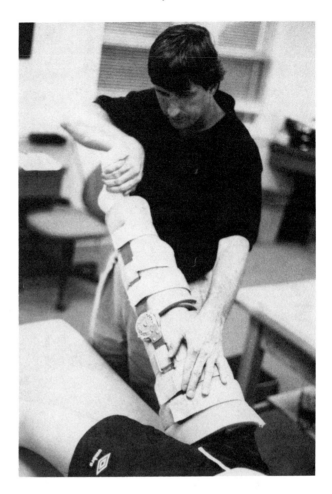

FIGURE 11-6. Postoperative flexion/adduction diagonal ROM exercise with knee in full extension in a cast/brace system.

ing on graft function, patellofemoral joint status, ROM, and neuromuscular (especially) quadricepts femoris muscle function.

Quadriceps femoris muscle exercises, as mentioned previously, are of great importance in the presence of PCL injuries. Patients progress from isometric contractions with manual and progressive resistive exercise (PRE) procedures to isotonic (concentric/eccentric) techniques. Whole-limb patterns in open, modified closed, and closed kinetic chain models are used (Figs. 11-6 to 11-8). Functional training in weight bearing begins as early as the fourth postoperative week, and even sooner in the presence of isolated nonoperative PCL injury. Included are balance, proprioception, strength, endurance, and stability exercises (Figs. 11-9 to 11-11). The PCL graft and patellofemoral joint are continually reassessed for adverse effects.

Progression and return to activity are much longer following postoperative reconstruction than in nonoperative cases. For the patient undergoing nonoperative management, several criteria are necessary for return to activity. Full active and passive knee ROM must be present. Neuromuscular function tested both qualitatively and quantitatively with manual, clinical, and functional techniques should closely reflect the motor status of the uninvolved lower extremity. Clinical experience has shown that results of isokinetic tests for quadriceps femoris and hamstring muscle peak torque, power, and work parameters should be within 10 percent of those for the uninvolved side. Good

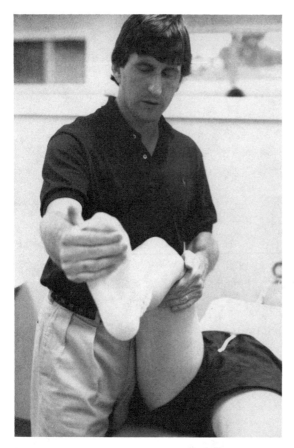

FIGURE 11-7. Passive extension/abduction ROM exercise with the knee close to full extension.

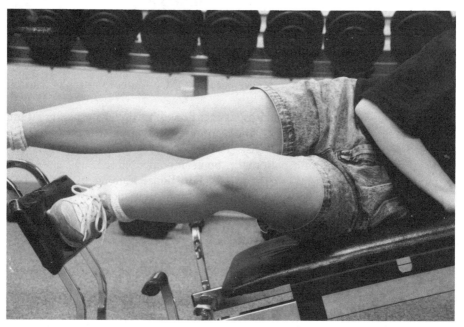

FIGURE 11-8. Incline leg press exercise with the postoperative knee in modified weight-bearing position. Placing the patient in a side-lying position with the left hip in slight adduction increases VMO muscle output. Note that the left tibia is in external rotation to avoid overstretching the posterolateral capsule. However, care must be given to avoid excessive external tibial rotation so as not to cause a posterolateral subluxation of the knee joint.

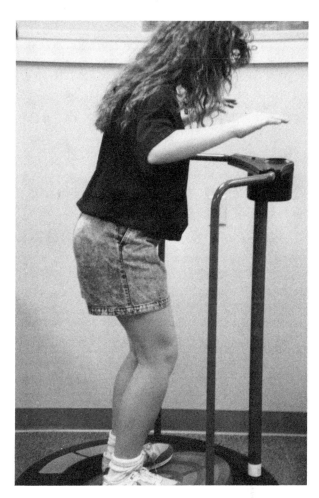

FIGURE 11-9. Balance training. Balance and proprioception can be facilitated through training on a platform system, beginning with bilataeral weight bearing and progressing to unilateral weight bearing on the involved extremity. (Kinesthetic Ability Training, BREG Inc., Vista, CA)

dynamic support of the patella during active tracking (gliding) along the femoral trochlear groove is an important goal, as is an asymptomatic patellofemoral joint. Altered patellar tracking can result in patellofemoral joint dysfunction after the patient returns to full activity. The vastus medialis obliquus (VMO) muscle should exhibit good muscle tone and should be recruited before the vastus lateralis (VL) muscle during active voluntary quadriceps femoris muscle contraction. Finally, there should be no active knee joint synovitis, effusion, or pain.

For patients with PCL reconstruction, an additional consideration is that the graft function should exhibit 5 mm or less posterior laxity compared with the uninvolved side.[1] Full participation in sports before graft maturation at 9 to 12 months following surgery has generally been contraindicated. Results of earlier return to activity have not been reported but an earlier return can be considered with close follow-up and strict criteria for progression. Some rehabilitation centers have been experimenting with accelerated rehabilitation programs similar to recently described ACL approaches, on an individual basis with consideration of pain swelling, stability, and neuromuscular control. Table 11-1 reviews the basic postoperative PCL program. The program is divided into four phases. The table includes approximate time frames for each phase, but actual patient progress depends on the rate of soft tissue healing (see Chapter 4) and the patient's ability to perform the exercises. Exercise phase I corresponds to the early stages

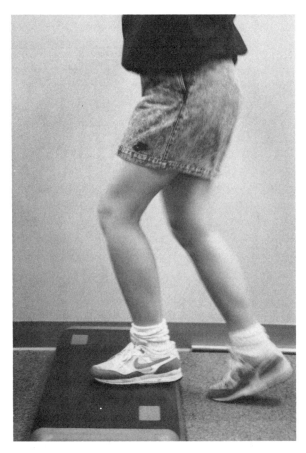

FIGURE 11-10. Forward/backward step-ups to generate quadriceps femoris–hamstring muscle cocontractions.

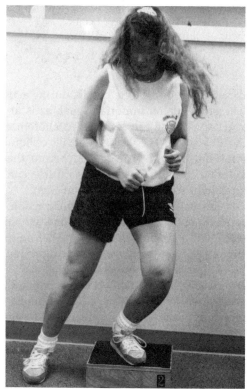

FIGURE 11-11. Plyometric training: lateral box jumping. Low-level plyometric or functional training in weight bearing can progress between 6 and 12 weeks.

314

TABLE 11–1
Rehabilitation Program Following PCL Reconstruction

Phase I: Weeks 1–4	1. Use ice, compression, and elevation to control effusion.
	2. Use a postoperative brace system to limit ROM to 0–40 degrees.
	3. Allow partial weight bearing with crutches as tolerated.
	4. Use passive and active assisted ROM exercise, including use of CPM for hospital inpatient.
	5. Use electrical muscle stimulation (EMS) to the quadriceps femoris muscle
	6. Use patellar mobilization techniques
	7. Prescribe straight leg raises (SLRs) and isometric exercise of the quadriceps femoris muscle.
	8. Prescribe exercises for strengthening the hip and lower trunk.
Phase II: Weeks 4–12	1. Replace the postoperative brace with a functional PCL brace.
	2. Progress patient to full weight bearing.
	3. Continue exercises aimed at restoring full ROM.
	4. Progress from isometric to isotonic exercise of the quadriceps femoris muscle.
	5. *No* resisted hamstring muscle exercises.
	6. Using caution, begin functional training exercises:
	Toe raises
	Minisquats
	Step-ups—forward, backward, lateral
	Leg presses
	Treadmill walking—forward, backward
	Balance training
	Stationary bicycle exercise
	Stationary ski track exercise
	Stairclimber exercise
Phase III: Weeks 12–24	1. Continue previous exercises.
	2. Begin isotonic, open kinetic chain hamstring muscle exercises.
	3. Continue low-level plyometric exercises for strength, endurance, proprioception, stabilization, balance and coordination. Emphasize techiques relevant to the patient's favored sports.
	4. Begin a program of moderate jogging.
Phase IV: Weeks 24–54	1. Continue and progress with the previous exercises.
	2. Continue progress toward reestablishing preinjury levels of function and activity.
	3. Complete the return to full activity. The patient must meet objective criteria of function to demonstrate completion of the rehabilitation program.

of healing (fibroplasia). The goals of this stage are to restore full ROM, prevent muscle atrophy, and protect the healing graft. Exercise phase II coincides with late fibroplasia and early maturation; goals include continued restoration of ROM and increased muscle strength. Near the end of phase II, the patient begins functional training exercises. Finally, phases III and IV continue to emphasize functional training to optimize muscle strength, endurance, proprioception, balance, and coordination. These phases feature a variety of closed kinetic chain exercises designed to simulate the functional needs of the patient.

CASE STUDIES

CASE STUDY 1

HISTORY

A 19-year-old intercollegiate soccer goalie had dived for a ball in front of the goal and collided with another player, who struck the goalie's left proximal tibia and displaced the bone posteriorly. The patient's foot was not planted at the time of injury. There was immediate severe pain, very little effusion, and inability to walk. His athletic trainer initially examined the knee, applied ice and compression, and placed the athlete in a non–weight bearing position on crutches and in a knee immobilizer. Two days later, the patient was seen by the orthopedist and a diagnosis was made of complete tear of the PCL. The diagnosis was later expanded to include posterolateral complex instability. The patient was then referred to physical therapy to begin rehabilitation.

CLINICAL EXAMINATION

On the initial examination the patient was asymptomatic with no pain or other complaints. No effusion was present in the knee joint. Patellofemoral joint exam was negative for instability, crepitus, and tenderness of peripatellar structures. However, there was atrophy of the VMO muscle with latent recruitment of the VMO muscle relative to the VL muscle, determined by palpation during an active contraction of the quadriceps femoris muscle. Also, lateral patellar tracking was noted during passive ROM of the knee joint. Stability testing revealed a markedly positive posterior tibial sag and posterior drawer test with 4.5 mm greater translation measured on the affected knee using instrumented testing. Posterolateral drawer test was also positive, and 5 mm greater displacement was seen in the involved than in the uninvolved knee. Varus stress tests were positive in both knee joint flexion and extension, with approximately 5 and 4 mm greater laxity, respectively, compared with the uninvolved knee. ROM was initially equal bilaterally for knee extension but limited to 100 degrees flexion actively and 115 degrees passively, with pain at end range. Medial and lateral meniscus tests were negative. Marked quadriceps femoris muscle dysfunction was found with clinical and manual tests. Moderate deficits were present with testing of the hip musculature, hamstring muscles, and lower leg muscles. The patient was partially weight bearing to tolerance at the time of the initial evaluation and he continued to wear his knee immobilizer to protect the secondary restraints to the PCL during early healing.

TREATMENT PLAN

Normally, a patient presenting with this type of injury—a complete tear of the PCL, with posterolateral laxity—has an unsatisfactory natural history. The late effects of a multiplanar laxity can be difficult to correct. Nonoperative care is usually not recommended; however, the patient expressed his desire to attempt nonoperative management to reduce the time of postoperative rehabilitation. Because his functional disability was not considered excessive and the patient was highly motivated for rehabilitation, the decision was made by the patient, his family, the surgeon, the physical therapist, and the athletic trainer to attempt nonoperative rehabilitation.

ASSESSMENT

Physical Therapy Problem List

1. Reduced active and passive knee flexion
2. Atrophy of the VMO muscle with altered recruitment pattern between the VMO and VL muscles
3. Altered (lateral) patellar tracking
4. Deficits of motor control in the major muscle groups in the involved extremity
5. Decreased functional status: partial weight bearing with crutches

Factors Affecting the Problems

1. Nonrepaired/nonreconstructed PCL
2. Secondary posterolateral instability, probably due to injury to arcuate complex
3. Young, athletic, well-motivated patient

REHABILITATION

Because this case was nonoperative, soft tissue healing of a potential graft was not considered when establishing the time frames of treatment. Therefore, the patient could be progressed at a much quicker pace than if this were a PCL-reconstructed knee. However, the injury to the arcuate complex needed to be considered and stresses reduced at least for 4 to 6 weeks along the posterolateral aspect of the knee joint. Because the patient was an athlete, treatment goals were established to restore a high level of function.

Initial Goals

1. Maximize full active and passive ROM
2. Increase quadriceps femoris muscle strength and facilitate recruitment of the VMO muscle
3. Increase strength in major muscle groups (especially the gastrocnemius muscle) in the involved lower extremity
4. Promote full weight bearing

Long-Term Goals

1. Maximize muscle function, including the hamstring muscles, in the involved extremity

2. Maximize cardiovascular fitness
3. Maximize lower extremity function, i.e., proprioception, balance, muscle flexibility, agility

Treatment

Therapeutic exercise techniques including proprioceptive neuromuscular facilitation (PNF), adjunctive PREs, and functional and isokinetic training were used to restore full neuromuscular function and provide dynamic stability to the knee. Electrical muscle stimulation (EMS) was helpful in augmenting neuromuscular recruitment and reeducation through the exercise techniques. Patellar mobilization techniques for stretching primarily the tight lateral structures (e.g., lateral retinaculum and iliopatellar band) were necessary. Cryotherapy following treatment assisted in control of postexercise synovitis or effusion.

Beginning with the initial treatment session and continuing until the end of week 2, the patient started on a series of PNF techniques and procedures including lower extremity flexion and extension diagonal patterns with the knee maintained straight. This approach created neuromuscular recruitment along the entire lower kinetic chain, especially the quadriceps femoris muscle, which is so crucial to the success for PCL management. Hip patterns were added to this program, with the knee maintained in extension to avoid overactivating the hamstring muscles. The hip patterns included extension/adduction/external rotation with knee extension and a linear hip/knee extension pattern. Hip adduction was applied with manual resistance and the patient in side-lying position. Strengthening of the hip adductors due to their fascial attachment to the VMO muscle facilitates recruitment of the VMO muscle. Manual resisted ankle plantarflexion was applied with the knee joint extended to isolate the gastrocnemius muscle. Isotonic reversal, a combination of isotonic and isometric techniques as described by Johnson and Saliba,[36] was applied to the knee joint through a pain-free arc of motion. In addition, the patient started on an inclined leg press (Total Gym, EFI, San Diego, CA), toe raises and wall-pulley hip PREs, in addition to straight leg raises (SLR), hip adduction, and leg extension PREs. By week 2, full ROM, both active and passive, was restored to the knee, with mild discomfort with overpressure at the end of flexion range. All neuromuscular deficits were reduced, and the patient was asymptomatic. The patient's immobilizer was discontinued in favor of a functional knee brace (Don Joy Four-Point PCL Brace, Don Joy, Carlsbad, CA), and full weight bearing was allowed.

Beginning with the third week of rehabilitation, the patient's functional training program was increased. This program included standing squats to 70 degrees (70-degree angle in a protective range to lower anteroposterior tibiofemoral joint translation); forward, backward, and lateral step-ups; balance board training; bicycling; and forward and backward treadmill walking. Backward treadmill walking is a safe method to recruit the hamstring muscles without creating a posterior tibial subluxation. The exercise is performed in a closed kinetic chain and produces cocontraction of the quadriceps femoris and hamstring muscles as well as compressive stability through the tibiofemoral joint. Manual techniques employed during the first 2 weeks were also continued but with more difficult positions and increasing resistance. Appropriate manual resistance through (1) isolated, open kinetic chain knee extension with the tibia in neutral and (2) external rotation and bridging of the hip with the patient supine were included in the program. Running was permitted by week 4 of this program. All functional training was done with the knee brace in place to control posterior tibial subluxation.

Reevaluation

By 6 weeks, full quadriceps femoris muscle and lower extremity neuromuscular function had been restored with manual, isokinetic, and functional techniques. Full active and passive ROM was present on bilateral comparisons. There was no pain at the end of knee flexion range. The patellofemoral joint was asymptomatic, and the patient's stability tests at the tibiofemoral joint remained unchanged. At this time he was discharged from treatment and began an ongoing rehabilitation program with his athletic trainer that emphasized functional training techniques compatible with his sport.

On subsequent follow-up visits, the patient had maintained a level of quadriceps femoris muscle function that tested isokinetically within 10 percent of the score of his uninvolved knee. At 10 months postinjury however, he presented with mild retropatellar crepitus; an instrumented posterior drawer test showed 2-mm greater posterior tibial sag than that of the uninvolved knee. He finished the final 2 years of his college eligibility as starting goalie, experiencing occasional patellar discomfort but no knee joint effusion, functional disability, or loss of ROM.

COMMENTS

This case represents a classically successful clinical scenario of the PCL deficient knee treated nonoperatively in an athlete. Unfortunately, the success of this patient represents only a small group of PCL patients. The long-term prognosis of this case is unclear, although we should assume that with a less vigorous athletic life-style after college, his situation should improve since activity modification has been shown to be important with nonoperative treatment success.

CASE STUDY 2

HISTORY

A 32-year-old stockbroker and recreational athlete presented with a locked, painful knee after arising from a kneeling position. The patient had initially injured his knee 5 years earlier when he slid into a catcher playing softball and received a blow to the anterior proximal tibia, driving the bone posterolaterally. At that time he had persistent effusion, pain at the lateral joint line, and a positive posterior drawer test.

Subsequent to the initial injury, he underwent a partial arthroscopic lateral meniscectomy but elected a 6-month nonoperative course of rehabilitation for PCL deficiency. After completion of rehabilitation, he was able to return to recreational sports but lacked confidence in the injured knee. The patient continued to experience recurrent meniscal locking, which he was able to self reduce with a rotation/extension maneuver. Patellofemoral joint discomfort also was present, particularly with prolonged sitting and when descending stairs.

CLINICAL EXAMINATION

Initial examination indicated a 6-mm greater posterior translation in the involved versus the uninvolved knee as measured with instrumented testing. The reverse pivot shift was positive. His external rotation test at both 30 and 90 degrees of flexion had 10 degrees greater rotation on the affected side in both test positions. A varus stress test at 30 degrees of knee flexion was 2 mm greater than the uninvolved side.

The patient's diagnosis included (1) displaced bucket handle tear of the lateral meniscus; (2) chronic PCL insufficiency; and (3) patellofemoral joint articular chondromalacia.

TREATMENT PLAN

Medical treatment options included (1) extensive lateral meniscectomy with the patient accepting the inherent risks of progressive articular damage of the lateral compartment and the patellofemoral joint; (2) lateral meniscal repair with a 4-to-6-week partial weight bearing and nonoperative PCL rehabilitation; and (3) lateral meniscal repair and PCL reconstruction (with a high-strength biologic graft substitute) that does not sacrifice the extensor mechanism.

The patient opted for a PCL reconstruction with lateral mensicus repair because of the progressive articular degenerative symptoms he had experienced for several months. Additionally, the patient was interested in having the best knee possible and wanted to avoid delaying surgery until his articular cartilage surfaces showed further irreversible damage.

This patient underwent an arthroscopically assisted PCL Achilles tendon allograft reconstruction placed through a femoral and tibial tunnel and secured in each bone tunnel by an interference screw (Fig. 11–12). Repair of the lateral meniscus buckethandle tear was performed with athroscopy and a small lateral incision. The patellofemoral joint had a large 12 × 12-mm area of chondral damage without exposed bone on the lateral patellar facet, and a lesion in the femoral sulcus. The cartilage along the medial femoral condyle was preserved. The lateral femoral condyle had a 7 × 5-mm chondral lesion.

IMMEDIATE POSTOPERATIVE REHABILITATION

Immediately following surgery the patient was placed on continuous passive motion (CPM) from 0 to 70 degrees in the recovery room. CPM was continued for the next 2 days while the patient was hospitalized. During the first postoperative week, he attained 90 degrees of knee flexion with the CPM. He was evaluated in the clinic 1 week after surgery.

PHYSICAL THERAPY EVALUATION

Active ROM measured 10 to 90 degrees; passive ROM measured from full extension to 90 degrees flexion. There was 1+ effusion in the knee joint. Significant atrophy was palpated in the VMO muscle and noted throughout the quadri-

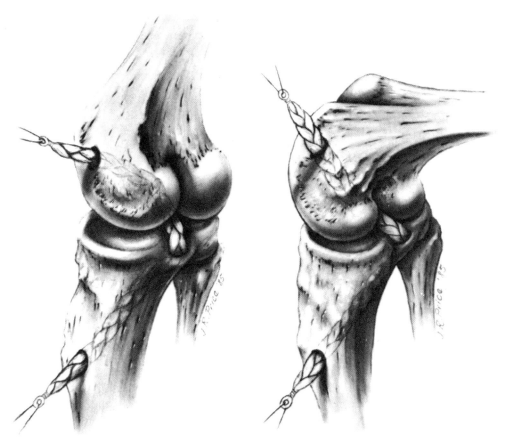

FIGURE 11–12. Synthetic PCL arthroscopically placed through femoral and tibial bone tunnels. (From Rosenberg, TD, Paulos, LE, and Abbot, PJ: Arthroscopic cruciate repair and reconstruction: An overview and descriptions of technique. In Feagin, JA [ed]: The Crucial Ligaments. Churchill Livingstone, New York, 1988, p 421, with permission.)

ceps femoris muscle, compared with the uninvolved side. The patient exhibited poor recruitment of his VMO muscle, and an active SLR resulted in an extensor lag (approximately 10 degrees). There was mild tenderness along the lateral joint line. The lateral retinaculum was tight to passive stretch. The arthroscopic surgical scars were almost healed, and tender. The patient was ambulating with touch-down weight bearing with crutches. He was wearing a hinged brace with ROM set from 0 to 60 degrees. The gastrocnemius and soleus muscles were atrophic and tight to passive stretch.

ASSESSMENT

Physical Therapy Problem List

1. Decreased active and passive ROM
2. Quadriceps femoris muscle atrophy and weakness
3. Atrophy and inhibition of the VMO with poor patellar dynamic stability

4. Tight lateral retinaculum with decreased gliding of the patellar medially
5. 1+ effusion of the knee joint
6. Weakness and tightness of gastrocnemius-soleus muscle group
7. Decreased weight bearing status to protect mensicus repair and PCL graft

Factors Affecting the Problems

1. Post–Achilles tendon allograft to reconstruct the PCL
2. Arthroscopically assisted technique
3. Lateral meniscus repair
4. Young, relatively active patient, intelligent and well motivated

Rehabilitation

The patient is 1 week post–PCL reconstruction, so that the graft has not yet healed (see Chapter 4) and the progression through rehabilitation will be partly guided by soft-tissue healing constraints. Exercises should be performed in positions that minimize retropatellar compressive forces (see Chapter 1) and pain. Healing constraints should also be guided by healing of the lateral meniscus repair, which usually requires a minimum of 5 months. However, this time course is highly variable and based on the surgeon's ability to adequately reduce and stabilize the meniscus. Healing time often extends beyond 12 months. Achilles tendon graft procured from donors can be larger and stronger than a patellar tendon autograft. Avoiding disruption of the patient's extensor mechanism with the allograft provides a significant advantage to the patient. However, care must be taken not to overstress the graft as it revascularizes and remodels. The patient is young and relatively active, so rehabilitation guidelines and time frames include functional exercises.

Initial Goals

1. Increase active/passive ROM
2. Resolve knee joint effusion
3. Optimize patellofemoral tracking and function
4. Increase strength of the quadriceps femoris muscle and improve motor recruitment of VMO muscle
5. Increase flexibility of the lateral retinaculum
6. Improve flexibility and strength of gastrocnemius and soleus muscles
7. Increase strength in all the major muscle groups of the involved extremity
8. Progress functional weight bearing status as graft and meniscus fixation improve

Long-Term Goals

1. Maximize active/passive ROM in the involved knee joint
2. Maximize muscle strength and muscle endurance in the involved lower extremity

3. Maximize balance/proprioception and muscle flexibility in the involved extremity
4. Maximize agility and cardiovascular endurance

Treatment

During the first week, the modalities included cryotherapy to reduce knee effusion, EMS over the VMO muscle to improve muscle recruitment, medial patellar mobilization to stretch the lateral retinaculum, and SLR to improve overall quadriceps femoris muscle strength. The patient was instructed in unassisted performance of ROM exercises with the brace removed.

During the first 4 postoperative weeks, lower extremity patterns were used with the knee maintained near full extension to facilitate the hip muscles with irradiation to the quadriceps femoris muscle. Walking in water and general bicycling for ROM were allowed at 3 weeks. The buoyancy of the water safely reduced stress through the tibiofemoral joint. By the end of the fourth week, weight bearing had progressed to 75 percent of full weight. Minisquats against a wall and toe raises were begun. Once the patient was able to perform an SLR without an extensor lag, the crutches were discontinued. All exercises were performed with the brace removed, although the patient continued to wear it during ambulation.

Reevaluation and Treatment

Between weeks 5 and 8, the patient had achieved 120 degrees active and 125 degrees passive knee flexion to full active knee extension. The brace was discarded. Isolated knee extension and leg press using PREs and manual techniques for concentric/eccentric quadriceps femoris muscle strengthening were added but in a limited arc (0 to 60 degrees), for two reasons: to minimize retropatellar pain and compressive stresses, and to allow further safe healing of the lateral meniscus. At week 5, hamstring isotonic concentric and eccentric exercises were allowed in the same arc of motion (0 to 60 degrees). Minisquats and leg press were continued, toe raises were added to strengthen the gastrocnemius muscle, and lower extremity flexibility training was initiated. At week 6, an instrumented laxity examination showed a 3-mm increase in posterior translation measurements for the involved side compared with the uninvolved.

After 8 weeks, rehabilitation emphasized endurance and advanced neuromuscular training. A stationary ski track and bicycle workouts were increased along with balance training. At 12 weeks, the patient discontinued formal therapy while continuing a program of quadriceps femoris strengthening and lower extremity neuromuscular functional training. An isokinetic test performed at the time of discharge from formal therapy indicated a quadriceps femoris power deficit in the range of 20 percent compared with the uninvolved side. The patient was fitted with a functional brace and instructed to begin jogging but to avoid cutting movements or jumping.

Long-Term Reevaluation

The patient was reevaluated in the clinic each month for 1 year postreconstruction. At 6 months an isokinetic retest indicated the quadriceps femoris bilateral power deficits were reduced to within 10 percent. The patient demonstrated no effusion or additional patellofemoral symptoms. He was instructed at that time in a functional program including sprinting, figure-eights, and jumping rope.

At 1 year postsurgery, the patient had a 3-mm greater posterior translation with instrumented testing, and full quadriceps femoris and lower extremity neuromuscular function via manual, clinical, functional and isokinetic evaluation. He had no episodes of effusion and an asymptomatic patellofemoral joint. He had returned to recreational basketball by 9 months postreconstruction.

COMMENTS

This patient represents the optimal case scenario of a surgically reconstructed PCL. Anatomic reconstruction of the PCL restores the normal kinematic axis of motion, which minimizes articular stress and deterioration. Further, by using an allograft as the PCL substitute, a larger, stronger graft can be used than one procured from the patient's own tissues. Allografts also negate the disadvantages of using a portion of the extensor mechanism, which is necessary for optimal patellar function as well as for controlling residual posterior laxity. Finally, the graft was placed arthroscopically with no significant dissection needed other than that for arthroscopic procedures. In one of the authors' (TDM) experience, there have been no cases of disease transmission or cruciate ligament rejections with allograft tissue in over 180 cases, although this issue remains controversial. This approach significantly decreases rehabilitation time and long-term problems.

CASE STUDY 3

HISTORY

While playing recreational basketball, a 25-year-old professional baseball player was injured when he overran the basket and struck a wall. On impact he struck the anterior tibia with the knee flexed at approximately 75 degrees. He experienced a crack, instant pain, and effusion. Immediately following the injury he was seen for aggressive nonoperative treatment of a PCL deficient knee. The treatment program was similar to the program outlined in case 1; the only difference was that this patient avoided a period of initial immobilization because he had to report to spring training relatively soon after the injury.

CLINICAL EXAMINATION

A mildly positive posterior drawer was found on the patient's initial exam, which was 7 days after injury. Instrumented testing measured a 2-mm greater posterior translation compared with the uninvolved knee. Valgus and varus stress tests at both 0 and 30 degrees were negative. Posterolateral drawer and rotation tests were mildly positive. Patellofemoral joint examination was negative for medial/lateral patellar subluxation, tenderness of peripatellar structures, and retropatellar crepitus. There was no effusion nor any ROM limitations. Quadriceps femoris muscle strength was surprisingly good, with only mild deficits including

VMO muscle atrophy and insufficiency. Gait was normal. Lateral meniscus testing (McMurray test; see Appendix, Fig. A−1) was positive. Medial meniscus evaluation was negative. The diagnosis made included (1) complete tear of the PCL; (2) mild posterolateral instability; (3) torn lateral meniscus; and (4) osteochondral fracture of the lateral femoral condyle and tibial plateau.

TREATMENT PLAN

The patient reported to spring training 2 weeks after his initial injury and continued his rehabilitation. At that time he elected to forgo surgical reconstruction of his PCL. He was participating as a pitcher on the AA level with diminished knee stability (but no "giving way") and mild, occasional effusion and patellofemoral joint pain. One month into the regular season he received a lateral blow during a bench-clearing brawl, with resultant pain, effusion, and increased functional disability from his initial evaluation. Arthroscopy was subsequently performed.

SURGERY

Surgery included arthroscopic examination with resection of a portion of the lateral meniscus. The patient was placed into a rehabilitation program emphasizing techniques detailed in case study 1, but he remained symptomatic. Five months later, reconstruction was recommended and the patient underwent surgery.

Arthroscopic findings included type III chondromalacia of the medial compartment, mild chondromalacia of the patella at the middle ridge, and complete PCL insufficiency. After arthroscopic inspection an anterior incision was made and the lateral third of the patellar tendon was obtained using bone from both the patella and tibial tubercle. The graft was secured with isometric placement (see Chapter 9) and stapled to secure fixation.

PHYSICAL THERAPY EVALUATION

Immediately after surgery the patient was placed into a CPM device set at 0 to 30 degrees of motion. A postoperative cast brace was maintained at 20 degrees flexion. Non−weight bearing ambulation on crutches was started immediately. He was instructed in quadriceps femoris muscle setting exercises and ankle pumps. The patient was evaluated in our clinic 1 week after surgery. At that time he had 0 degrees passive and +5 degrees active knee extension, and passive knee flexion to 55 degrees with 50 degrees of active knee flexion. He had 1 to 2+ knee joint effusion and tenderness along the lateral femoral condyle. There was reduced medial glide of the patella with tightness of the lateral retinaculum. The VMO muscle was atrophic to palpation. Contraction of the VMO was poor. Active SLR produced a 5-degree extensor lag. The gastrocnemius-soleus muscle group was atrophic and tight to passive stretch.

ASSESSMENT
Physical Therapy Problem List

1. Atrophy and muscle weakness of the quadriceps femoris muscles, particularly the VMO muscle
2. Tight lateral retinaculum with reduced patellar mobility and lateral patellar tracking
3. Knee joint effusion
4. Decreased active/passive ROM of the knee
5. Reactive lateral femoral chondromalacia
6. Weakness and dysfunction of the calf muscles
7. Decreased functional status with dependent ambulation

Factors Affecting the Problems

1. Involvement of secondary knee joint structures
2. Patellar tendon autograft
3. Staple fixation/isometric graft placement
4. Young professional athlete, highly motivated

REHABILITATION

The factors that affect this patient are similar to those described in Case Study 2. The use of a patellar tendon graft is among the strongest biologic substitutes. Bone-to-bone fixation at each end of the graft allows for earlier, aggressive rehabilitation. The problem with this autograft is that tissue is dissected from the patient's extensor mechanism, which increases the risk of patellofemoral joint dysfunction and quadriceps femoris muscle inhibition. In addition, staple fixation used in this reconstruction is not as strong as an interference screw (see Chapter 9). Therefore, periodic instrumented testing is important with this patient if an accelerated rehabilitation program is to be used. This patient is a professional athlete, and therefore his rehabilitation will ultimately involve high-level functional training.

Initial Goals

1. Eliminate effusion
2. Increase quadriceps femoris muscle strength and facilitate recruitment of the VMO muscle
3. Increase active/passive ROM of the knee
4. Improve extensibility of the lateral retinaculum and improve patellar mobility
5. Promote independent ambulation
6. Increase total leg strength

Long-Term Goals

1. Maximize strength of the muscles in the involved extremity
2. Maximize proprioception, balance, agility, and muscle flexibility

Treatment

Initial treatments were similar to those described in Case Study 2 and included ice to reduce knee tenderness and joint effusion, EMS to the VMO to improve muscle recruitment, medial patella glides to stretch the lateral retinaculum, and wall slides to improve dynamic ROM. SLR exercises were performed in four directions for hip flexion, hip abduction, hip adduction, and hip extension. These exercises were initiated with the patient standing, and as strength and motor control improved, the exercises were performed with the patient supine, side-lying, and prone. The emphasis was on low resistance and a high number of repetitions, to improve muscle strength and endurance. All exercises were performed out of the brace. The patient was instructed in partial weight bearing with crutches for the first 4 weeks. By the end of the third week, the patient had improved to 80 degrees of active and 90 degrees of passive knee flexion and full active knee extension. The postoperative brace was opened to allow full extension and 60 degrees flexion. At 6 weeks the postoperative brace was replaced with a functional brace without ROM stops (Donjoy Four-Point PCL Brace, Donjoy, Carlsbad, CA). The patient was not allowed independent ambulation without crutches until he could perform an SLR without an extensor lag, good graft fixation was evident, and synovitis was controlled.

Therapeutic techniques included the PNF patterns described in the previous case studies, with the knee remaining near full extension in the first 4 weeks. Following the third postoperative week, the patient began hip/knee extension techniques and mild manually resisted knee extension from 0 to 40 degrees. This arc of motion was progressed to 0 to 70 degrees by the sixth week. Toe raises, incline leg press, and minisquats were added between 4 and 6 weeks.

Reevaluation and Treatment

Following 6 weeks, the patient had full active and passive extension, and flexion to 105 degrees actively and 110 degrees passively. Exercises continued to emphasize improving quadriceps femoris muscle strength and avoiding resisted hamstring muscle strengthening. Bicycling, forward/backward treadmill walking, balance training, and step-ups were used as in the previous cases.

Second Reevaluation and Treatment

Instrumented testing at 6 weeks showed a 1-mm bilateral difference of posterior translation between the involved and uninvolved knee. Valgus, varus, and rotation tests showed no differences between knee joints. The patient experienced no episodes of joint effusion or patellofemoral joint symptoms, although the patella continued to track laterally due to residual tightness of the lateral retinaculum and weakness of the VMO muscle. Manual testing indicated marked weakness remaining in the quadriceps femoris, with mild hip/lower leg musculature deficiencies. Between 6 and 12 weeks, the patient continued strengthening with manual techniques and functional training. At 12 weeks, an isokinetic test indicated that bilateral deficits of power in the quadriceps femoris of 50 percent were present at both slow and fast angular velocities. The patient continued rehabilitation although he was now attending a gym to perform much of his training. However, he was instructed to jog only while wearing his functional brace, and to avoid cutting movements or jumping until his quadriceps femoris muscle deficits improved. Low-level plyometric training was initiated at this time.

At approximately 1 year he was finally able to reduce the quadriceps femoris neuromuscular deficits to within 20 percent of the uninvolved knee. He began a program of wind sprints, cutting, cariocas, and jumping rope. He showed no signs of effusion but experienced low-level patellofemoral joint dysfunction. His instrumented testing indicated a bilateral difference of 3 mm of posterior translation, which was slightly more than the 1-mm difference found at 3 months but remained within the acceptable level of graft strength proposed by Clancy.[1] He resumed baseball 1 year postreconstruction.

COMMENTS

This patient achieved a typical result from bone–patellar tendon–bone autograft. There were only mild patellofemoral complications including VMO muscle insufficiency, lateral patellar tracking, and retropatellar pain. The patient achieved good graft function, knee ROM, and muscle strength. Restoring quadriceps femoris muscle strength took up to a year, which may have reflected the inherent problem with harvesting a graft from the patient's extensor mechanism. In postoperative bone–patellar tendon–bone autograft reconstructions where graft stability is not as good as in this case, the quadriceps femoris muscle assumes a more important role as a dynamic posterior restraint. The therapist needs to be aware of the type of graft used by the surgeon. A reasonable expectation is that restoration of quadriceps femoris muscle strength will take longer when the patellar tendon autograft is used, as compared with a high-strength arthroscopically placed allograft. Conversely, the surgeon needs to know the preinjury status of the patient's quadriceps femoris muscle or whether the extensor mechanism was damaged along with the PCL. If a problem exists with the extensor mechanism, then the surgeon may want to avoid using a patellar tendon autograft.

SUMMARY

Posterior cruciate ligament injuries are much less common than ACL injuries. Because much less is known about the role of the PCL in the function of the knee than is known about the ACL, making decisions concerning surgical versus nonsurgical management of PCL deficient knees can be difficult. However, the advent of arthroscopy, advances in biologic substitutes, and emphasis on early and more aggressive rehabilitation has improved our ability to treat this usually chronic, functionally limiting problem. This chapter examined the decision-making process based on current knowledge derived from successfully treating patients with PCL injuries.

REFERENCES

1. Clancy, WG, Shelbourne, KD, and Zoellner, GB: Treatment of knee joint stability secondary to rupture of the posterior cruciate ligament: Report of a new procedure. J Bone Joint Surg [Am] 65:310, 1983.
2. Hughston, JC and Degenhart, TC: Reconstruction of the posterior cruciate ligament. Clin Orthop 164:59, 1982.

3. Baker, CL, Norwood, LA and Hughston, JC: Acute combined posterior cruciate and posterolateral instability of the knee. Am J Sports Med 12:204, 1984.
4. Cross, MJ and Powell, JF: Long-term followup of posterior cruciate ligament rupture: A study cf 116 cases. Am J Sports Med 12:292, 1984.
5. Dandy, DJ and Pusey, RJ: The long term results of unrepaired tears of the posterior cruciate ligament. J Bone Joint Surg [Br] 64:92, 1982.
6. Eriksson, E, Haggmark, T, and Johnson, RJ: Reconstruction of the posterior cruciate ligament. Orthopedics 9:217, 1986.
7. Fleming, RE, Blatz, DJ, and McCarroll, JR: Posterior problems in the knee: posterior cruciate insufficiency and posterolateral rotatory insufficiency. Am J Sports Med 9:107, 1981.
8. Fowler, PJ and Messich, SS: Isolated posterior cruciate injuries in athletes. Am J Sports Med 15:553, 1987.
9. Hughston, JC, et al: Acute tears of the posterior cruciate ligament: Results of operative treatment. J Bone Joint Surtg [Am] 62:438, 1980.
10. Insall, JN and Hood, RW: Bone-block transfer of the medial head of the gastrocnemius for posterior cruciate insufficiency. J Bone Joint Surg [Am] 64:691, 1982.
11. Lipscomb, AB and Anderson, AF: Surgical reconstruction of both the anterior and posterior cruciate ligaments. The American Journal of Knee Surgery 3:29, 1990.
12. Longenecker, SL and Hughston, JC: Long-term follow-up of isolated posterior cruciate injuries (abstr). Am J Sports Med 15:628, 1987.
13. Loos, WC, et al: Acute posterior cruciate ligament injuries. Am J Sports Med 9:86, 1981.
14. McCarroll, JR, et al: The posterior cruciate ligament injury. The Physician and Sportsmedicine 11:146, 1983.
15. Parolie, JM and Bergfeld, JA: Long-term results of non-operative treatment of isolated posterior cruciate ligament injuries in the athlete. Am J Sports Med 14:35, 1986.
16. Roth, JH, et al: Medial gastrocnemius tendon transfer to manage chronic posterior cruciate ligament insufficiency (abstr). Am J Sports Med 15:628, 1987.
17. Stanish, WD, et al: Posterior cruciate ligament tears in wrestlers. Can J Sports Sci 11:173, 1986.
18. Strand, T, et al: Primary repair in posterior cruciate ligament injuries. Acta Orthop Scand 55:545, 1984.
19. Tibone, JE, et al: Functional analysis of untreated and reconstructed posterior cruciate ligament injuries. Am J Sports Med 16:217, 1988.
20. Trickey, EL: Injuries to the posterior cruciate ligament: Diagnosis and treatment of early injuries and reconstruction of late instability. Clin Orthop 147:76, 1980.
21. Wirth, CJ and Jager, M: Dynamic double tendon replacement of posterior cruciate ligament. Am J Sports Med 12:39, 1984.
22. Hughston, JC: The absent posterior drawer test in some acute posterior cruciate ligament tears of the knee. Am J Sports Med 16:39, 1988.
23. Shelbourne, KD, et al: Combined medial collateral ligament-posterior cruciate rupture: Mechanism of injury. The American Journal of Knee Surgery 3:41, 1990.
24. Gollehon, DL, Torzilli, PA, and Warren, FR: The role of the posterolateral and cruciate ligaments in the stability of the human knee. J Bone Joint Surg [Am] 69:233, 1987.
25. Grood, ES, Stowers, SF, and Noyes, FR: Limits of movement in the human knee: Effect of sectioning the posterior cruciate ligament and posterolateral structures. J Bone Joint Surg [Am] 70:88, 1988.
26. Hughston, JC, et al: Classification of knee ligament instabilities. II. The lateral compartment. J Bone Joint Surg [Am] 58:173, 1976.
27. Hughston, JC, et al: Classification of knee ligament instabilities. I. The medial compartment and cruciate ligaments. J Bone Joint Surg [Am] 58:159, 1978.
28. Daniel, DM, et al: Use of quadricepts active test to diagnose posterior cruciate ligament disruption and measure posterior laxity of the knee. J Bone Joint Surg [Am] 70:386, 1988.
29. Hughston, JC and Norwood, LA: The posterolateral drawer test and external rotational recurvatum test for posterolateral rotatory instability of the knee. Clin Orthop 147:82, 1980.
30. Jackob, RP, Hassler, H, and Stacuble, HUI: Observations on rotatory instability of the lateral compartment. Acta Orthop Scand Suppl 52:191, 1981.
31. Shelbourne, KD, et al: Dynamic posterior shift test: An adjuvant in evaluation of posterior tibial subluxation. Am J Sports Med 17:275, 1989.
32. Engle, RP: Nonoperative posterior cruciate ligament rehabilitation. In Engle, RP (ed): Knee Ligament Rehabilitation. Churchill Livingstone, New York, 1991, p 145.
33. Rosenberg, TD, Paulos, LE, and Abbott, PJ: Arthroscopic cruciate repair and reconstruction: An overview and descriptions of technique. In Feagin, JA (ed): The Crucial Ligaments. Churchill Livingstone, New York, 1988, p 409.
34. Noyes, FR: Diagnosis and indications for PCL and posterolateral surgery. Presented at Annual Conference on Advances in the Knee and Shoulder, Cincinnatti, OH, April 1990.
35. Noyes, FR, et al: Biomechanical analysis of human ligament grafts used in knee ligament repairs and reconstructions. J Bone Joint Surg [Am] 66:344, 1984.
36. Johnson, G and Saliba, VJ: Proprioceptive Neuromuscular Facilitation I and II: Course Notes. Institute of Physical Art, San Anselmo, CA, 1990.

CHAPTER 12

Rehabilitation of Medial Capsular Injuries

Kevin E. Wilk, PT

Disorders of the knee are the most common problems confronting the sports physical therapist.[1] Ligamentous injuries to the knee account for 25 to 40 percent of all knee injuries[2,3] with sprains of the medial collateral ligament occuring most frequently.[1,4,5] Thus the medial collateral ligament (MCL), also referred to as the tibial collateral ligament (TCL), is a structure that receives much attention from the clinician.

Injuries to the medial capsule of the knee are especially common in sports. In football the TCL is the most commonly injured ligament.[6] Sprains of the knee account for 35 percent of all skiing injuries[7,8] and the TCL is the ligament most often involved. Injuries of the TCL can occur as a result of a blow to the lateral side of the knee or as a result of a twist or fall with the foot planted (Fig. 12–1). Therefore, this ligamentous injury occurs in contact sports such as football and wrestling and in noncontact sports such as skiing, basketball, soccer, and tennis.

Due to the common occurence of this injury, the sports medicine practitioner should understand the anatomy, biomechanics, and healing restraints of the medial capsule to allow successful rehabilitation to occur. This chapter addresses these basic and clinical science principles. In addition, two case studies are presented to illustrate problem-solving that uses the scientific rationale described in this chapter.

FUNCTIONAL ANATOMY

The medial aspect of the knee consists of both dynamic (musculature) and static (ligamentous) stabilizing structures. Considerable confusion exists concerning the structures that comprise the medial capsule of the knee. Warren and Marshall's[9] cadaveric dissections demonstrated three specific layers of the medial side of the knee (Fig. 12–2). Layer 1 includes the deep fascia overlying the vastus medialis, which extends from the patella to the popliteal fossa. The second layer comprises the superficial TCL.[9,10] This

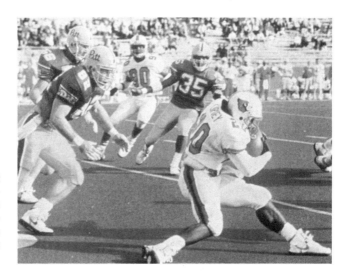

FIGURE 12-1. A noncontact injury to a football player resulting in a valgus force to the knee with tibial external rotation. The results may include injury to the TCL, ACL, or the extensor mechanism.

ligament is triangular, with a wide origin just below the adductor tubercle of the medial femoral condyle. This superficial ligament extends inferiorly and narrows to insert on the tibia 4 to 5 cm distal to the joint line just posterior and deep to the pes anserinus tendon insertion (Fig. 12-3).

Layer 3 consists of the capsule of the knee joint and contains the "deep" TCL, consisting of the meniscofemoral and the meniscotibial ligaments. These structures are just beneath the superficial TCL. This structure has a firm attachment to the medial

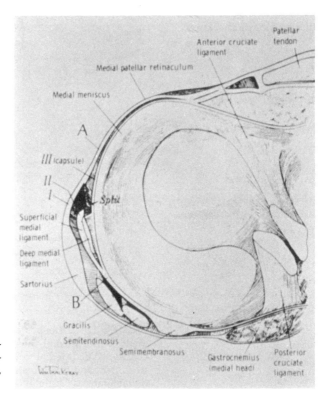

FIGURE 12-2. The medial compartment of the knee. (From Warren, LF and Marshall, JL,[9] p 56, with permission.)

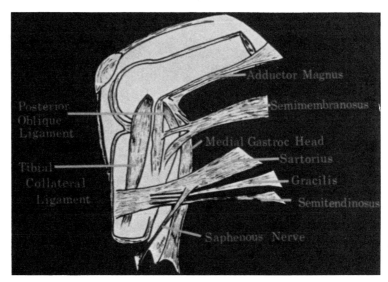

FIGURE 12-3. The medial or tibial collateral ligament (TCL). (Adapted from Wilk, KE and Clancy, WG: Medial collateral ligament injuries: Diagnosis, treatment, and rehabilitation. In Engle, RP [ed]: Knee Ligament Rehabilitation. Churchill Livingstone, New York, 1991, p 72.)

meniscus (Fig. 12-4). Posteriorly the oblique portion of the superficial TCL joins the deep portion of the TCL to form the posteromedial capsule. In addition, the semimembranosus tendon reinforces this region of the knee. Hughston and Eilers[11] have termed the thickness of this posteromedial corner the *posterior oblique ligament*. This structure is actually the capsular ligaments of layer 2 and 3 joining together to form the posteromedial corner of the knee.

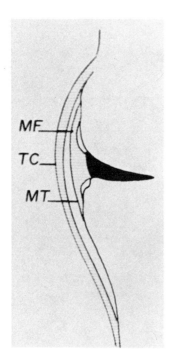

FIGURE 12-4. Deep medial capsular ligaments with attachment to the medial meniscus. (Adapted from Wilk, KE and Clancy, WG: Medial collateral ligament injuries: Diagnosis, treatment, and rehabilitation. In Engle, RP [ed]: Knee Ligament Rehabilitation. Churchill Livingstone, New York, 1991, p 72.)

In addition, a proximal portion of the superficial TCL attaches to the vastus medialis obliquus (VMO) portion of the quadriceps femoris muscle.[12,13] This attachment plays a role in neuromuscular control by providing feedback from the ligament to the muscle about intraligamentous tension.[13] The TCL possesses mechanoreceptors, such as Ruffini end-organs, pacinian corpuscles, and Golgi tendon organs, that contribute to joint proprioception.[14,15] Receptors in the TCL, anterior cruciate ligament (ACL), and the posterior horn of the medial meniscus initiate protective muscular contraction responses.[16,17] The reflex most often elicited consists of inhibition of the extensors and facilitation of the flexor muscle group.[18]

The dynamic stabilizers of the medial aspect of the knee consist of the pes anserine muscle group: the gracilis, sartorius, and semitendinosus muscles. In addition, the adductor magnus muscle is a significant stabilizer. The semimembranosus muscle has five points of insertion: (1) the posterior capsule over the medial meniscus; (2) the oblique fibers of the superficial TCL; (3) the oblique popliteal ligament; (4) the semimembranosus groove on the tibia; and (5) the posteromedial corner of the tibia near the joint line. The number of points of attachment indicates the muscle's importance in dynamic stabilization of the medial and posteromedial aspect of the knee (see Chapter 1).

BIOMECHANICS

Biomechanically, the superficial TCL acts as a primary valgus restraint. In addition, the ligament is taut throughout the joint range of motion (ROM) due to the semicircular pattern of its points of origin[19] (Fig. 12–5). The most anterior fibers of this ligament become taut as the knee flexes, then relax somewhat during extension. However, the entire substance of the TCL is maximally taut in full knee extension. This pattern demonstrates that the TCL is anterior to the instant center of motion of the knee.[19]

The TCL provides 78 percent of the resistance to valgus force when the knee is flexed at 25 degrees[20] (Fig. 12–6B). As the knee moves toward full extension, the posterior capsule provides 18 percent of the valgus restraint while the TCL's contribution decreases to 57 percent (Fig. 12–6A). In other words, as the knee moves toward full extension, the posterior and posteromedial aspects of the capsule become taut and prevent valgus translation; significant valgus opening in full extension therefore indicates an injury to the TCL as well as to the posteromedial and posterior aspects of the capsule.

Another TCL function is to limit external tibial rotation, especially as the knee approaches full flexion.[9,12,19,21] Selective tissue sectioning shows that when the deep portion of the TCL is cut, the increase in external rotation is minimal near full extension and increases with increased flexion.[19] Finally, the medial capsule is a secondary restraint to anterior translation when the ACL is absent. Therefore, in the ACL deficient knee the TCL acts as a stabilizer to anterior displacement of the tibia.

MECHANISM OF INJURY

The medial capsular ligaments are commonly injured in football secondary to a valgus force to the knee caused by contact or blow to the lateral aspect of the knee. This injury is often seen in linemen, especially defensive linemen, because of blocking

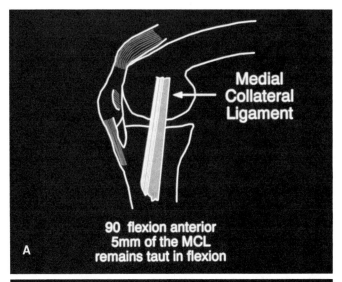

90 flexion anterior
5mm of the MCL
remains taut in flexion

A

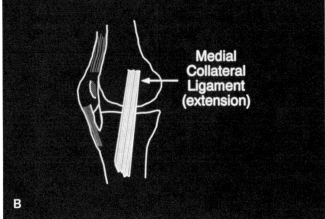

Medial
Collateral
Ligament
(extension)

B

FIGURE 12-5. *A*) TCL (MCL) with the knee at 90 degrees of flexion. The anterior fibers of the TCL remain taut in knee flexion. *B*) TCL (MCL) with the knee in full extension; the TCL is maximally taut. (Adapted from Wilk, KE and Clancy, WG: Medial collateral ligament injuries: Diagnosis, treatment, and rehabilitation. In Engle, RP [ed]: Knee Ligament Rehabilitation. Churchill Livingstone, New York, 1991, p 75.)

techniques designed to knock the legs out from under the rushing defensive lineman. Often the TCL is injured in conjunction with the ACL, as a result of a cutting maneuver, rotation of the knee, or a lateral blow. The combined injury of the TCL and ACL was often associated with tears of the medial meniscus. O'Donoghue described this injury as the "unhappy triad"[22-24] in 1959. Campbell[25] first described this combined injury in 1936. This combined knee injury involving the ACL, TCL, and medial meniscus was broadly acknowledged and accepted until a recent article by Shelbourne[26] disputed this occurrence. Shelbourne[26] reported on two groups of patients who underwent arthroscopic examination. One group consisted of patients with complete ACL disruption and grade II TCL sprains. The other group consisted of patients with complete ACL tears and complete TCL sprains. In both groups there was a higher incidence of lateral meniscal tears than of medial meniscal tears. These findings are consistent with other clinical observations.[27]

In addition, noncontact TCL injuries are also common and are due to valgus forces to the knee with tibial external rotation during a fall while skiing, playing soccer, or attempting to hit a low ball in tennis. This mechanism of TCL disruption is also seen

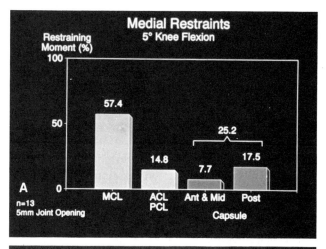

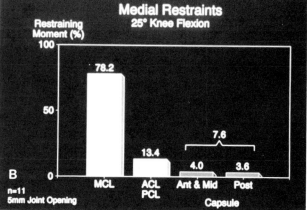

FIGURE 12-6. Comparative contributions to valgus force resistance at A) 5 degrees flexion and B) 25 degrees flexion. (From Grood, ES, et al: Ligamentous and capsular restraints preventing straight medial and lateral laxity in intact human cadaver knees. J Bone Joint Surg [Am] 63:1257, 1981, with permission.)

when an individual twists and falls away from the planted foot, causing a valgus and external rotation force to the knee that may lead to TCL, ACL, or extensor mechanism injury.

PHYSICAL EXAMINATION

Before the objective physical examination is initiated, a thorough subjective history should be taken to determine the mechanism of injury. The examiner should ask the patient to explain the injury, by prompting the patient to answer questions such as "Was a pop or tear felt or heard?" "Did swelling occur?" and "How long from the time of injury did it take for the swelling to occur?" The location of pain or tenderness, previous history of knee injuries, present activity level, and intended sports activities for the future are all pertinent items of information to gather at this point.

The physical examination starts with the assessment of swelling as determined by placing one hand on each side of the anterior surface of the knee and applying gentle pressure with one of the hands, as if pushing on the side of a water balloon. If swelling is present, the relaxed hand will feel the fluid move into it. The quantification of swelling is determined by an estimation of the amount of fluid present; mild swelling indicates about 25 ml or less, moderate swelling indicates 26 to 55 ml present, and severe swelling is represented by 56 ml or more.

Palpation of the knee is performed next. In association with TCL injuries, tenderness is often elicited over the adductor tubercle (the origin of the TCL) (Fig. 12–7). This point is often tender because this location serves as a dual origin for the TCL and the medial patellofemoral ligament, which is often injured with lateral patellar subluxation. To differentiate patellar subluxation from minor sprains of the TCL, palpation of the patella and patella facets, along with ligamentous tests, can clarify nature of the lesion. If the patella is painful upon palpation and valgus laxity is equal to that of the contralateral side, patellar subluxation should be suspected. Range of motion (ROM) following TCL injuries is often limited; full extension is usually painful, and knee flexion greater than 100 degrees can be extremely painful.

The ligamentous tests of the knee should begin with the Godfrey test (Fig. 12–8) to determine integrity of the posterior cruciate ligament (PCL). Second, the Lachman test should be performed to determine if the ACL has been injured (Fig. 12–9). The status of the PCL should be determined first to ensure accurate testing of the ACL. Next, a valgus stress test is performed to evaluate TCL integrity. The patient lies supine with the knee flexed to 25 to 30 degrees and netural tibial rotation (Fig. 12–10). To facilitate relaxation, the femur is stabilized with one hand and with the same hand the joint line is palpated. With the other hand on the distal tibia a valgus movement, or abduction is exerted. The medial joint space opening is estimated and the end feel or point is also evaluated. The findings are compared with those for the patient's contralateral normal knee. Ideally, the normal knee is evaluated first to acclimate the subject to the test and to avoid testing the involved extremity more than once.

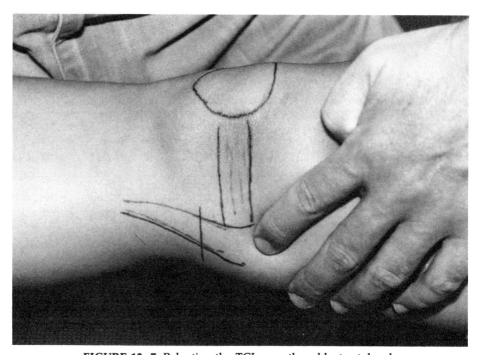

FIGURE 12–7. Palpating the TCL over the adductor tubercle.

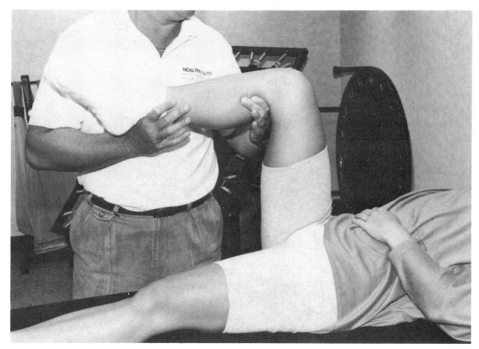

FIGURE 12-8. The Godfrey or sag test is used to determine the integrity of the PCL. With the knee flexed to 90 degrees, the examiner assesses the amount of posterior sag of the tibia on the femur.

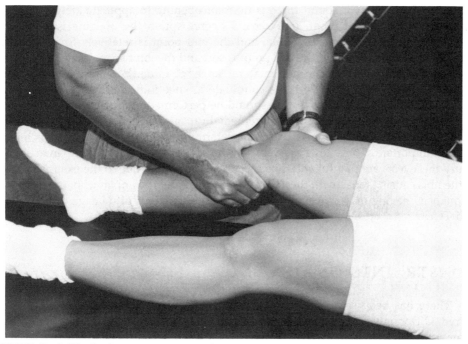

FIGURE 12-9. The Lachman test assesses the integrity of the ACL. The examiner, while imparting an anterior force to the proximal tibia with the knee in approximately 30 degrees of flexion, assesses the amount of excursion and the end feel.

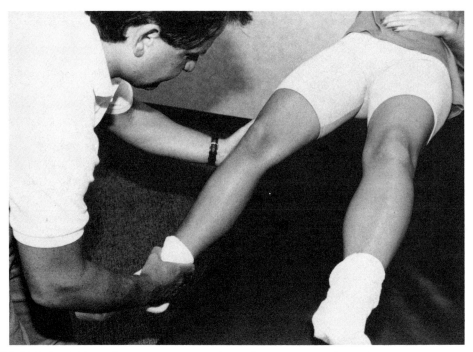

FIGURE 12-10. The valgus stress test is performed at approximately 30 degrees of knee flexion.

In first degree TCL sprain there is no joint opening to approximately 2 mm, and there exists a firm end point. In a second degree sprain the opening is 3 to 5 mm compared with the contralateral side, and the end point is relatively firm with slight give. In a third degree injury the end point is soft and the joint space opens more than 5 mm greater than that of the contralateral knee.[4,28] Grood[20] reported that a 5-mm increase in laxity compared with the contralateral knee indicated major TCL damage.

In addition, valgus stress testing should be performed at 0 degrees knee extension to determine the integrity of the posteromedial capsule. Specific tests such as McMurray's and Apley's tests, which are used to determine whether the meniscus is injured, are also important. These tests are depicted in the Appendix. Often with an acute TCL injury these tests are painful and thus cannot be performed due to the external rotation of the tibia causing tension on the TCL and eliciting pain. If complaints persist, magnetic resonance imaging may be useful in determining the extent of damage to the menisci and TCL.

CONSTRAINTS ON HEALING

There has been some controversy about whether an injured TCL should be repaired. O'Donoghue[29] reported that if a primary repair is not performed, the ends of the ligament may not remain in closed opposition and thus healing will be biomechanically inferior and prolonged. Several investigators have reported biomechanically stronger

TCLs in sutured canine knees compared with unsutured.[30-32] In a recent study, Woo and colleagues[5] reported their results after sectioning canine tibial collateral ligaments. The three groups studied were (1) no repair and immediate motion; (2) repaired and immobilized for 3 weeks; and (3) repaired and immobilized for 6 weeks. The tensile strength and biomechanical properties were analyzed at 6, 12, and 48 weeks postsectioning. The results indicated that the biomechanical properties of the nonrepaired ligaments exhibited the best results for all time frames. The investigators also reported that the longer the immobilization period (group 3), the lower the load to failure. In addition, the microscopic appearance of the repaired and nonrepaired ligaments appeared similar, and at 48 weeks was identical to the normal TCL. Numerous clinical studies have reported excellent results using a treatment protocol of immediate motion without surgical intervention.

Ellsasser[33] reported on clinical findings in 64 professional football players who sustained partial TCL sprains. All were treated nonoperatively and with mobilization; all patients returned to play in 3 to 8 weeks. Derscheid[34] recorded knee injuries during 4 academic years from 1974 to 1978. All TCL injuries were treated identically with motion and early exercise. The authors reported a return to participation in 10.6 days for grade I sprains and 19.5 days in grade II cases. Wilk[35] reported on 52 TCL sprains in athletes who were all treated with immediate motion, early weight bearing, and immediate exercise. The results indicated a return to sport activities after 9.2 days following a grade I sprain and 17.8 days after a grade II injury.

Thus, based on these studies and other clinical studies using both protocols (repair versus nonrepair) and immobilization versus immediate motion, most clinicians believe that following TCL sprains, the treatment of choice for isolated TCL sprains is no repair and immediate motion.[33-41] In addition, several authors have reported an enhanced healing response of the TCL by immediate motion and exercise.[37,41-44] Immediate motion and exercises provide a stimulus to the medial capsule, thus facilitating earlier and better healing of the injured structures.

The healing rate and mechanical properties of the TCL are altered and thus slowed in the absence of the ACL. Investigators have reported that the TCLs in knees with totally sectioned ACL showed less recovery than in those knee joints with intact ACLs.[40,45-47] Thus, in the case of ACL and TCL injuries, the recommended treatment is to reconstruct the ACL and apply immediate motion to promote healing of the injured TCL. We have experienced clinically that among such patients the rehabilitation process should be accelerated by comparison with patients with isolated ACL reconstruction.

The stages of TCL healing have been explained by several authors[48-51] and are phase 1 — acute inflammation, which occurs in the first 72 hours; phase 2 — repair and regeneration process, which begins at 48 to 72 hours, lasts up to 6 weeks, and is marked by collagen production; phase 3 — remodeling, which lasts at least 52 weeks (see Chapter 4). During this last phase the healing ligament continues to become stronger. The maximum return in strength appears to be approximately 70 to 75 percent of the preinjury level. The process is accelerated by motion and controlled stress to the torn ligament.

The optimal conditions for TCL healing are (1) maintenance of the torn fibers in close continuity; (2) intact and stable ACL and other supporting ligaments of the knee; (3) immediate controlled motion and stresses to the healing ligament; and (4) protection of the TCL against deleterious stresses (valgus and external rotation stresses) through the use of bracing and with patient compliance to promote the healing process.

REHABILITATION PROGRAM

The complete rehabilitation following an isolated TCL sprain can be divided into a four-phase rehabilitation program (Table 12–1). The rehabilitation program is based on five basic rehabilitation principles:

1. The effects of immobilization must be minimized.
2. Never overstress healing tissue.
3. The patient must fulfill specific criteria to progress.
4. The rehabilitation program should be based on current clinical and scientific research.
5. The rehabilitation program must be adaptable to each patient.

TABLE 12–1 Rehabilitation of Grade I, II, and III Isolated TCL Sprains

This program may be accelerated for grade I TCL/LCL sprains or may be extended depending on the severity of the injury. The following schedule serves as a guideline to help expedite returning an athlete to his preinjury state.

Please note that any increase in pain or swelling or loss of range of motion are signs that the progression of the program may be too rapid.

Phase 1: Maximal Protection

Goals

Early protected ROM
Prevent quadriceps atrophy
Decrease effusion/pain
A. Time of injury: Day 1
    1. Ice, compression, elevation
    2. Hinged brace, nonpainful ROM (or knee immobilizer if hinged brace not available)
    3. Crutches, weight bearing as tolerated
    4. Passive range of motion/active assisted range of motion exercise to maintain ROM
    5. Electrical muscle stimulation to quads, 8 hr per day (when possible)
    6. Isometrics quads, quad sets, 60 reps; 3 × day
       Straight leg raises (SLR), 3 sets of 15; 3 × day
B. Day 2
    1. 7-count SLR
    2. Hamstring setting
    3. Well leg exercises
    4. Whirlpool for ROM (cold for first 3–4 days, then warm)
    5. High-voltage galvanic stimulation to control swelling
    6. Continue above
C. Days 3–7
    1. Continue above
    2. Crutches, weight bearing as tolerated
    3. ROM as tolerated
    4. Eccentric quad work
    5. Bicycle for ROM stimulus
    6. Multi-angle isometrics with electrical stimulation
    7. Initial hip abduction, extension, 3 sets of 15
    8. Brace worn at night, brace during day as needed
    9. Balance drills in seated position

TABLE 12–1 Rehabilitation of Grade I, II, and III
Isolated TCL Sprains *(Continued)*

Phase 2: Moderate Protection

Criteria for Progression

1. No increase in instability
2. No increase in swelling
3. Minimal tenderness
4. PROM 10–100 degrees

Goals

Full painless ROM
Restore strength
Normalize ambulation (no assistive devices)
A. Week 2
    1. Continue strengthening program with PREs (knee ext/flex/leg press)
    2. Continue electrical muscle stimulation
    3. Continue ROM exercise
    4. Multi-angle isometrics with EMS
    5. Discontinue crutches
    6. Bicycle for endurance
    7. Water exercises, running in water forward and backward
    8. Full ROM exercises
    9. Flexibility exercises: hamstrings, quads, iliotibial band
    10. Proprioception training; balance drills
B. Days 11–14
    1. Continue as week 2
    2. PREs emphasis quads, medial hamstrings, hip adduction
    3. Initiate isokinetics, submaximal progressing to maximal fast contractile velocities
    4. Begin running program if full painless extension and flexion are present
    5. Stairmaster, stationary ski track, rowing machine
    6. Isokinetics, fast speed
    7. Exercise Tubing, high-speed training

Phase 3: Minimal Protection

Criteria for Progression:

1. No instability
2. No swelling/tenderness
3. Full painless ROM

Goals

Increase strength and power
A. Week 3
    1. Continue Strengthening Program
        Emphasis: Fast-speed isokinetics
                Eccentric quads
                Isotonic hip adduction, medial hamstrings
        4 Quad Program
        Knee extension (100–40 degrees)
        ½ squats
        Leg press
        Step-ups
        4 Endurance Program
        Bicycle 20 min
        Stationary ski track

continued

TABLE 12–1 Rehabilitation of Grade I, II, and III
Isolated TCL Sprains *(Continued)*

Pool running
Stairmaster
4 Stability Program
Balance/agility drills
Plyometrics
Exercise tubing, Hip/Hamstrings
Backward running
Running Program
Forward/backward running
Lateral shuffle/cariocas
Figure-eights/cutting

Phase 4: Maintenance

Return to Competition

1. Full ROM
2. No tenderness over TCL
3. No instability
4. No effusion
5. Muscle strength 85% of contralateral side
6. Quad strength = body weight (60%)
7. Proprioceptive ability satisfactory
8. Lateral knee brace

Maintenance Program

1. Continue isotonic strengthening exercises
2. Continue flexibility exercises
3. Continue proprioceptive activities
4. Continue 4 × 4 program
The above program may be accelerated for first degree TCL/LCL sprains or may be extended depending on the severity of the injury. The above schedules are guidelines only.
Again, note that any increase in pain or swelling or any loss of ROM are signs that one is progressing the program too quickly.

Source: Adapted from Wilk, KE and Clancy, WG: Medial collateral ligament injuries: Diagnosis, treatment, and rehabilitation. In Engle, RP (ed): Knee Ligament Rehabilitation. Churchill Livingstone, New York, 1991, pp 73–74.

These principles must be understood and followed as a treatment philosophy to ensure proper and complete healing.

In phase 1 the goals are to initiate immediate motion in a nonpainful arc of motion so that the deleterious effects of immobilization can be prevented and collagen synthesis and organization can be accelerated. Painful motion or too aggressive stretching may cause the healing collagen to be traumatized again and thus retard the healing process. Often a brace is used to protect the healing ligament. Early weight bearing is encouraged to stress the healing ligament and provides nourishment to the articular cartilage and subchondral bone. In addition, immediate quadriceps femoris muscle strengthening exercises are initiated to prevent muscular atrophy. The quadriceps femoris muscle will atrophy at a faster rate than the other muscles about the knee following a knee injury.[35,52,53] Electrical stimulation to the quadriceps femoris muscle is used to facilitate an increased muscular contraction, retard muscular atrophy, and provide reeducation to the muscle.[52,54-56] The reeducation of the muscle is designed to prevent "quadriceps femoris shutdown," which is the inability of the patient to perform an isometric quadriceps femoris muscle contraction or to exhibit quadriceps femoris muscle control. In addition, use of a bicycle or warm whirlpool can stimulate increasing range of motion.

In phase 2 the goals are to reestablish full nonpainful ROM and improve muscular strength. The strengthening exercises are accelerated. Isotonic exercises are implemented in the form of knee extensions, leg press, and hip exercises, especially hip adduction and hamstring curls. We also emphasize closed kinetic chain exercises such as minisquats, step ups, and use of Stairmaster (Stairmaster 400 PT, Randall Sports Medical Products, Kirkland, WA) (Fig. 12-11) and a stationary ski track. (Proprioception drills are emphasized to improve balance and agility [Fig. 12-12].) Pool exercises and pool running may also be initiated to improve total body conditioning and strengthening with minimal joint stress (Fig. 12-13).

Phase 3 is called the minimal protection phase. All exercises are progressed with a special focus on closed chain exercise, endurance exercise, balance activity, and high-velocity training. In addition, a running program is initiated with an emphasis on drills

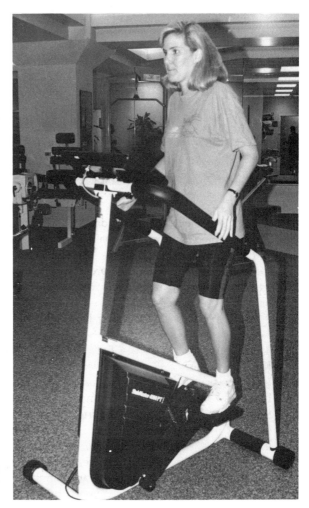

FIGURE 12-11. A patient using a stairclimber to perform a closed kinetic chain exercise.

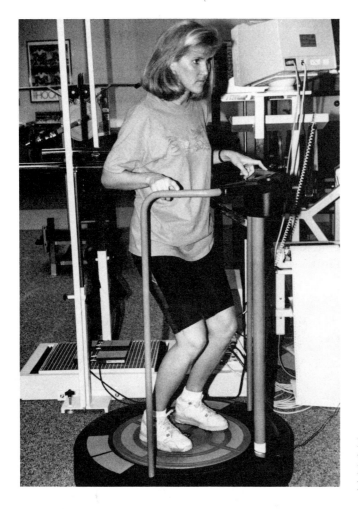

FIGURE 12-12. A patient using a balance device (BREG, Inc., Vista, CA) to perform a proprioception exercise.

and running specific to the demands of the patient's/athlete's life-style. Agility drills are begun to enhance coordination, balance, and neuromuscular control.

In the last phase, maintenance exercises are used when the athlete returns to his or her sport. However, an exercise program should be designed to continually increase strength and function, not merely to maintain strength. We have outlined the basic exercises in a 4×4 program. These exercises are designed to provide the stimulus to cause the continuation of muscular hypertrophy and endurance.

4 Quadriceps Program	*4 Endurance*
Knee extension	Bicycle
$\frac{1}{2}$ squats	Stairmaster
Leg press	Stationary ski track
Step-ups	Running program

4 Others	*4 Stability*
Hamstring curls	Balance/proprioceptive training
Hip strengthening	Backward running
Calf strengthening	Fast speed tubing
Ankle strengthening	Plyometrics

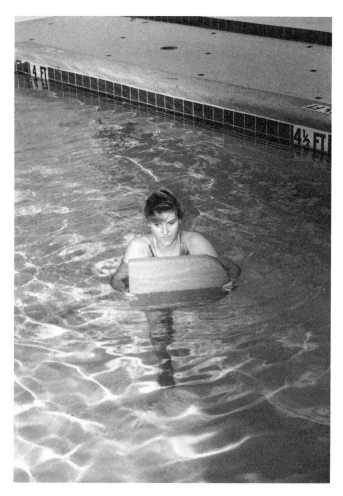

FIGURE 12–13. A patient performing a kicking exercise in water for total leg strengthening.

This rehabilitation program has been in use for 7 years with excellent success. Results from an ongoing clinical study including 115 isolated TCL injuries have shown a 98 percent success rate (patients have progressed through the program without major complications and returned to preexisting level of sport activities). The average return to sport after a grade I TCL injury is 9.2 days and for a grade II injury, 17.8 days.[35] Most of these individuals sustained their TCL injury during football (8 percent), skiing (6 percent) basketball (3 percent), wrestling (3 percent), and tennis (1 percent).

CASE STUDIES

CASE STUDY 1

HISTORY

A 23-year-old medical sales representative injured her right knee skiing 1 week prior to the evaluation. She reported that she was going downhill at a controlled moderate rate when her ski turned to the outside, resulting in external tibial rotation. She fell backward, causing a valgus stress to the knee. The patient reported a sharp pain on the medial side of her knee. She stated that she was able to ski down the hill very slowly. The knee became sore immediately, and she was unable to continue to ski. In addition, there was no swelling since the injury. She did not ski again but did some walking and biking, which resulted in increased soreness. She did not see a physician in Lake Tahoe, where the injury occurred. At the time of physical therapy evaluation her main·complaints were increased soreness with activities; inability to fully bend or straighten her knee; and an inability to play tennis, run, or swim.

EXAMINATION

Effusion	Minimal to none
Tenderness	Tender adductor tubercle (origin of TCL and medial patellofemoral ligament), slight tenderness posteromedial capsule, including joint line
Lachman test	Negative/firm end point
Drawer test	Negative/pain with knee flexion 90°
Pivot shift test	Not attempted
Valgus stress test 0°	Stable
Valgus stress test 25°	1+ with soft, painful end point
Varus stress test 0°	Stable
Varus stress test 25°	Stable
Patella apprehension	Trace positive, painful
Patella facet palpation	Slight tenderness on medial and lateral patellar facets superior and middle, no tenderness on the inferior facets
McMurray's test	Unable to perform/painful knee flex
ROM	20°–95°
Neurovasculature	Intact
Radiographs	Medial soft tissue effusion (mild)

Comments

Skiing is a common mechanism of TCL and ACL injuries due to knee position, increased force through the knee joint, and the long level arm of the skis. The facts that the patient did not hear a "pop" and that the Lachman test was stable indicated the ACL was probably spared and thus intact. Tearing the TCL rarely produces an audible "pop," but patients often report a tearing sensation.

That the patient is point tender on the adductor tubercle should reveal two facts. First, this site is the origin of the superficial TCL; therefore, tenderness may indicate a TCL sprain. Second, the adductor tubercle also serves as an origin of medial patellofemoral ligament. When the patella laterally subluxes, this structure is torn and tender. This patient's mechanism of injury—the knee flexed 25 to 30 degrees, external tibia rotation, and the body force moving to cause a valgus stress—can cause patella subluxation and TCL sprain. A careful and thorough screening is necessary to obtain a differential diagnosis. Such a diagnosis is often difficult to make in an acute situation and requires attention to detail and a thorough examination.

Differentiation of the two injuries occurs through four tests:

1. Valgus stress at 25° knee flexion — Joint opening that produces pain indicates TCL sprain.

2. Lateral glide test of patella — Produces a stretch on the medial patellofemoral ligament; if this structure is injured, the test will produce pain and increased patella translation, compared with the contralateral side.

3. Palpation of lateral facets — With patella subluxation the lateral facets are often tender on palpation.

4. ROM — With TCL sprains, both flexion and extension are limited; with patella subluxation only one motion is limited.

In addition, following patella subluxation there appears to be more knee joint effusion than in the presence of TCL sprains (especially grade I sprains). However, with grade II TCL sprains or grade III TCL sprains with ACL injury, knee joint effusion is always present.

Based on the evaluation, the patient probably sustained a grade I TCL sprain and a minor trauma to the medial patellofemoral ligament. In grade I TCL sprains the injury is to the superficial portion of the TCL structure; no injury is sustained to the deep TCL and no significant injury occurs at the posterior oblique portion of the TCL.

TREATMENT

Individuals who sustain grade I TCL sprains do extremely well with an aggressive, immediate motion rehabilitation program. In our ongoing study we have documented that competitive athletes returned to sports in 7 days postinjury when an isolated grade I sprain occurred. The recreational athlete required at least 3 weeks to return to cutting sports.

During the course of rehabilitation, if the patient is not improving and pain and swelling with occasional catching or locking persist, a return of the patient to the physician may be in order. These symptoms may indicate a meniscus tear that could have been sustained at the time of the TCL sprain but was not diagnosed because, due to pain, a thorough meniscal exam could not then be performed. If symptoms persist, a magnetic resonance imaging examination should be performed to determine the integrity of the medial meniscus and TCL.

This patient was placed on our isolated TCL sprain rehabilitation program. Grade I and II sprains can be successfully treated nonoperatively with excellent results.[33,34,40,53,57-59] Therefore, the keys to treatment are the accurate diagnosis of an isolated lesion (TCL sprain) and a rehabilitation plan that immediately incorporates motion to stimulate a healing response and organization of collagen fibers.[5,37,60] Controlled stress to the TCL produces a more rapid healing response and a stronger healed ligament.[5] Therefore, we choose to use a hinged brace or no brace rather than an immobilization brace.

REHABILITATION

Our rehabilitation program is outlined in Table 12-1. In phase 1 the goal is to provide a stimulus to the collagen tissue of the TCL through immediate motion. Therefore, we use both intermittent passive and active assisted ROM exercises through a nonpainful arc of motion. Proceeding through pain may cause microtrauma to the collagen tissue, which will produce an inflammatory response and thus slow the healing rate. Often a hinged brace is used to guard the healing TCL. The brace is often limited to 15 to 90 degrees; then ROM is progressed on an average of 5 degrees extension/10 degrees flexion every 5 to 7 days. Therefore, we anticipate full ROM by 21 days and in some cases as early as 14 days.

In addition, pain and inflammation in the knee joint result in atrophy of the quadriceps femoris muscle, especially the vastus medialis obliquus muscle. Therefore, isometric exercises are performed and supplemented with neuromuscular electrical stimulation to augment the voluntary contraction. The use of ice, compression, and elevation is beneficial to control inflammation. Crutches are rarely used in grade I TCL sprains but often used in grade II or III sprains. Most knees exhibit a minimal amount of genu valgum alignment of approximately 5 to 10 degrees, which is considered normal.[61] During ambulation the medial side of the joint undergoes minimal tensile stress, and thus early weight bearing forces are safe. If a patient exhibits significant genu valgum alignment of the knee (greater than 10 to 15 degrees), the medial compartment will receive a distraction force that may retard TCL healing. In these patients crutches may be used to minimize such stresses. Often these patients are placed in a double upright functional knee brace.

Phase 2 is for moderate protection. The goal of this phase is to improve the strength of the quadriceps, hamstrings, and hip adductor muscles. In addition, we want to obtain full, nonpainful ROM and promote the healing of the injured medial collateral ligament.

In this phase our isotonic program of knee extension, knee flexion, multidirectional hip machine, and multi-angle quadriceps muscle extensions is implemented. We emphasize closed kinetic chain exercises such as the leg press, step-ups, minisquats, and a stair-stepping machine (Stairmaster). In addition, proprioception drills are performed to assist in the rehabilitation for balance and to facilitate neuromuscular control. Also, the patient can begin an aquatic running program. This low-load functional progression is important before outside running and recreational sports are initiated.

In phase 3 the goals are to increase the patient's strength, power, and endurance and to begin a gradual return to functional sport activities. In this phase cardiovascular and neuromuscular control exercises are encouraged to improve endurance and coordination. Cardiovascular exercises are designed to increase blood flow to the heart and increase the exercise potential of the heart muscles. Cardiovascular exercises also help to increase the circulation of blood to the muscle, with the goal of improving muscular endurance. These exercises include high-velocity tubing exercises, Stairmaster, and stationary cycle. Exercises are designed to increase the potential of the skeletal muscles to perform work for a prolonged period of time. The patient is placed on our 4 × 4 program, which was discussed earlier.

Phase 4 prepares the patient to return to sport activities and includes return to competitive as well as maintenance programs. During this phase the patient should continue to improve her strength, endurance, coordination and skill. All patients should be told that they may feel slight pain along the TCL for up to 1 year after injury, particularly with extreme valgus stress to the knee joint.

This patient did extremely well on her program, and at 4 weeks postinjury returned to Lake Tahoe for spring skiing without a protective brace. She is presently involved in biking, aerobics, and swimming. On physical exam at 18 weeks postinjury, her knee joint was stable but with extreme valgus stress she noted minor point tenderness. This occurrence is not uncommon, and we have noted minor tenderness with valgus stress up to 6 to 8 months postinjury.

CASE STUDY 2

HISTORY

A 17-year-old high school senior running back was struck on the lateral side of the knee while his foot was planted and making a cut. The force was great enough to cause his foot to become dislodged from his shoe. The athlete also reported hearing a loud "pop" at the time of the contact. He was able to walk off the field with minor assistance. Evaluation on the field revealed a 1+ to 2+ Lachman test with soft end feel. On the sideline the player was evaluated again, and the results were as follows: valgus stress at 0 degrees (1+); valgus stress test at 25 degrees knee flexion (2+); varus stress at 0 degrees (1+); and varus stress at 25 degrees (1+). Lachman test indicated 2+ laxity with a soft end feel. That night the player was sent to our sports medicine emergency room for roentgenograms, placed in a knee brace locked at 30 degrees, instructed on partial weight bearing, and given isometric exercises. In addition, the patient was given a compression wrap to control joint effusion. He was also advised to elevate his leg and ice his knee. The athlete was seen 2 days later in the sports medicine clinic with his parents.

EXAMINATION

Effusion	Moderate
Tenderness	Adductor tubercle, tibial collateral ligament, medial and lateral joint line
Lachman test	1+ with soft end feel
Drawer test	Unable to flex to 90°
Pivot shift test	Unable to test due to patient's pain
Valgus stress 0°	1+
Valgus stress 25°	2+
Varus stress 0°	1+
Varus stress 25°	1+
Patella apprehension	Negative
ROM	20°–85° (pain with full extension/flexion)
Neurovascular status	Intact
Radiographs	Normal, soft tissue swelling medially

Comments

Valgus stress to the knee from an external blow is a common mechanism of injury for the TCL. With the foot planted (joint compression) and a rotatory force occurring as in making a cut, this often involves the joint surfaces, the medial and lateral menisci, and the posteromedial capsule. The ACL is often involved in contact injuries that couple rotation and a valgus stress. The fact that the player heard a "pop" implicates the ACL, which should be carefully screened to ensure it is not also injured. Injuries to the ACL and the medial capsule are treated differently from isolated TCL injuries. This patient was a young, healthy, active male who wanted to play collegiate sports, particularly football. Thus an accurate diagnosis is necessary so that surgery (if required) can be performed as soon as possible to ensure adequate rehabilitation time before the next season.

The patient was examined in the sports medicine office. Results were similar to those of the field examination, with a few exceptions. The patient's ROM (20 to 80 degrees) appeared slightly less than at the time of injury. In addition, the patient could not elicit a quadriceps muscular contraction, such as a quad set. The swelling appeared to be slightly increased. The Lachman test revealed 1+ laxity with a soft end point. The anterior drawer test was also positive, with 1+ laxity; the posterior drawer test was negative. Valgus stress test was 2+ with a painful end point that was soft. Valgus stress test at 0 degrees exhibited minimal opening (1+), and varus stress at 0 degrees indicated 2+ opening. The pivot shift test was attempted but, due to pain and swelling, the test could not be performed. The patient received a KT-2000 (Medmetric Inc., San Diego, CA) instrument test, which indicated the injured side exhibited 4 mm greater translation at 20 lb compared with the uninjured side, and 5 mm greater translation at 30 lb.

Based on the manual examination, KT-2000 results, and mechanism of injury, the diagnosis was made of an ACL tear, partial TCL sprain and a possible medial meniscus lesion. Thus, the patient was encouraged to undergo an arthroscopic examination of his knee to determine the extent of the injury with particular attention to the ACL, medial meniscus, and medial capsule. Prior to surgery, magnetic resonance imaging was performed to document tissue injuries. The results indicated a partial ACL injury, soft-tissue swelling of the medial capsule of the knee, and a posterior horn tear of the lateral meniscus.

TREATMENT

The options were fully explained and discussed with the family. The posterior lateral meniscus tear needed to be either excised or repaired. The tear of the ACL, although partial, appeared to involve greater than 50 percent of the ligament. Injuries that large usually become complete tears in active individuals. Such a combination of injuries takes a considerable time to rehabilitate in a nonoperative protocol, and the prognosis for return to full sports participation was unsure. Based on the discussion, the family chose to have the arthroscopic examination and to have the menisci and the ACL repaired, if needed. The patient was scheduled for surgery in 10 days and was sent to physical therapy for preoperative instruction and exercises.

Preoperative Physical Therapy

This patient was seen in physical therapy for instructions regarding postoperative exercises and self-care (Table 12–2). A preoperative KT-2000 test was per-

TABLE 12–2 Preoperative Protocol for Anterior Cruciate Ligament/Patellar Tendon Autograft (ACL/PTG) Reconstruction

A. Protocol explained to patient
1. Importance of rehabilitation program and the role the patient must play in the program are explained.
2. Importance of cooperation for successful program is explained.
3. Patient is motivated to excel and continue rehab. program.
4. Patient information/data collected for further analysis.
B. Preoperative instructions
1. Instructions on neuromuscular stimulation (electrical stimulation) given to patient.
2. Instructions on rehab. brace (patient fitted for postoperative brace)
3. Counseling on mechanism of injury, pathomechanics of reinjury, and importance of activity modification
C. Preoperative tests
1. Laxity testing (KT-2000 testing)
2. Strength testing (if possible)
3. ROM measurements
4. Girth measurements
D. Strengthening program is outlined.
1. Isometric exercises are explained and demonstrated.
2. Straight leg raises
3. Self ROM exercises
4. Hip abduction/adduction exercises
5. Intermediate ROM exercises
E. Therapist establishes relationship with patient and accessibility to patient for any questions or problems that may occur.
F. Patient views instructional video.

formed to document laxity. He was fitted for a postoperative brace, instructed on use of muscle stimulation for the quadriceps femoris muscle, and instructed on crutch walking. The patient and family also viewed an instructional video on the surgical technique and the rehabilitation exercises to be used postsurgery. The time frames and milestones regarding walking, running, sports activities, and other functional activities were fully discussed.

Quadriceps femoris muscle exercises, such as quadriceps muscle sets, straight leg raises (SLRs) and multi-angle isometric knee extension at 90, 60, and 40 degrees were shown and explained to the patient. In addition, hip abduction/adduction movements and hamstring muscle curls were demonstrated for the patient to perform at home. The muscle stimulator was used at home on the quadriceps femoris muscles during active exercise to retard the quadriceps muscular atrophy. The brace was locked from 20 to 90 degrees, a ROM that was nonpainful to the patient. He was encourged to perform daily ROM exercises to provide a mechanical stimulus to the healing TCL. Crutch walking with weight bearing as tolerated was implemented. The patient was seen 3 times weekly before surgery with the goals of (1) decreasing joint effusion; (2) retarding muscular atrophy; (3) reestablishing normal range of motion; and (4) improving his functional status.

Surgery

The patient was taken to the operating room, where general anesthesia was induced endotracheally and the patient's knee stability examined. Results showed a 2+ Lachman test; 2+ anterior drawer; and a positive pivot shift (see Appendix, Fig. A–9, for explanation of pivot shift test). A diagnostic arthroscopy was performed, which revealed a large horizontal tear of the lateral meniscus, a torn ACL, and partial medial capsule damage. A 10-mm-wide bone–patellar tendon–bone graft was harvested with 25-mm bone plugs on each side. An inferolateral patellar portal was made and the arthroscope was introduced into the knee joint. A notchplasty was performed along the medial aspect of the lateral femoral condyle.

There was a horizontal cleavage tear of the posterior horn of the lateral meniscus. Due to the size, location, and direction of the tear a repair probably would have minimal success. Therefore, a partial lateral meniscectomy was performed. The medial compartment was investigated and the meniscus was found to be completely intact. The articular surfaces of both the medial and lateral compartments were normal. The patellar compartment was normal as well. The medial capsular ligament complex exhibited moderate tearing of the deep portion of the meniscofemoral ligament complex. Examination of the posteromedial capsule showed no sign of trauma. Given the site and extent of the medial capsular complex, conservative treatment would probably yield an excellent result.

The sites for the tibial and femoral tunnel were determined and checked for isometricity (see Chapter 9). Both the tibial and femoral tunnels were drilled through the previous attachment site of the ACL, and the bone–patellar tendon–bone graft was passed through the tibial tunnel into the femoral tunnel under direct vision of the arthroscope. The graft was then secured using a Kurasoka (interference) screw. The tibial bone graft was then secured over a post following drilling and measurement of the hole through a cortical screw. The tendon was tied about the post, and under direct vision the graft was placed under excellent tension with no evidence of impingement.

The tourniquet was then deflated at 82 minutes. Drains were placed, one intra-articular and one underneath the skin incision, and the skin incision was closed. Later the patient was returned to his own hospital room and placed on continuous passive motion (CPM) from 0 to 90 degrees and ice packs for the night.

Postoperative Care and Rehabilitation

Postoperative care for the ACL reconstruction using a patellar tendon autograft (ACL/PTG) is outlined in Table 12–3 and further described in Chapter 9. The postoperative rehabilitation of a patient who has had an ACL reconstruction using a patellar tendon autograft (PTG) with concomitant partial lateral meniscectomy and who sustained an TCL tear that was not repaired is treated like an isolated ACL/PTG protocol. The main difference is that the patient receiving an isolated ACL reconstruction and exhibiting no other pathology is allowed to ambulate with knee motion at 6 weeks (for the first 6 weeks, ambulation is performed with the knee locked at 0 degrees of extension). This particular patient is allowed ambulation with motion at 4 weeks because of the TCL injury. Motion in the patient with an ACL reconstruction and unrepaired medial capsule injury is more difficult to obtain than in the patient with an isolated ACL reconstruction. This is due to the increased scarring of the medial capsule with its excellent blood supply. These patients also exhibit increased pain, and initially a more concerted effort is made to stimulate the quadriceps femoris musculature, in particular the vastus medialis obliquus muscle. CPM is used for a longer period, in most cases for 6 to 8 weeks. The use of motion is the key to the healing of the TCL injury; thus early motion is encouraged.

TABLE 12–3 Postoperative Rehabilitation for Anterior Cruciate Ligament/Patellar Tendon Autograft (ACL/PTG) Reconstruction

I. Immediate Postoperative Phase (1–7 days)

Day 1

Brace — Brace locked in 0-degree extension immediately after surgery.
Weight bearing — Two crutches as tolerated (less 50%)
Exercise:
Ankle pumps
Passive knee extension to 0 degrees
SLRs
Quad sets, glut sts
Hamstring stretch
Muscle stimulation — Electrical stimulation to quads (4 hours per day) during quad sets
CPM — 0 to 90 degrees as tolerated
Ice and elevation — Ice 20 minutes out of every hour and elevate with knee in extension

Days 2–4

Brace — Brace locked at 0 degrees
Weight Bearing — Two crutches as tolerated
ROM — Patient out of brace 4–5 times daily to perform self ROM.
Exercises:
Multi-angle isometrics at 90, 60, 30 degrees (for quads)
Intermittent ROM exercises continued
Patellar mobilization
Ankle pumps
SLRs (all 4 directions)
Standing weight shifts and minisquats [(0–30 degrees)ROM]
Hamstring curls
Continue quad sets/glut sets
Muscle stimulation — Electrical stimulation to quads (6 hours per day) during quad sets,
    multi-angle isometrics, and SLRs
CPM — 0 to 90 degrees
Ice and elevation — Ice 20 minutes out of every hour and elevate with knee in extension

Days 5–7

Brace — EZ Wrap brace locked at zero degrees
Weight bearing — Two crutches as tolerated
ROM — Patient out of brace to perform ROM 4 to 5 times daily.
Exercises
Multi-angle isometrics at 90, 60, 30 degrees
Intermittent ROM exercises
Patellar mobilization
Ankle pumps
SLRs (all 4 directions)
Standing weight shift and minisquats (0–30 degrees)
Passive knee extension
Hamstring curls
Active knee extension 90–40 degrees
Muscle stimulation — Electrical muscle stimulation (continue 6 hours).
CPM — 0–90 degrees
Criteria for discharge from hospital:
Quad control (ability to perform quad sets)
Good patellar mobility
Minimal effusion
ROM (0–90 degrees)

continued

TABLE 12–3 Postoperative Rehabilitation for Anterior Cruciate
Ligament/Patellar Tendon Autograft (ACL/PTG) Reconstruction *(Continued)*

II. Maximum Protection Phase (2–6 weeks)

Goals:
Absolute control of external forces and protection of graft
Nourish articular cartilage
Decrease fibrosis
Stimulate collagen healing
Decrease swelling
Prevent quad atrophy

Week 2

Goals — Prepare patient for ambulation without crutches
1. Brace — Brace locked at 0 degrees. Patient continues to perform self ROM.
2. Weight bearing — As tolerated 50% or greater
   (goal: to be off crutches by the end of week 2.)
3. KT-2000 arthrometry test performed (15 lb.)
4. Exercises:
   Multi-angle isometrics at 90, 60, 40 degrees
   Leg raises (all 4 planes)-initiate PRE (not to exceed 1 lb per week)
   Hamstring curls
   Knee extensions 90–40 degrees; Initiate PRE (not to exceed 1 lb per week)
   Mini squats (0–40 degrees)
   Intermittent full ROM (4–5 times daily)
   Patellar mobilization
   PROM
   Calf stretching
   Proprioception training
   Well leg exercises
5. Swelling control — ice, compression, elevation

Week 4

1. Brace — Brace locked at 0 degrees; continue to perform self ROM.
2. Full weight bearing — No crutches; one crutch if necessary
3. KT-2000 test performed
4. Exercises:
   Same as week 2
   Initiate bicycle for ROM stimulus and endurance
   Initiate eccentric quads 40–100 degree ROM; initiate PREs
   PROM exercises (0–120 degrees)
   Pool walking
   Stairmaster
   Stationary ski track

III. Controlled Ambulation Phase (6–8 weeks)

Goals — Control forces during walking
Brace — Discontinue locked brace. Brace opened 0–125 degrees

Week 6

1. Full weight bearing without crutches with brace
   Criteria for full weight bearing:
   AROM 0–115 degrees
   Quad strength 60%–70% of contralateral side
   No change on KT-2000 test
   Decreased effusion
2. ROM 0–125 degrees and greater
3. Continue exercises of 4 weeks:

TABLE 12–3 Postoperative Rehabilitation for Anterior Cruciate Ligament/Patellar Tendon Autograft (ACL/PTG) Reconstruction *(Continued)*

Initiate swimming, pool running, lateral movements
Stretching program
Hamstring PREs
4. Increase closed kinetic chair rehab
5. Increase proprioception training

Week 8

1. Discontinue post operative brace
2. Exercises — Continue PREs
3. KT-2000 test

IV. Moderate Protection Phase (10–15 weeks)

Goals:
Protect patellofemoral joint's articular cartilage
Maximal strengthening for quads, lower extremity

Week 12

Begin isokinetic, 100–40 degrees ROM
Continue minisquats with tubing (0–45 degrees)
Initiate lateral step-ups
Initiate pool running (forward and backward)
Emphasize eccentric quad work
Bicycle for endurance (30 min)
Begin walking program
KT-2000 test
Isokinetic muscular test
Proprioception test

Week 14

PREs for all lower extremity musculature
Vigorous walking program with brace
Continue exercises from week 12

V. Light Activity Phase (3–4 months)

Goals:
Developpment of strength, power, endurance
Begin to prepare for return to functional activities
1. Exercises:
   Begin running program
   Straight line to figure eights and then to cuttng
   Agility drills
   Continue balance drills
   Continue isokinetics midrange (90–40 degrees), intermittent speed
   Continue minisquats/lateral step-ups
   Continue high-speed isokinetics, full ROM
2. Tests:
   Isokinetic tests 16 weeks
   KT-2000 test (prior to running program)
   Functional tests (prior to running program)
3. Initiate plyometric training (5 months)
Criteria for running:
Isokinetic test intepretation satisfactory
KT-2000 unchanged
Functional test 70% of contralateral leg (see Appendix, Fig. A–12, showing functional hop test)

continued

TABLE 12–3 Postoperative Rehabilitation for Anterior Cruciate
Ligament/Patellar Tendon Autograft (ACL/PTG) Reconstruction *(Continued)*

VI. Return to Activity

Advanced rehabilitation and return to competitive sports
Goals — Achieve maximal strength, further enhance neuromuscular coordination and
endurance.
1. All exercises accelerated
2. KT-2000 Test
3. Isokinetic test prior to return

6-Month Follow-up

KT-2000 arthrometry test
Isokinetic test
Functional test

12-Month Follow-up

KT-2000 arthrometry test
Isokinetic test
Functional test

On the day after surgery, the patient was brought to the inpatient physical therapy department, where electrical muscle stimulation was applied to the quadriceps femoris muscle during isometric quadriceps femoris muscle exercises. Passive extension of the knee joint to 0 degrees was emphasized along with hip abduction/adduction exercises. The patient was encouraged to ambulate, weight bearing as tolerated, with the brace locked at 0 degrees.

CPM was applied from 0 to 90 degrees for approximately 10 hours per day. Drains were removed 24 to 48 hours after surgery. By the second to third postoperative day, patella mobilization techniques were performed to ensure proper patella motion. The patient performed minisquats (from 0 to 30 degrees) and also weight shifting activities. The patient was encouraged to use the uninvolved leg to assist the operated knee through the ROM of 0 to 90 degrees at least 5 times daily.

The hospital stay after this type of surgery is generally 3 to 4 days. Before discharge from the hospital the patient must fulfill 4 criteria: (1) PROM 0 to 90 degrees; (2) good patella mobility; (3) quadriceps femoris muscle control (able to do quadriceps femoris muscle set and SLR); and (4) minimal effusion. Before discharge, written instructions are given regarding the exercise program, and wound care, ambulation, and the ACL protocol. The patient is encouraged to maintain compression on the knee, with ice and elevation whenever possible to control postoperative effusion.

This patient was seen 7 days after surgery in the outpatient physical therapy facility with the physician. At this time the treatment program was outlined and a team approach was presented to the patient, and his family by the physician and therapist.

At week 2 the patient was ambulating at least 75 percent and weight bearing as tolerated with crutches and the brace locked at 0 degrees. (Most patients are off crutches at 14 days). He performed multi-angle quadriceps femoris muscle isometrics, quadriceps muscle sets, SLR, knee extensions from 90 to 40 degrees and minisquats at 0 to 30 degrees. In addition, intermittent passive range of motion

(PROM) from 0 to 100 degrees, patellar mobilizations, hamstring muscle curls, and hip SLRs in all four directions were undertaken. Drills to enhance proprioception and balance were emphasized. In addition, a patient who receives an acute ACL reconstruction (within 24 days of injury) has a greater risk of developing arthrofibrosis. For that reason and because of the accelerated healing rate of the TCL, ROM exercises were emphasized.

During week 4 bicycle riding was initiated for ROM stimulus. Pool walking, minisquats, and leg press exercises were implemented. Serial knee arthrometer tests (KT-2000) were performed every 2 weeks to ensure graft stability during the course of rehabilitation. At 4 weeks postoperatively the brace was unlocked to allow motion during ambulation and assist in the prevention of arthrofibrosis.

By week 6, this patient's PROM was 0 to 125 degrees. At this time use of the brace was discontinued. In addition, swimming, Stairmaster, stationary ski track, and a special emphasis on closed kinetic chain exercise such as leg press, step-ups, minisquats, and walking were all initiated. The goal of the closed kinetic chain exercises was to increase joint compressive forces, thus minimizing the anteroposterior translation.

The light activity phase began at 3 months following surgery. An isokinetic test, knee arthrometer test, and balance test were performed before a running program was begun. This patient's KT-2000 arthrometry test indicated the operative knee was 1 mm tighter than the contralateral side. The isokinetic test indicated a quadriceps femoris muscle deficit of 26 percent compared with the contralateral side; hamstring muscles were of equal strength bilaterally. The involved quadriceps femoris muscle to body weight was 62 percent, which we considered excellent for 3 months after surgery.[62] Agility drills, a running program, and balance drills were then begun. This patient was encouraged to gradually increase functional activities, beginning with straight line running (forward/backward) and progressing to lateral movements and cutting.

Usually an athlete can return to competitive sport activities at approximately 6 to 7 months postoperatively. Before returning to practice, the athlete is evaluated by the physician and therapist to determine whether the athlete requires a functional brace. Often we will apply a brace for 1 year postoperatively, especially with interior football linemen who receive blows to the legs repeatedly. We believe the brace may give the patient an increased proprioception awareness of knee position and may assist in maintaining awareness of the limb. In addition, the brace provides the patient with a sense of added protection to the knee.

COMMENTS

These two case studies illustrated two specific and contrasting TCL injuries. The first case discussed an individual who sustained a grade I TCL sprain in a noncontact fashion during snow skiing. In that case we were challenged to differentiate between the TCL sprain and the presence of a patellar subluxation injury. The clinical examination showed no appreciable increase in patellar mobility or increased tenderness of the patellar facets. The clinical laxity testing of the TCL indicated a slight increase in translation and noticeable tenderness. That patient was treated successfully with our nonoperative TCL sprain rehabilitation program and returned to skiing and sports within 4 weeks of the initial injury.

The second case was slightly less challenging and appears more straightforward. This individual sustained a contact injury to the TCL and ACL due to a valgus stress. Several facts can be learned from this case. First, TCL sprains in the presence of an ACL disruption do poorly conservatively, and eventually the ACL must be reconstructed, enabling the TCL to heal. Second, when rehabilitating this type of patient the clinician must be aware of the increase in the healing response, due to the injury to the medial capsule; thus motion must be emphasized. This intensive motion plan is suggested to prevent the presence of arthrofibrosis. Finally, acutely performed ACL reconstructions also exhibit a greater incidence of arthrofibrosis; thus motion is given special emphasis, especially passive knee extension.

SUMMARY

There are several key points to consider when treating medial capsular injuries of the knee. First, early intervention in the form of early motion, immediate quadriceps femoris muscle exercises, and weight bearing is critical to the success rate. Second, swelling should be reduced quickly to prevent quadriceps femoris muscle atrophy and quadriceps femoris muscle shutdown. Third, a criteria-based protocol should be used, because every patient is different and thus each heals at a slightly different rate. Also, individually designed exercises and drills should be used. Finally, an accurate and complete evaluation must be performed to determine the correct diagnosis. Successful treatment of TCL injuries is dependent on determining whether an isolated lesion exists. In the presence of associated pathology, such as injury to the ACL, the healing rate of the TCL will be slowed, due to additional stress placed on the medial capsule to stabilize the knee.

REFERENCES

1. Nicholas, JA and Hershman, EB: The Lower Extremity and Spine in Sports Medicine. CV Mosby, St Louis, MO, 1986, p 657.
2. Dehaven, KE and Litner, DM: Athletic injuries: Comparison by age, sport, and gender. Am J Sports Med 14:218, 1986.
3. Powell, J: 636,000 injuries annually in high school football. Athletic Training 22:19, 1987.
4. Ellison, AE: Skiing injuries. Clin Symp 29:543, 1977.
5. Woo, SL-Y, et al: Treatment of the medial collateral ligament injury. II. Structure and function of canine knee in response to differing treatment regimens. Am J Sports Med 15:22, 1987.
6. Blyth, CF and Mueller, FO: Football injury and survey: Part I. The Physician and Sportsmedicine 2(9):45, 1974.
7. Earle, AS: Ski injuries. JAMA 180:285, 1962.
8. Moritz, JR: Ski injuries: Statistical and analytical study. JAMA 121:97, 1943.
9. Warren, LF and Marshall, JL: The supporting structures and layers of the medial side of the knee: An anatomical analysis. J Bone Joint Surg [Am] 61:56, 1979.
10. Brantigan, OC and Voshell, AF: The mechanics of the ligaments and menisci of the knee joint. J Bone Joint Surg [AM] 23:44, 1941.
11. Hughston, JC and Eilers, AF: The role of the posterior oblique ligament and repairs of acute medial (collateral) ligament tears of the knee. J Bone Joint Surg [Am] 55:923, 1973.
12. Müller, W: The knee: Form, Function, and Ligament Reconstruction. Springer-Verlag, New York, 1983.
13. Indelicato, PA: Injury to the medial capsuloligamentous complex. In Feagin, JA (ed): The Crucial Ligaments. Churchill Livingstone, New York, 1988, p 197.
14. Andrew, BL: The sensory innervation of the medial ligament of the knee joint. J Physiol (Lond) 123:241, 1954.
15. Barrack, RL and Skinner, HB: The sensory function of knee ligaments. In Daniel, DM, Akeson W, and

O'Connor J (eds): Knee Ligaments: Structure, Function, Injury and Repair. Raven Press, New York, 1990, p 95.

16. Arnoczky, SP: Anatomy of the anterior cruciate ligament. Clin Orthop 172:19, 1983.
17. O'Connor, BL: The mechanoreceptor innervation of the posterior attachments of the lateral meniscus of the dog knee joint. J Anat 138:15, 1984.
18. Skoglund, ST: Joint receptors and kinesthesis. In Iggo, A (ed): Handbook of Sensory Physiology, Vol 2, Somatosensory System. Springer-Verlag, New York, 1973, p 111.
19. Warren, LF, Marshall, JL, and Girgis, F: The prime static stabilizer of the medial side of the knee. J Bone Joint Surg [Am] 56:665, 1974.
20. Grood, ES, et al: Ligamentous and capsular restraints preventing straight medial and lateral laxity in intact human cadaver knees. J Bone Joint Surg [Am] 63:1257, 1981.
21. Warren, LF and Marshall, JL: Injuries of the anterior cruciate and medial collateral ligaments of the knee: A long-term follow-up of 86 cases. II. Clin Orthop 136:197, 1978.
22. O'Donoghue, DH: Surgical treatment of injuries to the ligaments of the knee. JAMA 169:142–151, 1959.
23. O'Donoghue, DH: Analysis of end results of surgical treatment of major injuries to the ligaments of the knee. J Bone Joint Surg [Am] 37:1, 1955.
24. O'Donoghue, DH: Surgical treatment of fresh injuries to the major ligaments of the knee. J Bone Joint Surg [Am] 32:721, 1950.
25. Campbell, WC: Repair of the ligaments of the knee. Surg Gynecol Obstet 62:964, 1936.
26. Shelbourne, KD and Nitz, PA: The O'Donoghue triad revisited: Combined knee injuries involving anterior cruciate and medial collateral ligament tears. Am J Sports Med 19:474, 1991.
27. Clancy, WG: Personal communication, March 1991.
28. Daniel, DM: Diagnosis of a ligament injury. In Daniel, DM, Akeson, W, and O'Connor, J (eds): Knee Ligaments: Structure, Function, Injury and Repair. Raven Press, New York, 1990.
29. O'Donoghue, DH: Surgical treatment of fresh injuries to the major ligaments of the knee. J Bone Joint Surg [Am] 32:721, 1950.
30. Clayton, ML and Weir, CR: Experimental investigations of ligamentous healing. Am J Surg 98:373, 1959.
31. Clayton, ML, Miles, JS, and Abdulla, M: Experimental investigation of ligamentous healing. Clin Orthop 61:148, 1968.
32. Korkala, O, Rusanen, M, and Groblad, M: Healing of experimental ligament rupture. Arch Orthop Trauma Surg 102:179, 1984.
33. Ellasasser, JC, Reynolds, FC, and Omohundro, JR: The Non-operative treatment of collateral ligament injuries of the knee in professional football players. J Bone Joint Surg [Am] 56:1185, 1974.
34. Derseheid, GL and Garrick, JG: Medial collateral ligament injuries in football: Non-operative management of grade I and II sprains. Am J Sports Med 9:365, 1981.
35. Wilk, KE and Corzatt, RD: Non-operative rehabilitation of grade I & II sprains of the medial collateral ligament in athletes. Paper presented at Combined Sections Meeting, American Physical Therapy Association, Washington, DC, February 1988.
36. Frank, C, et al: Physiology and therapeutic value of passive joint motion. Clin Orthop 185:113, 1984.
37. Vailas, AC, et al: Physical activity and its influence on the repair process of medial collateral ligaments. Connect Tissue Res 9:225, 1981.
38. Goldstein, WM and Barmada, R: Early mobilization of rabbit medial collateral ligament repairs: Biomechanical and histologic study. Arch Phys Med Rehabil 65:239, 1984.
39. Indelicato, PA: Non-operative treatment of complete tears of the medial collateral ligament of the knee. J Bone Joint Surg [Am] 65:323, 1983.
40. Fetto, JF and Marshall, JL: Medial collateral ligament injuries of the knee: A rationale for treatment. Clin Orthop 132:206, 1978.
41. Woo, SL-Y, et al: The biomechanical and morphological changes in the medial collateral ligament of the rabbit after immobilization and remobilization. J Bone Joint Surg [Am] 69:1200, 1987.
42. Tipton, CM, Mathies, RD, and Martin, RK: Influence of age and sex on strength of bone-ligament junctions in knee joints of rats. J Bone Joint Surg [Am] 60:230, 1978.
43. Tipton, CM, et al: The influence of physical activity on ligaments and tendons. Med Sci Sports Exerc 7:165, 1975.
44. Woo, SL-Y, et al: Tensile properties of the medial collateral ligament as a function of age. J Orthop Res 4:133, 1986.
45. Ohland, KJ, et al: The effect of partial and total transection of the anterior cruciate ligament on medial collateral ligament healing in the canine knee. Transcriptions in Orthopedics Research Society 14:322, 1989.
46. Forbes, I, et al: The biomechanical effects of combined ligament injuries on the medial collateral ligament. Transcriptions in Orthopedics Research Society 13:186, 1988.
47. Woo, SL-Y, Young, EP, and Ohland, KJ: The effects of transection of the anterior cruciate ligament on healing of the medial collateral ligament. J Bone Joint Surg [Am] 72:3, 382, 1988.
48. Frank, CB, Schachar, N, and Dittrich, D: Natural history of healing in the repaired medial collateral ligament. J Orthop Res 1:179, 1983.
49. Jack, ER: Experimental rupture of the medial collateral ligament of the knee. J Bone Joint Surg [Br] 32:396, 1950.

50. Laws, G and Walton, M: Fibroblastic healing of grade III ligament injuries. J Bone Joint Surg [Br] 70:390, 1988.
51. Woo, SL-Y and Tkach, LV: The cellular and matrix response of ligaments and tendons to mechanical injury. In Leadbatter, WB, Buckwalter, JA, and Gordon, SL (eds): Sports Induced Inflammation: Clinical and Basic Science Concepts. American Academy of Orthopedic Surgeons, Chicago, 1989, pp 189–204.
52. Eriksson, E and Haggmark, T: Comparison of isometric muscle training and electrical stimulation supplementing isometric muscle training in the recovery after major knee ligament surgery. Am J Sports Med 7:3, 169, 1979.
53. Hastings, DE: Non-operative treatment of complete tears of the knee joint. Clin Orthop 147:22, 1980.
54. Delitto, A, Rose, SJ, and McKower JM: Electrical stimulation vs. voluntary exercise in strengthening thigh musculature after anterior cruciate ligament surgery. Phys Ther 68:5, 660, 1988.
55. Lossing, I, et al: Effects of electrical muscle stimulation combined with voluntary contractions after knee ligament surgery. Med Sci Sports Exerc 20:93, 1988.
56. Morrissey, MC, Brewster, CE, and Shields, CL: The effects of electrical stimulation on the quadriceps during post-operative knee immobilization. Am J Sports Med 13:40, 1985.
57. Balkors, B: The course of knee ligament injuries. Acta Orthop Scand Suppl 198:42, 1982.
58. Goshall, RW and Hansen, CA: The classification, treatment and follow-up evaluation of medial collateral ligament injuries of the knee. J Bone Joint Surg [Am] 56:1316, 1974.
59. Holden, DL, Eggert, AW, and Butler, JE: The non-operative treatment of grade I and II medial collateral ligament injuries to the knee. Am J Sports Med 11:340, 1983.
60. Tipton, CM, et al: Influence of exercise of strength of medial collateral knee ligaments of dogs. Am J Physiol 218:894, 1970.
61. Kapandji, IA: The Physiology of the Joints, Vol 2, Lower Limb. Churchill Livingstone, New York, 1970, p 72.
62. Wilk, KE, et al: Anterior cruciate ligament reconstruction rehabilitation: A six month follow-up of isokinetic testing recreational athletes. Isokinetic Exercise Science 1:1, 36, 1991.

CHAPTER 13

Rehabilitation of Lateral Compartment Injuries

Michael J. Wooden, MS, PT, OCS

Injuries to the lateral aspect of the knee, although less common than those involving the anteromedial aspect, are often debilitating and present a challenge to the patient, surgeon, and physical therapist. Improvements in surgical technique and an understanding of knee function and mechanics have served to decrease morbidity and return the patient to normal function more quickly.

This chapter provides a brief description of lateral knee capsuloligamentous injuries, an overview of general rehabilitation principles, and two case studies, each with specific rehabilitation chronologies and procedures. A selected bibliography is provided for the reader interested in seeking further information on this topic.

ANATOMY

Chapter 1 of this book contains a thorough discussion of knee anatomy. Some key anatomic points specific to lateral injuries are reviewed here. Figures 1–10 and 1–21 illustrate the structures that support the lateral aspect of the knee. These include[1-4]:

- The *arcuate complex,* which is composed of the fibular collateral ligament, the posterior one-third aspect of the lateral capsule or *"arcuate ligament,"* the popliteus tendon, and the lateral head of the gastrocnemius.
- The meniscofemoral ligament of Wrisberg
- The fabellofemoral ligament
- The iliotibial band (ITB)
- The anterior and posterior cruciate ligaments

These structures primarily resist varus stresses—for example, in a medial blow to the knee—but also offer most of the resistance to rotational and hyperextension forces

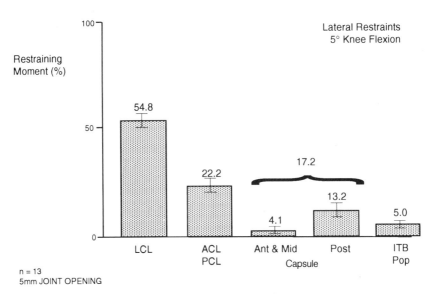

FIGURE 13-1. Comparative contributions to lateral restraint of the various lateral structures. (From Grood, ES, et al: Ligamentous and capsular restraints preventing straight medial and lateral laxity in intact human cadaver knees. J Bone Joint Surg [Am] 63(8):1263, 1981, with permission.)

(Fig. 13–1). Depending on the mechanism of injury, these tissues are stretched or torn, creating lateral instabilities in various combinations.

CLASSIFICATION OF LATERAL INSTABILITIES

Straight Lateral Instability

Structures involved: The fibular collateral ligament (FCL), the middle third of the lateral capsule, the posterior third of the lateral capsule, and the posterior cruciate ligament.[4,6]

Mechanism: A blow to the medial aspect of the knee with the foot fixed to the ground and the knee near extension.

Total disruption in this injury is uncommon but the ligament and capsule can be stretched or partially torn, sometimes in combination with meniscal tears.[4,6]

Anterolateral Rotary Instability

Structures involved: The middle third of the lateral capsule and, often, the antero-medial band of the anterior cruciate ligament (ACL). The ITB may also be damaged.[4,7,8]

Mechanism: Forceful flexion and internal rotation of the tibia on a fixed foot. The movement causes an anterior subluxation of the tibia in an internal rotation direction, as the ITB is forced anterior to the axis of knee joint rotation. There may be a lateral blow to the knee, but the injury can also occur in a noncontact situation.[4,7,8]

This injury occasionally occurs in combination with an acute tear of the ACL. More commonly, the injury is associated with a laxity of the lateral capsule and ACL deficiency and becomes a recurrent condition, with spontaneous subluxation and reduction during activity.[7]

Posterolateral Rotary Instability

Structures involved: The arcuate complex and sometimes, the lateral head of the gastrocnemius muscle. The posterolateral band of the ACL may also be injured, contributing to further laxity.[4-6]

Mechanism: A blow to the anterior aspect of the knee with the leg in external rotation, resulting in a "rotational recurvatum" subluxation.[9]

SPECIAL TESTS FOR LATERAL KNEE INSTABILITIES

The literature is replete with information regarding the evaluation and diagnosis of knee injuries. There are some inconsistencies and disagreements among authors, and no single test should be the determining factor. Table 13-1, adapted from several sources,[2,4,8,10,11] represents a consensus on which tests are most helpful in arriving at the type of injury. These tests may not be particularly useful in the rehabilitation process but are of critical importance to the physical therapist or athlete trainer involved in acute injury evaluation.

GENERAL PRINCIPLES OF REHABILITATION

Many protocols for knee rehabilitation can be gained from reviewing the literature.[12-14] Such treatment guidelines should be followed provided they are tailored to the specific needs and demands of each patient.[12] Clearly the rehabilitation goals for a football player hoping to return to play differ from those for a more sedentary individual. Communication of the rehabilitation goals and time frames among the surgeon, rehabilitation specialist, third-party payer, patient's family, and of course, the patient should be established and maintained throughout the course of treatment. A misunderstanding of these goals may result in frustration and delay in the patient's return to function. Treatment planning following surgery must also be predicated on the type of

TABLE 13-1 Special Tests for Lateral Knee Instabilities

| Special Test | Structure | | | | | |
	FCL	Lateral Capsule	Arcuate Complex	ITB	PCL	ACL
Varus at 0 degrees	X*	X	X	X	X	
Varus at 30 degrees		X				X
Apley's distraction (internal rotation)	X	X				
External rotation/ recurvatum			X			
Pivot shift		X	X			X
ALRI†		X	X			
PLRI‡			X			

*Possible positive sign
†Anterolateral rotary instability
‡Posterolateral rotary instability

procedure used. Thus the physical therapist must communicate with the surgeon to ascertain the type of approach; what tissues are repaired, moved, or augmented; what movements must be avoided in the early stages; and the status of secondary knee joint restraints.

The rehabilitation program should follow a functional progression. A series of exercises and activities are formulated to simulate motor requirements of the patient's preinjury functional level. The program will include open and closed kinetic chain exercises, muscle strength, power and endurance training, agility drills, proprioception and coordination training, and flexibility exercises. Chapter 5 describes the principles and rationale of the exercise progression.

Malone[12] recommends using treatment phases which consider the stage of healing and maintenance of function, and into which specific treatments are incorporated, as depicted in Table 13–2. Notice that time frames have not been established; these will vary according to several factors:

1. Tissues injured
2. Surgical procedure, if any, including the type of repair or reconstruction, the type of tissue graft used, and whether arthroscopy or arthrotomy was used
3. Position and duration of immobilization
4. The status of secondary restraints
5. The patient profile including the initial evaluation, age, preinjury activity levels, and functional (including sports) goals
6. Response to treatment

The therapist's initial evaluation must provide a comprehensive data base from which treatment plans and goals are formulated and against which subsequent progress is measured. Throughout the course of treatment each session should include:

Test — Treat — Retest — Modify Treatment

In this way the patient is monitored not only for progress but also for potential adverse responses to treatment, such as increases in pain, swelling, and reactivity.

TABLE 13–2 Phases of Knee Rehabilitation

Phase	Concerns	Treatment/Activity
1	Inflammation Tissue healing Maintenance of function	Controlled AROM
2	Tissue maturation Strength/endurance Protection	Controlled ROM Progressive weight bearing
3	Maturation Basic function Skill reacquisition	Light activity and function Submaximal PRE
4	Functional progression Return to skill arena Return to competition	Advanced rehabilitation Return to function
5	Maintenance	Continued rehabilitation

Source: Adapted from Malone, T: Surgical overview and rehabilitation process for ligamentous repair. In Mangine, RE (ed): Physical Therapy of the Knee. Churchill Livingstone, New York, 1988, p 164, with permission.

The use of treatment phases, establishment of a data base, and constant observation for response to treatment will help to individualize the rehabilitation process. The following case studies are presented as examples of this process, including use of the phases outlined in Table 13–2.

CASE STUDIES

CASE STUDY 1: PARTIAL TEAR OF THE FIBULAR COLLATERAL LIGAMENT WITH TORN POSTERIOR HORN OF THE LATERAL MENISCUS

The purpose of this case study is to outline conservative treatment and rehabilitation of a traumatic lateral knee injury.

HISTORY

This patient was a 17-year-old man who presented with a 3-week history of left knee joint pain, stiffness, and swelling since injuring himself at work. He described the mechanism as his having slipped on a wet floor; the foot slipped backward as the knee flexed and internally rotated forcefully. He was seen that day by his family physician, who aspirated slightly bloody fluid from the knee and referred the patient to an orthopedic surgeon. Subsequent examination revealed:

• Positive McMurray's sign for the lateral compartment
• Pain, but no instability on varus stress of the fibular collateral ligament with the knee in extension
• Grade I–II instability on varus stress test of the fibular collateral ligament with the knee flexed to 30 degrees
• Magnetic resonance imaging (MRI) findings suggestive of torn posterior horn, lateral meniscus, and partial tear of the fibular collateral ligament

The patient was then referred to physical therapy, 3 weeks after the injury. He had been placed in an extension splint, which he had been wearing constantly except while showering.

Subjectively, the patient reported knee stiffness, pain on attempts at ambulation without the splint, and inability to do "leg lift exercises" because of pain. He reported no significant previous history, and was otherwise healthy. He was not taking medication and reported no known allergies. He had not missed any time from school, and his immediate goal was to return to his part-time job in a fast-food restaurant. Although he was on his feet for long periods at work, his duties were relatively light. He did not participate in sports, and his only form of exercise was occasionally riding a bicycle.

EVALUATION

A summary of significant findings on physical therapy examination was as follows:

- Full weight bearing in the splint
- Minimal effusion with no rebound (ballottement) of the patella
- Tenderness on moderately deep palpation of the fibular collateral ligament, posterolateral aspect of the capsule, and the posterior horn of the lateral meniscus
- Knee passive range of motion (PROM): 8 to 85 degrees
- Simultaneous pain and tissue resistance at end-range flexion and extension
- An extension lag of several degrees, that is, the patient was unable to maintain full available extension during straight leg raising
- Minimal quadriceps femoris muscle isometric contraction, with no palpable contraction of the vastus medialis obliquus muscle (VMO)
- loss of thigh girth of 0.75 in (4 in above midpatella)
- Inability to perform one straight leg raise (SLR) without the splint
- Fair + (3+/5) hamstring muscle strength in knee flexion
- Because of pain, special ligament and cartilage tests, previously documented by the orthopedist, were deferred.
- Patellar mobility in superior-inferior and lateral medial glides was not restricted or painful.
- The hip and ankle joints were pain free and exhibited normal ROM and muscle strength.

ASSESSMENT

Based on these findings and the working diagnosis, the following problems, with rehabilitation goals, were outlined:

1. Decreased PROM with moderate reactivity secondary to the injury, effusion, and subsequent immobilization of the knee joint in extension
   Goals: Reduce pain and reactivity with modalities. Increase active/passive ROM in the knee joint, respecting the reactivity
2. Weakness of the quadriceps femoris muscles, especially the VMO muscle, secondary to joint effusion and the period of immobilization; moderate weakness of the hamstring muscles
   Goals: Increase quadriceps femoris and hamstring muscle strength beginning with isometric contractions progressing to resistive exercises as tolerated. Quantify weakness with an isokinetic dynamometer muscle test when the patient is ready for maximum effort muscle contractions
3. Poor tolerance to basic quadriceps femoris muscle exercises
   Goal: Increase tolerance through decreased pain and proper instruction
4. Reliance on the splint for ambulation
   Goal: "Wean" from splint over a period of 1 to 2 weeks once he could perform an SLR, bear weight without pain or sensation of instability, and provide adequate patellar control

TREATMENT

The patient was followed regularly 2 to 3 times per week. Compliance was excellent, and his progression through treatment was outlined as follows:

Week 1 (Phase 1)

The initial treatment consisted of:

1. Phonophoresis with 10 percent hydrocortisone ointment, an anti-inflammatory agent, to the posterolateral aspect of the knee joint to reduce pain and inflammation[15,16]
2. Medium-frequency stimulation (MFS) to the quadriceps muscles with a Mettler System 207 unit (Mettler Electronics Corp., Anaheim, CA). Parameters chosen were 2,500-Hz tetanizing current[15,17] with a 10-second stimulation followed by a 50-second rest. Electrodes were placed over the femoral triangle and the VMO muscle. As a muscle reeducation exercise the patient was instructed to contract the quadriceps femoris muscles maximally during each stimulus, which assisted in the recruitment of muscle fibers during each contraction.[15] The patient reported mild discomfort under the electrodes but was able to perform the muscle contractions.
3. Sitting knee joint extensions with a 1-lb weight, which was estimated to be 50 percent of the patient's 1 maximum repetition (MR). The actual MR was not attempted because of pain. The 1-lb weight was only slightly uncomfortable. A protocol of five sets of 10 repetitions was established as a baseline strength-return program.[18] The patient was able to contract concentrically and eccentrically from 90 degrees flexion to about 10 degrees from full extension.
4. Standing hamstring muscle curls with 5 lb. A program of five sets of 10 repetitions was established as above.
5. PROM exercises with physiologic grade II+ oscillations at end-range flexion and extension, to decrease pain and increase mobility[19]
6. Cold packs for 15 minutes to reduce treatment-induced soreness
7. Home exercises of SLRs and quadriceps femoris muscle isometric contractions in full available knee joint extension were reviewed, and patient was encouraged to walk without the brace as tolerated.

Week 2

By the third visit, the patient could perform an SLR independently; quadriceps femoris muscle isometric contractions were still difficult but painless. Passive extension was 0 degrees, but there was still an extensor lag on active knee joint extension. Palpable contractions of the VMO muscle were noted. There was minimal pain at end-range knee joint flexion, which had improved to 108 degrees. The patient reported no significant pain or swelling following treatment. He was able to walk painlessly without the splint, with no tendency for the knee joint to relax reflexively or buckle; therefore, the splint was discontinued. Phonophoresis was discontinued but MFS to the VMO muscle was continued because of the persistent extensor lag. Five minutes of short-arc, back and forth motion of the knee joint on the exercise bike was added. Flexion mobilizations were continued, using grade IV oscillations.

Week 3 (Phases 2 and 3)

On the sixth visit PROM was 0 to 125 degrees and nearly painless. The active knee joint extensor lag was resolved, and visible contraction of the VMO muscle was noted. The patient was now pedaling full arc on the bike with moderate resistance. Submaximal-effort isokinetic exercises of knee joint extension and flexion on the MERAC (Universal Equipment Co., Cedar Rapids, IA) dynamometer were added (10 repetitions × five sets). Submaximal-effort isokinetic exercise was chosen to reduce patellofemoral joint and tibiofemoral joint reaction forces while still allowing the quadriceps femoris and hamstring muscles to contract against resistance through the available knee joint ROM.[20] Also submaximal-effort isokinetic resistance selectively recruits type I muscle fibers, which have been shown to atrophy in knee joint dysfunction.[20-22]

On the eighth visit excellent tolerance to all exercises was noted; the patient reported no pain following exercise sessions, and there was no warmth or effusion of the knee joint, which would have indicated an adverse inflammatory response to the exercise. Therefore, a maximal-effort isokinetic test, comparing the quadriceps femoris and hamstring muscles of the injured and noninjured lower extremities, was performed on the MERAC (Fig. 13–2). Parameters studied were peak torque (PT), peak-torque to body-weight ratio (PT:BW), average peak torque (APT), and average power (AP), at preset speeds of 90 and 200 degrees per second. The results were as follows:

Muscle	Parameter	Deficit at 90 degrees per second	Deficit at 200 degrees per second
Left quadriceps femoris	PT	40%	24%
	PT:BW	40%	24%
	APT	23%	21%
	AP	23%	19%
Left hamstring	All of above	None	None

At this time there was no longer an extensor lag, PROM was full, and there were no signs of an inflammatory reaction to treatment. Therefore, MFS, mobilization, and cold pack treatments were discontinued. A new goal to reduce the quadriceps femoris muscle deficits to less than 15 percent in all measured parameters was established. To achieve this goal the exercise program was modified to include:

• 10 minutes on the exercise bike, full effort with moderate resistance
• Progressive resistive exercises (Figs. 13–2 through 13–5):

Eccentric leg presses @ 40 lb, 10 reps × five sets
Eccentric leg extensions @ 10 lb, 10 reps × five sets
Hamstring muscle curls @ 10 lb, 10 reps × five sets

Resistance was increased to an estimated 75 percent of MR.[18]

• Because deficits in muscle function were found at low and high speeds, multispeed isokinetic exercise was begun using a velocity spectrum protocol (modified from Davies[20]):

Speeds: 90—120—150—180—210—240—240—210—180—150—
120—90 degrees/second

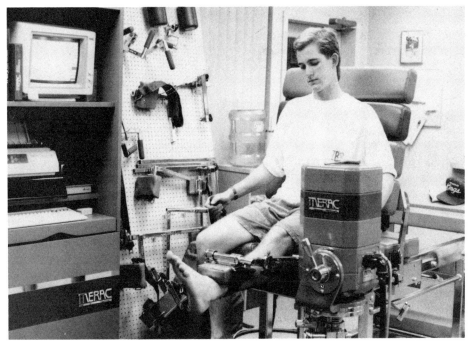

FIGURE 13-2. Isokinetic testing of the left quadriceps femoris and hamstring muscles.

Repetitions: 10 at each speed

Total: 120 repetitions, with maximal effort contractions to load the quadriceps femoris and hamstring muscles maximally throughout the ROM. Using isokinetic exercise at low and high speeds is thought to effect increases in strength and power, respectively, and the high numbers of repetitions were to improve muscular endurance.[18,19]

- *Plan*: Retest on the MERAC after 6 workouts, and adjust the protocol accordingly.

Week 4 (Phase 4)

Continued good exercise tolerance was exhibited subjectively and objectively. Exercise biking was increased to 20 minutes. Isokinetic exercise repetitions were increased to 15 at each speed (total of 180 repetitions). Five minutes of closed kinetic chain simulated stair climbing on the Stairmaster (Randall Sports Medicine Products, Kirkland, WA) was begun. To maximize quadriceps and hamstring muscle activity, cadence was 120 steps per minute and the patient was instructed to use only minimal handrail support.[23]

Week 5 (Phase 4)

To promote power and endurance, repetitions on the MERAC were gradually increased to 20 repetitions at each speed. Time on the Stairmaster was also gradually increased to 10 minutes at 120 steps per minute. On the 14th visit the isokinetic test was repeated with the following results:

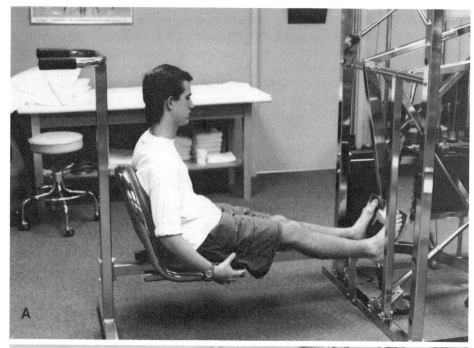

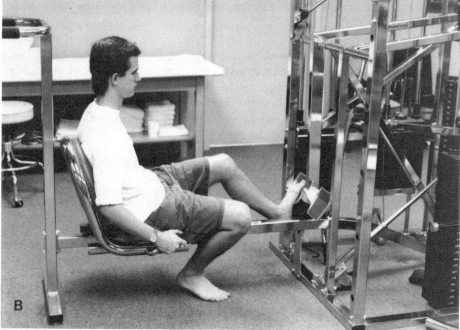

FIGURE 13-3. Leg presses. *A)* The patient lifts the weights with both legs. *B)* The patient lowers the weight eccentrically with the involved (left) leg.

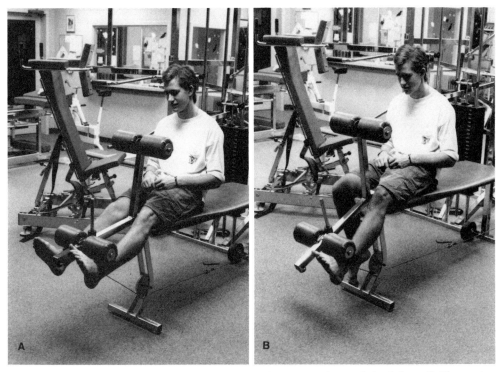

FIGURE 13-4. Knee extensions. *A)* The patient lifts the weights with both legs. *B)* The patient lowers the weight eccentrically with the involved (left) leg.

Muscle	Parameter	Deficit at 90 degrees per second	Deficit at 200 degrees per second
Left quadriceps femoris	PT	18%	11%
	PT:BW	17%	10%
	APT	14%	9%
	AP	14%	10%
Left hamstring	All of above	None	None

The patient had full, painless active and passive ROM, no pain on walking or stair climbing, and nearly all quadriceps femoris muscle deficits were reduced to less than 15 percent. He had been back at work for about 3 weeks without difficulty. Physical therapy was therefore discontinued, because all goals had been met. The patient was advised to return in 1 month for another isokinetic muscle test to ensure maintenance of muscle strength gains. He was to resume all activities, including riding his 10-speed bike.

Week 10 (Phase 5)

The patient returned for the MERAC retest, which indicated that deficits on all criteria were reduced to less than 5 percent. He reported no problems with any activities and, by this time, had been released from the care of the orthopedist.

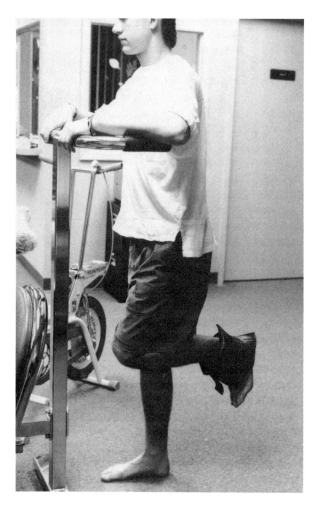

FIGURE 13-5. Standing hamstring curls.

COMMENTS

This case study presented the evaluation and rehabilitation of a patient with a traumatic injury to the fibular collateral ligament and lateral meniscus. With no history of locking, and with findings suggestive of a Grade I–II injury, a nonsurgical approach was taken, which is supported in a recent study by Kannus.[14] Conservative management was further justified by the patient's functional goals, which did not include a return to sports or heavy activity. This patient progressed uneventfully, and all preset functional goals were met within 10 weeks of beginning physical therapy. If surgery had been required for meniscectomy, meniscal repair, or repair of the lateral ligament, implications for rehabilitation would have differed significantly. Failure to respond to treatment, or worsening of symptoms during the course of treatment, might have necessitated eventual surgical intervention. The reader is referred to Chapter 14 for a discussion of rehabilitation after meniscal surgery.

The following case deals with a surgical repair of the lateral aspect of the knee in an individual with significantly different needs and goals.

CASE STUDY 2: ANTEROLATERAL ROTARY INSTABILITY WITH RECURRENT TIBIAL SUBLUXATION; PARTIAL TEAR OF THE ANTERIOR CRUCIATE LIGAMENT

HISTORY

This patient was a 17-year-old high school football player who originally injured his left knee during his sophomore year. He was a defensive back, and he recalled the injury as a blow to the "back and outside" aspect of the knee when an opposing lineman attempted to block him. The blow apparently forced the knee into valgus and flexion as the lower leg rotated internally. He reported having missed 3 or 4 weeks of the season, during which time the pain, stiffness, and swelling subsided and he did "strengthening exercises." He returned to play the final two games in a brace given to him by the team trainer. He felt he was at "80 percent" but experienced occasional "clunking sensations" along with moderate lateral knee joint pain when flexing and extending the knee.

The following year, during preseason practice, he experienced increased pain and more frequent subluxing sensations, and by the third week of practice was unable to continue. Subsequent evaluation by an orthopedic surgeon revealed:

- Grade I–II positive pivot shift test, which reproduced the pain and the clunking sensation
- Positive anterolateral rotary instability (ALRI) test: anterior drawer with the tibia in internal rotation
- Pain and mild instability with a varus stress at 30 degrees flexion
- MRI results suggestive of a partial (less than 25 percent of the anteromedial portion) tear of the ACL; both menisci appeared to be intact

A diagnosis of ALRI with recurrent subluxation, secondary to chronic laxity of the lateral capsule, along with a partial ACL tear was made. The patient underwent surgery for lateral "minireconstruction" as described by Andrews and associates.[24] This extra-articular procedure involves division of the ITB with tenodesis of this structure to the lateral femoral condyle (see Chapter 10). Splitting of the ITB provides tightness of the anterior fibers in flexion and the posterior fibers in extension. Tenodesis to the femur maintains the ITB posterior to the axis of knee joint rotation, reducing the tendency for the lateral tibial plateau to sublux anteriorly. A major advantage of the extra-articular procedure is to reduce postoperative fibrosis and contracture and increase the rate of rehabilitation compared with that of intra-articular procedures[12,24] (see Chapter 10). The procedure provides stability to the anterolateral aspect of the knee joint and, by preventing subluxation, allows healing of the partially torn ACL. Because less than 25 percent of the ACL was torn, the minireconstruction was used.[25]

Following surgery the patient was placed in a cylinder cast in 30 degrees flexion and was instructed in leg-raise exercises and non–weight bearing crutch ambulation. Four weeks later the cast was replaced with a rehabilitation brace that allowed 15 degrees to 90 degrees flexion. At that time he was referred to physical therapy with the precautions to avoid passive knee joint extension and internal tibial rotation to protect the tenodesis; knee joint extension and internal rotation performed too soon could separate the ITB from the lateral femoral condyle.

EVALUATION

The patient presented with complaints of knee joint stiffness and difficulty performing SLRs now that the immobilizing cast had been removed. He had begun minimal partial weight bearing with crutches. He listed as his immediate goals the return of knee joint mobility and strength, and a desire to "get rid of the crutches." His long-term goal was to return to football by the beginning of the next season, which was 11 months away. A summary of significant objective findings was as follows:

- PROM (out of the brace): 22 to 78 degrees, with moderate pain at end-ranges
- Active ROM (AROM): 30 to 65 degrees
- F − SLR with an extensor lag of 8 degrees
- Minimally palpable contraction of the VMO muscle
- F+ hamstring muscle strength
- 1+ knee joint effusion
- Decreased passive mobility of the patella in medial-lateral and superior-inferior glides (compared with the opposite limb)
- Decreased skin mobility, especially along the lateral surgical scar
- Hip joint and ankle joint complex were normal for ROM and muscle strength

ASSESSMENT

Based on the evaluation, the following problems and goals were defined:

1. Decreased PROM subsequent to surgery and immobilization of 4 weeks
   Goal: Increase ROM using only active extension to protect the mini-reconstruction
2. Precaution against internal rotation of the tibia
   Goal: Avoid internal rotation during exercise
3. Decreased patellar mobility
   Goal: Increase patellar mobility to assist in gains in knee joint ROM[26]
4. Decreased quadriceps femoris and hamstring muscle strength, secondary to injury, surgery, and immobilization
   Goal: Increase muscle strength, progressing from isometric contractions to PREs and isokinetic exercise (Quantify muscle strength with an isokinetic dynamometer when exercise tolerance indicates the patient is ready for maximal-effort contractions.)
5. Ambulation limited to partial weight bearing with crutches
   Goal: Progress to full weight bearing when active extension is at least − 5 degrees and the quadriceps femoris muscle is strong enough to support weight bearing and provide adequate patellar control (i.e., the knee does not "give way")
6. Decreased skin mobility
   Goal: Mobilize the skin with transverse friction massage to prevent skin contracture

The patient was followed regularly with excellent compliance, attendance, and motivation.

Week 1 (Phase 1)

For exercise and electrical muscle stimulation parameters, refer to Case 1. The initial treatment consisted of:

1. MFS to the quadriceps muscles along with isometric contraction of the quadriceps femoris muscles for muscle reeducation.
2. Active knee joint extension in sitting, lifting the weight of the brace only, inasmuch as the patient was unable to lift any additional weight.
3. Active hamstring muscle curls in standing, again lifting only the weight of the brace.
4. Instruction in SLRs, quadriceps femoris muscle isometric contractions, and active knee joint extension and flexion (as above) to be done twice daily at home. The brace was worn for all exercises; the patient was instructed to maintain external tibial rotation while exercising.
5. Patellar mobilizations using thumb contacts in superior, inferior, medial, and lateral glides.[27] Because there was minimal pain, grade IV mobilizing oscillations were used.[19]
6. Transverse friction massage to the surgical scar and surrounding skin, performed for 3 to 5 minutes.[28]
7. Following treatment, a cold pack was applied for 15 minutes to reduce the chance of treatment-induced soreness, swelling, and inflammation.

Weeks 2 to 4

By the end of week 3, VMO muscle contraction was palpable and firm, and the extensor lag was nearly resolved. Therefore, MFS to the quadriceps femoris muscles was discontinued.

By week 4, AROM and PROM were from 15 to 90 degrees to the limits of the brace. A 2-lb weight was added for active knee joint extension, and 4 lb were added for active knee joint flexion. Patellar mobility was improved but still limited compared with the right knee joint, so patellofemoral joint mobilization was continued. The patient complained of moderate soreness lasting 2 to 4 hours after most treatment sessions; therefore, cold packs were continued. Despite the temporary soreness, there were no signs of increased tibiofemoral or patellofemoral joint reactivity at the start of subsequent sessions; therefore, the progression of strengthening and mobilization was continued.

At the end of week 4 (8 weeks postsurgery), the patient returned to the orthopedist for reevaluation. The brace ROM stops were increased to 5 to 90 degrees, and the patient was told to increase weight bearing in the brace as tolerated. The therapist was advised to begin careful passive knee joint extension to − 5 degrees.

Weeks 5 to 8 (Phase 2)

Based on the orthopedic reevaluation and continued good tolerance, treatment was amended as follows:

1. Passive mobilization into extension with anterior tibial glides, and continued superior glides of the patella.[26] Resistance preceded pain; thus reactivity appeared to be low, and grade IV and IV+ mobilizing oscillations were continued.
2. PREs were continued with added resistance: 5 lb for extension, 8 lb for flexion (again, refer to Case 1 for progression).
3. Submaximal-effort quadriceps femoris and hamstring muscle isokinetic exercises were begun. The patient was positioned on the MERAC apparatus and, to protect the repair, an extension "stop" at -30 degrees from full knee joint extension was programmed into the dynamometer. Using the video monitor for visual feedback the patient was instructed to maintain knee joint extension torque to less than 15 ft-lb, and flexion to less than 10 ft-lb. This submaximal-effort activity was sufficient to provide resistance throughout the available knee joint range yet seemed to be minimal enough to prevent anterior shearing of the tibia. As with PREs, the patient was advised to maintain external tibial rotation. The initial MERAC workout consisted of four sets of 10 repetitions at a speed of 90 degrees per second. To improve muscle endurance, 1 set of 10 repetitions was added with each session up to a maximum of 10 sets.
4. Ten minutes on a stationary bicycle ergometer, with minimal resistance, to encourage knee joint ROM.

This program continued through week 8 (12 weeks postsurgery), at which time active and passive knee joint ROM were from 2 to 125 degrees. Skin and patellofemoral mobility were full, and there was no extension lag. The patient was fully weight bearing in the brace. At this time he returned to the orthopedist, who discontinued the brace and advised progression to maximum effort on the MERAC with an extension stop to further protect the repair.

Week 9 (Phase 3)

Because skin, tibiofemoral-joint, and patellofemoral-joint ROM were approaching normal limits, mobilization and friction massage were discontinued, with the expectation that continued resistive exercises would continue to increase knee joint extension. Cold applications were also discontinued, because the patient was having minimal posttreatment soreness and no indications of joint reactivity.

The exercise protocol at this time included:

1. Leg presses, concentric and eccentric, four sets of 10 repetitions with 40 lb resistance
2. Knee joint extensions, concentric and eccentric, four sets of 10 repetitions with 10 pounds resistance
3. Maximal-effort isokinetic quadriceps femoris and hamstring muscle contractions; 10 sets of 10 repetitions at 200 degrees per second, with an extension stop at -15 degrees. A speed of 200 degrees per second was chosen, theoretically to reduce potential joint reaction forces.
4. The patient was able to step up on a 10-inch stool painlessly with the involved leg. Therefore, lateral and front step-ups were added to the program.

This program continued through week 11, with monitoring at each session for pain, effusion, and skin warmth as potential signs of increased knee joint reactivity. There were no positive signs.

Week 12

The patient was 4 months postsurgery, with good tolerance to maximal-effort isokinetic exercise evident. A comparative test for PT, PT:BW, APT, and AP (see Case 1) was administered, with the results listed as follows:

Muscle	Parameter	Deficit at 90 degrees per second	Deficit at 200 degrees per second
Left quadriceps femoris	PT	46%	33%
	PT:BW	46%	33%
	APT	39%	26%
	AP	41%	31%
Left hamstring	PT	24%	19%
	PT:BW	24%	16%
	APT	21%	18%
	AP	22%	17%

Because the test indicated significant deficits at low and high speeds, the isokinetic protocol was changed to a multi-speed protocol (see Case Study 1), incorporating speeds from 90 to 240 degrees per second, with the higher speeds more closely reflecting functional angular velocities.[20] Isokinetic exercises, PREs, bicycle ergometry, and step-ups were continued for another 4 weeks. In light of the continued good tolerance to step-ups, simulated stair climbing on the Stairmaster was begun to increase the amount of closed kinetic chain activity. The patient would not begin jogging until the above bilateral deficits were reduced to 10 percent or less.[12]

Week 16 (Phase 4)

A retest on the MERAC indicated reduction of strength deficits in most parameters to 7 to 12 percent. Therefore, the patient was allowed to begin jogging on level surfaces. He was fitted for a derotational knee brace, which he would soon use during sprinting, cutting, jumping, and other functional activities. Isokinetic exercise was discontinued, but the patient maintained PREs at his school's weight room. His independent program for the ensuing month was outlined as follows:

1. To increase further quadriceps and hamstring muscle strength, continued PREs using free weights, Universal Gym and Nautilus equipment at the school, 3 times per week. Leg presses, leg extension, and leg curl exercises were emphasized.
2. To promote closed kinetic chain function and to improve cardiovascular fitness, the patient was to use the Stairmaster or a bicycle ergometer for up to 30 minutes per day, 5 days per week. This program could be substituted with riding a 10-speed bike, weather permitting.
3. Jogging at the school track, three or four times per week. He began with one quarter mile (3 to 4 minutes), and was to increase gradually by adding no more than one quarter mile per session. To reduce the chance of overuse or microtrauma injury, he would jog only on days he did not lift weights.

The patient was told to return to the clinic in 4 weeks for reassessment, including a MERAC retest. He was to discontinue activity and return immediately if pain, stiffness, or swelling developed.

Week 20 (Phase 5)

The patient was 6 months postsurgery. Given his athletic participation goals, this time marked a crucial point as the rehabilitation process entered phase 5. Reevaluation revealed painless knee joint ROM of 0 to 130 degrees. Isokinetic retest indicated quadriceps femoris and hamstring muscle deficits of less than 15 percent in all parameters. Therefore, there was less need for active, "hands-on" physical therapy, but a great need for maintenance of mobility and muscle strength and for progression to functional exercises and activities. By this time, he had received the knee brace. Functional knee braces play a controversial role in prevention of reinjury, but wearing a brace might at least give the patient confidence during more advanced activities.

He reported excellent tolerance to the jogging and exercise program, experiencing only occasional, brief soreness. While wearing the brace, the patient was to begin sprinting, cutting maneuvers, single-leg hopping, lateral running, and backward running to simulate football activities. These activities, along with the weight lifting, biking, and running, were increased as tolerated and were to be continued until spring football practice, in about 3 months. He was to return to the clinic for evaluation of functional activities in 1 month, or sooner if knee problems arose.

Week 24

The patient reported no problems with the knee joint. He demonstrated full ability to perform the functional tasks listed above. He was advised to continue these and the weight-lifting program indefinitely. Physical therapy was discontinued.

COMMENTS

This patient presented with a history of chronic, recurrent ALRI, which was treated with an extra-articular, lateral "minireconstruction." Surgical treatment was selected because the recurrent subluxation became a painful and debilitating problem, interfering with sports participation. In clear contrast to Case Study 1, this patient's specific needs required protracted phases 4 and 5 that emphasized functional activities in anticipation of return to football. He progressed through the phases of rehabilitation carefully and successfully, and he was able to return for his senior year of football 11 months after the surgery. All rehabilitation goals were met.

SUMMARY

The two cases presented have shown differences, not only in types of injury but also in goal setting and treatment planning based on their specific demands. Certainly, not all cases of knee joint injury progress as uncomplicatedly as they did, and the reader should realize that both patients were healthy, well-motivated teenagers. Even in these types of patients, however, complications may occur. Regardless of the patient's age or the type of injury, the rehabilitation process described should help the clinician in the problem-solving process of treatment progression based on frequent reevaluation and treatment modification.

ACKNOWLEDGMENTS

I wish to thank Bruce Greenfield for his patience and guidance, and the manuscript reviewers for their constructive criticisms. I am particularly grateful to Tab Blackburn for his indispensable input.

REFERENCES

1. Blackburn, TA and Craig, E: Knee anatomy: A brief review. Phys Ther 60(12):1556, 1980.
2. Mangine, R and Heckman, T: The knee. In Sanders, B (ed): Sports Physical Therapy. Appleton & Lange, Norwalk, CT, 1990, p 423.
3. Seebacher, JR, et al: The structure of the posterolateral aspect of the knee. J Bone Joint Surg [Am] 64(4):536, 1982.
4. Hughston, JC, et al: Classification of knee ligament instabilities. I. The lateral compartment. J Bone Joint Surg [Am] 58(2):173, 1976.
5. Grood, ES, et al: Ligamentous and capsular restraints preventing straight medial and lateral laxity in intact human cadaver knees. J Bone Joint Surg [Am] 63(8):1257, 1981.
6. Davies, GJ, Wallace, LA, and Malone, T: Mechanisms of selected knee injuries. Phys Ther 60(12):1590, 1980.
7. Bassett, F: Anterolateral rotatory instability of the knee. Phys Ther 60(12):1635, 1980.
8. Slocum, DB and Larson RL: Rotatory instability of the knee. J Bone Joint Surg [Am] 50:211, 1969.
9. Andrews, JR: Posterolateral rotatory instability of the knee: Surgery for acute and chronic problems. Phys Ther 60(12):1637, 1980.
10. Magee, DJ: Orthopaedic Physical Assessment. WB Saunders, Philadelphia, 1987, p 266.
11. Hoppenfeld, S: Physical Examination of the Spine and Extremities. Appleton-Century-Crofts, New York, 1976, p 171.
12. Malone, T: Surgical overview and rehabilitation process for ligamentous repair. In Mangine, RE (ed): Physical Therapy of the Knee. Churchill Livingstone, New York, 1988, p 163.
13. Paulos, LE, Wnorowski, DC, and Beck, CL: Rehabilitation following knee surgery: Recommendations. Sports Med 11(4):257, 1991.
14. Kannus, P: Nonoperative treatment of grade II and III sprains of the lateral ligament compartment of the knee. Am J Sports Med 17(1):83, 1989.
15. Kahn, J: Principles and Practices of Electrotherapy. Churchill Livingstone, New York, 1987, p 89.
16. Kleinkort, JA and Wood, F: Phonophoresis with 1% versus 10% hydrocortisone. Phys Ther 55:1320, 1975.
17. Owens, JE and Malone, T: Treatment parameters of high frequency electrical stimulation as established on the Electro-Stim 180. Journal of Orthopaedic and Sports Physical Therapy 4(3):162, 1983.
18. Sanders, MT: Weight training and condition. In Sanders, B (ed): Sports Physical Therapy. Appleton & Lange, Norwalk, CT, 1990, p 239.
19. Maitland, GD: Peripheral Manipulation, ed 2. Butterworth & Co, Boston, 1977, p 52.
20. Davies, GJ: A Compendium of Isokinetics in Clinical Usage and Rehabilitation Techniques, ed 3. S & S Publishers, Onalaska WI, 1987.
21. Edstrom, L: Selective atrophy of red muscle fibers in long-standing knee joint dysfunction: Injuries of the anterior cruciate ligament. J Neurol Sci 11:551, 1970.
22. Haggmark, T, Jannson, E, and Erikson, E: Fiber type, area and metabolic potential of the thigh muscle in man after knee surgery and immobilization. Int J Sports Med 2:17, 1981.
23. Wooden, MJ, et al: EMG activity of selected muscle groups in post-knee surgery patients during simulated stair climbing activity. Unpublished material. Emory University, Atlanta, 1991.
24. Andrews, JR, et al: Surgical repair of acute and chronic lesions of the lateral capsular ligamentous complex of the knee. In Feagin, JA (ed): The Crucial Ligaments. Churchill Livingstone, New York, 1988, p 429.
25. Noyes, FR, et al: Partial anterior cruciate ligament tears: Progression to complete ligament deficiency. J Bone Joint Surg [Br] 71:825, 1989.

26. Noyes, FR, Wojtys, EM, and Marshall, MT: The early diagnosis and treatment of developmental patella infera syndrome. Clin Orthop 265:241, 1991.
27. Wooden, MJ: Mobilization of the lower extremity. In Donatelli, RA and Wooden, MJ (eds): Orthopaedic Physical Therapy. Churchill Livingstone, New York, 1988, p 624.
28. Cyriax, J and Russell, G: Textbook of Orthopaedic Medicine, Vol 2, ed 9. Balliere Tindall, London, 1977, p 11.

SUGGESTED READINGS

American Academy of Orthopaedic Surgeons: Symposium on the Athlete's Knee: Surgical Repair and Reconstruction. CV Mosby, St. Louis, 1980.

Cross, MJ and Crichton, KJ: Clinical Examination of the Injured Knee. Gower Medical Publishing, London, 1987.

Daniel, DW, Akeson, WH, and O'Connor, JJ (eds): Knee Ligaments: Structure, Function and Repair. Raven Press, New York, 1990.

Edgerton, VR, et al: Morphological basis of skeletal muscle power output. In Jones, NL (ed): Human Muscle Power. Human Kinetics Publishers, Champaign, IL, 1986.

Müller, W: The Knee: Form, Function and Ligament Reconstruction. Springer-Verlag, Berlin, 1983, p 76.

Nicholas, JE and Hershman, EB (eds): The Lower Extremity and Spine in Sports, Vols 1 and 2. CV Mosby, St. Louis, 1986.

Wolf, SL: Clinical Decision Making in Physical Therapy. FA Davis, Philadelphia, 1985.

CHAPTER 14

Rehabilitation of Meniscal Injuries

Judy L. Seto, MA, PT
Clive E. Brewster, MS, PT

Our understanding of the importance of the menisci in the biomechanics of the knee has steadily progressed since 1968, when Jackson[1] wrote, "The exact function of that structure (meniscus) is still a matter of some conjecture." At that time it was usual to remove the entire substance if any doubt existed regarding the integrity of the meniscus. Today we know that the menisci are not optional or expendable structures but in fact have an integral role in normal knee joint mechanics. The menisci contribute to normal knee joint mechanics by providing load-bearing capabilities, shock absorption, joint stability and congruity, lubrication, protection against capsular and synovial impingement, load transmission, stress reduction of the articular cartilage, and nutrition and by limiting the extremes of flexion and extension.[2-6] This chapter presents a program for rehabilitation after meniscectomy and meniscal repair based on current knowledge of knee biomechanics; the principles discussed are illustrated in relevant case studies.

ANATOMY

The menisci are C-shaped wedges of fibrocartilage located between the tibial plateau and femoral condyles. The menisci contain 70 percent type I collagen, as opposed to hyaline cartilage, which consists predominately of type II collagen.[5,7] The larger semilunar medial meniscus is more firmly attached than the loosely fixed, more circular lateral meniscus. The anterior and posterior horns of both menisci are secured to the tibial plateaus. Anteriorly the transverse ligament connects the two menisci; posteriorly the meniscofemoral ligament helps stabilize the posterior horn of the lateral meniscus to the femoral condyle.[8] The coronary ligaments loosely connected the peripheral meniscus rim to the tibia.[8,9] Although the lateral collateral ligament passes in close proximity, the lateral meniscus has no attachment to this structure. The joint capsule attaches to the entire periphery of each meniscus but more firmly adheres to the medial meniscus. The deep medial ligament, a thickening at the midpoint of the joint capsule, firmly attaches the medial meniscus to the femur and tibia. An interruption in the joint capsule's attachment to the lateral meniscus, forming the popliteal hiatus, allows the popliteus tendon to pass through to its femoral attachment site.[10] Contraction by the popliteus during knee flexion pulls the lateral meniscus posteriorly, avoiding entrapment within the joint space. The medial meniscus does not have a direct muscular connection but may be influenced by the semimembranosus muscle's attachment to the joint capsule. These muscular connections allow the menisci to move. The medial meniscus may shift a few millimeters, while the less stable lateral meniscus may move at least 1 cm.[11]

Bullough and associates[12] and Shrive and colleagues[13] report that the collagen fibers of the meniscus are oriented in a circumferential pattern. When a compressive force is applied in the knee joint, a tensile force is transmitted to the menisci. The femur attempts to spread the meniscus anteroposteriorly in extension and mediolaterally in flexion. The peripheral rim of the meniscus, with its strong attachments to the tibia and femur, maintains a tensile force (hoop tension). The joint capsule and surrounding collateral ligaments assist the menisci to preserve their structure. Shrive and colleagues[13] studied the effects of a radial cut in the menisci's peripheral rim during loading. In joints with intact menisci, the force was applied through the menisci and articular cartilage. However, a lesion in the peripheral rim disrupted the normal mechanics of the menisci and allowed it to spread when a load was applied. The load was now distributed directly to the articular cartilage. In light of these findings, it is essential to preserve the peripheral rim during partial meniscectomy to avoid irreplaceably disrupting the structure's hoop tension capability.

Blood Supply

The blood supply to the menisci is limited to their peripheries; each structure's central region is avascular. The medial and lateral geniculate arteries anastomose into a perimeniscal capillary plexus supplying the synovial and capsular tissues of the knee joint. The vascular penetration via this capsular attachment is limited to 10 to 25 percent of the peripheral widths of the medial and lateral meniscal rims.[10,14,15] Renstrom and Johnson[5] reported a 20 percent decrease in the vascular supply by age 40, which may be attributed to weight bearing over time. Arnoczky[14] suggests that the blood supply to the meniscus has not altered but that the complexity of the meniscus itself reduces the structure's capability of using the available blood supply.

The presence of a vascular supply to the meniscus is an essential component in its potential for repair. The blood supply must be able to support the inflammatory response normally seen in wound healing (see Chapter 4). In a study using canine subjects, Arnocsky[14] reported that after an injury in the vascularized peripheral rim, a fibrin clot rich in inflammatory cells formed. A fibrinous scaffold was formed that allowed vessels from the perimeniscal capillary plexus and a proliferative vascular pannus from the "synovial fringe" to penetrate the fibrous scar. Fibrovascular scar tissue formed in the lesion, blending with the surrounding fibrocartilage. Cabaud and associates[16] reported that several months elapsed before the scar tissue assumed the appearance of normal fibrocartilage.

Arnoczky[14] proposed a classification system that categorizes lesions in relation to the meniscal vascular supply. An injury resulting in lesions within the blood-rich periphery is called a *red-red tear*. Both sides of the tear are in tissue with a functional blood supply, a situation that promotes healing. A tear encompassing both the peripheral rim and central portion is called a *red-white tear*. In this situation, one end of the lesion is in tissue with good blood supply, while the opposite end is in the avascular section. A *white-white tear* is a lesion located exclusively in the avascular central portion; the prognosis for healing in such a tear is poor. Repair of lesions in the red zone has yielded good results. Stone and colleagues[17] examined patients 2 to 6 years after meniscus repair. Seventy-four percent of patients who had repairs performed within 0 to 3 mm of the synovial meniscal junction had good to excellent results. This zone corresponds with the vascularized red-red zone. Recent reports describe techniques for manufacturing a vascular access channel from the peripheral vasculature, to improve the chances of tissue in the central region to repair itself. These lesions may then heal via the natural progression of fibrovascular scar proliferation as in normal meniscal healing.

BIOMECHANICS

The menisci follow the motion of the femoral condyle during knee flexion and extension. Shrive and colleagues[13] presented a model of normal meniscal function. During extension the femoral condyles exert a compressive force displacing the meniscus anteroposteriorly (Fig. 14–1). As the knee moves into flexion, the condyles roll backward onto the tibial plateau. The menisci deform mediolaterally, maintaining joint congruity and maximal contact area. Attachment of the popliteus tendon to the lateral meniscus actively pulls the structure posteriorly. During flexion the lateral meniscus is passively pulled posteriorly by the meniscofemoral ligament and actively pulled posteriorly by contraction of the popliteus muscle.[9] The small degree of medial meniscus movement is controlled by the short superficial and deep medial ligaments. As the knee flexes, the femur externally rotates on the tibia and the medial meniscus is pulled forward.[9]

The menisci directly influence the transmission of forces, distribution of load, amount of contact force, and pressure distribution patterns.[13,18–20] The articular cartilage covers relatively the same amount of surface area medially and laterally, 11.98 ± 0.56 cm² and 11.24 ± 0.48 cm², respectively. However, the medial and lateral menisci are not

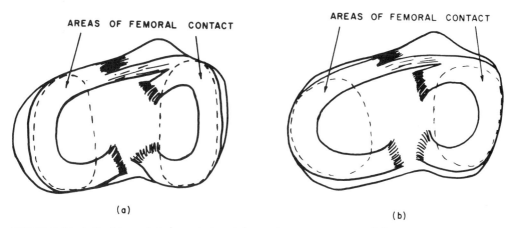

AREAS OF FEMORAL CONTACT   AREAS OF FEMORAL CONTACT

(a)   (b)

FIGURE 14–1. Position of the menisci and femoral contact areas in full extension (*a*) and full flexion (*b*). (From Shrive, NG, O'Connor, JJ, and Goodfellow, JW: Load-bearing in the knee joint. Clin Orthop 131:282, 1978, with permission.)

equal in the surface area they occupy, 7.3 ± 0.82 cm^2 and 8.63 ± 0.63 cm^2, respectively.[21] Kurosawa and associates[20] classified the load bearing patterns of normal knees into three phases. The *incongruous phase* consists of loads less than 500 N. The femoral condyles contact the menisci, and deformation occurs primarily at the meniscal and articular cartilage levels. The *congruous phase* involves loads greater than 1,000 N. As the menisci spread to the peripheral areas, most of the articular cartilage is in contact with the femoral condyles. Deformation takes place at the interface of the menisci, cartilage, and the subchondral bone. Loads approximately 750 N comprise the *intermediate phase*. When a load is applied, the uncovered articular cartilage and both menisci are compressed by the femoral condyles.[18-20] The menisci assist in distributing the load across the tibial plateus.

The contact area was examined by Fukubayashi and colleagues,[18] using a casting technique. When a force of 1,000 N was applied during loading of the knee joint, the menisci were found to occupy 70 percent of the contact area, with the medial compartment supporting 25 percent more than the lateral compartment. As the load increased, the difference gradually decreased with equal load distribution to the medial and lateral tibial plateaus. With the menisci removed, the contact areas significantly decreased in both compartments by more than 50 percent. The medial side continued to provide 30 percent more contact area than the lateral side. Walker and Erkman[19] supported this finding of reduced contact area following meniscectomy. They measured the normal contract area on each femoral condyle to be 6 cm^2. After meniscus removal the contact area was reduced to 2 cm^2. These studies show that the menisci act to significantly increase the tibiofemoral contact areas.

Pressure distribution patterns and levels were also examined during the presence or absence of menisci. In normal knee joints, the highest pressure points are located in the uncovered articular cartilage in the medial compartment and are equally distributed on the lateral meniscus and lateral articular surfaces of the lateral compartment.[18,19] This finding and the fact that the lateral meniscus covers a significantly larger surface area than the medial meniscus suggest that the lateral meniscus assumes a greater role in pressure distribution. In addition, the peak pressures doubled after menisci removal while the contact area decreased by one half. The areas of peak pressure remained within the same contact areas. Radin and co-workers[22] used photoelasticity on a model simulating the properties of the meniscus to evaluate stress distribution patterns of the knee. When the medial meniscus was excised, the stresses on the lateral compartment were unaltered. In the medial compartment, however, the stresses on the femur doubled and increased six to seven times on the tibial plateau. The forces became concentrated rather than distributed. Removal of the central two thirds of the medial meniscus moderately increased the stresses on the medial compartment. With retention of the peripheral one-third rim, the peripheral and middle portions of the compartment are protected.[23,24] Thus the menisci assist in transmitting stresses across a larger surface area and reduce the concentration of pressure on the articular cartilage and subchondral bone.[21]

MENISCAL INJURIES

Meniscal injuries, particularly sports-related ones, usually involve damage due to rotational force. A common mechanism of injury is a varus or valgus force directed to a flexed knee. When the foot is planted and the femur internally rotated, a valgus force applied to a flexed knee may cause a tear of the medial meniscus. A varus force on a flexed knee with the femur externally rotated may lead to a lateral meniscus lesion. The medial meniscus is more firmly attached than the relatively mobile lateral meniscus, and this may result in a greater incidence of medial meniscus injury.[25]

Degenerative changes have been demonstrated following total meniscectomies, indicating the importance of the menisci.[8,26-28] Fairbank[27] conducted a radiologic study following total meniscectomies and found three distinct changes. Varying degrees and combinations of anteroposterior ridge formation on the femoral condyle, generalized flattening of the femoral articular surface, and joint-space narrowing were seen. These changes were evident as early as 5 months after surgery and gradually became more prominent with time. McGinty and associates[24] examined 89 knees after total meniscectomy and found joint-interval narrowing and condylar flattening. Shrive and colleagues[13] found changes in the shape of the tibial and femoral condyles in response to pressure distribution changes. Kurosawa and co-workers[21] studied 14 specimens with and without intact menisci and measured changes in the load deflection and load contact areas. Sclerosis, or flattening of the subchondral bone, was discovered following meniscectomy. This was attributed to the increased localized concentration of stresses on the subchondral bone during static and dynamic loading.

Although degenerative alterations may occur after complete meniscectomy, the relationship between meniscal tears and the incidence of osteoarthritis is not conclusive. At one time, physicians and rehabilitation specialists believed that leaving a torn meniscus would lead to osteoarthritic damage necessitating removal of the entire structure. Studies have shown, however, that leaving degenerative menisci in place affords more articular cartilage protection than does complete meniscectomy.[29] Fahmy and colleagues[26] inspected knees from subjects of necropsies and amputations for osteoarthritic changes and meniscal pathology. They found that meniscal tears were not indicative of a definite course leading to degeneration. Although 42 percent of the medial and 52 percent of the lateral meniscus tears showed articular surface changes, 26 percent and 71 percent of the normal medial and lateral menisci, respectively, also demonstrated articular surface changes. In fact, 7 percent of the compartments with normal medial menisci had gross osteoarthritic changes. In addition, 14 percent and 33 percent of the torn medial and lateral menisci, respectively, exhibited normal articular surfaces. Noble and Hamblen[30] supported these findings and discovered similar results when examining osteoarthritic changes in subjects following horizontal cleavage lesions. Fifty percent of the subjects with normal articular cartilage had normal menisci. However, 38.5 percent of the severely degenerated compartments also showed normal menisci, and 18.4 percent of the normal compartments contained menisci with horizontal cleavage tears. In other words, degenerative changes did not consistently occur with torn menisci; normal menisci also demonstrated abnormalities in the articular surface. In fact, the articular cartilage underneath the degenerative menisci was found to be better preserved than the cartilage in unprotected areas. These results indicate that normal menisci do not ensure against articular changes and that torn menisci do not doom the knee joint to degeneration.

An alternative to total meniscectomy is partial meniscectomy. Removing the lesion alone while preserving as much as possible of the fibrocartilage may afford the best possible protection of the underlying articular surfaces. Follow-up studies of partial and total meniscectomy report fewer degenerative changes, greater satisfactory results, and faster recovery time among patients undergoing partial meniscectomies.[28,31] Northmore-Ball and associates[28] report patients with arthroscopic and open meniscectomies returned to sports 6.1 and 10.8 weeks after surgery, respectively. Persons receiving a total meniscectomy returned to sports in 13.7 weeks. In addition, 90 percent of the subjects with arthroscopic and 85 percent of the subjects with open partial meniscecto-mies reported excellent and good results (i.e., no symptoms or minor symptoms such as aching or swelling after vigorous activity but no disability). Total meniscectomy patients had more complaints of symptoms, with only 68 percent rating their knees as excellent or good. Cox and associates[31] compared the results of partial versus total meniscectomy among 12 dogs. Animals with total meniscectomies showed the greatest degenerative changes, consisting of pitting erosion and/or fibrillation of the articular surfaces of the medial tibial plateau and medial femoral condyle. Other symptoms of great severity in total meniscectomy subjects included increased synovial fluid and synovial inflamma-tion and thickening.

EVALUATION

A thorough subjective history will help the examiner to choose the appropriate clinical tests for the physical examination. A complete understanding of the exact mechanism of injury will point to the type of meniscal involvement to look for. Initial symptoms may include acute joint-line pain, joint effusion, locking, and giving way. Acute joint-line pain may occur as a result of stretching of the coronary ligaments holding the meniscus to the rim of the tibial plateau. This symptom, however, does not rule out capsular or ligamentous involvement.

A meniscal lesion does not always present with significant joint effusion. Only the peripheral region has a vascular supply, and only tears in that region will cause bloody fluid to be seen upon aspiration; tears in the avascular central section do not show this sign. Damage to the joint capsule, cruciate ligaments, or collateral ligaments may produce bloody fluid without indicating the extent of meniscal damage.

Locking is a common symptom after meniscal lesion and usually occurs at 20 to 45 degrees of joint extension.[25] If a torn fragment has been trapped within the joint, extension may feel limited against a rubbery resistance. Joint effusion or capsular involvement may also mimic signs of locking. A more reliable indicator of meniscal lesion is a click or snap after the joint unlocks.

The patient may also report a sensation of giving way after a meniscal tear. In true meniscal lesions the fragment becomes momentarily lodged in the knee joint, causing a sense of buckling. It is important to distinguish this finding from the sensation of giving way due to joint instability (e.g., anterior cruciate ligament tear) or buckling secondary to decreased quadriceps femoris muscle activity.

Clinical Examination

During clinical examination, the examiner should use the uninvolved leg as the norm for comparison with qualitative and quantitative findings of the involved leg. The examiner should look for effusion and signs of atrophy and check the state of healing of the incision. Assess the gait pattern, looking for deviations or compensatory movements. The patient may have difficulty fully extending the knee if the motion is blocked by a meniscal tear. Full flexion, as in squatting, may be painful or impossible due to a tear. Marked atrophy of the quadriceps femoris muscle, especially the vastus medialis oblique (VMO) segment, is sometimes an indication of long-standing meniscal injury, because the patient may be avoiding or unable to achieve full extension, and it is at or near full extension that most tension is required of the VMO muscle.[32]

Girth (circumference) measurements allow for a general assessment of effusion and atrophy. Swelling within the knee joint is grossly measured by a girth measurement taken at the joint line. Measurements taken at 5 cm and 20 cm proximal to the base of the patella, and 15 cm distal to the apex of the patella, can indirectly indicate atrophy in the VMO, quadriceps femoris, and calf muscles, respectively. It is difficult, however, to determine the exact contribution of soft-tissue mass to a girth measurement.

The amount of effusion does not indicate the presence or absence of a meniscal lesion. Aspiration of bloody fluid, however, is a sign of disrupted blood vessels in the peripheral meniscus, cruciate ligaments, or collateral ligaments. Localized palpable tenderness at the joint line is often present with meniscal lesion, because the coronary ligaments are irritated. The joint lines should be assessed for palpable pain, but the location of the tenderness is not a sure sign of the type of lesion. The examiner should use stability tests for anterior, posterior, and varus-valgus motion to rule out additional soft-tissue involvement. Several special tests may be used to assess meniscal involvement (Table 14–1). A negative or positive result of any test does not by itself establish the presence of a meniscal lesion, but along with the other objective findings, such a test result can help to differentiate a meniscal tear from other possible knee injuries.

TESTS OF MENISCAL INVOLVEMENT

Apley Test[25,33]

This test is used to distinguish between meniscal and ligamentous involvement. With the prone patient's knee flexed at 90 degrees and the leg stabilized by the examiner's knee, the examiner distracts the knee while rotating the tibia internally and externally (Fig. 14–2A). Pain during this maneuver indicates ligamentous involvement. The examiner then compresses the knee while again internally and externally rotating the tibia (Fig. 14–2B). Pain during this maneuver indicates meniscal tear.

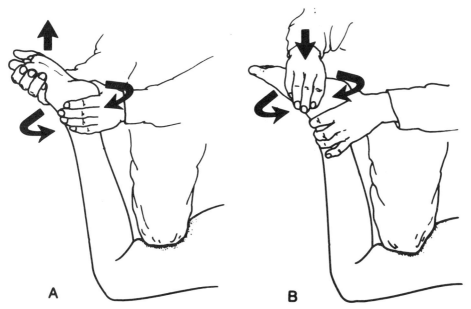

FIGURE 14–2. Apley's test. *A)* Distraction. *B)* Compression. (From Magee,[33] p 293, with permission.)

TABLE 14–1 Tests of Meniscal Involvement

Test	When Indicated	Position	Theory	Positive Test
Apley test	Differentiate between meniscus and ligament involvement	Prone. Knee flexed 90 degrees. Distract knee joint while internally and externally rotating tibia. Compress knee joint while internally and externally rotating tibia.	Distraction with rotation stresses ligamentous lesion. Compression with rotation stresses meniscal lesion.	Pain with distraction (ligament) or compression (meniscus) indicates a lesion.
Bragard's sign	Localized anterior joint line point tenderness	Supine or sitting. Palpate anteromedial joint line with knee extended and external rotation, or anteriolateral joint line with knee extended and internal rotation.	Flexion with internal or external rotation displaces the lesion forward.	Palpable pain at anteromedial or anterolateral joint line indicates meniscal lesion.
"Bounce home" test	Unable to fully extend knee joint	Supine. Knee fully flexed and then passively extended.	A lesion will block motion into complete extension.	Extension blocked or rubbery or springy end feel.
Childress' test	Pain with squatting	"Duck walk" in squatted position.	A lesion will block motion or elicit pain.	Motion blocked or painful during duck walk.
McMurray test	Detect middle or posterior horn meniscus tears	Supine. Hip and knee fully flexed. Extend knee while internally or externally rotating tibia.	"Snap" produced as torn meniscus rides over femoral condyle.	Audible or palpable snap or click with extension and internal rotation (lateral meniscus lesion) or external rotation (medial meniscus lesion).

Test	Positive Sign	Position/Procedure	Mechanism	Findings
Merke's sign	Pain with rotation in standing	Stand. Knees extended. Rotate trunk.	Lesion displaced during rotation.	Medial side pain with internal rotation (medial meniscus lesion); lateral side pain with external rotation (lateral meniscus lesion). No rotation with extension. Possible meniscus or cruciate ligament tear blocking rotation.
Modified Helfet test	Decreased tibial rotation	Sitting with knee flexed 90 degrees. Extend knee.	At 90 degrees knee flexion, tibial tubercle in line with midline of patella. As knee extends, tibia rotates and tibial tubercle in line with lateral border of patella.	
O'Donoghue test	Pain with tibial rotation	Supine. Knee flexed 90 degrees. Internally and externally rotate twice, then fully flex knee and repeat rotations.	Capsular irritation or meniscal lesion.	Pain at 90 degrees or full flexion during rotation indicates meniscus tear or joint capsule irritation.
Payr's sign	Pain with sitting cross-legged	Cross-legged sitting. Downward pressure applied along medial aspect of knee.	Posterior horn lesion displacement	Medial compartment pain with pressure.
1st Steinmann's sign	Anterior joint line point tenderness	Supine. Hip and knee flexed 90 degrees. Tibia quickly and forcefully internally and externally rotated.	Sudden rotation displaces meniscus into joint, pulling on lesion.	Pain in medial side with external rotation (med meniscus lesion) or lateral side with internal rotation (lateral meniscus lesion).
2nd Steinmann's sign	Anterior joint line point tenderness	Sitting. Knee flexed 90 degrees. Palpate along anteromedial joint line. Passively extend, then flex knee.	Meniscus displaced posteriorly when knee is extended and anteriorly when flexed.	Point tenderness shifts more posteriorly toward the collateral ligament with flexion.

Bragard's Sign[25]

This test may be used if anterior joint-line point tenderness is present. To test for a medial lesion, the examiner extends and externally rotates the tibia; this maneuver will displace a meniscal lesion forward, if one exists. Palpable tenderness along the anterior medial joint line is reduced with flexion and internal rotation, so reported pain when the examiner palpates along the anterior lateral joint line during extension and external rotation tends to verify the existence of a lateral meniscal lesion.

"Bounce Home" Test[33]

The patient is supine with his or her heel cupped in the examiner's hand. The examiner fully flexes the knee and then passively extends the knee (Fig. 14–3). If the knee does not reach complete extension or has a rubbery or springy end feel, the knee may be blocked by a torn meniscus.

Childress Test[34]

The examiner instructs the patient to squat with the knee fully flexed and attempt to "duck walk." If the motion is blocked, a meniscal lesion is indicated. Pain in this position, however, may indicate either a meniscal tear or patellofemoral joint involvement.

McMurray Test[25,33]

This test demonstrates tears of the middle or posterior horn of the meniscus. With the patient supine and the hip and knee fully flexed, the examiner applies a valgus force and externally rotates the tibia while extending the knee (Fig. 14–4A). An audible or palpable pop or snap indicates a medial meniscus tear. Lesions of the lateral meniscus are tested by applying a varus force and internally rotating the tibia during knee extension (Fig. 14–4B). The snap is produced as the torn fragment rides over the femoral condyle during extension. A snap in extreme flexion is indicative of a posterior horn tear; a click at 90 degrees of flexion indicates a lesion in the middle section of the meniscus.

Merke's Sign[25]

The examiner instructs the patient to stand with knees extended and to rotate the trunk. This movement causes compression of the menisci. Medial compartment pain during internal rotation of the tibia indicates a medial meniscal lesion. Lateral compartment pain occurring during external rotation of the tibia indicates a lateral meniscal lesion.

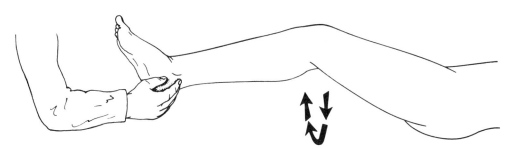

FIGURE 14–3. "Bounce home" test. (From Magee,[33] p 292, with permission.)

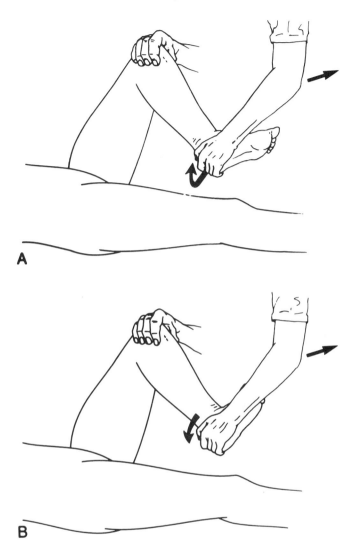

FIGURE 14-4. McMurray test. *A)* Testing for medial meniscus lesion. *B)* Testing for lateral meniscus lesion. (From Magee,[33] p 292, with permission.)

Modified Helfet Test[33]

The examiner instructs the patient, while sitting on the edge of a table with the knee flexed 90 degrees, to extend the knee (Fig. 14-5). If knee mechanics are normal, the tibial tuberosity will be seen in line with the midline of the patella in full flexion; during extension, the tibia rotates and the tibial tubercle moves into line with the lateral border of the patella. Failure of the tibia to rotate during extension indicates a meniscal lesion or cruciate ligament involvement.

O'Donoghue Test[33]

With the patient prone, the examiner flexes the knee 90 degrees. The examiner rotates the tibia internally and externally twice, then fully extends the knee and repeats the rotations. Increased pain during rotation in either or both knee positions indicates a meniscal tear or joint capsule irritation.

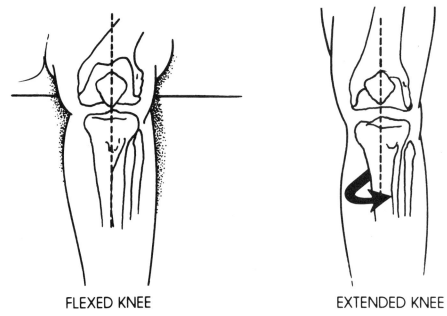

FLEXED KNEE   EXTENDED KNEE

FIGURE 14-5. Modified Helfet test (negative test shown). (From Magee,[33] p 293, with permission.)

Payr's Sign[35]

With the patient sitting cross-legged, the examiner exerts downward pressure along the medial aspect of the knee (Fig. 14-6). Medial knee pain indicates a posterior horn lesion of the medial meniscus.

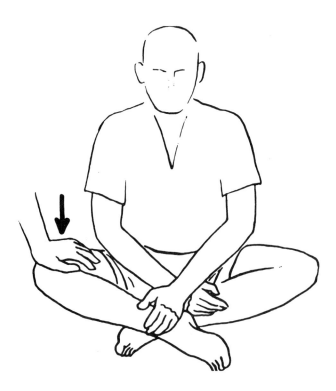

FIGURE 14-6. Payr's sign. (From Ricklin et al,[25] p 20, with permission.)

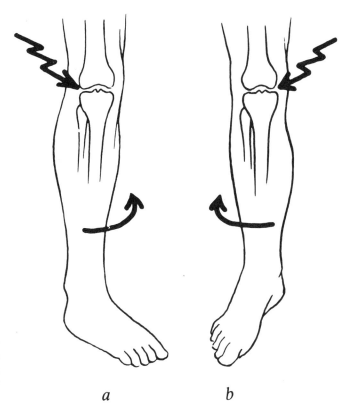

FIGURE 14-7. First Stein-mann's sign: *a*) Lateral menis-cus lesion. *b*) Medial meniscus lesion. (From Ricklin et al,[25] p 21, with permission.)

a   *b*

First Steinmann's Sign[25]

With the supine patient's knee and hip flexed at 90 degrees, the examiner forcefully and quickly rotates the tibia internally and externally. Pain in the lateral compartment with forced internal rotation indicates a lateral meniscus lesion (Fig. 14–7a). Medial compartment pain during forced external rotation (Fig. 14–7b) indicates a lesion of the medial meniscus.

Second Steinmann's Sign[25,33]

This test is indicated when point tenderness is located along the anterior joint line. When the examiner moves the knee from extension into flexion (Fig. 14–8), the menis-cus, along with its lesion, is displaced posteriorly. The point of tenderness also shifts posteriorly toward the collateral ligament.

REHABILITATION

The protocols for patient rehabilitation after partial meniscectomy and meniscus repair take into consideration both biomechanical principles and the results of physical examination. Factors such as the extent and location of the lesion, amount of articular cartilage degeneration on weight bearing surfaces, duration of injury, and joint stability affect the speed and aggressiveness of the rehabilitation program. There is no preset duration for any phase of rehabilitation described in this section, and phases may overlap depending upon the patient's progress and symptoms. The protocols should be adjusted to each patient's status, progress, and goals.

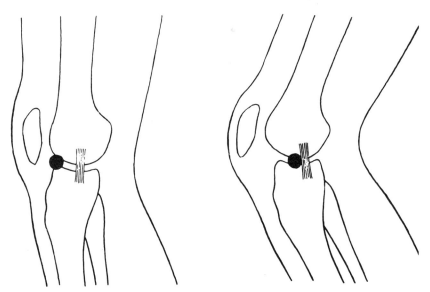

FIGURE 14-8. Second Steinmann's sign. Point tenderness shifts posteriorly along the anterior joint line when the knee is passively extended and then flexed. (From Ricklin et al,[25] p 19, with permission.)

Meniscectomy

INITIAL PHASE

When the patient first reports to outpatient physical therapy 4 to 7 days after surgery, he or she is usually bearing full weight or as much weight as tolerated on the involved leg, depending on the amount of cartilage removed and the degree of articular cartilage involvement. Modalities are used as needed to decrease pain or swelling, including heat/ice contrasts, ice alone, transcutaneous electrical nerve stimulation (TENS), electric galvanic stimulation, and phonophoresis. As needed, the patient should perform such lower-musculature flexibility exercises as hamstring, quadriceps femoris, hip flexor, hip adductor, and calf muscle stretches. Each range of motion (ROM) exercise should be held for 30 seconds and repeated five times. Each strengthening exercise should be done in two sets of 10 repetitions unless otherwise noted.

At this stage, the emphasis should be placed on overcoming any limitations to ROM. To increase passive flexion ROM, the patient should do wall slides: Lying supine with the involved leg placed on the wall, with a towel between foot and wall to decrease friction (Fig. 14-9A), the patient allows gravity to pull the foot downward, causing the knee to flex. The patient uses the uninvolved leg to control the speed of descent and to push the involved leg back up into extension (Fig. 14-9B). The patient need not use the quadriceps muscle of the involved leg for this exercise but can use the muscle if there is no pain. The patient should do one set of 20 repetitions, trying to increase ROM gradually with each repetition.

After the patient attains 110 to 115 degrees of flexion, he or she may substitute heel slides for supine wall slides to increase flexion ROM: Seated on a smooth surface (e.g., floor) with the back against a stable object and a towel underneath the foot to reduce friction, the patient actively flexes until he or she can reach the towel, then pulls the

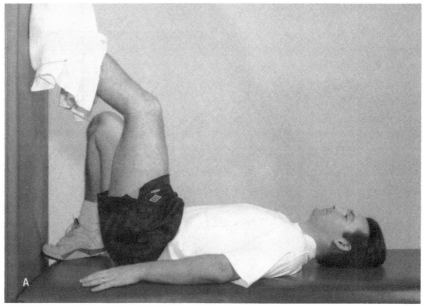

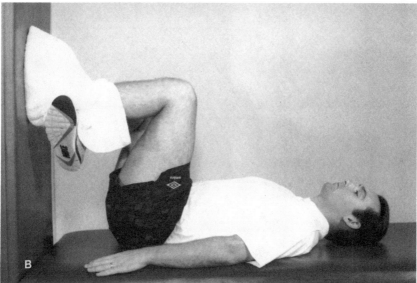

FIGURE 14-9. Supine wall slides: *A*) starting position. *B*) Flexed position.

towel to achieve further, passive ROM (Fig. 14–10A). Once the ankle can be grasped, the patient pulls on it, if ROM allows, to increase knee flexion (Fig. 14–10B). This position permits more leverage for increasing ROM.

To increase extension ROM, the patient can perform gel slides to increase extension ROM: The patient sits on a smooth surface with the uninvolved leg fully extended and the involved leg flexed. Placing a lubricant, such as a gel, under the heel of the involved foot to facilitate the motion, the patient actively extends the knee, holds the stretch for 5 to 10 seconds, and then flexes the knee, withdrawing the foot (Fig. 14–11). This exercise, repeated 20 times, permits cyclic extension of the knee.

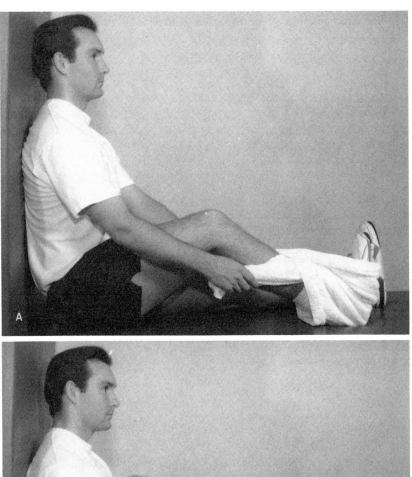

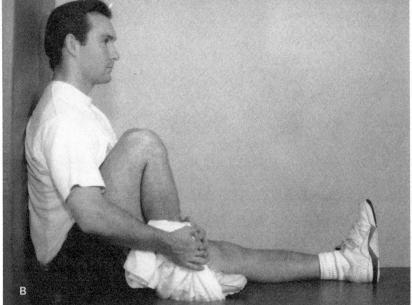

FIGURE 14-10. Heel slides. *A)* Starting position. *B)* Flexed position.

Isometric hip adduction exercise strengthens the adductor muscles, which will help to keep the adductor tendon taut and may influence the VMO muscle. The horizontal fibers of this muscle originate from the medial intermuscular septum and distal hip adductor tendons and insert into the suprapatellar tendon[36]; therefore, strengthening this muscle may in turn improve patellar tracking and reduce the possibility of patello-femoral joint problems.

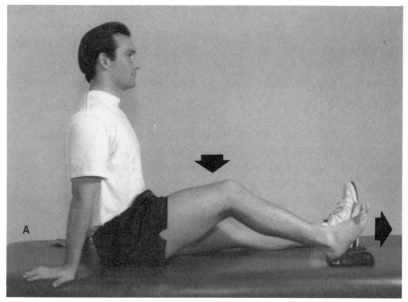

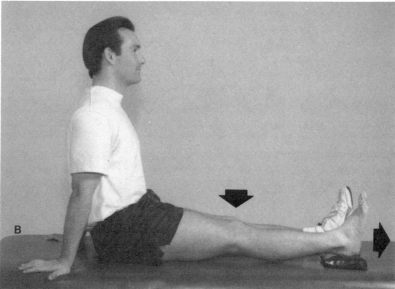

FIGURE 14–11. Gel slides to increase extension range of motion. A) Starting position. B) Extended position.

Sets of isometric quadriceps muscle exercises assist in strengthening the quadriceps muscle, especially the VMO segment. The patient extends the hip while contracting the quadriceps muscle. A small bolster may be placed under the knee to support the knee if full extension is not possible or if there is pain. Electrical muscle stimulation may be used to help retrain poorly contracting VMO or quadriceps femoris muscles.

Short-arc quadriceps femoris muscle exercises strengthen the quadriceps femoris muscle (Fig. 14–12). Sitting with the involved knee supported in 45 degrees of flexion by a bolster, the patient extends the hip into the bolster while extending the knee, maintaining this cocontraction for 10 seconds, then relaxing for 5 seconds.

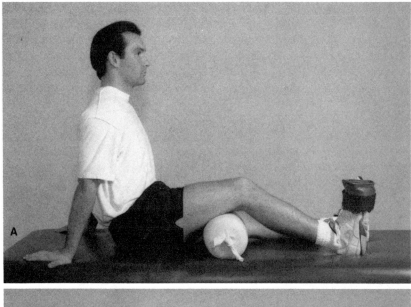

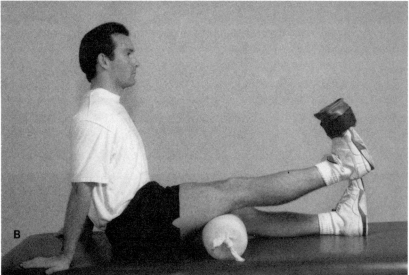

FIGURE 14-12. Short arc quadriceps femoris exercise. *A*) Starting position. *B*) Extended position.

Additional exercises to strengthen the lower-extremity musculature such as the hamstrings, hip adductors, hip abductors, and calf muscles are included in the program. The patient can begin isotonic hamstring-muscle strengthening exercises when he or she can flex the knee to at least 80 to 90 degrees. Hip abduction may begin when there is adequate VMO muscle contraction and strength; if quadriceps femoris muscle strength is decreased, there may be lateral tracking of the patella. If the patient begins hip abduction exercises before the quadriceps femoris muscle is strong enough, the exercises may contribute to increased lateral tracking. The tensor fasciae latae muscle inserts into the iliotibial band distally. This fascial sheath blends into the intermuscular septum and attaches to the supracondylar tubercle, patella, patellar ligament, and Gerdy's tubercle.

Although contraction of the tensor fasciae latae muscle will not increase iliotibial band tension, tightness of this fascial sheath may contribute to lateral patellar tracking.[35]

Depending on weight bearing ability and other symptoms, the patient can begin toe raise exercises. If there is articular cartilage degeneration, however, such exercises may increase the compressive forces on the remaining articular cartilage and underlying subchondral bone. This exercise may be performed standing or seated. Proper foot placement is important, as it influences the stresses at the knee. Supination of the foot causes tibial external rotation and a varus force at the knee joint, resulting in increased pressure in the medial compartment. Pronation causes tibial internal rotation, a valgus force at the knee joint, and increased lateral compartment pressure.

Stationary bicycling may begin when the patient attains 115 to 120 degrees of knee flexion. This exercise increases joint lubrication, which helps to improve ROM. Tension and resistance should be adjusted according to the patient's complaints of pain or effusion. If the patient's ROM is not adequate, bicycling may cause forced motion and increased pressure, irritating the knee.

INTERMEDIATE PHASE

The patient should have achieved full ROM by this phase. Modalities are continued as their need is indicated by symptoms. Continue flexibility and strengthening exercises, increasing resistance as tolerated. The patient may progress to isokinetic strength and endurance training.

Speeds greater than 200 degrees per second and six to nine sets of 10 repetitions are recommended for strength training exercises. Endurance training exercises should be performed at 300 degrees per second for 30 to 60 seconds. Exercise at lower speeds and higher resistance is not recommended because of the resulting high stresses within the patellofemoral joint.

The patient may also begin closed kinetic chain exercises during this phase. If the quadriceps femoris muscle is strong enough (i.e., if the patient can lift 10 lb during short-arc quadriceps femoris muscle exercise) the running program may begin. The first stage of the running program is jogging in place on a trampoline. Unless pain or swelling occurs, the patient gradually progresses to jogging for 10 to 15 minutes.

ADVANCED PHASE

During the advanced phase, the patient continues to progress in strength training exercises while beginning to return to sports activities. Track running may begin when the patient is able to run on the treadmill for 10 to 15 minutes at a pace of 7 to 8 minutes per mile (depending upon the patient's previous activity level). Once mileage on the track has reached 2 to 3 miles, agility drills and drills appropriate to the specific sport may begin.

Meniscus Repair

The program for rehabilitation following meniscus repair is similar in principle to that following meniscectomy. There are, however, more limitations on the patient's weight bearing status, and the duration of each phase of rehabilitation is expected to be longer, to allow for healing. Full weight bearing will be postponed until 4 to 6 weeks after surgery, to reduce the tensile and compressive forces on the repair site. During the initial phase of rehabilitation, more attention should be paid to applying modalities to decrease pain and effusion. ROM exercises are performed, but with caution, to avoid delaying the healing process. Mobilization of the patella may be required to ensure proper mechanics of the patellofemoral joint. Stretching exercises include calf stretches to reduce the possibility of Achilles tendinitis or shin splints when (gradually) the patient resumes weight bearing on the involved leg. Ankle ROM exercises may also be required to maintain adequate ankle ROM before weight bearing begins.

Open kinetic chain strengthening exercises may begin during the initial phase, but caution must be used and the exercises reduced or suspended if the patient reports pain. Isokinetic training should not begin until the patient is able to lift 10 lb on the short-arc quadriceps muscle exercise. The running program may begin when the quadriceps femoris and hamstring muscles of the involved leg have reached approximately 70 percent of the strength of the same muscles of the uninvolved leg, as demonstrated by an isokinetic strength test.

CASE STUDIES

CASE STUDY 1

History

The patient was a 46-year-old businessman and recreational athlete with a 9-month history of left knee pain. The patient did not remember any specific mechanism of injury but recalled playing softball during that time and had noticed medial joint-line pain the next day. The pain gradually subsided but reappeared when he tried to run. Patient refrained from running for 2- to 3-week periods but experienced pain each time he attempted to resume running. The patient sought medical attention when the knee became aggravated by impact activities and the pain would not completely subside with rest.

INITIAL EXAMINATION

The physician's physical examination revealed quadriceps femoris atrophy of 1 cm when girth was measured. Stability tests (e.g., pivot shift, anterior drawer, Lachman, varus test, valgus test) were all negative. The patient exhibited a positive McMurray test with an audible pop. No effusion was observed. Hip, knee, and ankle ROM were all found to be within normal limits. Roentgenograms were taken and were unremarkable. Palpable tenderness was elicited along the posterior medial joint line. A magnetic resonance imagining (MRI) scan was scheduled to rule out a meniscal tear.

The MRI revealed a full-thickness horizontal tear of the posterior horn of the medial meniscus. The lesion reached the tibial surface centrally and passed through to the peripheral third. The lateral meniscus, posterior cruciate, articular cartilage, and collateral ligaments were all normal. However, the anterior cruciate ligament appeared attenuated, possibly due to chronic injury.

SURGICAL TREATMENT

The patient underwent a partial medial meniscectomy with 40 percent of the posterior horn removed; a stable peripheral rim was left. Fifty percent of the medial femoral condyle displayed grade I changes. Postoperative follow-up 1 week later showed no evidence of infection, inflammation, or drainage. Physical therapy was recommended at this time, with medical follow-up in 3 weeks.

PHYSICAL THERAPY

Physical therapy treatment sessions began 9 days after surgery. The patient reported no pain with activities of daily living but felt discomfort at the arthroscopic portal sites when he descended stairs or walked down an incline. The patient stated that he had been fully weight bearing since his surgery and had been walking for exercise 3 to 4 miles per day without any problems. No anti-inflammatory or pain medication was used after surgery. The patient had no prior history of knee injury.

Evaluation

Range of motion: Flexion ROM on the uninvolved side was measured to be 150 degrees actively and passively. The involved side showed a flexion ROM deficit of 50 degrees actively and 45 degrees passively, with empty end feels as compared with the uninvolved side. Extension of the uninvolved side was 0 degrees both actively and passively. On the involved side extension was −5 degrees actively and +5 degrees passively.

Atrophy: Girth measurements revealed a 2.2-cm deficit, and a 1.5-cm deficit at 20 and 5 cm above the base of the patella, respectively, when compared with the uninvolved leg. A 1.4-cm calf deficit was measured at 15 cm distal to the apex of the patella.

Stability tests: Stability tests could not be conducted secondary to splinting by the patient. However, examination during surgery indicated no ligament damage and normal stability.

Patella: No patellar crepitus or restriction in mobility was noted in the medial, lateral, cephalad, or caudal directions.

Effusion: Mild effusion was observed using the ballottement test (see Chapter 8).

Tone: Quadriceps femoris and VMO muscle tone were assessed to be Fair−.

Palpation: Palpable tenderness was only elicited at the arthroscopic incision portals.

Assessment

The patient appeared to be recovering status after a partial medial meniscectomy with no complications or complaint of pain with activities of daily living (ADLs). ROM appeared to be limited by normal apprehension following surgery and mild effusion. No blocking, catching, locking, or restriction was noted. The patient's chief problems were assessed to be:

1. Decreased ROM, especially flexion
2. Decreased strength, especially of the quadriceps femoris muscle
3. Mild effusion.

To summarize, the patient's chief problems were atrophy, decreased quadriceps strength, and decreased ROM. The patient would benefit from strengthening and ROM exercises. Due to the amount of quadriceps femoris and VMO atrophy, sufficient quadriceps femoris strength should be of concern so that secondary problems involving the patellofemoral joint do not occur.

Factors Affecting the Problems

The patient is a highly motivated, competitive recreational athlete. A possible problem could be proper modification of ADLs, allowing adequate time for strengthening to occur and thereby reducing the stress applied to the knee joint. Grade I articular cartilage changes are already evident on 50 percent of the medial femoral condyle. The patient's age does not appear to be a major limiting factor as the patient has remained active and has no previous knee injury. Attenuation of the anterior cruciate ligament as seen in surgery may play a future role in degenerative changes in the knee if instability develops over time.

Goals

1. Full flexion ROM
2. Minimum of 80 percent quadriceps femoris and hamstring strength as compared with the uninvolved side
3. Eliminate effusion
4. Return to previous activities such as running

Treatment

The patient attended physical therapy three times a week for 3 weeks before returning to the physician for a follow-up examination. Each session was approximately 1 hour in duration.

Week 1. Strengthening exercises were performed consisting of isometric hip adduction, isometric quadriceps femoris sets, short-arc quadriceps femoris, hamstring curls, hip adduction, and toe raises. Towel slides were performed to increase flexion ROM. A stationary bicycle was used to increase lower-extremity strength and endurance. Ice was applied at the end of each session as a prophylactic measure to reduce possible swelling and discomfort following exercise.

First Reassessment. No evidence of effusion noted. The patient had 140 degrees passive flexion, a 10-degree deficit when compared with the uninvolved leg. The patient progressively increased the resistance on all exercises and was without complaint of pain or effusion with the rehabilitation program or ADLs.

Week 2. The patient progressed in all exercises, increasing resistance as tolerated. Eccentric quadriceps femoris strengthening exercises were initiated when the patient was able to lift 10 lb during the short-arc quadriceps femoris exercise. When the patient reached a level of 15 lb with short-arc quadriceps femoris and 25-lb eccentric quadriceps femoris exercises, he was allowed to begin jogging in place on a trampoline. This was the first phase of the running program. The trampoline is believed to be less stressful with smaller compressive forces as compared with running on a treadmill or outdoors.

Second Reassessment. The patient had no symptoms related to increased progression of strengthening exercises and advancement to trampoline jogging. The program was continued as tolerated, with an isokinetic strength test scheduled at the end of the third week. If the patient was without problems, he would progress to the treadmill, which coincided with his being 1 month postsurgery.

Week 3. The patient steadily increased his quadriceps femoris strength, lifting 25 lb during short-arc quadriceps femoris exercises and 45 lb during eccentric quadriceps femoris exercise. Calf strengthening exercises gradually increased to 100 lb without problems. The patient progressed to treadmill running at 6 mph without complaint.

Final Deposition. The patient performed an isokinetic strength test at speeds of 240 — 180 — 120 degrees per second, and endurance was tested at 300 degrees per second. At the time this patient was treated, we used isokinetic speeds less than 200 degrees per second, but presently we use speeds greater than 200 degrees per second for strength training and testing. Average peak torque was measured at 85 percent quadriceps femoris and 91 percent hamstrings, when compared with the uninvolved side. At this time the patient was recommended to be discharged from physical therapy and was instructed in a home exercise program and running progression. The patient belonged to a gym where weight equipment, stationary bicycle, and treadmill were available. Follow-up conversation with the patient 6 months after discharge revealed no symptoms or complaints of pain. The patient had resumed running and playing golf without limitation.

CASE STUDY 2

HISTORY

The patient was a 49-year-old male fireman who had injured his right knee. While at work the patient was ascending stairs and felt a small click in his right knee. The patient felt some irritation during the next few days, which gradually improved. He subsequently felt his status deteriorate and progressively become worse over the next 2 days.

INITIAL EXAMINATION AND TREATMENT

The physician's physical examination revealed −20 degrees extension and 90 degrees flexion. No effusion was evident. Marked tenderness was noted along the tibial collateral ligament. No instability was noted upon examination. Roentgenograms were taken and were unremarkable. The physician's impression was of possible tibial collateral ligament involvement. The recommended course of treatment was cortisone injection, anti-inflammatory medication (Indocin), ice to decrease pain, and non–weight bearing status using crutches. Reassessment was scheduled in 3 weeks.

Three weeks later, the patient reported immediate relief and 80 percent improvement following the injection. Slight tenderness at the tibial collateral ligament region was found upon palpation. The patient's ambulatory status had improved. Physical therapy was recommended at this time for instruction in a home exercise program.

INITIAL PHYSICAL THERAPY
Evaluation

The patient reported that he was now fully weight bearing and that his symptoms had decreased with the anti-inflammatory medication. The patient also stated that he had run during 2 days coinciding with the time frame that his pain became worse. His chief complaints were moderate tenderness upon palpation at the distal aspect of the right tibial collateral ligament. His recreational activities include running two to three times per week, 2 miles per session, and weight lifting three times per week.

Range of motion: Passive extension ROM was −5 degrees in both knees. Passive flexion ROM with the involved knee was 140 degrees and 150 degrees in the uninvolved knee.

Stability tests: No laxity was noted upon testing for anterior, posterior, varus, or valgus instability.

Tone: Good + quadriceps and VMO tone was observed in both thighs.

Flexibility: Hamstring tightness was measured by a straight leg test: 90 degrees left and 80 degrees right.

Palpation: There was moderate palpable tenderness over the tibial collateral ligament just distal to the joint line.

Treatment

The treatment consisted of two sessions. The patient was instructed in strengthening exercises consisting of isometric hip adduction, isometric quadriceps femoris sets, short-arc quadriceps femoris sets, hip adduction, isometric hamstring sets, toe raises, and hamstring curls. One treatment of ultrasound with Myoflex, an analgesic cream, was directed to the area of palpable tenderness over the tibial-collateral ligament. No change in medial joint-line area pain was noted upon reassessment during the second visit. Ice was applied as a prophylactic measure following exercise to reduce possible swelling and discomfort. The patient was instructed in a home program consisting of the above exercises and was discharged from physical therapy.

CONTINUING MEDICAL TREATMENT

One month after the second physical therapy visit, the physician reevaluated the patient. The patient reported relief and dramatic improvement after the cortisone injection, followed by intermittent episodes of increased pain requiring him to use crutches during ambulation. An MRI scan was scheduled to rule out a possible meniscus lesion.

The MRI scan revealed a tear of the medial meniscus. The patient had been without any mechanical symptoms and had improved with his present course. The physician recommended the patient continue his present home exercise program and perform an isokinetic strength and endurance test in 1 month. The patient's status would be reassessed in 1 month, and if improvement was not complete, a partial meniscectomy would be considered.

One month later, the patient's isokinetic test showed 84 percent quadriceps femoris strength and 90 percent hamstring strength as compared with the uninvolved side. Overall the patient continued to show improvement but had intermittent symptoms of popping and clicking, which, however, had not limited his ADLs. Physical examination showed some popping, clicking, and crepitus, with diminished discomfort along the medial joint line. The physician's recommended course of action was to continue his present home exercise program and reassess his status in 6 weeks.

Ten weeks later the physician reevaluated the patient, who continued to complain of pain and discomfort along the medial aspect, a sensation of buckling with turning, and decreased strength. A diagnostic operative arthroscopy was scheduled at this time, with possible medial meniscectomy.

An arthroscopic partial medial meniscectomy was performed 2 months later, and a complex tear in the posterior third of the medial meniscus was found. Additional operative findings included grade II articular changes in 20 percent of the medial and odd patellar facets, and grade I articular changes in 100 percent of the lateral tibial plateau. The articular cartilage of the medial compartment, femoral condyles, cruciate ligaments, and lateral meniscus were found to be normal upon examination.

One week after the surgery, the patient was progressing smoothly with no evidence of infection, inflammation, or drainage. His ROM was 80 degrees flexion and −10 degrees extension, with slight swelling observed. Physical therapy was recommended at this time.

POSTOPERATIVE PHYSICAL THERAPY

Postoperatively, the patient was fully weight bearing and his chief complaints were stiffness and intermittent sharp, shooting pain along the medial joint line. His symptoms were aggravated by descending stairs, less so when ascending stairs. Presently patient was not taking any anti-inflammatory or pain medication.

Evaluation

Range of motion: On the uninvolved side, the patient's flexion ROM was 140 degrees both actively and passively, and the extension ROM was 0 degrees actively and +5 degrees passively. Flexion ROM on the involved side was 90 degree actively and 100 degrees passively, and extension ROM was −10 degree actively and −5 degree passively.

Girth measurements: No significant difference was measured in thigh or calf girth.

Stability tests: These could not be performed secondary to patient splinting. Arthroscopic surgery indicated normal cruciate ligaments.

Patella: Mild crepitus was noted on the involved side.

Effusion: Mild swelling was noted during the ballottement test.

Tone: Fair+ quadriceps femoris and poor+ VMO muscle tone was observed.

Palpation: Palpable tenderness was elicited at the medial joint line and rated as 4 on a pain scale of 0 (no pain) to 10 (maximum pain).

Assessment

The patient was recovering normally after partial medial meniscectomy following chronic medial meniscus tear. The only complaint of pain with ADLs was during stair climbing. ROM appeared to be limited by normal apprehension following surgery and mild effusion. No blocking, catching, locking, or restriction was noted. The patient's chief problems were assessed to be:

1. Decreased ROM, especially flexion
2. Mild effusion
3. Palpable medial joint-line tenderness
4. Decreased quadriceps femoris and hamstring muscle strength, as demonstrated by isokinetic testing

Factors Affecting the Problems

The patient was a highly motivated fireman in excellent health. A potential problem was modification of activities and restriction of running to allow adequate time for strength development and recovery from the surgery. Degenerative changes were evident in the articular surfaces of the patella and lateral compartment, which may cause symptoms at a later time. The patient had intermittent symptoms of joint-line pain, clicking, and popping for the past 7 to 8 months with ADLs. Although girth measurements were normal, decreased quadriceps femoris and hamstring muscle strength was evident with isokinetic testing and from subjective reports of decreased strength. There is no direct correlation between strength and girth measurements. Objective strength measures using an isokinetic test indicated 16 percent quadriceps femoris and 10 percent hamstring muscle deficits. The patient was working as a fireman while continuing to attend physical therapy, and thus, depending on his work activities, irritation of the knee joint was possible.

Goals

1. Full ROM
2. Eliminate effusion
3. Eliminate medial joint line pain
4. Quadriceps femoris and hamstring muscle strength equal to the uninvolved side
5. Return to full duty as a fireman without restriction

Treatment

The patient attended physical therapy two or three times per week, each session 1 to 1½ hours in duration.

Treatments 1 to 7. Supine wall slides and gel slides were performed to increase flexion and extension ROM, respectively. Strengthening exercises consisted of isometric hip adduction, quadriceps femoris/hamstring muscle cocontraction, short-arc quadriceps femoris sets, hip adduction, hip extension, toe raises, and stationary bicycling. Ice was applied at the conclusion of each session to decrease potential swelling and minimize possible soreness. Electrical muscle stimulation was used for two sessions for reeducation of the VMO muscle.

Physical Therapy Reassessment. One month after surgery, the patient had full extension and a deficit of 5 degrees flexion ROM. He had no complaint of medial joint line pain with ADLs, and no effusion was noted. The patient was able to lift 15 lb during short-arc quadriceps femoris exercises and 50 lb during eccentric quadriceps femoris exercises. The plan for the patient's course of treatment was to continue the strengthening program as tolerated and progress to a running program, beginning with jogging on a trampoline.

Physical Therapy Treatment and Reassessment. Ten weeks after surgery, the patient had steadily progressed with increased resistance in all strengthening exercises. He was able to lift 40 lb during short-arc quadriceps femoris exercises, 55 lb during eccentric quadriceps femoris exercises, and 50 lb during hamstring curls. The patient advanced to treadmill running up to 7.2 mph for 10 minutes prior to progressing to track running. He began running 1 mile, gradually progressing to 2 to 2½ miles. However, upon return to physical therapy after a 2-week absence, the patient complained of increased medial joint line soreness and pain with a valgus force due to performing construction and gardening activities (i.e., squatting, kneeling, shoveling) at home. He also reported increasing his running to 4 to 5 miles outdoors. No effusion or swelling was noted. However, there was palpable tenderness at the medial joint line and infrapatellar tendon. The patient had no complaints of pain with resistive exercises or stationary bicycling. An isokinetic strength test measured the average peak torques of the quadriceps femoris and hamstring muscles as 66 percent and 88 percent, respectively.

The treatment plan consisted of continuing strengthening exercises as tolerated, decreasing running to 1½ miles, and the use of TENS and phonophoresis with 1 ml dexamethasone cream (Hexadrol) and 1 ml of 4 percent topical xylocaine to reduce medial joint line pain.

Physical Therapy Treatment and Reassessment. Three months after surgery, the patient continued his strengthening program as tolerated and running was limited to 1½ miles. Two treatment sessions using TENS and one session using phonophoresis with 1 ml Hexadrol and 1 ml of 4 percent topical xylocaine reduced the medial joint-line area pain. The patient had no complaints of pain during ADLs or exercises.

Final Disposition. Four months after surgery, the patient progressed to running 2¼ miles without symptoms. An isokinetic strength test was performed, revealing 62 percent quadriceps and 108 percent hamstring muscle average peak torque as compared with the uninvolved knee. The patient was recommended to be discharged from physical therapy at this time and to continue exercises independently. He had weight equipment available to him and was instructed in his home exercise program with emphasis on quadriceps femoris muscle strengthening exercises. Physician reevaluation 6 weeks later reported that the patient was running 4 to 5 miles three to four times per week, with occasional soreness. An isokinetic test performed 7 months after surgery showed the average peak torque of the quadriceps femoris and hamstring muscles as 75 percent and 91 percent, respectively. The patient was without limitations and was released to full duty without restrictions.

SUMMARY

A rehabilitation program following meniscectomy and meniscus repair was presented. Attention should be given to the stability of the lesion, location of the lesion with respect to vascularity, and biomechanical changes when deciding on surgical or conservative treatment. The primary goal following meniscectomy is to protect the remaining articular cartilage and underlying subchondral bone while strengthening the lower-extremity musculature to reduce knee joint stresses. The same considerations apply to repaired menisci, with gradual weight bearing for 3 to 4 weeks after surgery to protect the repair and allow healing to occur.

REFERENCES

1. Jackson, JP: Degenerative changes in the knee after meniscectomy. BMJ 2:525, 1968.
2. Gershuni, DH, Hargens, AR, and Danzig, LA: Regional nutrition and cellularity of the meniscus: Implications for tear and repair. Sports Med 5:322, 1988.
3. Grana, WA, Connor, S, and Hollingsworth, S: Partial arthroscopic meniscectomy. Clin Orthop 164:78, 1982.
4. MacConaill, MA: The movements of the bones and joints. III. The synovial fluid and its assistants. J Bone Joint Surg [Br] 32:224, 1950.
5. Renstrom, P, and Johnson, RJ: Anatomy and biomechanics of the menisci. Clin Sports Med 9:523, 1990.
6. Welsh, RP: Knee joint structure and function. Clin Orthop 147:7, 1980.
7. DeHaven, KE: The role of the meniscus. In Ewing, JW (ed): Articular Cartilage and Knee Joint Function: Basic Science and Arthroscopy. Raven Press, New York, 1990, p. 103.
8. McBride, ID and Reid, JG: Biomechanical considerations of the menisci of the knee. Can J Sports Sci 13:175, 1988.
9. Last, RJ: The popliteus muscle and the lateral meniscus. J Bone Joint Surg [Br] 32:93, 1950.
10. Arnoczky, SP and Warren, RF: Microvasculature of the human meniscus. Am J Sports Med 10:90, 1982.
11. Brantigan, OC and Voshell, AF: The mechanics of the ligaments and menisci of the knee joint. J Bone Joint Surg 23:45, 1941.
12. Bullough, PG, et al: The strength of the menisci of the knee as it relates to their fine structure. J Bone Joint Surg [Br] 52:564, 1970.
13. Shrive, NG, O'Connor, JJ, and Goodfellow, JW: Load-bearing in the knee joint. Clin Orthop 131:279, 1978.
14. Arnoczky, SP: Arthroscopic surgery: Meniscal healing. Contemporary Orthopaedics 10:31, 1985.
15. Arnoczky, SP and Warren, RF: The microvasculature of the meniscus and its response to injury: An experimental study in the dog. Am J Sports Med 11:131, 1983.
16. Cabaud, HE, Rodkey, WG, and Fitzwater, JE: Medial meniscus repairs: An experimental and morphological study. Am J Sports Med 9:129, 1981.
17. Stone, RG, Frewin, PR, and Gonzales, S: Long-term assessment of arthroscopic meniscus repair: A two- to six-year follow-up study. Arthroscopy 6:73, 1990.
18. Fukubayashi, T and Kurosawa, H: The contact area and pressure distribution pattern of the knee: A study of normal and osteoarthritic knee joints. Acta Orthop Scand 51:871, 1980.
19. Walker, PS and Erkman, MJ: The role of the menisci in force transmission across the knee. Clin Orthop 109:184, 1975.
20. Kurosawa, H, Fukubayashi, T, and Nakajima, H: Load-bearing mode of the knee joint: Physical behavior of the knee joint with or without menisci. Clin Orthop 149:283, 1980.
21. Ahmed, AM and Burke, DL: In-vitro measurement of static pressure distribution in synovial joints. I. Tibial surface of the knee. J Biomech Eng 105:216, 1983.
22. Radin, EL, De Lamotte, F, and Maquet, P: Role of the menisci in the distribution of stress in the knee. Clin Orthop 185:290, 1984.
23. Casscells, SW: The torn meniscus, the torn anterior cruciate ligament, and their relationship to degenerative joint disease. Arthroscopy 1:28, 1985.

24. McGinty, JB, Geuss, LF, and Marvin, RA: Partial or total meniscectomy: A comparative analysis. J Bone Joint Surg [Am] 59:763, 1977.
25. Ricklin, P, Ruttimann, A, and Del Buono, MS: Meniscus Lesions: Diagnosis, Differential Diagnosis and Therapy, ed 2. Thieme Medical Publishers, New York, 1983, p 16.
26. Fahmy, NRM, Williams, EA, and Noble, J: Meniscal pathology and osteoarthritis of the knee. J Bone Joint Surg [Br] 65:24, 1983.
27. Fairbank, TJ: Knee joint changes after meniscectomy. J Bone Joint Surg [Br] 30:664, 1948.
28. Northmore-Ball, MD, Dandy, DJ, and Jackson, RW: Arthroscopic, open partial, and total meniscectomy: A comparative study. J Bone Joint Surg [Br] 65:400, 1983.
29. DeHaven, KE: Decision-making factors in the treatment of meniscus lesions. Clin Orthop 252:49, 1990.
30. Noble, J and Hamblen, DL: The pathology of the degenerate meniscus lesion. J Bone Joint Surg [Br] 57:180, 1976.
31. Cox, JS, et al: The degenerative effects of partial and total resection of the medial meniscus in dogs' knees. Clin Orthop 109:178, 1975.
32. Lieb, FJ and Perry, J: Quadriceps function. J Bone Joint Surg [Am] 50:1535, 1968.
33. Magee, DJ: Orthopedic Physical Assessment. WB Saunders, Philadelphia, 1987, p 292.
34. Bose, K, Kanagasuntheram, R, and Osman, MBH: Vastus medialis oblique: An anatomic and physiologic study. Orthopedics 3:880, 1980.
35. Jakob, RP, Hassler, H, and Staeubli, H-U: Observations on rotatory instability of the lateral compartment of the knee. Acta Orthop Scand Suppl 191:6, 1981.
36. Raskas, D and Lehman, RC: Meniscal injuries in athletes: Pinpointing the diagnosis. The Journal of Musculoskeletal Medicine 5:18, 1988.

CHAPTER 15

Rehabilitation after Total Knee Replacement

Brenda Greene, MMSc, PT, OCS

Physical therapists frequently treat patients who have undergone total knee arthroplasty (TKA). Some clinicians feel TKA treatment is routine and self-evident; but when treatments are analyzed, we realize little information exists to guide us in our decisions. The experienced clinician uses the minimal knowledge base available to make effective clinical decisions. This chapter examines the knowledge base necessary for physical therapists to offer safe and effective treatment of patients following TKA. The first part of the chapter briefly discusses the medical management of patients after TKA, and the second portion addresses physical therapy management decisions within the context of case studies.

INDICATIONS FOR TOTAL KNEE ARTHROPLASTY

The primary indications for TKA are pain and instability.[1] Stiffness and deformity in the presence of pain and/or instability are also indications for TKA.[1] The most common diagnoses that result in pain, instability, stiffness, and deformity of the knee joint are osteoarthritis and rheumatoid arthritis. The age of the patient undergoing a TKA will vary depending on the surgeon's preference and the patient's diagnosis. Generally the patient with rheumatoid arthritis seeking a TKA will be younger than the osteoarthritis patient seeking a TKA. The age of the osteoarthritis patient seeking a TKA will depend on the amount of degeneration and the patient's activity level. Individuals who seek TKAs usually demonstrate the following characteristics: aged 60 or older except for rheumatoid arthritis patients, who are often younger than age 60; arthritis symptoms in other joints; and chronic joint pain resulting in decreased activity level and decreased muscle strength. All of these characteristics may become factors that affect the outcome of TKA surgery and rehabilitation.

CLASSIFICATION OF TOTAL KNEE ARTHROPLASTY PROSTHESES

Knee prostheses can be classified in several different ways. One classification system consists of two categories, surface replacements and constrained prostheses.[2,3] Figure 15–1A shows an anterior view and Figure 15–1B a medial view of a femoral and tibial surface replacement prosthesis. Figure 15–2A shows an anterior view and Figure 15–2B a medial view of a constrained prosthesis. Note the central post between the femoral and fibial components for stability. The most common prostheses, surface replacements, provide new articular surfaces of a metal alloy or plastic.[2,3] The surgical procedures for surface replacement prostheses may retain or sacrifice the anterior cruciate ligament, posterior cruciate ligament, or both. The surgical procedures for the constrained prosthesis sacrifice the cruciate ligaments (and possibly the collateral ligaments) but create stability by prosthetic design.[2] The design involves a type of post, linking the femoral and tibial components, that provides inherent stability.

The method of fixating the prosthesis to the bone (with or without cement) will influence the course and aggressiveness of rehabilitation. Recently, porous-coated, cementless prostheses have been developed to avoid long-term looosening that is problematic in younger, active patients with cemented prostheses.[4] The theoretical basis for

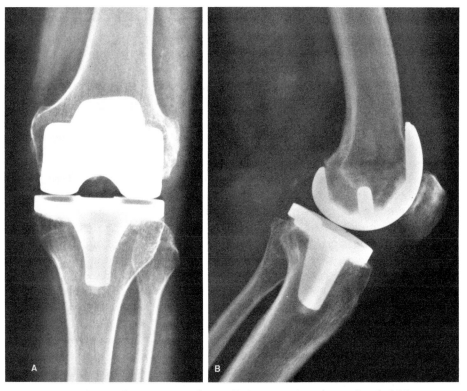

FIGURE 15–1. Surface replacement prosthesis. *A*) Anterior view, femoral and tibial components. *B*) Medial view, femoral and tibial components.

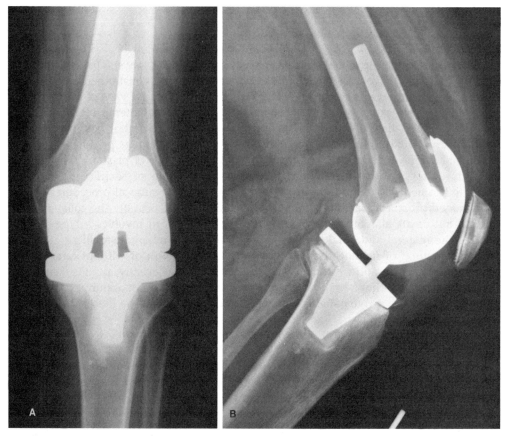

FIGURE 15-2. Constrained prosthesis. *A*) Anterior view. *B*) Medial view. In both views, note the central post linking the femoral and tibial components.

cementless, porous-coated fixation is based on the concept of facilitating bony ingrowth to the prosthesis. The undersurface of the prosthesis is a porous material, with pores the approximate size of the cancellous bone matrix that is apposed to bone. Because of the dynamic nature of bone, the conditions are appropriate for bony ingrowth to occur into the porous prosthesis. This direct biologic fixation between bone and prosthesis may improve stress distribution to the bone.[5] Another reported benefit of ingrowth fixation is preservation of a maximal amount of bone stock in the event that a TKA revision is required.[5] The long-term benefit of the cementless approach is unknown. Debate in the medical community persists regarding the existence of short-term benefits. Bourne[6] reported the cementless method to be no better at fixation than the cemented method. The significance of cemented or noncemented fixation with respect to postsurgical rehabilitation is that a longer protective phase is usually recommended with the cementless method to allow for secure bony fixation.[7,8] Weight bearing on the extremity with a cementless prosthesis is limited for 6 to 12 weeks.[7,8] Bourne and associates recommend 50 percent weight bearing in the first 6 weeks, then over the next 6 weeks an increase to full weight bearing with one external support.[7]

MEDICAL MANAGEMENT

Postoperative medical management revolves around preventing the major possible complications, namely (1) thromboembolic disease; (2) disorders of wound healing; and (3) range of motion (ROM) limitations.[9] The incidence of deep vein thrombosis after total knee arthroplasty is reported to be 50 to 70 percent.[9,10] One to 2 percent of TKA patients develop symptomatic pulmonary emboli (PE) and 0.1 to 0.4 percent of all TKA patients develop fatal pulmonary emboli.[9] Theoretically, the larger the clot and the more proximal the location, the greater the risk of pulmonary emboli. The popular prophylaxis regimen includes anticoagulation therapy (aspirin, low-dose Coumadin, low-dose heparin) and intermittent compression stockings.[9,11]

Wound healing is reported to be a problem in 10 to 20 percent of TKA patients.[9] The standard incision is midline on the skin and through the medial portion of the extensor mechanism and capsule.[11] Risk factors that increase the likelihood of wound healing problems include: poor nutrition, obesity, diabetes, and smoking.[9] Early motion via continuous passive motion (CPM) machine or physical therapy has been associated with both improved wound healing[9,12] and delayed wound healing.[13] The parameters of passive motion application—such as amount of motion, rate, and hours of usage— likely affect whether wound healing is delayed or not. One study looked at the effect of the initial ROM settings of the CPM machine and the subsequent daily machine ROM increases on the viability of the wound edges.[14] Viability of wound edges was measured via transcutaneous oxygen tension. The results were that beyond 40 degrees of flexion the oxygen tension rapidly decreased. Based on these findings, the recommended protocol for CPM use is 40 degrees flexion for the first 3 postoperative days, then increased up to 20 degrees each day until 90 degrees is reached. The findings did demonstrate that using a rate of 1 cycle per minute, the oxygen tension did return to normal during the extension phase of CPM. The complication of delayed wound healing will impede the physical therapist's inpatient goals of increasing knee joint ROM and returning the patient to an appropriate functional level. We should be aware of patients at risk for delayed wound healing, and be careful to detect and report evidence of delayed wound healing.

We do not know if the findings regarding CPM relate to passive or assisted range of motion performed by physical therapists. Because passive range of motion (PROM) may produce effects at the wound similar to those of CPM, including decreased oxygen tension at the wound, prolonged flexion stretch should perhaps be avoided during the early stages of wound healing. Research to test this hypothesis is needed before guidelines on PROM in healing wounds can be given.

REHABILITATION CONSIDERATIONS

The primary goal of post surgical rehabilitation is the restoration of full, painless ROM. No definitive answer exists for why some patients have difficulty gaining ROM postsurgically and other patients do not. Possible risk factors associated with restricted ROM include: reduced ROM prior to arthroplasty[15]; patient motivation[15]; inflammatory reaction[9]; and patient apprehension.[9] Given the extensive amount of soft-tissue disruption and soft-tissue healing, ROM is a critical issue following TKA. The etiology of limited motion is probably multifactorial. Initially, when movement of a healing area is painful, patients will naturally avoid movement and thereby avoid pain. Second, during soft-tissue healing a random deposition of collagen occurs[16] unless mechanical stress is applied. The result of the random deposition of collagen is abnormal cross-link formation between collagen fibers and the development of adhesions in the connective tissue, thereby limiting motion.[16] Applying mechanical stress to the newly formed collagen fibers should help the collagen to orient to the direction of the stress, prevent formation of abnormal cross-links, and result in a mobile scar.[16] Applying mechanical stress should also (1) modulate synthesis of proteoglycans and collagen; (2) maintain a critical inter-fiber distance; (3) influence the deposition of newly synthesized collagen fibers in such a manner as to resist tensile stresses; and (4) prevent the development of anomalous cross-links.[17] Methods of applying mechanical stress include active, active assistive, and passive exercises in physical therapy and CPM.

In many facilities, CPM has become a routine procedure in the postoperative management of patients who have undergone total knee arthroplasty. The CPM machine may be implemented in the recovery room directly after surgery, or 2 to 3 days postoperatively. The rationale for waiting a few days to begin CPM is to allow for initial wound healing.[9] If the TKA patient does not gain 75 to 90 degrees of knee joint flexion ROM before hospital discharge, a manipulation under anesthesia will frequently be performed.[9,15]

Claims of positive results from CPM use include greater ROM by the time of hospital discharge[12,14]; greater ultimate ROM gained[12,14]; decreased hospital stay[9,12,14]; decreased pain[12]; decreased incidence of wound complications[9,12]; and decreased incidence of thromboembolic disease.[12] The benefit of decreased incidence of thromboembolic disease has not been supported by two separate researchers.[10,18] Other negative reports contradictory to the above findings are delayed wound healing[13] and decreased extension ROM.[19]

The exact optimal dosage of CPM (i.e., length of time on the unit) is not known. An early study that reported beneficial effects of CPM had patients in the CPM units for 20 hours per day.[12] Improvements in ROM similar to those reported in the earlier studies have not been found with two 2-hour treatments[19] and three 1-hour treatments.[20] Another study compared a group of TKA patients using CPM for 20 hours per day and a group of TKA patients using CPM for 5 hours per day.[21] The conclusion was that no statistically significant difference in knee joint flexion ROM existed between the groups, but a trend toward increased knee joint flexion ROM was demonstrated in the 20-hour-per-day group. Comparison of the above results suggests that the optimal length of time on CPM is at least 5 hours per day, although further study is needed for a more precise determination.

CASE STUDIES

The purpose of the case studies is to provide examples of the problem-solving process and clinical decisions made for two different TKA patients. The theoretical rationale and research data (when available) for the clinical decisions made are included.

CASE STUDY 1

Overview

Identify the patient's problem:

Limited functional activity

Identify characteristics of the problem:

Soft-tissue healing
Restricted left knee joint flexion and extension ROM
Limited strength in muscles of the left hip and knee joints
Gait requiring an assistive device
Postsurgical pain

Identify factors affecting the problem:

Patient is 51 years of age
Diagnosis—osteoarthritis, left knee
Systems other than musculoskeletal system are uninvolved
Left TKA surface replacement (tibial, femoral, and patellar components); porous-coated, noncemented fixation
Patient is motivated to return to employment

Determine a method to resolve the problem:

Therapeutic exercise program to increase strength in the knee flexor and extensor muscles; hip abductor, adductor, flexor, and extensor muscles
Therapeutic exercise program to increase flexion and extension ROM in the knee joint
Neuromuscular electrical stimulation to the quadriceps femoris muscle during the first 2 weeks of physical therapy to facilitate coordinated, strong muscle contractions
Cryotherapy to decrease pain and inflammation

Evaluate effectiveness of the method of resolution:

Ongoing subjective, goniometric, circumferential, and manual muscle test measurements

Modify management:

Therapeutic exercise program adjusted and modalities added or deleted based on reevaluation findings

HISTORY

Mr. W. was a 51-year-old man with severe tricompartmental osteoarthritis (OA) of the left knee joint. In tricompartmental OA, degeneration is noted in the articulations between both the medial and lateral tibiofemoral compartments as well as the patellofemoral compartment or joint.[22] Mr. W. had been treated conservatively with nonsteroidal anti-inflammatory drugs and physical therapy in the past, with little improvement. His right knee joint was also intermittently painful and roentgenograms demonstrated degenerative joint changes. He had no other significant medical history.

Mr. W. lived in a two-story house with his wife. He had been employed for 25 years with the phone company, and for most of those years he was involved in a great deal of repetitive knee flexion activity (telephone pole climbing). Having retired from the phone company, he worked part-time in lawn maintenance. He enjoyed golfing during his leisure time. He estimated walking 1 to 2 miles per day.

Mr. W. underwent a left surface replacement TKA replacing the tibial, femoral, and patellar components. The prosthesis was porous-coated and noncemented for bony ingrowth fixation. Postoperative care in the hospital consisted of routine antibiotics and anticoagulation medication, CPM 12 to 14 hours per day, transcutaneous electrical neuromuscular stimulation (TENS) for pain, physical therapy for range of motion exercises, strengthening exercises, and gait training with crutches (20 to 30 lb partial weight bearing on the left). Mr. W. was discharged to his home on the 10th postoperative day and began outpatient physical therapy 2 weeks post-TKA.

Mr. W. presented with OA, a typical diagnosis for knee arthroplasty. He was a bit young for such severe degeneration, but his work involved a great deal of repetitive knee flexion, which likely contributed to the early degenerative changes in his knee joints. He also demonstrated degenerative changes in his right knee joint, which could worsen during the protective period of the left knee. Fortunately, no other peripheral or spinal joints demonstrated degeneration; therefore, wrist, shoulder, and ankle joints should sustain the additional stress during the protective period of the left knee.

The porous-coated, noncemented implant was chosen because the patient is young and active. Presumably Mr. W. had good bone stock previously because he was young, healthy, and active; thus the bone was likely to be successful in growing into the implant, creating a stable long-term fixation. However, his relatively high activity level could result in wear of the prosthesis necessitating a revision. Hopefully more bone stock should be preserved without the use of cement if a revision is required in the future.

Soft-tissue healing had already been affected by use of CPM. The newly forming collagen being laid down in the capsule and skin had been given mechanical stress to improve flexibility. Two weeks postsurgery the pain should have decreased but may still require intervention. He appeared well motivated and interested in returning to his prior functional level without the severe left knee joint pain.

Based on information from the history and the interview, Mr. W.'s primary problem was limited function secondary to the healing left total knee arthroplasty. Anticipated characteristics of the limited function were soft-tissue healing, limited ROM of the left knee joint, limited strength of the left knee joint musculature, gait requiring an assistive device, and postsurgical pain.

Factors affecting Mr. W.'s outcome were those described previously: his age, diagnosis, type of prosthesis, soft-tissue healing, activity level, and motivation. Mr. W. would be expected to have a favorable outcome or resolution of his primary problem because he was young and had only two joints involved in the degeneration. His soft-tissue healing and flexibility had already been positively affected by the use of CPM. He would probably require protected weight bearing with crutches for 6 to 12 weeks due to bony ingrowth fixation. Mr. W.'s activity level would have to be addressed during rehabilitation in an effort to preserve the life of the prosthesis and minimize the progression of degeneration in the right knee joint.

PHYSICAL THERAPY

Initial Evaluation

Subjective: Achy pain in the left knee, rated 4/10. Pain increases with activity and decreases with rest. Intermittent right knee joint pain, occurs several times per week, rated 2/10 when present.

Structure: Weight appropriate for height.

Circumferential Measurements	Right	Left
10 cm above knee joint line	47 cm	41 cm
4 cm above knee joint line	36 cm	37 cm
Knee joint line	36 cm	40 cm
Midcalf	30.5 cm	30 cm

Palpation: Mildly increased skin temperature of the left knee joint. Closed, mobile scar. Mild diffuse edema. Negative ballottement test for joint effusion.

Active ROM: Left knee 5 to 90 degrees, left hip and ankle functional. Right knee 0 to 120 degrees.

Passive ROM: Left knee 0 to 97 degrees, right knee 0 to 125 degrees.

Strength: Left hip 4/5 all motions. Left knee extension 3−/5 (5 degrees extension lag). Left knee flexion 4/5. Left ankle dorsiflexion and plantarflexion 5/5.

Assessment

The following physical therapy problems were found:

1. Limited function based on history and assisted gait
2. Limited ROM in left knee joint flexion and extension
3. Limited strength in the quadriceps femoris muscles, hamstring muscles, and all muscles about the hip joint.

Treatment

In an effort to maintain and increase Mr. W.'s strength and ROM, the first priority of treatment was to instruct him in a home exercise program. This program consisted of quadriceps femoris isometric muscle setting (quad sets), straight leg raises, hamstring isometric muscle setting (ham sets), and sitting active knee flexion. Physical therapy treatments in the first week consisted of (1) neuromuscular electrical stimulation, (2) progressive resistive exercises, (3) active and passive knee joint flexion stretch, and (4) cold pack applied to the knee joint.

1. *Neuromuscular electrical stimulation (NMES) to the quadriceps femoris muscle.* Medtronic Respond II device (Medtronic, San Diego, CA). Stimulation parameters: Waveform — asymmetric biphasic square wave; pulse width — 300 microseconds; frequency — 35 pps; on time 10 seconds, off time 15 seconds; intensity — tetanic contraction. Electrodes were placed over the motor points for vastus medialis and rectus femoris muscles. Electrical stimulation was used during quad set, straight leg raise, and terminal extension exercises.

Mr. W. needed assistance in achieving functional quadriceps femoris muscle activity. Evidence in support of this assessment includes: (1) left knee joint extension lag; (2) decreased knee joint extension strength, and (3) decreased thigh circumference. An *extension lag* is defined as a "condition in which active range of motion into knee extension is less than passive range of motion into knee extension."[23] An extension lag is not an uncommon finding in patients who have undergone TKA, especially in TKA patients who have also been treated with CPM. Two reports in the literature document a greater extension lag in TKA patients who used CPM.[19,24] Decreased quadriceps femoris muscle activity may be the result of muscle atrophy or the result of reflex muscle inhibition due to pain[25,26] and effusion.[27,28]

Because Mr. W. was not reporting a great deal of pain and he demonstrated mild diffuse extracapsular swelling, the muscle weakness was assessed to be primarily from muscle atrophy.

Obtaining full active knee joint extension is a necessary goal for efficient function. An upright knee joint position of as little as 5 degrees of flexion requires a quadriceps muscle force of 30 percent body weight to stabilize the knee.[29] With increasing knee flexion, increased knee extensor force is required for stabilization. Increased knee flexion in stance also produces increased compressive forces on the patella.[29,30] Perhaps the lack of full knee extension contributes to early wear of the patellar component of the prosthesis.

One of the proposed outcomes of NMES is muscle facilitation and reeducation in postoperative orthopedically involved patients.[31] A study that reported improved muscle contraction after knee surgery[32] lends support for the use of NMES. In TKA patients, use of NMES was demonstrated to be effective in decreasing the extensor lag when combined with CPM during the postoperative hospital phase.[33] Stimulation parameters used in the reported study were the following: waveform — asymmetric biphasic; pulse width — 300 microseconds; frequency — 35 pps; on time 15 seconds. The electrical stimulation was used for three hourly sessions during the extension phase of the CPM machine. Even though Mr. W. was no longer on CPM, use of NMES with similar stimulation parameters should still be beneficial to decrease the extension lag.

2. *Progressive resistive exercises to the hip abductor, adductor, flexor, and extensor muscles.* Exercises consisted of straight leg raises into flexion, extension, abduction, and adduction.

Functional strength in the hip musculature is needed for normal gait, work, and recreational activities. Mr. W. demonstrated a strength deficit in the muscles about the left hip joint. Given his age and prior activity level, he should have achieved normal strength in the muscles about the left hip joint. Progressive resistance exercises to these muscles is an accepted approach to increase muscle strength.[34,35]

3. *Manual active assisted and passive knee joint flexion stretch.* The patient is positioned sitting on the edge of a plinth with the hip stabilized (Fig. 15-3).

Active assisted exercises into knee joint flexion will result in inhibition of the antagonist (quadriceps femoris muscle) and facilitation of the agonist (hamstring muscles).[36] Provided that Mr. W. could relax, increased passive knee joint flexion could have supplemented the active assisted exercises. The decision of when to use passive stretching and how much stretching is effective comes from clinical experience and should be guided by the patient's signs and symptoms.

The most effective and least harmful method of passive stretching is to provide a low-load, prolonged stretch.[37,38] Application of a low-load, prolonged stretch involves taking the joint to the end of the comfortable range of motion and maintaining the stretch for at least 1 minute. Active contraction in the antagonistic muscles should not be present. The theoretical basis for low-load, prolonged passive stretch is to use enough time to affect the viscous, plastic components of connective tissue and therefore provide a permanent lengthening.[39] The phenomenon of a continued tissue deformation under a constant load is referred to as *creep* and is the result of viscoelastic properties of the connective tissue.[40]

Heat and contract-relax techniques may be used adjunctively with passive stretching. The reported effects of heat are increased circulation, pain threshold

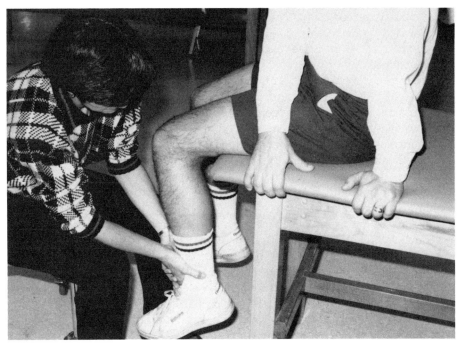

FIGURE 15-3. Active knee flexion to the patient's end range followed by a low-load passive stretch into knee flexion.

elevation, altered muscle spindle firing rates, and increased tissue extensibility when combined with stretch.[41,38] Studies on the effect of heat and prolonged stretch in rat tail tendon demonstrated a significant lengthening with stretch and heat; the elongation benefit was even greater if the load was maintained during the cooling phase.[42] No heat was chosen for Mr. W. because he demonstrated a reasonable amount of knee joint flexion at 2 weeks postoperatively. Hold-relax to the hamstring muscles (agonists) was occasionally employed. The neurophysiologic rationale for this technique is reciprocal inhibition of the quadriceps femoris muscle via agonist muscle spindles.[43] Contract-relax or hold-relax techniques to the quadriceps femoris muscle (antagonists) would also have been effective to gain joint ROM, but in consideration of soft-tissue healing these techniques were deferred during the first 2 weeks.

4. *Cold pack applied to the knee joint at the end of the treatment session.* Duration of cryotherapy was 10 minutes.

Mr. W. demonstrated increased skin temperature and swelling around the left knee joint. Warmth and swelling are two signs of local inflammation. Short-duration cryotherapy is a standard treatment for inflammation because of its physiologic effects. The reported effects of cold are pain threshold elevation, arteriole vasoconstriction, and a decrease in metabolism and vasoactive agents, resulting in reduced inflammation.[44,45]

Reevaluation—week 1: At the end of the first week, active ROM was increased to 5 to 105 degrees. Circumferential measurements were the same, and there was no increase in reports of pain. Evidence of increased mobility without increased tissue irritation dictated a continuation of the same plan.

Reevaluation—week 2: At the end of the second week, active ROM was increased to 0 to 112 degrees. Circumferential measurement at midpatella (42.5 cm) was decreased by 0.5 cm. Quadriceps femoris muscle strength was 3/5.

Based on decreasing swelling, increasing ROM, and increasing strength, the weights on the resistive exercises were increased and use of NMES was discontinued.

Reevaluation—week 3: At the end of the third week, active ROM was 0 to 110 degrees. Mr. W. reported more pain in the left knee joint. He also reported being more active at home (i.e., going shopping). Circumferential measurements at midpatella increased to 43 cm.

Increased activity at home and perhaps in physical therapy resulted in increased inflammation. The plan was to rest more at home, continue with the exercises in physical therapy, and add approximately two treatments of high-voltage electrical stimulation (80 pps, negative polarity, electrodes placed over the joint) with cryotherapy.

One of the proposed effects of high-voltage electrical stimulation is edema reduction.[46] The specific mechanisms by which high-voltage electrical stimulation effects edema reduction have not been identified. However, proposed theoretical mechanisms for edema reduction following high-voltage electrical stimulation are that (1) negatively charged current of the electrical stimulation repels negatively charged serum proteins and prevents protein leakage into the interstitium[47]; (2) lymphatic uptake of proteins and fluid is enhanced[46]; and (3) permeability of microvessels to plasma proteins is reduced.[48]

Reevaluation—week 4: At the end of the fourth week, active ROM was 0 to 118 degrees. Circumferential measurement at midpatella was 42.5 cm, a decrease of 0.5 cm. Quadriceps femoris muscle strength was 3/5. Mr. W. was 6 weeks postoperative and was cleared by the physician for full weight bearing. Gait without any assistive device resulted in a significant antalgic gait pattern, so a straight cane was dispensed. He was instructed in its proper use.

Mr. W. had made progress in physical therapy, but based on his need for an assistive device during ambulation and his strength limitations, physical therapy was continued three times per week for 2 more weeks.

Over the next 2 weeks, resistive exercises were progressed and weight bearing exercises such as the leg press and 20-degree wall slides were added (Fig. 15–4). A gradual walking program was initiated for independent home use. Mr. W. was instructed in joint protection principles for his knee. Use of a stool or power weeder was recommended during lawn maintenance activities to minimize the prolonged deep squatting. One-legged standing balance was assessed and was found to be decreased on the left. The patient was started on short-arc lunge exercises for balance and proprioception retraining (Fig. 15–5).

Reevaluation—week 6: At the end of 6 weeks, active ROM was 0 to 120 degrees. Strength in the muscles about the hip joint was normal except for the abductor and flexor muscles, which were 4/5. Mr. W. was assessed to ensure he was correctly executing his home exercise program consisting of straight leg raises

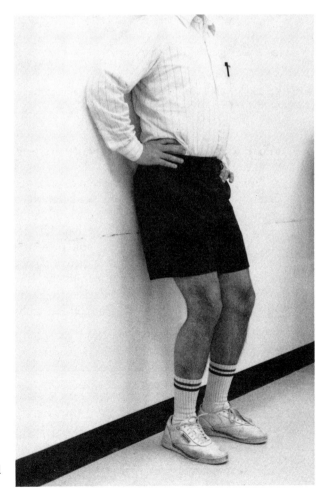

FIGURE 15–4. Wall slide, a closed kinetic chain exercise.

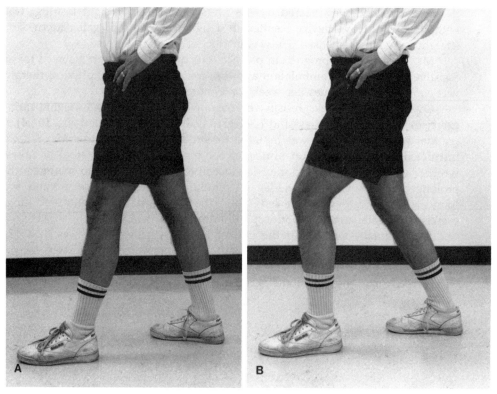

FIGURE 15-5. Small arc lunge exercises for balance and proprioception retraining. *A*) Beginning position. *B*) Ending position.

into flexion, adduction, and abduction; wall slides; and terminal knee joint extension.

Physical therapy was decreased to once per week to assess his progress and to determine when independent ambulation without use of the cane could commence.

Reevaluation — week 8: Mr. W. had 120 degrees of functional knee joint flexion, his pain was minimal but still present at times, and he could ambulate smoothly without deviations or assistive devices. After 8 weeks of physical therapy (14 sessions, 10 weeks postoperatively), Mr. W. was doing well on his own. He was independent in a home exercise program and able to walk approximately ½ mile per day. Mr. W. was discharged from physical therapy.

CASE STUDY 2

OVERVIEW

Identify the patient's problems:

Limited functional activity
Laterally subluxing patella

Subsequent loosening of the prosthetic components
TKA revision and lateral release

Identify characteristics of the problems:

Diffuse knee joint and proximal tibial pain
Recurrent effusions of the left knee joint
Ambulation with a walker
Limited strength in muscles of the left hip and knee joints, especially the vastus medialis muscle
Restricted knee joint flexion ROM

Identify factors affecting the problems:

Patient is 66 years of age
Diagnosis—OA, left knee joint; OA, right hip and knee joints
History of hypertension controlled by medication, otherwise other systems uninvolved
Left TKA surface replacement (tibial, femoral, and patellar components), porous-coated, cemented
Patient is overweight

Determine a method to resolve the problems:

Thermal and electrical modalities to decrease the inflammatory reaction, effusion, and pain in the left knee joint
Therapeutic exercise program to increase vastus medialis strength and to maintain and increase active ROM of the left knee joint
Orthotic with a lateral pad to assist medial patellar tracking

Evaluate effectiveness of the method of resolution:

The initial signs of treatment effectiveness will be a decrease in the inflammatory response. Circumferential measurements, palpation, and subjective assessments are methods to evaluate the inflammatory response. Later signs of treatment effectiveness are improved vastus medialis muscle strength and decreased lateral patellar subluxation. See the next section for methods of evaluating vastus medialis muscle strength and patellar subluxation. In Mrs. M.'s case, physical therapy treatments were not successful until after further surgical intervention.

Modify management:

Physical therapy management was aimed at improving the muscle imbalance causing lateral patellar subluxation. However, due to the inflamed state of the tissues, modifications in exercise intensity and modality application depended on the tissue response.

HISTORY

Mrs. M. was a 66-year-old woman with severe OA in the left knee and resultant mild valgus deformity. Increasing pain and crepitus in the left knee brought her to the orthopedist. Her past history indicated OA in the right hip and a right femoral supracondylar fracture treated with open reduction internal fixation 6 years previously. Since the fracture treatment, her right leg has been 2.5 cm shorter than the left. Medical history was positive for hypertension controlled by Inderal. She lived in a two-story home with her daughter, son-in-law, and two grandchildren (ages 10 and 12). Prior to her surgery she assisted in cooking and cleaning.

Mrs. M. underwent a left surface-replacement TKA to replace the tibial, femoral, and patellar components. The prosthesis was porous-coated and cemented. Postoperative care in the hospital consisted of routine antibiotics and anticoagulation medication; and physical therapy for ROM exercises, strengthening exercises, and gait training with a walker. No CPM was used. Mrs. M. was discharged to her daughter's home on the 15th postoperative day. Mrs. M. was instructed in home exercises, but no physical therapy was prescribed. Five weeks after her operation, she was referred to physical therapy with the diagnosis of status post–left TKR with lateral patellar subluxation.

Mrs. M. presented with OA, a typical diagnosis for knee arthroplasty. In contrast to Mr. W., Mrs M. was older, had greater involvement in other joints (OA of the right hip and knee joints), and had a mild genu valgus deformity, which was corrected with the TKA surgery. Based on the diagnosis, history, and interview, Mrs. W.'s primary problems were her laterally subluxing patella, limited functional ability, and pain.

Mrs. M.'s lateral patellar subluxation was most likely caused by an insufficient vastus medialis muscle or abnormal lateral structures.[49] In general, factors associated with lateral patellar subluxation are an increased Q angle, patella alta, lateral insertion of the patellar tendon, a laterally tilted patella, and hypoplasia of the vastus medialis muscle.[50,51] Mrs. M.'s valgus deformity likely contributed to an increased valgus vector of the quadriceps femoris muscle and lateral patellar subluxation.

Measurement of the amount of lateral patellar subluxation or vastus medialis activity is difficult. Visual observation will determine whether subluxation is present, but quantifying the amount of subluxation is typically not done clinically. One report in the literature measured the lateral displacement force of the quadriceps femoris muscle on the patella via a hand-held dynamometer during maximal voluntary contraction.[51] The method to quantify the amount of vastus medialis muscle activity is electromyography (EMG). Because the therapist did not have access to EMG, the best measurement of vastus medialis activity was indirectly through lateral patellar subluxation. Manual muscle test of the knee joint extensor muscles will give information regarding overall quadriceps femoris isometric muscle strength, and circumferential measurements will give information regarding overall thigh atrophy.

Factors affecting Mrs. M.'s outcome were those described previously: her age; diagnosis (including OA of the uninvolved hip and knee joints); hypertension controlled by medication; type of prosthesis; and overweight status. To compensate for her leg length discrepancy, she had been previously fitted with a shoe lift. Because of her hypertension and medication, vital signs were monitored. Due to OA involvement in joints other than the surgical joint, exercises and activities were monitored for their possible effect on nonsurgical joints. Mrs. M. was informed of the stressful effect of extra weight on her joints and her recent implant. However, given her age and activity level, the likelihood of her weight decreasing was small. Prognosis for return to prior functional level was good; however, due to multiple joint involvement, delayed physical therapy, and joint effusions, the time required to complete rehabilitation would likely be longer than 3 months.

PHYSICAL THERAPY

Initial Evaluation

Subjective: Mrs. M. occasionally had a sensation of the patella "slipping." She had diffuse achy pain around the left knee joint extending from the tibial tubercle to the superior patella, rated 7/10. The pain was present daily and decreased with rest and at night to 4/10.

Vital signs: Blood pressure, heart rate, and respirations were within normal limits.

Structure: Overweight (5 feet, 4 inches tall; weight 155 lb).

Circumferential Measurements	Right	Left
10 cm above knee joint line	47 cm	41 cm
4 cm above knee joint line	36 cm	37 cm
Knee joint line	36 cm	40 cm
Midcalf	30.5 cm	30 cm

Observation: There was muscle atrophy resulting in a "hollow" area over the vastus medialis muscle, and erythema around the left knee joint. Mrs. M. ambulated with a walker. She was cleared for full weight bearing but demonstrated decreased stance time on the left and decreased step length bilaterally.

Palpation: Mild warmth and effusion around the left knee joint. Healed scar. Positive ballottement test due to intracapsular effusion.

Active ROM: Left knee 5 to 90 degrees, obvious lateral subluxation of the patella during active knee extension; left hip and ankle functional. Right knee 0 to 115 degrees, right hip lacking 15 degrees to full extension, ankle dorsiflexion to neutral.

Passive ROM: Left knee 0 to 95 degrees, right knee 0 to 120 degrees. Good patellar mobility medially.

Strength: Results were as follows:

	Right	Left
Hip abduction	3/5	3/5
Hip adduction	3+/5	3+/5
Hip extension	4/5 (in limited range)	4/5
Hip flexion	3/5	3/5
Knee extension	4/5	3−/5 (5 degrees extensor lag)
Knee flexion	4/5	3/5
Ankle dorsiflexion	4/5	4/5
Ankle plantarflexion	4/5	4/5

Special tests: Ober's test for iliotibial band tightness was positive bilaterally.

Assessment

The following physical therapy problems were found:

1. Left knee joint effusion
2. Limited strength in the quadriceps femoris muscles, especially the vastus medialis muscle allowing lateral patellar subluxation
3. Limited ROM in left knee joint flexion and extension
4. Pain
5. Limited function

Treatment

The treatment priority for Mrs. M. was to decrease the effusion. While not in physical therapy she was instructed to wear a compressive stocking, elevate the leg higher than her heart, and ice the knee 15 minutes out of every hour whenever possible. Her home exercise program consisted of quadriceps femoris muscle sets, straight leg raises, hamstring muscle sets, and sitting active knee flexion. Physical therapy treatments in the clinic in the first 2 weeks consisted of the electrical stimulation, cold pack application, therapeutic exercise, and active ROM.

1. *High-voltage electrical stimulation* (80 pps, negative polarity, electrodes over the knee joint).
2. *Cold pack* applied to the knee joint during electrical stimulation and at the end of the treatment session.

Frequency of the treatment was recommended at three times per week, but Mrs. M. was only able to attend therapy two times per week.

Mrs. M. demonstrated signs of knee joint effusion and decreased quadriceps femoris muscle strength. Decreased quadriceps femoris muscle strength may result from atrophy or from reflex muscle inhibition due to pain[25,26] and effusion.[27,28] Because intra-articular swelling and pain were present, decreased quadriceps femoris muscle activity was attributed to pain and effusion. The implication of these findings for Mrs. M.'s treatment was that pain and effusion must be addressed before significant strength gains would be seen. In addition to ice, compression, and elevation, electrical stimulation may be used to decrease the inflammatory response and/or effusion. The two most popular mechanisms of decreasing swelling with electrical stimulation are (1) activation of the muscle pump to provide intermittent compression of the lymphatic vessels, thus enhancing absorption of interstitial fluid[52]; and (2) enhancing lymphatic uptake of proteins and fluid by creating a negatively charged electrical field around the injured tissue[47] (see Case Study 1, Reevaluation—week 3).

3. *Therapeutic exercise* consisting of isometric quadriceps femoris muscle contraction sets at multiple angles (15, 30, and 45 degrees of knee joint flexion) and straight leg raises on the left. Stretching of the hamstring muscles and tensor fasciae latae muscle on the left. Resistive hip adduction, flexion and extension bilaterally.

Strength gains from isometric exercise have been shown to be specific to the angle at which the muscle is exercised, with an overflow of 15 degrees in each direction.[53] Because isometric exercises were employed and strength improvements throughout the ROM were desired, use of multiple angles was required. Second, when the joint is placed in the loose-pack position (approximately 30 to 40 degrees of knee flexion), less intra-articular pressure will exist; therefore, less quadriceps femoris inhibition will result from joint capsule tension receptors due to joint distension. Three research studies that support this theory found decreased inhibition of the quadriceps femoris muscle at 30 degrees[54,55] and 40 degrees[56] compared with full knee joint extension.

Strengthening of the hip joint adductor muscles only (and not the abductor muscles) was chosen because of the imbalance between the vastus medialis and vastus lateralis muscles and because of evidence of lateral patellar subluxation. Hip joint adduction may increase the activity of the vastus medialis as measured by EMG,[57] which should improve medial patellar tracking. Stretching to the hamstring muscles and tensor fasciae latae was also aimed at restoring muscle balance. Because of Mrs. M.'s history of OA in the right hip, exercises were also initiated for the right side.

4. *Active ROM into knee joint flexion and extension.* Due to the joint effusion, passive ROM was not emphasized for fear of irritating the joint. But the need to maintain ROM was addressed through active ROM.

Reevaluation—week 2: At the end of the second week, circumferential measurements at the knee joint line were unchanged. Warmth, erythema, and palpable joint effusion were still present. Lateral patellar subluxation during active knee joint extension was present.

Treatment priority was still to decrease the effusion. Mrs. M.'s home follow-up program of ice, compression, and elevation was reviewed. Electrical stimulation was altered for activation of the muscle pump. NMES (Medtronics Respond II) was provided at 35 pps; on time 10 seconds, off time 25 seconds; electrodes placed over motor points for vastus medialis and rectus femoris muscles; intensity to mild muscle contraction. The therapeutic exercise program continued with an increase in repetitions as tolerated. No weight was added due to the effusion. Mrs. M was also fitted with a knee support with a patellar cut-out and pad located laterally to assist in medial patellar tracking.

Reevaluation—week 4: At the end of the fourth week, Mrs. M. was still ambulating with a walker. She reported a slight decrease in the intensity of knee pain (now rated 6/10). Active ROM was increased slightly to 5 to 95 degrees, with obvious lateral patellar subluxation during extension. Passive ROM was increased slightly to 0 to 100 degrees. Her knee joint was still warm, with palpable effusion.

Mrs. M. saw her physician and had the knee joint aspirated. The cultures were negative for infection. After the knee joint effusion was decreased and she was tolerating high repetitions of her exercises, the resistance for her exercises was progressively increased. NMES for muscle-pump and quadriceps femoris muscle strengthening was continued.

Reevaluation—week 6: Mrs. M. reported that the knee joint pain was primarily over the proximal tibia and less over the knee joint. Mild warmth over the knee joint persisted. Active ROM increased to 0 to 100 degrees with obvious lateral patellar subluxation. Strength in muscles about the left and right hips increased to the 4/5 range except abduction, which was 3 + /5 bilaterally.

Treatment continued with emphasis on hip adduction exercises and NMES to the vastus medialis muscle only. A home program of NMES was initiated 4 hours per day. Standing terminal knee joint extension exercises with NMES were added.

Reevaluation—week 8: Mrs. M.'s status was essentially the same as 2 weeks earlier. Physical therapy was discontinued. Mrs. M. continued on a home exercise program consisting of NMES during terminal knee joint extension, straight leg raise, and hip adduction exercises. At this time the therapist did not know that loosening of the prosthetic components was a problem. However, 1 month later when Mrs. M. underwent surgical revision, the femoral and tibial components were recemented due to loosening. She also received a surgical release of the vastus lateralis muscle and lateral retinaculum to improve the lateral patellar subluxation. She was discharged from the hospital after 2 weeks. Three weeks postoperatively she returned to outpatient physical therapy.

Evaluation Following Second Surgery

Subjective: Overall, greatly improved compared with prior to the revision. Mild pain (3/10) over the vastus lateralis region during end range flexion and extension and during maximum isometric extension contraction.

Vital signs: blood pressure, heart rate, and respirations within normal limits.

Structure: The following data were recorded:

Circumferential Measurements	Right	Left
10 cm above knee joint line	47 cm	41 cm
4 cm above knee joint line	36 cm	36 cm
Knee joint line	36 cm	37 cm

Observation: There was atrophy of the vastus medialis muscle, indicating quadriceps muscle weakness. The incision was closed. No warmth or erythema, but mild diffuse swelling about the left knee joint was present. The patient ambulated independently with a walker but demonstrated decreased stance time on the left and decreased step length bilaterally.

Active ROM: Left knee 10 to 95 degrees. Occasional mild lateral subluxation of the patella during extension.

Passive ROM: Left knee 0 to 97 degrees.

Strength: Results were as follows:

	Right	Left
Hip abduction	3+/5	3+/5
Hip adduction	4/5	4/5
Hip extension	4/5	4/5
Hip flexion	3/5	3/5
Knee extension	4+/5	3−/5 (10 degrees extensor lag)
Knee flexion	4/5	3+/5
Ankle dorsiflexion	4/5	4/5
Ankle plantarflexion	4/5	4/5

Assessment

Mrs. M. had less pain and joint effusion after her revision. She also demonstrated improved medial patellar tracking, but worsened extension lag.

Physical therapy problems:

1. Limited strength in the quadriceps femoris muscles, especially the vastus medialis muscle
2. Limited ROM in left knee joint flexion and extension
3. Limited function

Treatment

The therapeutic exercise program described previously was reinstituted. The primary objective of the exercise program was to improve the vastus medialis muscle strength and eliminate the extension lag. Because swelling and pain were no longer problems, the primary cause of the extension lag was assessed to be muscle weakness. Again, Mrs. M. was on a home exercise program and was able to attend physical therapy only twice per week.

Reevaluation—week 2: Active ROM improved to 5 to 105 degrees in the left knee joint. Mild occasional lateral patellar subluxation was still present, but no warmth or swelling.

The resistance of the exercises was progressively increased. Single-leg standing balance and stationary bike exercises were initiated. The patient progressed to short-arc wall slides.

Reevaluation: Mrs. M. continued in physical therapy for an additional $2\frac{1}{2}$ months. Upon discharge she was ambulating with a straight cane for short distances and without any assistive device in the house. She did not have any consequential gait deviations. Her knee extension strength increased to 4/5, with rare lateral patellar subluxations. She returned to her previous functional level. She was independent in a home exercise program consisting of short-arc wall slides, hip adduction, and stretching to the tensor fasciae latae and hamstring muscles.

Mrs. M. achieved her physical therapy goals of improved functional level. She did not make good progress in physical therapy until her problem of prosthetic loosening was addressed. The lateral patellar subluxation also improved after surgical intervention. Although the second surgery initially resulted in a regression, it allowed her overall greater rehabilitation potential.

SUMMARY

Physical therapy management of patients who have undergone total knee arthroplasty is often very rewarding. Knowledge of the type of prosthesis implanted, type of fixation used, and any complications the patient encountered facilitates effective physical therapy treatment. Use of the problem-solving method in physical therapy management will assist the therapist in recognizing commonalities and differences among patients who have undergone TKA. Identification of commonalities among patients will promote efficient treatments, and identification of differences will promote individualized programs. The problem-solving process in clinical decision making can be efficient and effective.

ACKNOWLEDGMENTS

Special thanks to Jeri Krause, PT, Marguerita Goins, PT, and Walt Carpenter, MD.

REFERENCES

1. Savastano, AA: Total Knee Replacement. Appleton-Century-Crofts, New York, 1980, p 31.
2. Insall, JN: Surgery of the Knee. Churchill Livingstone, New York, 1984, p 598.
3. Scott, WN: Total Knee Revision Arthroplasty. Grune & Stratton, Orlando, FL, 1987, p 3.
4. Hungerford, DS, Krackow, KA, and Kenna, RV: Total Knee Arthroplasty: A Comprehensive Approach. Williams & Wilkins, Baltimore, 1984, p 71.
5. Bushul, M, Hastings, DE, and Bogoch, E: Porous-coated anatomic total knee replacement: A clinical and radiographic review. In Niwa, S, Paul, JP, Yamamoto, S (eds): Total Knee Replacement. Springer-Verlag, Tokyo, 1988, p 175.
6. Bourne, RB, Rorabeck, CH, and Nott, L: A prospective comparison of the cemented kinematic II and cementless PCA total knee replacements. In Niwa, S, Paul, JP, and Yamamoto, S (eds): Total Knee Replacement. Springer-Verlag, Tokyo, 1988, p 49.
7. Bourne, RB, Rorabeck, CH, and Nott, L: A prospective comparison of the cemented kinematic II and cementless PCA total knee replacements. In Niwa, S, Paul, JP, and Yamamoto, S (eds): Total Knee Replacement. Springer-Verlag, Tokyo, 1988, p. 58.
8. Stulberg, DS and Stulberg, BN: The biological response to uncemented total knee replacements. In Rand, JA and Dorr, LD (eds): Total Arthroplasty of the Knee. Aspen Publishers, Rockville, MD, 1987, p. 164.
9. Ecker, ML and Lotke, PA: Postoperative care of the total knee patient. Orthop Clin North Am 20:55, 1989.
10. Goll, SR, Lotke, PA, and Ecker, ML: Failure of continuous passive motion as prophylaxis against deep venous thrombosis after total knee arthroplasty. In Rand, JA, and Dorr, LD (eds): Total Arthroplasty of the Knee. Aspen Publishers, Rockville, MD, 1987, p 299.
11. Insall, JN: Surgery of the Knee. Churchill Livingstone, New York, 1984, p. 646.
12. Coutts, RD, Toth, C, and Kaita, JH: The role of continuous passive motion in the rehabilitation of the total knee patient. In Hungerford, DS, Krackow, KA, and Kenna, RV (eds): Total Knee Arthroplasty: A Comprehensive Appoach. Williams & Wilkins, Baltimore, 1984, p 126.
13. Insall, JN: Surgery of the Knee. Churchill Livingstone, New York, 1984, p. 648.
14. Johnson, DP: The effect of continuous passive motion on wound-healing and joint mobility after knee arthroplasty. J Bone Joint Surg [Am] 72:421, 1990.
15. Insall, JN: Surgery of the Knee. Churchill Livingstone, New York, 1984, p 658.
16. Arem, AL and Madden, JW: Effects of stress on healing wounds. I. Intermittent noncyclical tension. J Surg Res 20:93, 1976.
17. Woo, S, et al: Connective tissue response to immobility: correlative study of biomechanical and biological measurements of normal and immobilized rabbit knees. Arthritis Rheum 18:257, 1975.
18. Lynch, PA, et al: Deep venous thrombosis and continued passive motion after total knee arthroplasty. J Bone Joint Surg [Am] 70:11, 1988.
19. Nielsen, PT, Rechnagel, K, and Nielsen, SE: No effect of continuous passive motion after arthroplasty of the knee. Acta Orthop Scand 59:580, 1988.
20. Gose, JC: Continuous passive motion in the postoperative treatment of patients with total knee replacement. Phys Ther 67:39, 1987.
21. Basso, DM and Knapp, L: Comparison of two continuous passive motion protocols for patients with total knee implants. Phys Ther 67:360, 1987.
22. Johnson, RP: Mechanical disorders of the knee. In McCarty, DJ (ed): Arthritis and Allied Conditions. Lea & Febiger, Philadelphia, 1989, p 1398.
23. Sprague, R: Factors related to extension lag at the knee joint. Journal of Orthopedic and Sports Physical Therapy 3:178, 1982.
24. Ritter, MA, Gandolf, VS, and Holston, KS: Continuous passive motion versus physical therapy in total knee arthroplasty. Clin Orthop 244:239, 1989.
25. Young, A, et al: The effect of intraarticular bupivicaine on quad inhibition after meniscectomy. Med Sci Sports Exerc 15:154, 1983.
26. Arvidsson, I, et al: Reduction of pain inhibition on voluntary muscle activation by epidural analgesia. Orthopedics 9:1415, 1986.
27. deAndrade, JR, Grant, C, and Dixon, AJ: Joint distension and reflex muscle inhibition in the knee. J Bone Joint Surg [Am] 47:313, 1965.
28. Spencer, JD, Hayes, KC, and Alexander, IJ: Knee joint effusion and quadriceps reflex inhibition in man. Arch Phys Med Rehabil 65:171, 1984.
29. Perry, J, Antonelli, D, and Ford, W: Analysis of knee-joint forces during flexed-knee stance. J Bone Joint Surg [Am] 57:961, 1975.

30. Hungerford, D and Barry, M: Biomechanics of the patellofemoral joint. Clin Orthop 144:9, 1979.
31. Baker, L: Clinical uses of neuromuscular electrical stimulation. In Nelson, RM and Currier, DP (eds): Clinical Electrotherapy. Appleton & Lange, Norwalk, CT, 1987, p 122.
32. Eriksson, E and Haggmark, T: Comparison of isometric muscle training and electrical stimulation supplementing isometric muscle training in the recovery after major knee ligament surgery. Am J Sports Med 7:169, 1979.
33. Haug, J and Wood, LT: Efficacy of neuromuscular stimulation of the quadriceps femoris during continuous passive motion following total knee arthroplasty. Arch Phys Med Rehabil 69:423, 1988.
34. Spielholz, N: Scientific basis of exercise programs. In Basmajian, J and Wolf, S (eds): Therapeutic Exercise, ed 5. Williams & Wilkins, Baltimore, 1990, p 58.
35. Kisner, C and Colby, L: Therapeutic Exercise: Foundations and Techniques. FA Davis, Philadelphia, 1990, p 68.
36. Kandel, ER and Schwartz, JH: Principles of Neural Science. Elsevier North-Holland, New York, 1985, p 319.
37. Light, KE, et al: Low-load prolonged stretch vs. high-load brief stretch in treating knee contractures. Phys Ther 64:330, 1984.
38. Warren, CG, Lehmann, JF, and Koblanski, JN: Heat and stretch procedures: An evaluation using rat tail tendon. Arch Phys Med Rehabil 57:122, 1976.
39. Sapega, A, et al: Biophysical factors in range of motion exercises. The Physician and Sportsmedicine 9:57, 1981.
40. Nordin, M and Frankel, V: Basic Biomechanics of the Musculoskeletal System. Lea & Febiger, Philadelphia, 1989, p 68.
41. Michlovitz, SL: Thermal Agents in Rehabilitation. FA Davis, Philadelphia, 1990, p. 92.
42. Lehmann, JF, et al: Effect of therapeutic temperatures on tendon extensibility. Arch Phys Med Rehabil 51:481, 1970.
43. Sullivan, PE, Markos, PD, and Minor, MAD: An Integrated Approach to Therapeutic Exercise. Appleton & Lange, Norwalk, CT, 1982, p 139.
44. Michlovitz, SL: Thermal Agents in Rehabilitation. FA Davis, Philadelphia, 1989, p. 66.
45. Knight, K: Cryotherapy: Theory, Technique, and Physiology. Chattanooga Corporation, Chattanooga, TN, 1985, p 17.
46. Alon, G: High Voltage Stimulation: A Monograph. Chattanooga Corporation, Chattanooga, TN, 1984, p 15.
47. Newton, RA: High voltage pulsed galvanic stimulation: Theoretical bases and clinical applications. In Nelson, RM and Currier, DP (eds): Clinical Electrotherapy. Appleton & Lange, Norwalk, CT, 1987, p 176.
48. Reed, B: Effect of high voltage pulsed electrical stimulation on microvascular permeability to plasma proteins: A possible mechanism in minimizing edema. Phys Ther 68:491, 1988.
49. Fox, TA: Dysplasia of the quadriceps mechanism: Hypoplasia of the vastus medialis muscle as related to the hypermobile patella syndrome. Surg Clin North Am 55:199, 1975.
50. Hughston, JC: Subluxation of the patella. J Bone Joint Surg [Am] 50:1003, 1968.
51. Bohannon, RW: Effect of electrical stimulation to the vastus medialis muscle in a patient with chronically dislocating patellae. Phys Ther 63:144, 1983.
52. DeDominico, G and Alon, G: High voltage stimulation: An Integrated Approach to Clinical Electrotherapy. Chattanooga Corporation, Chattanooga, TN, 1987, p 132.
53. Knapp, JJ, et al: Non-specific effects of isometric and isokinetic strength training at a particular joint angle (abstr). Med Sci Sports Exerc 12:120, 1980.
54. Krebs, DE, et al: Knee joint angle: Its relationship to quadriceps femoris activity in normal and post arthrotomy limbs. Arch Phys Med Rehabil 64:441, 1983.
55. Stratford, P: Electromyography of the quadriceps femoris muscles in subjects with normal knees and acutely effused knees. Phys Ther 62:279, 1981.
56. Shakespeare, DT, et al: The effect of knee flexion on quadriceps inhibition after meniscectomy. Clin Sci 65:64, 1983.
57. Hanten, W and Schulthies, S: Exercise effect on electromyographic activity of the vastus medialis oblique and vastus lateralis muscles. Phys Ther 70:9, 1990.

Miscellaneous Special Tests of the Knee

Malton A. Schexneider, MMSc, PT, OCS

The goals of clinical examination include the determination of the mechanism of injury (microtrauma and/or macrotrauma), identification of the tissue(s) involved, extent of tissue involvement, assessment of functional status, and the establishment of rehabilitative goals. Determination of tissue involvement and functional status is predicated on the clinician's knowledge of anatomy, biomechanics, and the ability to sense subtle changes in the anatomic/biomechanical interrelationship. To differentiate the various anatomic structures that may be involved in a particular condition, various tests have been designed to assess the components of static, dynamic, and neural influences of a particular region. These clinical tests are intended to isolate a specific structure or structures that are predominantly involved in the regulation or integration of functional movement.

Within the scope of knee examination, the examiner is provided with numerous choices of clinical tests designed to assess the static, dynamic, and neural integrity of knee function. Specific tests are chosen based upon mechanism of injury, clinical signs and symptoms, and the clinician's ability to perform the test in a reliable fashion. The preceding chapters have identified numerous special tests designed to determine ligamentous and meniscal involvement, along with tests designed to elicit symptoms arising from the cumulative effects of microtrauma. This section reviews and describes the application of the commonly used tests and the structures each test assesses. Tests have been classified into those assessing, meniscal and patellofemoral integrity, ligamentous integrity, and the integrity of other structures around the knee.

TESTS FOR THE DETERMINATION OF MENISCAL AND PATELLOFEMORAL DYSFUNCTION

McMurray Test (Fig. A – 1)[1-3]

Position:	Patient supine with operator standing on the patient's involved side.
Test:	Operator flexes patient's hip and knee and internally or externally rotates the tibia on the femur. While maintaining the internal or external rotation, a varus or valgus force is respectively applied at the joint line as the operator extends the knee and palpates the medial or lateral joint space. The test is considered positive if the patient experiences pain during the maneuver and/or an audible or palpable "click" within the joint is sensed by the operator.

Structures Tested:	External rotation and valgus force
	        Medial meniscus
	Internal rotation and varus force
	        Lateral meniscus

Apley's Compression Test (Fig. A – 2A)[2,3]

Position:	Patient prone with knee flexed to 90 degrees.
Test:	Operator applies a vertically directed force through the

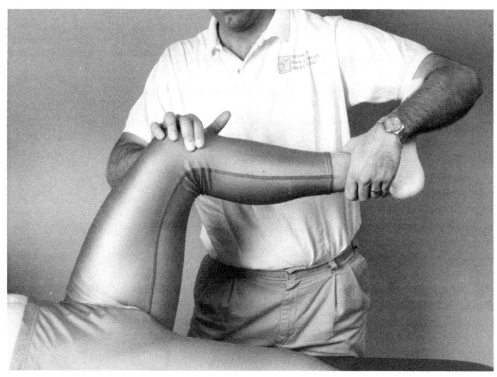

FIGURE A-1. McMurray test.

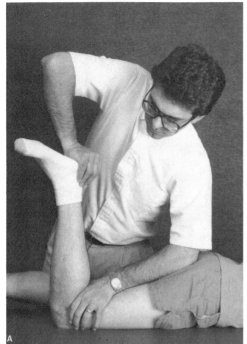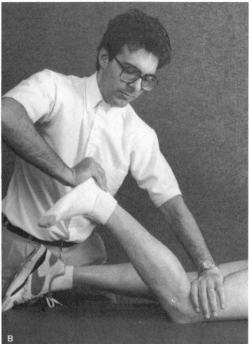

FIGURE A-2. *A*) Apley's compression test. *B*) Dynamic version.

patient's heel while maintaining the tibia in either internal or external rotation on the femur. The test is considered positive if pain is elicited during the maneuver.

Structures Tested: Posterior horns of the medial or lateral meniscus

Apley's Compression Test, Dynamic Version (Fig. A–2B)[1]

Position: Patient prone with knee flexed to 90 degrees.

Test: Operator applies a vertically directed force through the patient's heel while maintaining the tibia in either internal or external rotation on the femur. While maintaining this force, the operator passively extends the patient's knee through the range of motion. The test is considered positive if pain is elicited during the maneuver.

Structures Tested: Entire surface of the medial or lateral meniscus

Patellofemoral Grinding Test (Fig. A–3)[1,2,3]

Position: Patient supine with knee flexed to approximately 20 degrees.

Test: Using the web space of his top hand, operator contacts the superior aspect of the patella. Operator maintains a cau-

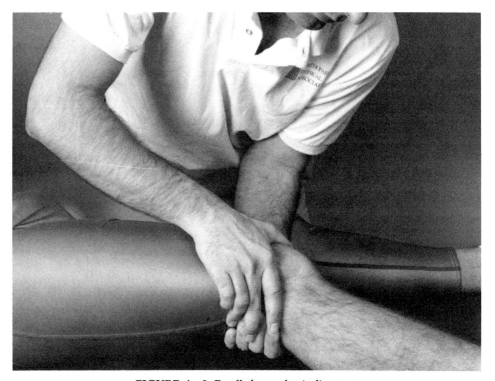

FIGURE A-3. Patellofemoral grinding test.

	dally directed force, and patient is asked to actively contract his quadriceps muscle. Operator assesses patient's apprehension to the test and pain reproduction.
Structures Tested:	Joint surfaces of the patellofemoral joint

TESTS FOR THE DETERMINATION OF LIGAMENTOUS INTEGRITY

Varus and Valgus Stress Test (Fig. A-4)[1-4]

Position:	Patient supine with operator standing on the side to be tested.
Test:	Operator abducts the lower extremity and flexes the knee to approximately 30 degrees while keeping the posterior aspect of the thigh on the table. Operator places thumb and index fingers of palpating hand over the medial and lateral joint lines. Using his thigh to create a fulcrum, operator abducts or adducts the tibia on the femur and senses for excessive laxity in the medial or lateral joint spaces. With a valgus stress, care should be taken to begin the maneuver in a varus position; whereas varus testing should begin in the neutral position, keeping in mind that

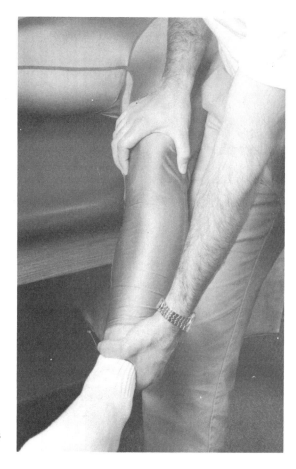

FIGURE A-4. Varus and valgus stress test.

there is approximately 9 mm of physiologic laxity in the lateral joint space. The knee is then fully extended and the above procedure repeated. With the knee extended, no movement should be discerned.

Structures Tested: Valgus stress at 30 degrees of flexion
   Medial capsule, tibial collateral ligament
Valgus stress at full extension
   Medial capsule, tibial collateral ligament, anterior and posterior cruciate ligaments, posteromedial capsule
Varus stress at 30 degrees of flexion
   Lateral capsule, lateral collateral ligament
Varus stress at full extension
   Lateral capsule, lateral collateral ligament, anterior and posterior cruciate ligaments, posterolateral capsule

Noyes' Flexion Rotation Drawer Test (Fig. A-5)[2]

Position: Patient supine with the operator maintaining the patient's involved lower extremity in a neutral anatomic position.

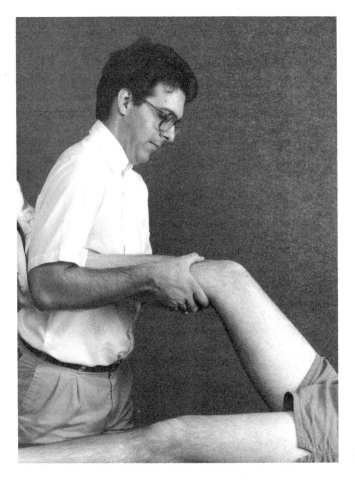

FIGURE A–5. Noyes' flexion rotation drawer test.

Test: The operator grasps the proximal aspect of the patient's tibia while cradling the lower aspect of the leg between his or her side and medial aspect of the upper arm. While passively carrying the knee into flexion, the operator applies a posteriorly directed force through the proximal aspect of the tibia. A positive test is indicated when the tibia is felt to reduce or "jerk" into a posterior and medial direction at approximately 10 degrees flexion.

Structures Tested: Anterior cruciate ligament, arcuate complex

Sag Test (Fig. A–6)[2]

Position: Patient supine with hip and knee placed in 90 degrees of flexion.

Test: Operator places a straightedge on a line running from the distal pole of the patella to the tibial tubercle. Operator observes for any evidence of the tibia "sagging" posteriorly on the femur, indicating laxity of the posterior cruciate/capsule complex.

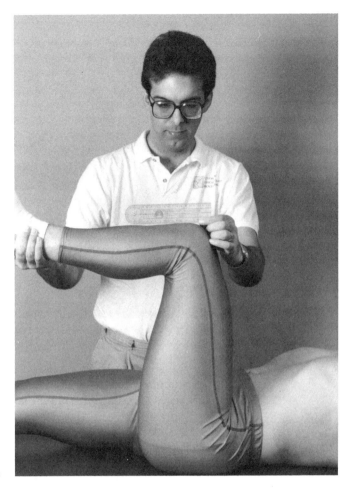

FIGURE A–6. Sag test.

Structures Tested: Integrity of the posterior cruciate ligament and the posterior capsule

Anterior/Posterior Drawer Test (Fig. A–7)[1-4]

Position: Patient supine with knee flexed to 90 degrees and foot firmly on table. Operator sits on the toes of the patient's bent leg and grasps the proximal aspect of the tibia, with his or her thumbs resting on the joint line anteriorly and index fingers palpating the medial and lateral hamstring tendons posteriorly.

Test: Operator gently translates the tibia anteriorly, palpating for a "stepping" at the joint line between the tibial plateau and femoral condyles, and for a ligamentous end feel. At all times during the maneuver, the hamstring tendons must remain in a relaxed state. A posteriorly directed translation is then performed, sensing for a similar stepping sensation and end feel. The test is considered positive

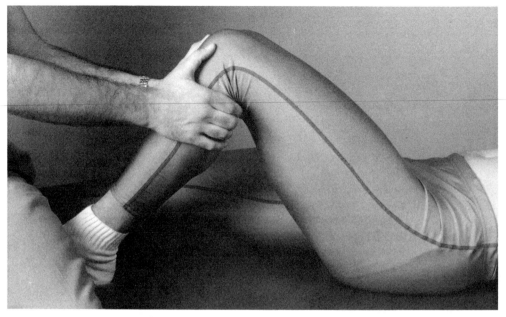

FIGURE A-7. Anterior/posterior drawer test.

if excessive translation is observed or a "boggy" end feel is encountered. False-positive results with the anterior drawer will be encountered if the tibia is subluxed posteriorly prior to testing. Therefore, a sag test (posterior cruciate/posterior capsule laxity) should be performed prior to performing an anterior drawer test.

Structures Tested: Anterior drawer
Anterior cruciate ligament, anterior portion of the medial and lateral tibiomeniscal ligaments, posterior cruciate ligament
Posterior drawer
Posterior cruciate ligament, posterior capsule

Lachman Test (Fig. A–8A)[1,2,4]

Position: Patient supine with operator standing on the side to be tested. Operator's top hand supports the thigh in about 20 to 30 degrees of flexion, while the bottom hand reaches over the medial aspect of the tibia and grasps the posterior and proximal aspect of the tibia with the thumb resting on the tibial tubercle.

Test: While stabilizing the femur with the top hand, the operator directs an anterior translation of the tibia on the femur, palpating for a definitive ligamentous end feel. The test is considered positive if excessive translation is observed or a "boggy" end feel is encountered.

Structures Tested: Integrity of the anterior cruciate ligament

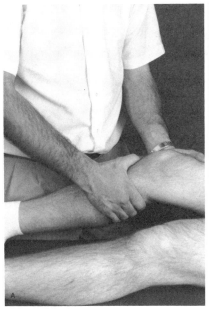

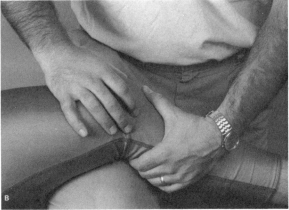

FIGURE A-8. *A*) Lachman test. *B*) Modified Lachman test.

Modified Lachman Test (Fig. A-8B)[1,2,4]

Position:	Patient supine with knee flexed over operator's thigh (approximately 20 to 30 degrees). Operator places top hand above the patella with thumb and index finger palpating the medial and lateral joint line, while the palm of the hand rests on the anterior aspect of the lower thigh. The bottom hand reaches over the medial aspect of the tibia and grasps the posterior and proximal aspect of the tibia with the thumb resting on the tibial tubercle.
Test:	While stabilizing the femur with the top hand, operator directs an anterior translation of the tibia on the femur, palpating for displacement at the joint line and a definitive ligamentous end feel. The test is considered positive if excessive translation is observed or a "boggy" end feel is encountered.
Structures Tested:	Integrity of the anterior cruciate ligament

Lateral Pivot Shift Test (Fig. A-9)[2,4]

Position:	Patient lies supine with the hip and knee slightly flexed. The operator stands on the side to be tested, grasping the patient's foot with one hand and the posterior aspect of the fibula with his or her other hand.
Test:	The operator internally rotates the tibia on the femur to approximately 20 degrees. While the operator applies a valgus force through the knee, the knee is passively carried

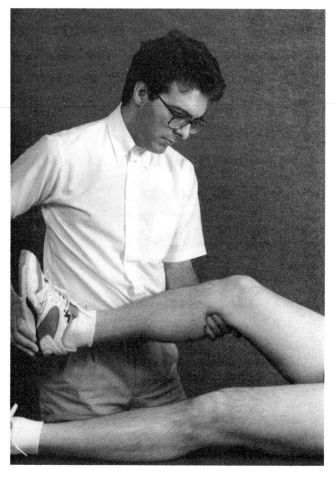

FIGURE A-9. Lateral pivot shift test.

into 20 to 40 degrees of flexion. Indications of a positive test would be the sensation of a "giving way" or "thud" as the tibia is posteriorly and medially reduced to its normal anatomic position.

Structures Tested: Anterior cruciate ligament, arcuate complex, lateral capsule

KT-2000 Arthrometer* Test (Fig. A–10)[5]

Position: Patient supine with knee flexed to 25 degrees over a firm bolster.

Test: The operator uses an arthrometer designed to measure the displacement (in millimeters) of the tibia in either an anterior or posterior direction. The patient is supine in a relaxed position. The lower extremity is supported with a thigh support above the superior pole of the patella. A footrest can be used to support the foot below the lateral

---

*Med-Metric Company, San Diego, CA.

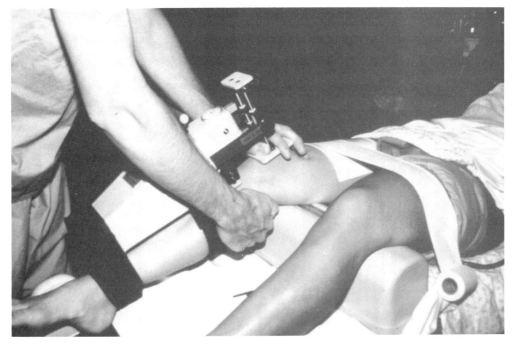

FIGURE A-10. KT-2000 arthrometer test.

malleoli. Care must be taken to maintain neutral rotation of the tibia. The arthrometer is positioned along the crest of the tibia, with the V-shaped undersurface of the arthrometer aligned to the tibial crest. The most proximal portion of the patellar sensor pad is positioned even with the inferior patellar pole, and not on the patellar tendon. To test for tears of the anterior cruciate ligament, the examiner applies two to three posterior pushes to set the tibia in a starting position. (For testing of the posterior cruciate ligament, the examiner would apply two to three anterior pulls before testing.) The tibia is then pulled anteriorly, and readings are taken at 15, 20, and 30 lb force. Three trials are performed with each force, with the average displacement recorded. Anterior displacement beyond 3 to 5 mm would indicate an insufficient anterior cruciate ligament, whereas posterior displacement beyond 3 to 5 mm would indicate posterior cruciate insufficiency.

Structures Tested: Anterior cruciate ligament, posterior cruciate ligament

OTHER SPECIAL TESTS

Noble's Compression Test (Fig. A–11)[6]

Position: Patient supine with hip and knee flexed to 90 degrees

Test: The operator applies constant pressure to the lateral femoral condyle while slowly extending the knee. If pain is

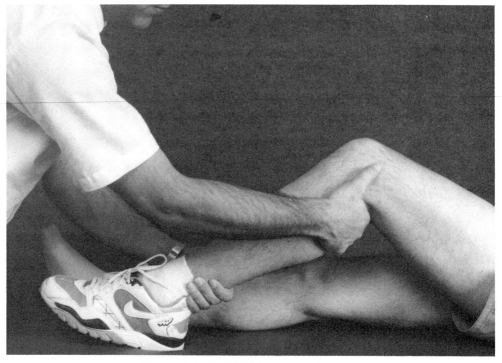

FIGURE A-11. Noble's compression test.

elicited from the pressure of the operator's thumb when
the knee reaches 30 degrees of flexion, the test is considered positive for iliotibial band friction syndrome.

Structures Tested: Iliotibial band

Functional Hop Test (Fig. A–12)[7]

Position: Beginning in standing position, the patient performs four
functional tests.

Tests: 1. *Single hop for distance.* Patient hops on involved and
uninvolved lower extremity. Distance recorded is average
taken of two repetitions.
2. *Timed hop.* Patient hops on involved and uninvolved
lower extremity for 6 meters while being timed. The test is
performed twice and an average taken of the two scores.
3. *Triple hop for distance.* Patient performs three consecutive hops on involved and uninvolved lower extremity.
The test is performed twice, and an average taken of the
two scores.
4. *Crossover hop for distance.* Patient performs three consecutive hops on involved and uninvolved lower extremity
across a 1.5-cm line. The maximum distance covered in
three hops is calculated. The test is performed twice with

Single Hop for Distance

Timed Hop

Triple Hop for Distance

Cross-over Hop for Distance

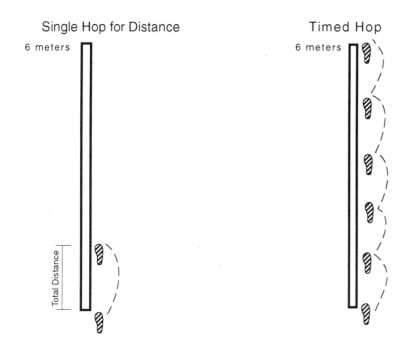

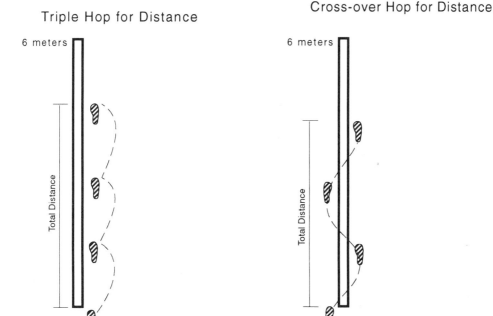

FIGURE A–12. Functional hop test. (Adapted from Noyes FR, Barber SD, and Mangine, RE: Abnormal lower limb symmetry determined by function hop tests after anterior cruciate ligament rupture. Am J Sports Med 19:513, 1991, with permission.)

the average taken of the two scores. Differences between involved and uninvolved lower extremities are calculated. Calculated differences of less than 85 percent between involved and uninvolved lower extremity are considered abnormal.

Structures Tested: Functional status of anterior cruciate deficient knees

One-Leg Stork Test (Fig. A–13)[2,8]

Position: Patient standing.

Test: The patient is asked to place the sole of the foot of the uninvolved lower extremity on the medial aspect of the knee of the involved lower extremity. The test is considered positive if the patient is unable to retain his or her balance for 14 seconds.

Structures Tested: Neural stabilizers of the knee joint

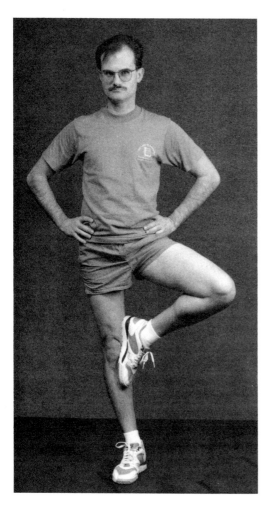

FIGURE A–13. One-leg stork test.

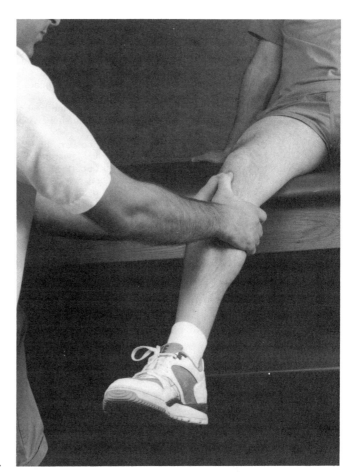

FIGURE A–14. Hoffa test.

Hoffa Test (Fig. A–14)[5]

Position:	Patient seated with knee flexed to 90 degrees
Test:	Operator places fingers over the infrapatellar tendon and applies an anterior-posterior pressure as the patient actively extends his or her knee. This maneuver prevents the fat pad from becoming prominent during extension and results in pain if the region is symptomatic.
Structures Tested:	Impingement of infrapatellar fat pad

ACKNOWLEDGMENTS

Special thanks to Jim Boudreaux for his participation in modeling for each of the special tests. Also, special thanks to Dean Lavenson for his time and expertise in photographing each of the tests.

REFERENCES

1. Davies, GJ and Larson, R: Examining the knee. The Physician and Sportsmedicine 6(4):49, 1978.
2. Davies, GJ, Malone, T, and Bassett, FH: Knee examination. Phys Ther 60(12):17, 1980.
3. Hoppenfeld, S: Physical Examination of the Spine and Extremities. Appleton-Century-Crofts, New York, 1976.
4. Poole, RM and Blackburn, TA: Dysfunction, evaluation, and treatment of the knee. In Donatelli, RA and Wooden, MJ (eds): Orthopaedic Physical Therapy. Churchill Livingstone, New York, 1989, p 493.
5. Walters, J: Personal communication, February, 1992.
6. Magee, DJ: Orthopedic Physical Assessment. WB Saunders, Philadelphia, 1987, p 250.
7. Noyes, FR, Barber, SD, and Mangine, RE: Abnormal lower limb symmetry determined by function hop tests after anterior cruciate ligament rupture. Am J Sports Med 19(5):513, 1991.
8. Wallace, L: Rehabilitation following patellofemoral surgery. In Davies, GJ (ed): Rehabilitation of the Surgical Knee. CyPress, Ronkonkoma, NY, 1984, p 45.

Index

An "F" following a page number indicates a figure; a "T" indicates a table.

I

Iatrotropic stimulus, 70
Ice. *See* Cryotherapy; RICE regimen
Iliopatellar band, 26
  tightness of, 182
Iliotibial band, 26, 26F, 155
  pivot shift and, 289, 290F. *See also* Extra-
    articular reconstructions
  proximally based, extra-articular reconstruction
    using, 293, 295–297, 296F
  stretching of, 161, 161F
  tightness of, 182
Iliotibial band friction syndrome (ITBFS), 155
  case study of, 159–162, 161F, 162F
  extrinsic factors in, 155
  flexibility tests in, 59, 155, 156F
  leg length discrepancy and, 151
  special tests for, 59
  subtalar joint pronation and, 148
  training surfaces and, 142
Iliotibial tract, 25–26, 26F
Imbalance, reflex sympathetic, intra-articular
  reconstructions and, 273–274
Immobilization
  fibroblastic stage of healing and, 100
  inflammatory stage of healing and, 90
  intra-articular reconstructions and, 254T,
    256–257, 257F
    complications of, 273
  negative effects of, 113
Incline leg press exercise, posterior cruciate
  ligament injuries and, 312F
Incongruous phase of load bearing, 384
Inertial exercise, advantages and disadvantages
  of, 120T
Inflammation. *See also specific disorder; specific
  location*
  microtrauma injuries and, 139–140
  rheumatoid arthritis and, 207
Inflammatory stage of healing, 88, 90–92
  therapeutic considerations during, 92
Infrapatellar bursae, 10F, 11, 153
Infrapatellar fat pad, 11
Infrapatellar plica, 9, 10F
Infrapatellar tendon, 179F
Injury. *See* Trauma; *specific type*
Innervation. *See* Nerve supply
Insertional site failure, 87–88
Instability. *See also* Stability
  lateral, 362–379. *See also* Lateral instabilities
  total knee arthroplasty for, 410. *See also* Total
    knee arthroplasty (TKA)
Instrument stability testing, 60, 62
Intercondylar notch, 6
  tibial spine and, 6
Interference screw, graft fixation using, 251
Intermediate phase of load bearing, 384
Interstitial fluid, 158
Intra-articular reconstructions, 245–246
  allografts in, 102. *See also* Grafts
  arthrotomy in, arthroscopically assisted
    procedures versus, 246–247
  autografts in, 101, 103F. *See also* Grafts
  case studies of, 274–284, 283F
  complications following, 272–274

rehabilitation of
  ambulation in, 260, 262, 262F
  CPM devices in, 257–258, 258F
  derotation braces in, 272
  functional exercise in, 270F, 270–271, 271F
  general guidelines for, 254T–255T, 254–272
  healing potential during, 253–254
  identification of problems in, 254, 256
  immobilization in, 256–257, 257F
  lower extremity conditioning in, 268–270,
    269F
  progression in, 256
  return to activity and, 271–272
  ROM exercise goals in, 258–260, 259F–261F
  strengthening exercises in, 262–268,
    264F–267F
  surgical factors in, 246–253, 248T, 249T
  secondary injuries and, 252–253
  soft-tissue healing and, 101, 102F, 103F
  synthetics in, 102, 104. *See also* Grafts
  timing of, related surgical procedures and, 252
Iontophoresis, ITBFS treatment with, 160
Isokinetic exercise
  advantages and disadvantages of, 120T,
    123–124, 124T
  arthritis and, 221
    osteoarthritis, 229–230
  lateral compartment injury and, 368, 369F, 376
  patellofemoral joint dysfunction and, 192
Isometric exercise. *See also* Exercise
  advantages and disadvantages of, 120T
  arthritis and, 219–220
  intra-articular reconstructions and, 268–270,
    269F
  meniscectomy and, 396–397
  total knee arthroplasty and, 426–427
Isometry, graft placement using, 252
Isotonic exercise
  advantages and disadvantages of, 120T
  arthritis and, 220
  intra-articular reconstructions and, 263, 264F
  patellofemoral joint dysfunction and, 192
ITBFS. *See* Iliotibial band friction syndrome

J

Jogging, microtrauma and. *See also* Microtrauma
  incidence of, 140
Joint reaction forces. *See also* Compressive forces;
  Shear forces; Tensile forces
  patellofemoral, 37–38
Joint stability. *See* Stability

K

Kinematics, 33–34
  functional, tibiofemoral joint and, 36–37
Kinesthetic exercises, 119
Kinesthetic status, assessment of, 57–58
Kinetic chains, 34
Knee, functional anatomy of, 3–39. *See also*
  Functional anatomy of knee
Knee dips, intra-articular reconstructions and,
  266F, 267
Knee evaluation, sequential, 43–64. *See also*
  Sequential evaluation